Computed Tomography of the Brain and Orbit
(EMI SCANNING)

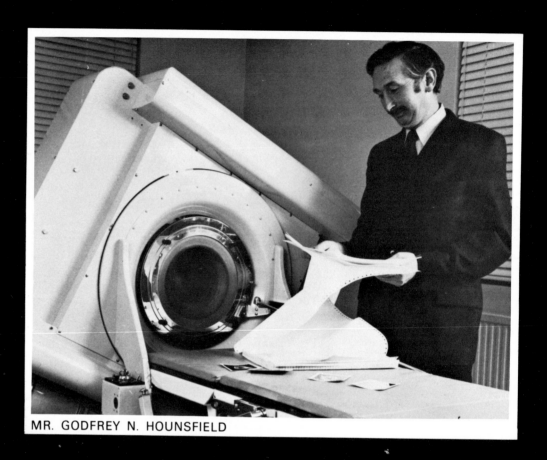

MR. GODFREY N. HOUNSFIELD

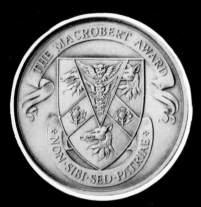

The MacRobert Award 1972

The MacRobert Award, which has been described as the Nobel Prize for engineering, consists of £25,000 and a Gold Medal presented annually by the Council of Engineering Institutions on behalf of the MacRobert Trusts. The Award is made for successful technological innovation which has contributed (or will contribute) to the national prestige and prosperity of the United Kingdom. The rules allow the prize to be made to a team of no more than five people or to an individual making an outstanding contribution to engineering, the physical technologies or to the application of the physical sciences.

Computed Tomography of the Brain and Orbit

(EMI SCANNING)

PAUL F. J. NEW, M.D., F.A.C.R.

Chief of Neuroradiology Service, Department of Radiology
Massachusetts General Hospital
Associate Professor of Radiology
Harvard Medical School

WILLIAM R. SCOTT, M.D.

Acting Associate Professor of Radiology
Stanford University Medical Center

The Williams & Wilkins Company/Baltimore, Maryland

Made in the United States of America

Library of Congress Cataloging in Publication Data

New, Paul F   J
    Computed tomography of the brain and orbit (EMI scanning)

    Includes index.
    1.   Brain—Diseases—Diagnosis.   2.   Tomography. I. Scott, William Robert, 1939–
joint author. II. Title. |DNLM: 1. Brain—Radiography. 2. Orbit—Radiography.   3. To-
mography, Radiographic. WL141 N532c|
RC386.5.N48   616.8′04′754   75-14178
ISBN 0-683-06455-X

Composed and printed at the
Waverly Press, Inc.
Mt. Royal and Guilford Aves.
Baltimore, Md. 21202, U.S.A.

DEDICATION

To my wife, Ann

P. F. J. N.

Preface

This book is based on slightly more than one and a half year's experience with a remarkable and fundamentally new technique of x-ray examination of soft tissues.

Essentially the product of a concept and of the work of Mr. Godfrey Hounsfield of the Central Research Laboratories of EMI Ltd., this British x-ray scanning system substitutes scintillation counters for x-ray film as the primary detector, and utilizes computer technology. By these means, sensitivity in detection of photon attenuation is increased by roughly two orders of magnitude compared with x-ray film.

The problem of determining the image in a plane, derived from attenuation along discrete paths through a plane of an object, was first solved by Radon in 1917 (57A). The application of this technique for radiological examinations was introduced by Cormack in 1963 (13A). In 1961, Dr. W. H. Oldendorf (48), a practicing clinical neurologist, lamenting that the soft tissues within the cranium were so nearly homogeneous in radiodensity that the brain was completely invisible on plain film examination, described experiments utilizing a gamma-ray source and a collimated scintillation counter to detect discontinuities in a rotating model. The beam was passed through the object in such a way that a point within the object was monitored. The point was then moved, and changes in radiodensity of the point were detected and displayed as the point scanned through a plane within the object. The system was shown to be theoretically capable of producing a cross-sectional display of radiodensity discontinuities within an irregular object such as the head. However, no biological system was studied. Oldendorf commented upon the far greater count rates that could be obtained from x-ray sources compared with the radioisotope sources, but he did not pursue the matter. A mechanical scanner having some resemblance to the EMI scanner was pioneered by Dr. D. E. Kuhl of Philadelphia for the purposes of applying tomographic principles to nuclear imaging (34, 35). Mr. Hounsfield, with great ingenuity, elaborated these basic concepts and coupled radiation physics with computer technology in such a way as to provide a novel and practical method of data retrieval.

Once it was demonstrated that Hounsfield's system was capable of successful *direct imaging* of details within soft tissue structures, it was logical to apply the method in the first instance to imaging of the cranial contents. As these contents are so well shielded by bone and contain no naturally occurring contrasting substances such as fat planes or gas as in the chest and abdomen, they are completely invisible until revealed, essentially *indirectly*, by the use of intravascular or intrathecal contrast agents.

Had Hounsfield's invention proved capable of no more than a realistic demonstration of the gross size and position of the major cerebral ventricles, its success as a clinical tool would have been assured. That the EMI scanner is capable of providing so very much more than this information, indeed direct information concerning the structure of normal and abnormal tissues, accounts for the rapidity with which the method has gained widespread interest and acclaim.

The introduction of computed tomography (CT) must be compared in significance with the introductions of cerebral pneumography by Walter Dandy and cerebral angiography by Egas Moniz, but its importance surpasses those vital contributions to neuroradiological diagnostic methods to the extent that its use will not result in the morbidity (and still occasional mortality) associated with those traditional methods. Such morbidity has been a significant, although steadily decreasing, deterrent to the early use of these methods in investigation.

In one step we have moved into an era in which it is frequently possible to obtain more definitive information regarding many forms of intracranial disease without hazard or discomfort to the patient than can be provided by the most refined forms of angiography and pneumography, methods that have been developed painstakingly over decades. It is in an attempt to satisfy a widespread interest that this book has been prepared. Although the relatively short experience with the method and the inevitable rapidity of development of this new technique may militate against extended usefulness of this work, we believe that there exists a significant need for a convenient source of information summarizing the principles, present equipment, and basic techniques of examination.

This work should be of value to neuroradiologists, neurologists, neurosurgeons, psychiatrists, ophthalmologists, and ophthalmologic surgeons, whether in training or in practice. Application of CT to the study of other areas of the body is an inevitable and important step to be made in the not too distant future. Therefore, general radiologists should find this an interesting prologue.

An attempt has been made to provide evidence of the value, limitations, and present state of the art of computed tomographic scanning in cranial neuroradiological diagnosis. The future of the method is rich with promise and, undoubtedly, technological improvements will come apace.

Paul F. J. New, M.D., F.A.C.R.
Boston

Acknowledgments

The author gratefully acknowledges the assistance of his colleagues in Neuroradiology and in the Neurological and Neurosurgical Services of the Massachusetts General Hospital, who have given generously of their time in discussion of various aspects of many of the cases illustrated in this work.

Mr. John Hatton, EMItronics Inc., has provided considerable assistance and valuable advice throughout the period of my involvement with the new scanning method.

Particular recognition is given to the kindness of Dr. James Ambrose, Consultant Neuroradiologist, Atkinson Morley's Hospital, for giving so freely of his time and knowledge during my visits to Britain to obtain advance information on many aspects of EMI scanning, prior to the first installation in North America and during initial testing of the "high-resolution" modifications 1 year later. I am also indebted to him for the majority of the 160 x 160 matrix scans illustrating normal anatomy in Chapter 5.

I wish to express my sincere thanks to Dr. William H. Sweet, Chief of the Neurosurgical Service at the Massachusetts General Hospital and Professor of Neurosurgery at Harvard Medical School, for his constant support and encouragement over many years and to Dr. Juan Taveras, Radiologist-in-Chief, Massachusetts General Hospital and Professor of Radiology, Harvard Medical School, without whose foresight in arranging for early acquisition of an EMI scanner this book might well not have been written.

My thanks are also due to Mr. Godfrey Hounsfield, Head of Medical Systems, Section of Central Research Laboratories, EMI Ltd.; to Dr. Saul Aronow, Physics Research Section, Department of Radiology, Massachusetts General Hospital, for clarification of many details in the physics and computer technology; to the dedicated technologists and secretaries of the Neuroradiology Section of the Department of Radiology, Massachusetts General Hospital; and to Mrs. Edith Tagrin, Head of the Medical Art Department, Massachusetts General Hospital, for her valuable assistance in preparing many of the illustrations.

Many of the angiographic studies quoted in the text were performed by or under the supervision of Dr. Glenn Roberson, Assistant Radiologist, Massachusetts General Hospital and Assistant Professor of Radiology, Harvard Medical School. He is largely responsible for the uniformly high quality of these studies.

The neuropathological studies recorded in this work were performed in the Charles S. Kubik Laboratories of the Massachusetts General Hospital; and the very significant contributions made by many neuropathologists, notably Dr. E. P. Richardson, Associate Professor of Neuropathology, Harvard Medical School, Dr. Fred H. Hochberg, and Dr. J. Philip Kistler are acknowledged with pleasure.

Finally, I wish to thank Miss Paula Halpin and Miss Selma Surman, who prepared the typescript, and the editorial staff of The Williams & Wilkins Co. for their encouragement and advice.

P. F. J. N.

Contents

Part
ONE

CHAPTER 1

Historical Background

In 1967 Godfrey Hounsfield, who had led the design team on the EMIDEC 1100, the first British solid-state business computer, was engaged in the investigation of pattern recognition and computer storage techniques at the Central Research Laboratories of EMI. He was engaged in determining methods by which information on a pattern could be stored and was seeking to develop techniques for computer reading of the written word. It was known that information concerning the constituents of a given pattern could be stored in many forms other than as values on a television-type raster, the conventional approach.

The accuracy with which these forms of information could be transformed from one state to another was also studied, together with the efficiency of the process of transformation. During this work it became clear that there were many areas in which large amounts of information could theoretically be made available but where the techniques used for retrieval were so inefficient that a large proportion of the available data was completely wasted.

In considering areas that could benefit most markedly from improved methods of information retrieval, it was realized that x-ray examination was especially suitable for closer study. Owing mainly to superimposition of details of three-dimensional structures on a two-dimensional x-ray film and the relative insensitivity of x-ray film emulsions in discriminating between materials of closely similar attenuation coefficients, a very substantial amount of useful information contained in a transmitted x-ray photon beam is not recovered by conventional techniques.

Mr. Hounsfield therefore investigated the application of multidirectional scanning and more efficient forms of data retrieval to this field. It can be shown that, when a given number of x-ray photons passes through a body, they are capable of revealing a calculable amount of information about the density of the constituent tissues. The basic assumption in the EMI research program was that measurements taken of x-ray transmissions through a body from all possible directions would contain the information on all the constituents of that body. It was appreciated that the results would be very difficult to interpret, but nonetheless the information would require only a mathematical solution, using a computer to perform the calculations. The information could then be presented in the conventional raster form, and the results would contain all the information necessary to produce a three-dimensional picture.

In formulating practical methods of presenting the results to the diagnostician, it was decided that the most convenient form would be to divide them, as in the principle of tomography, into pictures representing a series of "slices." Collectively, these would give a three-dimensional representation of the tissue structures. This approach also meant that the transmission readings taken through the body could be limited to single planes (Fig. 1.1). Each beam path is therefore part of a series of simultaneous equations from which a picture can be constructed.

In order to prove that the mathematical solution was practical, tests were carried out using a computer. A picture was interpreted as a series of numbers in a matrix, and the computer was programmed to calculate the values of the equivalent transmission readings taken through the object at many angles of scan. The process was then carried out in reverse, so that the picture was reconstructed from the values of the transmission readings previously obtained. The success of this work led to experiments on a mechanical scanning system that measured the transmission of gamma rays through a number of inanimate objects (Fig. 1.2).

At this stage, it was recognized that the significance of the experiments being conducted should be brought to the attention of the Department of Health and Social Security, from which enthusiastic support was received.

Experiments continued with the mechanical system but, because of the low intensity of gamma radiation, the

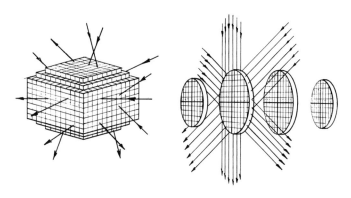

POSSIBLE PATHS OF READINGS THROUGH OBJECT.

FIG. 1.1. Possible paths of photon transmissions through an object. The computer-oriented system is shown on the *right*. X-ray photons are passed through the plane of the slice via its edges. In this case the whole path length of the x-ray beam would pass through the slice and therefore the transmission readings obtained would be confined to the slice. Under these conditions, the solution would not be affected by external unknowns, an important fact to recognize. (Reprinted by permission of EMI Ltd.)

machine had to be left operating 9 days to produce one picture! It took a large computer 2½ hours to process the readings. The computer was required to solve the equivalent of 28,000 simultaneous equations and was programmed in Fortran. The best accuracy achieved during these experiments was of the order of 4%, which was inconsistent with the maximum theoretical value (½%). In consequence, the method of interpolation between picture points was modified and subsequent experiments were carried out using x-rays (Fig. 1.3). Results much closer to the theoretical maximum were eventually achieved, although the process was still unacceptably slow, requiring at least 1 day to produce a picture.

Specimens of human tissue were obtained for evaluation of the machine. In the course of this work and in cooperation with Dr. James Ambrose, Consultant Radiologist at Atkinson Morley's Hospital, Wimbledon, England, readings were taken of a specimen of human brain. There was considerable elation when the pictures processed from these readings revealed that not only was the tumor in the specimen clearly isolated but that it was also possible to discriminate between grey and white matter. This was an exciting confirmation of the theoretical premises on which the investigation had been based.

However, further analysis of the results revealed that the formalin used to preserve the specimens had enhanced the readings to give an atypical result. Fresh bullock brains were then used to check the experimental results, and, although the variations in tissue density

were less pronounced, it was confirmed that a large amount of anatomical detail, such as the ventricles and the pineal, was readily discernible. Tests were also carried out on sections from the area of the kidneys of pigs, and this work also produced encouraging results (Fig. 1.4).

The results achieved on specimens of brain tissue indicated that it would be feasible to develop a practical machine for clinical use in radiology and that the technique would make an immediate and important contribution in the field of neuroradiology.

A specification for a brain machine incorporating the new technique was submitted to the Department of Health and Social Security, and, with their cooperation, design and development were completed in August 1970.

The first machine was installed at Atkinson Morley's Hospital in September 1971 under the guidance of Dr. Ambrose. The processing time for each picture was reduced to 20 minutes on an ICL 1905 computer by using

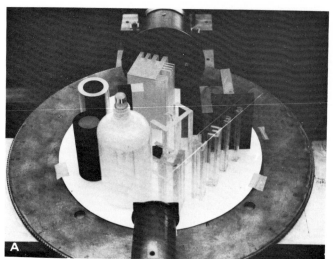

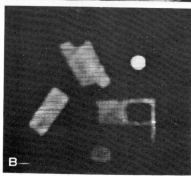

FIG. 1.2.
A. Experimental scanning system using gamma rays. An americium gamma source was used and the radiation was measured by computing techniques. (Reprinted by permission of EMI Ltd.)
B. The first picture produced by the gamma ray system. (Reprinted by permission of EMI Ltd.)

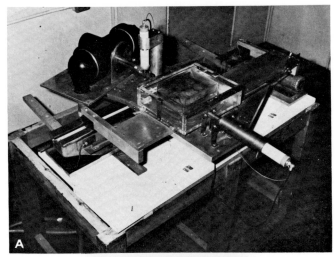

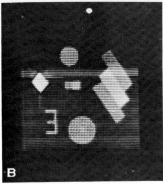

FIG. 1.3.
A. Experimental scanning system using x-rays to study brain tissue specimens. (Reprinted by permission of EMI Ltd.)
B. The first picture produced by this system, using Plexiglas objects. (Reprinted by permission of EMI Ltd.)

machine code instead of Fortran, and it was originally intended to pass the data on each patient's examination over a telephone data link for processing by a remote computer. Further work on improved processing techniques made it possible to carry out the computation in less than 5 minutes on site, using a minicomputer, and this facility is now incorporated as an integral part of the system.

The new system of x-ray section scanning was first reported by Ambrose and Hounsfield in 1972 and described at the annual congress of the British Institute of Radiology in April of that year. In the following month, computerized transverse axial scanning was described for the first time in the United States by Mr. Hounsfield and the initial clinical results were discussed by Dr. James W. D. Bull at Dr. M. Schechter's postgraduate course in neuroradiology in New York in May 1972. News of this most exciting advance spread rapidly, and it was not long before orders for the equipment were placed by the Mayo Clinic and by the Massachusetts General Hospital. Installations were made in these two medical centers in June and July 1973, and clinical application of the method was initiated at the Massachusetts General Hospital at the beginning of August 1973.

The anticipated rapid and enthusiastic acceptance of the method by the clinical staff at the Massachusetts General Hospital was realized to a level unprecedented by the introduction of any other new radiological technique. To date (December 1974), approximately 3000 patients have been studied by this technique at the Massachusetts General Hospital.

As the value and wide applicability of the new method were increasingly documented by the numerous presentations by Ambrose and others at scientific meetings and by papers reporting the early results, it became widely

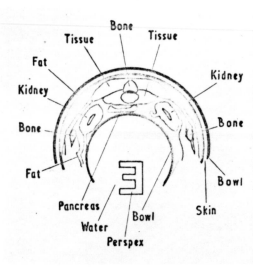

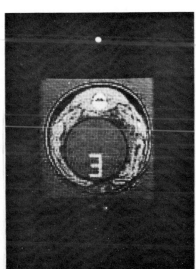

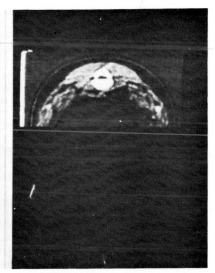

FIG. 1.4. Test x-ray scans through pig sections. (Reprinted by permission of EMI Ltd.)

realized that the new type of brain scanning was to become firmly established as an integral part of the armamentarium of neuroradiological diagnosis. At the time of writing, approximately 30 installations are in operation in North America. Dr. A. K. Ommaya, Deputy Chief of Surgical Neurology, National Institute of Neurological Diseases and Stroke, published an early report of computerized axial tomography of the head following initial experience during two visits to London in the fall of 1972, and he returned to London in the spring of 1973 at the invitation of Dr. James Ambrose and Mr. Allan Richardson, F.R.C.S., Director of Neurosurgery at Atkinson Morley's Hospital. During several weeks, he undertook quantitative calibration studies of x-ray absorption in phantoms and neural tissues. These results and those of early clinical computed tomographic (CT) scanning at the Mayo Clinic and Massachusetts General Hospital were reported at the Boston postgraduate course in neuroradiology in September 1973. James Ambrose and Hillier Baker reported on preliminary results with the new scanner at the annual meeting of the Radiological Society of North America later that year.

A "users group" was informally set up towards the end of 1973, and the contributions by this group, which met for 1½ days at the end of May 1973, formed the basis of the first Symposium on Computerized Axial Tomography at the Montreal Neurological Institute, under the sponsorship of Dr. Romeo Ethier. (Of the many alternative names for the technique, the consensus at this meeting was that Computed Tomography was the most satisfactory.) Another short symposium devoted entirely to the subject was organized by Dr. Michael Huckman at Presbyterian-St. Luke's Hospital, Chicago, Illinois, in October 1974. An International Symposium and Course in Computed Tomography, sponsored by the senior author and Dr. Juan M. Taveras, was held in Bermuda in March 1975.

Following the demonstration of feasibility by Hounsfield and EMI, Dr. Robert Ledley of Georgetown University devised and constructed a prototype scanner capable of scanning the entire body. Although the time required to complete a scan, being similar to that of the EMI cranial scanner, militates against scans having the same accuracy as those obtained in the head when respiratory, cardiac, and gastrointestinal motion are involved, this equipment, known as the ACTA scanner (18, 37, 58), provided sufficient promise to spur development of scanners specifically designed to overcome the special problems. These are particularly those of physiological motion and tissue bulk encountered in scanning of the trunk.

At the Bermuda Symposium, Hounsfield announced the introduction of a new EMI scanner, designed for scanning of the torso, with individual section-scanning times of 20 seconds. The initial scans obtained with this equipment revealed startling clarity and detail in the chest and abdomen. At the same meeting, Dr. Ralph Alfidi gave a presentation based upon results with the prototype DELTA body scanner developed by Ohio Nuclear. Although the body scans produced with this unit, installed at the Cleveland Clinic, had been obtained with scan times of approximately 7 minutes, the results clearly indicated the enormous clinical potential of the method. More recently, improved DELTA scans have been obtained by reducing scan time to approximately 2 minutes.

Of particular interest to neuroradiologists is the potential for cross-sectional scanning of the spine and of pathological lesions developing within or encroaching upon the spinal canal.

In addition to the above, a number of well-known manufacturers of radiological equipment and others are working intensively to develop improved equipment for cranial scanning and for general body scanning. Federal support for basic and applied research in the entire field of reconstruction tomography has grown rapidly. It is to be expected, therefore, that technical advances in these fields will be made with considerable rapidity.

The MacRobert Award (£25,000 and Gold Medal) was awarded to Mr. Hounsfield in 1972 for his "epoch-making" development.

CHAPTER 2

General Description of the EMI Scanner: Operational Notes

The basic equipment comprises ten units (Fig. 2.1): patient table, scanning unit, x-ray control unit, computer cabinet unit, viewing unit, line printer unit, motor generator, high-voltage generator, cooling oil pump, and teletype.

PATIENT TABLE

This is a modification of an Elema-Schönander hydraulically adjustable special procedure patient table (Fig. 2.2). Vertical adjustment is obtained by foot pedal. The table is capable of being locked against horizontal movement by application of brakes to the rollers. At present, the tabletop is not capable of tilting. A handwheel provides smooth horizontal movement of the tabletop. When the tabletop is coupled to the headbox of the scanning unit, rotation of the handwheel causes horizontal movement of the tabletop, patient, and headbox together, permitting adjustment of the patient in relation to the x-ray beam and, therefore, of the level of tissue section to be scanned. A scale is provided on the scanner assembly for reference in selection of scan levels. A canvas strap with elastic cords is provided. With the patient's knees flexed, this strap is applied to the buttocks and upper thighs to provide counterpressure to the pressure of water in the headbox, when it is filled, and to assist in immobilization. Slides allow adjustment of the position of the strap along the length of the patient table.

A second canvas strap, also horizontally adjustable, permits the patient's legs to be lightly secured to ensure maintenance of knee flexion.

A hydraulic chair, capable of tilting and of changing the degree of body and lower extremity flexion, has recently become available as an alternative to the table.

SCANNING UNIT

The scanner gantry (Fig. 2.2) supports the x-ray tube. This is a modified fixed anode radiation therapy tube, oil cooled and with a focal spot size of 12 x 2.25 mm nominal. The mean x-ray beam length can be altered to scan tissue slices of 13 or 8 mm in thickness by the selection of collimator diaphragms located near both the x-ray tube and the detectors that can readily be interchanged. On the opposite side of the gantry are two precisely aligned sodium iodide crystal photomultiplier detectors, each of which monitors one-half of the x-ray beam, so that each scanning sequence provides data regarding contiguous tissue slices, each optionally of 13 or 8 mm thickness. Beam width is nominally 3 mm and beam length is 26 or 16 mm, depending on choice of collimator. A ruled glass graticule is fixed to the detector assembly. As it moves, it interrupts a light beam to provide 160 (240)* timing signals during a single parallel traverse of the beam and detectors across the waterbox and head, resulting in 160 (240) individual photon transmission measurements. Very precise alignment of the graticule is required for accuracy of measurements.

A precisely machined Plexiglas (Perspex) rectangular waterbox is situated in the central space of the scanning gantry and rotates with the gantry. The beam path through the waterbox (vide infra) is 27 cm, and the box is approximately 18 cm deep. A water pump permits filling and emptying of this headbox via flexible hoses. The

---

* The basic data given refer to the originally supplied 80 x 80 matrix. As of October 1974, a higher resolution system has been made available as an optional modification that can be applied to existing equipment in a short time. This system uses a 160 x 160 matrix and a new computer program. Figures in parentheses will refer to the 160 x 160 matrix modification.

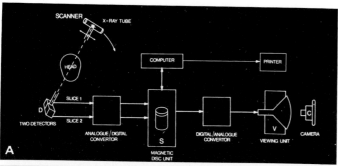

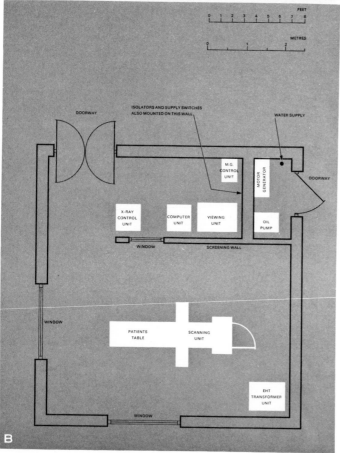

FIG. 2.1.

A. BLOCK DIAGRAM OF THE PRINCIPAL UNITS of the EMI scanner system. During scanning, the data are semiprocessed and put onto a disc buffer store. After completion of the first scan, this information is fully processed by the computer and automatically placed on a magnetic disc. (Reprinted by permission of EMI Ltd.)

B. EXAMPLE OF INSTALLATION LAYOUT. An area of 600–800 square feet is desirable for the suite. The scanning room should be equipped with a sink, instrument counter, and storage cabinets for drugs, syringes, needles, swabs, adhesive tape, phantoms, and other accessories. The control area requires adjustable lighting (preferably with dimmer switches) to provide for low light level viewing of the cathode ray tube and higher levels for examination of photographs and printout data. X-ray film illuminators are a convenience. Air conditioning is generally needed to control heat generated by the electrical components. The motor generator supplying the H. T. generator and the pump assembly should be housed in a separate small room because of the noise they generate (maximum, approximately 80 decibels at 1 meter). This room must be ventilated to remove heat generated (approximately 1.5 kW of heat). Film storage in a cool area, storage for printout paper, a table for viewing printouts, and racks for displaying Polaroid scan photographs are most desirable. Adjacent office space, a patient waiting room, and file storage for records are needed. Separate access to the control room and scanning room is important. (Reprinted by permission of EMI Ltd.)

waterbox is sealed on the patient surface by a circular metal rim and rubber O-ring seated in a circular metal flange that is attached to the waterbox and in a mating stationary circular flange, thus forming a rotatable water-tight seal. Removable collars carrying a thin plastic cylinder or cone can be inserted into the front orifice of the water tank (Fig. 3.3).

Four knurled knobs secure a metal ring to the flange. The ring carries a latex rubber head bag and the cone or cylinder insert and provides a water-tight seal. The latex bag is molded in the form of a cap, which normally projects into the waterbox, within the plastic cone or cylinder. Four tabs are attached to the interior of the latex cap to assist in drawing the cap down over the

lower part of the patient's head as the waterbox is gradually filled during the positioning procedure.

Single Scan Sequence

The x-ray beam makes a traverse of the waterbox and its contents (Fig. 2.3). Following completion of the traverse, the gantry indexes 1° and the traverse is repeated in the opposite direction. This sequence is repeated until 180 traverses have been completed. Each point in the waterbox and its contents has thus been scanned 180 times, over an arc of 180°. Two contiguous slices have been scanned, from which two pictures will be generated. During the scan sequence, the photon detectors have monitored the beam quality after passage

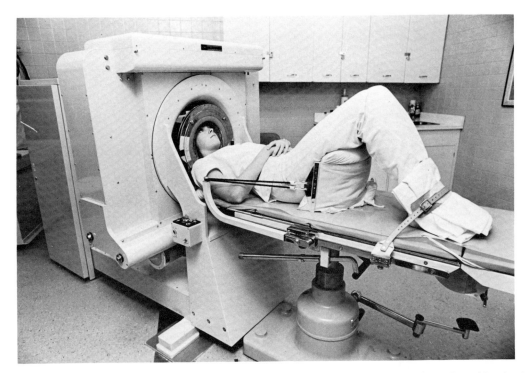

FIG. 2.2. "PATIENT" IN POSITION ON THE ADJUSTABLE TABLE. A canvas strap with adjustable elastic cords provides counterpressure against the pressure of the water-filled box. The maintenance of the required knee flexion is aided by the second strap at the ankles. A comfortable position should be assured to minimize the possibility of movement during cranial scanning. The head is shown placed within the rubber cap projecting into the waterbox. The scanner gantry carrying the x-ray tube and photon detectors surrounds the waterbox.

through the box and water and through other materials within the waterbox. Thus, for each traverse, eventual calculations of photon attenuations produced by materials within the waterbox will be referenced against attenuation produced by water alone plus other fixed materials. In addition to the two x-ray beams that go through the waterbox, a third beam from the x-ray tube goes through an absorber equivalent to 27 cm of water and is measured by a third scintillation detector. This is a reference beam, and each of the 180 (240) readings in a traverse is compared to its reading at the moment of measurement.

In normal operation, the scan sequences are initiated with the x-ray tube in the lowermost position, and the subsequent rotation of the gantry is from this point to the viewer's left when standing behind the unit and looking towards the top of the patient's head. This direction of scanning provides a picture that represents a view from the top of the patient's head with the face uppermost (brow up). The direction of the scanning rotation can be altered to run in an arc to the right, but this results in pictures that are inverted (patient's face lowermost, brow down). In addition, the scan may be started at any angle from normal to normal +89°, with a corresponding alteration in picture orientation.

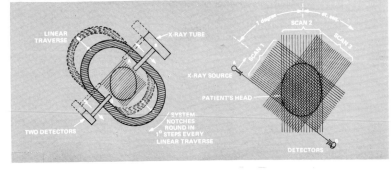

FIG. 2.3. DIAGRAMMATIC REPRESENTATION OF SCANNING SEQUENCE, which comprises a series of 180 parallel traverses of the accurately aligned x-ray beam and two photon detectors, with 1 degree rotation of the gantry after each linear sweep. Each block of tissue in each of the two simultaneously scanned sections (slices) will have been scanned 180 times at the completion of a scan sequence, and the photon transmission measurements obtained are averaged for each small tissue block. The readings are digitized and fed to the computer, which solves 28,800 simultaneous equations for each slice to derive absorption (attenuation) values in each block. (Reprinted by permission of EMI Ltd.)

Waterbox

The upper and lower surfaces of the Plexiglas water-box should be kept clean, and care should be taken that no dirt is allowed to lie on the surfaces. It has been found that a single layer of Scotch tape placed on the upper surface of the Plexiglas in the path of the beam is sufficient to produce a recognizable artifact. Photon-dense material on the surface (such as a spot of oil) is capable of producing dramatic artifacts, which appear in the form of circular bands in the central area of the scan.

Gas bubbles allowed to accumulate within the water-box can produce striking artifacts capable of producing severe scan degradation. For this reason, the use of deaerated water in the water reservoir is desirable. The addition of a biostatic agent to the water is advised to inhibit growth of algae, and the water should be changed every few months. Whenever the waterbox is emptied into the reservoir for the purpose of changing the cylinder, cone insert, or headbag or for other reasons, care must be taken during the waterbox refilling cycle to expel as much air as possible from the waterbox through the outflow holes. Any material coming into contact with the water in the box should be thoroughly cleaned before insertion, including the surface of a new head bag.

Scan Time

The time required for a single complete scan sequence is approximately 4½–5 minutes. By means of a selector switch in the scanning unit, alternative scanning speeds can be set to obtain approximate scanning times of 6½, 8½, or 11½ minutes. At the normal scan speed of 4½ minutes, 10^5 photons pass through each slot in the detector graticule during each measurement during a horizontal sweep. Increasing the scan time provides a proportionate increase in the number of photons passing through each slot. This will decrease quantum noise but increases the possibility of scan degradation by motion of the patient.

X-RAY CONTROL UNIT

This is remote from the scanning unit and contains the necessary controls and interlocks for operating the scanning unit and x-ray tube (Fig. 2.4). A warm-up period of 15 minutes is required after overnight shut down, with progressive increase in tube loading until the maximum setting of 140 kV and the usual operating milliamperage of 33 is reached in order to keep the x-ray tube free of gas. If equipment stands idle for 4 or more hours during the day, warm-up procedure should be repeated using half of the usual recommended times in the EMI Operator Instruction Manual, to which reference should be made for details of operating procedure.

Detector sensitivity can be varied when necessary, as for example when 8-mm slice collimators are used ((the readings on the level meters *PICTURE 1*, *PICTURE 2*, and *REFERENCE* (A25) (Fig. 2.4B) will be approximately halved and photomultiplier detector output voltage will need to be adjusted to increase detector sensitivity)). Also, change of scanning speed will require adjustment of detector sensitivity. Detector sensitivity is set by scanning a completely filled waterbox and adjusting the sensitivity rotary switches so that the three meters (one for each of the 2 sections and one for water reference) peak in the green area during the scanning. The over-range indicator on the control panel will be illuminated if there is an excess of air around the patient's head. This may also happen if the patient moves. The computer will continue to accept the readings, although the picture may be of poor quality. At this point, the operator has the option of aborting the scan. Experience in the use of equipment will enable appropriate decisions in this regard with reference to the clinical condition of the patient.

The x-ray control panel also carries the high-voltage supply for the photomultiplier tubes. Since this voltage controls the amplification of the photomultiplier tubes, it is set in conjunction with the sensitivity controls described above to keep all 3 meters in the green area. The voltage showed rarely needs to be changed.

COMPUTER

The heart of the computational system of the scanner is a dedicated computer that is programmed to require minimal attention by the operator. This small computer, a Nova 820 (Data General Corporation), has a 16 bit words and 24,000 word core. Associated with it is a Diablo disc drive, the magnetic cartridge discs of which carry programs and data. A Teletype machine allows input of control words and a Tally line printer provides fast hard-copy readouts of numerical data. The Teletype and Tally are also used to communicate with the computer for special information processing and for trouble shooting.

The great convenience of the machine arises from the use of discs. Each magnetic disc can record about 1½ million 16 bit words. Part of each disc is used for programs, and the remainder is used for recording images being processed and completed pictures. There are 12 buffers, each of which can hold semiprocessed data from a scan section awaiting processing. The capacity is 60 (36) processed sections. Since each disc carries all the program information necessary for operating, the loading procedure for a new disc is simple. Changes in programs may be made by simple rewriting on the existing discs. A most useful feature is that damage to one disc affects only that disc. The computer program of the 80 x 80 matrix system uses an iterative algorithm to process the pictures. The principal of this algo-

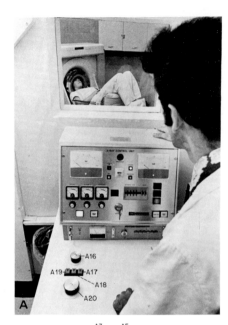

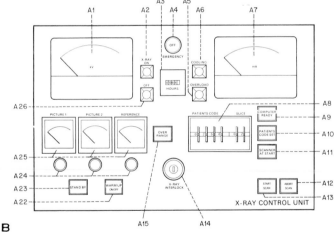

FIG. 2.4.

A. Technologist at the x-ray control unit monitoring the over range warning lamp and the photomultiplier signal level reference meters and observing the patient being scanned.

B. THE X-RAY CONTROL UNIT.

A1. KV Meter. Meter for indicating the voltage applied to the X-ray tube.

A2. X-ray On. Warning lamp indicating that the X-ray tube is energized.

A3. Hours. Indicates the cumulative running time of the X-ray tube in hours and tenths.

A4. Emergency Off. Press button that cuts power from all scanning circuits and the X-ray tube and must be used only in an emergency.

A5. Overload. Warning lamp that is illuminated if the X-ray tube overload trip operates.

A6. Cooling. Indicator lamp showing that the cooling oil pump is operating.

A7. mA Meter. Meter indicating the current through the X-ray tube.

A8. Patient's Code and Slice. Thumb wheels for setting up the patient's code and slice (see *A10*).

A9. Computer Ready. Indicator lamp that is illuminated when the computer status is such that it will accept information from the scanner.

A10. Patient's Code Set. Illuminated push button switch that has to be pressed after setting the patient's code on the thumb-wheel switches (*A8*).

A11. Scanner at Start. Indicator lamp showing that the scanner is at the start position.

A12. Abort Scan. Illuminated push button switch used to stop scanning and switch off the X-rays should the scanning sequence need to be abandoned.

A13. Start Scan. Illuminated push button switch for starting the X-ray scanning sequence.

A14. Over Range. Warning lamp indicating over-ranging of the detectors.

A15. X-ray Interlock. A key switch operated by the interlock key.

A16. mA Control. Varies the current through the X-ray tube.

A17. 140kV⎫
A18. 120kV⎬ Push buttons to select the appropriate X-ray tube voltages.
A19. 100kV⎭

A20. kV Control. Varies the voltage applied to the X-ray tube.

A21. Photomultiplier Power Supply ON/OFF Switch. To switch on or off the photomultiplier power supply unit.

A22. Warm-up ON/OFF. Illuminated push button switch that controls the X-ray tube warm-up procedure.

A23. Stand-by ON/OFF. Illuminated push button switch controlling the scanning circuits.

A24. Detector Sensitivity Selectors. Three 11-way rotary switches adjusting the sensitivity of the slice A, slice B, and reference photomultipliers.

A25. Pictures 1 and 2 and Reference. Meters indicating the signal level from the integrators for each of the three photomultipliers.

A26. X-ray Off. Indicator lamp showing X-rays off.

(Reprinted by permission of EMI Ltd.)

rithm is that, initially, each measured value of attenuation is assumed to come from a uniform distribution along the line of the x-ray beam. As successive readings are taken, these values are shifted to match the new readings. This procedure is repeated, cycling around and around the readings until the estimated matrix of attenuation values is statistically consistent with the observed numbers. This iteration is a long process, so that, even with a reasonably fast computer and with a program written in a fast machine language, it still requires approximately 4–5 minutes to process a scan section. With the 160 x 160 matrix system, the computer program is based on convolutional methods and computation can also proceed while the scanner is in operation. Reconstructed images are available for viewing in less than 30 seconds following completion of a scan sequence.

It should be kept in mind that the mathematical methods of information processing are in a state of rapid development and change. Improvement in the forms of higher speed, better resolution, less sensitivity to artifacts, and better storage capabilities can be expected in the near future.

Although the computer is the key element in the data processing, there are a number of electronic circuits especially built for the system that perform part of the processing and control. These are contained in a rack on the main computer unit.

Data Processing

During scanning, the data are semiprocessed and put onto a disc buffer store (Fig. 2.1). After the first scan has been completed, this information is fully processed by the computer and automatically placed on the magnetic disc. The processing light (*C10*) on the computer control panel (Fig. 2.5) will be illuminated while processing is in progress.

If the scan/view switch (*C3*) is set to the view position while a slice is being processed, the processing of this slice will be completed but no more processing will be carried out. Thus, computer processing cannot proceed while the viewer is being operated, although it can continue while scanning proceeds. The lack of ability of the present equipment to permit viewing (and analysis) while the scanner is in operation, or while processing of the data is proceeding, has proved to be a significant limitation in our attempts to arrange efficient operation of the machine in patient scanning and in economical use of the radiologists' time. With the original program and matrix, the computer takes 8 minutes to process the data pertaining to a pair of slices (4–5 minutes per slice) after each scan. The problem is eased with the installation of a new program and 160 matrix system, since the new program and increased computer core permits the completion of the processing of two slices less than ½

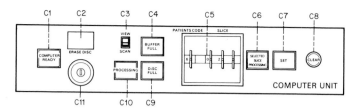

FIG. 2.5. COMPUTER CONTROL UNIT.

C1. Disc Ready. Warning light indicating readiness of disc and computer unit to commence operation.

C2. Erase Disc. Illuminated push button switch to erase information stored on disc store.

C3. View/Scan. Selector switch to allow the processed information to be viewed. In the scan position it allows information to be processed and/or scanning to be carried out.

C4. Buffer Full. This warning lamp is illuminated when the maximum number (12) of unprocessed slices has accumulated in the buffer store.

C5. Patient's Code and Slice. Thumbwheel selectors used for setting the last digit of a patient's code for priority processing.

C6. Selected Slice Processing. Indicator lamp that is illuminated while the slice set by the thumbwheel selectors (*C5*) is being processed.

C7. Set. Illuminated press button switch that reads in the code set by *C5* when depressed.

C8. Clear. Push button pressed to clear the code setting on *C6* if it is no longer to be processed out of turn.

C9. Disc Full. Warning lamp that is illuminated when the number of scans completed fills the disc store section with processed slices.

C10. Processing. Indicator lamp that is illuminated while slices are being processed by the computer.

C11. Key Switch. This accepts the interlock key for disc erasure.

(Reprinted by permission of EMI Ltd.)

minute after scan completion. With the 80 x 80 matrix system, each magnetic disc can carry data of up to 60 processed slices. With the new program, the capacity of the magnetic disc is reduced to approximately 36 slices.

It should be noted that, with the 80 x 80 and 160 x 160 systems, processing of slices proceeds during operation of the scanner, subsequent to the *initial* scan. Processing of information can be deferred, but only up to the point that the buffer becomes filled to its capacity of 12 unprocessed slices. Scanning may be commenced again when there is sufficient space in the buffer.

Scans may be processed out of sequence by setting the patient's code and slice numbers on the computer control thumbwheels (Fig. 2.5, *C5*) to show the last digit of the patient's code, the scan number, and either slice A or B. The computer will complete processing of the current slice and then operate on the selected slice. After the selected slice has been processed or the clear button (*C8*) is pressed, the computer will continue to process the remaining slices in normal order. This facility will not be necessary, of course, with the high-definition system, and these controls will become inoperative or may be used for other functions.

VIEWER

This unit incorporates a cathode ray tube (CRT) on which is presented an analogue display of the absorption data of each tissue slice (Fig. 2.6). The presentation is in the form of a grey scale, in which brightness is proportional to the x-ray absorption coefficient of the material in each picture point of the scan. In the display, the most radiodense materials appear as peak white, and the least dense appear as full black. One tissue slice is viewed at a time. With the scan obtained in the usual manner, the picture is presented as though the observer was viewing from the top of the patient's head, with the patient in the brow-up position. The computed tomographic (CT) scan code number is presented at the top of the picture followed by the slice designation (1A, 1B, 2A, etc.) originally set on the x-ray control unit at the time of scanning.

At the bottom of the CRT display is a horizontal grey scale to permit adjustment of the viewing and photographic white and black level basic controls (which, once adjusted, should be left undisturbed). Generally, optimum photographic records are obtained when the two darkest rectangles are barely distinguishable from each other and the two lightest zones are readily distinguishable.

As noted under "Computer," the viewer cannot be used while processing of information by the computer is proceeding. If the view/scan switch (C3) on the computer control panel is set to view, processing of a slice underway will be continued to completion before any slice is displayed on the viewer. The last processed slice will be displayed initially. To select other slice pictures, the selector switch (B9) can be used to hunt sequentially through a series in the order in which they are carried on the magnetic disc, in forward or reverse directions. The slices are stored on the disc in a continuous loop so that the slice preceding the first slice on the disc is the last one on the disc.

The form of the data display on the CRT is set up by operation of the window width (B10) and the window level (B13) controls.

Window Width

This control (B10) in effect permits selection of the range of absorption values (units) between black and peak white displayed on the CRT and, therefore, of the degree of contrast (latitude in the display of absorption data) (Figs. 2.7, 2.8, and 2.9). In the routine display modes, window width may be selected in a series of steps from 20–100, resulting in a progressive diminu-

tion of effective contrast of the display as the range of absorption values included in the display is progressively increased as higher window widths are set.

Modification of Window Width Control

At our request, an additional control was installed on the MGH viewer replacing the window 100 terminal with a separate control knob permitting continuous variation of window width between the 20 and the *MEASURE* settings (see below). In practice, the best differentiation of pathological tissue with an absorption range very similar to adjacent normal tissues is obtained with a window width setting in this additional range, but window widths 5 and 10 have proved to be sufficient additional widths for most such lesions.

Window Level

The window level control (B30) sets the level of the center of the range selected by the window width control to any desired point on the scale of x-ray absorption coefficients (Fig. 2.7 and 2.10). The basic range provided is ±50 units. This may be extended to ±500 units by moving the switch B12 to the ×10 position.

With the basic range setting of ±50 units, choice of window width and window level settings is dictated by the material under examination and is chosen to give the best apparent display of tissue detail. With the 80 x 80 matrix, the window width setting we prefer is usually 20 and the window level generally is in the range of 12–18. Under these conditions, cerebrospinal fluid appears black, bone appears white, and brain tissue appears as various shades of grey. With experience, the best settings can be achieved rapidly.

MEASURE Position of Window Width Control (M)

This position of the window width control effects a window width of less than unity and enables the x-ray absorption coefficient at any desired point in the picture to be measured. This position of the control is used, therefore, for detailed analysis of absorption data. At this setting, numerical values for absorption in any picture point on the CRT display can be obtained. As the window level is increased using control B13, when the point under examination just changes from white to black, the absorption value of the point can be read off the scale on the window level control. The same absorption measurement of any given point can also be obtained by progressive lowering of the window level control. The level on the scale at which the point just changes from black to white gives the absorption value for the point (see scale of units used in machine calibration in Fig. 2.10). In practice, most substances under investigation will be spread over a number of picture points and all will show a range of absorption

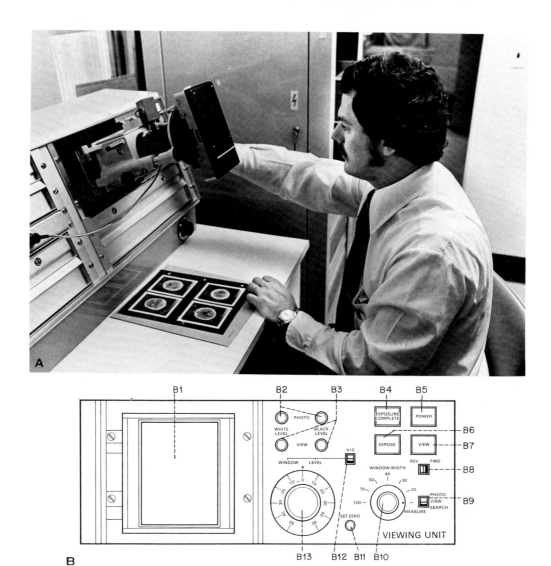

FIG. 2.6.

A. VIEWING UNIT. Processed scan data are presented on the cathode ray tube in the form of pictures, in which light intensity is directly proportional to calculated photon absorption at each point. The display can be modified extensively by the operator and numerical absorption values can be obtained for any tissue block. Values so obtained are those presented numerically on the paper printout of the scan. An attached Polaroid camera is being used to provide permanent scan records, a set of which are shown on the counter.

B. VIEWING UNIT CONTROL PANEL.

B1. Viewer. Cathode ray tube screen on which the processed results are displayed.

B2. White and Black Levels-Photo. Preset controls set to give the correct reproduction of the black and white levels and grey scale on the photograph.

B3. White and Black Levels-View. Controls used to give the correct display of black and white levels and grey scale on the cathode ray tube screen.

B4. Exposure Complete. This indicator lamp is illuminated 3 seconds after the expose button (*B6*) is pressed and indicates that the picture is ready for development.

B5. Power. Push on/push off switch controlling the power to the viewer unit.

B6. Expose. Push button that may be depressed when illuminated to expose the film in the camera.

B7. View. Push on/push off switch to allow results to be displayed.

B8. Reverse/Forward. Biased switch to select the preceding or succeeding slice in sequence.

B9. Photo-View-Search Selector. The up position causes the expose button (*B6*) to be illuminated. The central position is used for normal viewing. The search (down) position allows continuous sequencing of successive slices in conjunction with the forward and reverse selector (*B8*).

B10. Window Width. This control selects the range of X-ray absorption values that will give black to peak white on the display.

B11. Set Zero. This control presets the zero setting of the window level control.

B12. ×10. When this switch is in the up position, the scale of the window level (*B13*) is multiplied by 10.

B13. Window Level. This control sets the midpoint of the range selected by the window width control (*B10*) to any desired point on the scale of X-ray absorption values.

WINDOW WIDTH AND WINDOW LEVEL RELATED TO DISPLAY

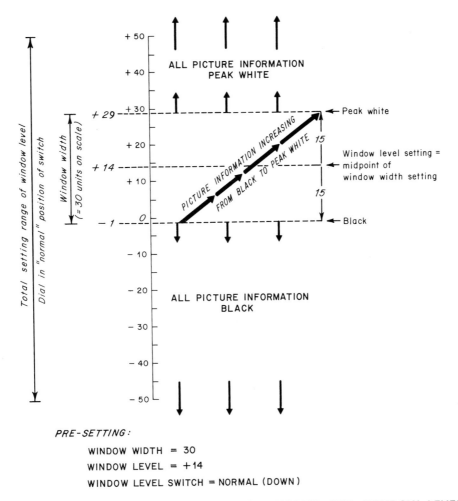

PRE-SETTING:

WINDOW WIDTH = 30
WINDOW LEVEL = +14
WINDOW LEVEL SWITCH = NORMAL (DOWN)

FIG. 2.7. DIAGRAM ILLUSTRATING EFFECT OF WINDOW WIDTH AND WINDOW LEVEL IN RELATION TO DISPLAY. With the basic range setting on switch *B12* (normal), the range of the scale is ±50 units. The window width control setting determines the range of absorption values displayed on the CRT. In this example, the window width is set at 30; there are 30 units between black and peak white on the display. Window level (the level of the middle of the selected window width) has been set at +14, and therefore absorption numbers lower than −1 (14 − 15) will appear as black and numbers higher than +29 (14 + 15) will appear as peak white. Numbers between −1 and 29 will appear as shades of grey, darker for the lower numbers and lighter for the higher numbers.

To set the viewing unit view black and white level controls (*B3*) and set zero (*B11*).

a. Set selector (*B9*) to view.

b. Set the window level (*B13*) to +50.

c. Turn the black level fully anticlockwise.

d. Turn the white level fully anticlockwise.

e. Wait until the corners of the display disappear.

N.B. As images persist, it is necessary to make adjustments slowly.

f. Turn the black level clockwise until the corners of the display just reappear.

g. Turn the white level clockwise until the second step on the grey scale at the bottom of the display appears.

h. The black and white levels may need further slight adjustment. The aim is to obtain even steps of intensity change along the grey scale.

i. Set the window level control (*B13*) to 0 and the normal/×10 switch (*B12*) to Normal.

j. Set the window width control (*B10*) to Measure.

k. Adjust the set zero (*B11*) until the corners of the display just change from black to white. The set zero control is not operative on the ×10 range.

(Reprinted by permission of EMI Ltd.)

15

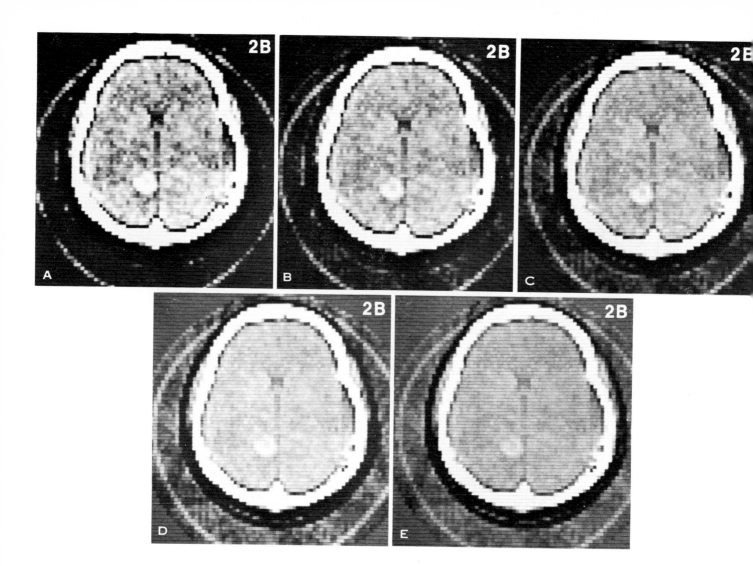

FIG. 2.8

A–E. EFFECT OF WINDOW WIDTH SELECTION ON "CONTRAST" OF CRT DISPLAY. This series of Polaroid photographs of the CRT display was taken with a window level setting of 18. The slice was scanned at approximately 30° to Reid's base line, passing through the inferior portions of the frontal horns and third ventricle anteriorly and through the cerebellum, a short distance above the fourth ventricle, posteriorly. The rounded high absorption (*white*) area in the left paramedian portion of the cerebellum represents the cross-section of a cerebellar hematoma, measuring approximately 2 cm in diameter. **A,** taken with a window width setting of 20 (20 units between black and peak white); **B,** at a window width of 30; **C,** at a setting of 40; **D,** at a setting of 50; **E,** at a setting of 75. Note the progressive decrease in contrast of the image as the window width is increased to include a larger number of units between black and peak white in the display. The choice of window widths for display (and photography) is subject to individual preference, but it should be noted that, the wider the window width, the greater the suppression of details of variation in absorption data; in general, it is advisable to choose the lowest window compatible with a coherent appearance of the picture. Wider window widths at times may provide an optimal display of the recorded data, for example, when "noise" is excessive. Increased noise levels are produced when there is very high beam absorption as by dense bone in the region of the skull base, and particularly when movement has occurred during scanning. High noise levels are produced when very dense material (such as Pantopaque, large surgical clips, shunt valves, hair grips, and prosthetic metal plates or mesh), or very low density material, such as peri- or intracranial gas, is included in the scanned slice. In general, the wider the window required to produce a coherent appearance of the display, the greater is the noise level in the scan. As the window width is increased and the range widened to include lower absorption values, the low absorption zone of the air trapped in the hair of the patient becomes progressively more visible and is best seen in **E**. While the presence of some air around the head does not produce obvious degradation of the scan, it is advisable to minimize possible adverse effects by placing a stockinette cap over the patient's head before insertion into the head bag to reduce the amount of air when the patient has a luxuriant head of hair (see Chapter 3). The narrow zone of greater density bounding the air shadow represents the headbag. Outside this is the approximately circular contour of the plastic head cylinder and, finally, the circular contours marking the perimeter of the zone of the waterbox included in the scan. *The latter is constant at 23.4 cm and should measure 8.0 cm on the CRT display when the machine is properly calibrated (21.8 cm with the 160 x 160 matrix system).* Each square on the CRT display measures 23.4/8.0 = 2.94 mm using the 80 x 80 matrix (or approximately 1.5 mm with the 160 x 160 matrix).

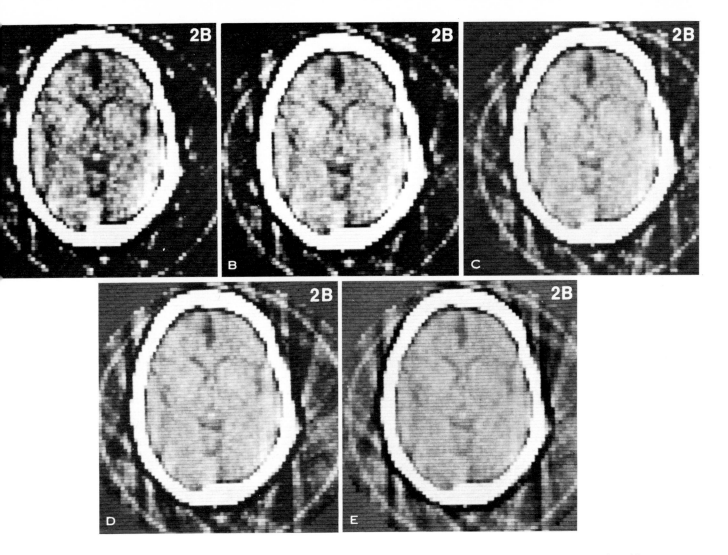

FIG. 2.9.

A–E. EFFECT OF WINDOW WIDTH SELECTION ON THE APPEARANCE OF THE CEREBRAL VENTRICLES AND SUBARACHNOID SPACES. This scan was obtained on a patient with cerebral cortical atrophy. The lateral and third ventricles are not enlarged, but there is marked widening of the frontal portion of the longitudinal fissure and some enlargement of the subarachnoid spaces over the external surfaces of the frontal lobes. The sylvian cisterns and quadrigeminal and superior cerebellar cisterns are somewhat enlarged also. This series of Polaroid pictures was obtained with a window level setting of 18. Window width setting in **A** was 20, in **B** was 30, in **C** was 40, in **D** was 50, and in **E** was 75. Note the progressive decrease in contrast with the larger window widths. There was some lateral head motion during this scan as evidenced by the vertical alternating white and black bands adjacent to the outer aspect of the skull. This motion increased the noise in the scan, and the optimal window width display is obtained at 30 or 40 rather than at 20. The slightly higher absorption of the caudate nuclei and putamina can be distinguished at window widths 20 and 30, but can barely be distinguished at window width 40, and is suppressed at wider windows. The change in appearance of the calcification in the pineal and the decreasing discrimination of the CSF-containing spaces with the wider windows should be noted. The artifacts in the regions of the water in the headbox are more clearly shown because the wider window settings include more of the lower absorption values.

values. Generally, it is simple to obtain the peak absorption values of the tissue or other material under examination, but the lowest absorption value of the material may be more difficult to define precisely. An attempt to find the lower absorption level of the range involves making a judgement regarding the endpoint of the enlargement of the area of the material or tissue and the dividing line between this and surrounding normal tissue or other material as the window level is slowly brought lower. Note should always be taken of the possibility of partial volume phenomena (see Chapter 4).

Range of Absorption Values

Several factors can be involved in causing all substances scanned to have a range of absorption (attenuation) coefficients: (1) heterogeneity of x-ray beam; (2) quantum noise; (3) nonhomogeneous absorption in different areas of substance; and (4) partial volume phenomenon.

Setting of Viewing Unit

To view black and white level controls (*B3*) and to set 0 (*B11*):
A. Set selector (*B9*) to view.
B. Set the window level (*B13*) to +50.
C. Turn the black level fully anticlockwise.
D. Turn the white level fully anticlockwise.
E. Wait until the corners of the CRT display disappear. (Note that, owing to persistence of images of the CRT, it is necessary to make adjustment slowly).
F. Turn the black level clockwise until the corners of the CRT display just reappear.
G. Turn the white level clockwise until the second step on the grey scale at the bottom of the display disappears.
H. The black and white levels may need further slight adjustment. The aim is to obtain even steps of intensity change along the grey scale.
I. Set the window level control to 0 and the normal/×10 switch (*B12*) to Normal.
J. Set the window width control to Measure.
K. Adjust the set 0 (*B11*) until the corners of the display just change from black to white. The set 0 control is not operative on the ×10 range.

Photography of the CRT Display

Photographic records may be obtained of the CRT display, normally using a Polaroid camera and Polaroid film (100 series). This film is automatically processed in 15 seconds. Processing for less than 15 seconds reduces the contrast of the print, but an increase in processing time of up to 1 minute or somewhat more does not appreciably affect the appearance of the print.

Initial Photographic Setup

When the preset controls have been set up to give a satisfactory display in the view mode, the selector (*B9*) is set to *PHOTO*. The Polaroid camera shutter is set to B and the aperture is set to 16 as an initial setting. The camera on its mount is swung into position and is fastened using the over-center catch.

The exposure control (*B6*) is pressed, and when the exposure complete indicator (*B4*) has illuminated, the print is pulled from the camera. After the required period for development, the print is peeled off and coated. The photograph should then be checked to ensure that it has the same appearance as does the display in the view mode. If it does not, the photo black and white presets of *B2* and the iris setting of the camera are adjusted to obtain this condition. Once the controls *B2* have been set properly, they rarely require readjustment.

Note that, while there is a considerable advantage in the rapid print production of the Polaroid method, the need for coating of prints adds appreciably to the burden of work when a large number of photographic records is required. ((A new Polaroid black and white film (Type 107C) that requires 30-second processing but does not require subsequent fixation has been tested and has proven satisfactory for the purpose of obtaining permanent records of scans in our preliminary experience.))

Photographic Records

The number of photographic records of each case obtained will vary widely according to the type of case and the choice of the individual.

At the Massachusetts General Hospital, it has been the practice to undertake complete analyses of the scans of each case at the outset. This procedure was determined by our desire to explore the full potential of the analytical method, and the decision was influenced by the lack of a permanent record of the scan data on magnetic tape. Digital printout of each slice provides a form of permanent record, but, as will be discussed, the digital record is much less satisfactory for clinical work than are CRT viewing and analysis of data. Since the magnetic disc (Diablo) is capable of storing data of only 60 slices (equivalent to the record of 7.5 patients at an average of four scans, i.e., eight slices per patient) and since our stock of magnetic discs has been limited (8–10 at different times), records on discs have had to be erased after a few days. With the 160 x 160 matrix, each magnetic disc will hold data of only about 36 slices. Conversion of the digital data on the printout to a magnetic disc record is a very tedious process and therefore is not generally practical.

For the above reasons, it has been our practice to obtain between 16 and 32 Polaroid print records per case, depending on the complexity of the problem. At a present cost of $2.89 per Polaroid 8-exposure cartridge, this represents a cost of between $5.78 and $11.56 in film per case, to which must be added the cost of time involved in making and annotating (with window width and level figures) the photographic records. In our practice, basic routine photographic recording includes a print of the "best quality" CRT display of each slice and a photograph of each slice obtained with an M setting of 11 or 12 to provide a general representation of cerebrospinal fluid-containing spaces (including partial volume areas of CSF spaces), supplemented by several photographs at different M settings to record the general absorption range and the extent of any pathological process identified on each relevant slice. In addition, to record in more detail the analysis of pathological lesions and questionable areas of absorption, it has been our practice to draw diagrams of slices, outlining suspected or obvious lesions, and to insert the absorption ranges of obvious or suspected pathology.

Although the availability of a permanent record in the form of magnetic tape now provides the highly desirable opportunity to review in additional detail any scan for clinical or investigative purposes, it is undoubtedly good discipline to proceed as though no such permanent record will be available and to obtain the most complete analysis and record possible at the outset.

While it is recognized that this philosophy makes the interpretation of a CT scan as painstaking as that of a cerebral angiogram or pneumoencephalogram, it is our belief that the diagnostic information contained in a CT scan is sufficiently large in amount and potentially informative to make this approach essential to sound neuroradiological practice.

While CT scanning can be used as a highly informative survey method of investigation, its potential value is so much greater that we feel that efforts should not be spared in obtaining the maximum possible amount of information from the data obtained. It is believed that only by this approach will there be realization of the full potential benefit of this form of examination in reducing the requirement or duration of hospitalization and the need for invasive procedures.

ABSORPTION SCALES AND DATA

An arbitrary scale of absorption values forms the basis of EMI scan measurements. The absorption of water is taken as the reference level 0. The normal intracranial soft tissues occupy a narrow absorption band (approximately 4% in width) centered at a level of about 3% (Fig. 2.10A). For this reason, a working scale of 5 times the basic scale is used (Fig 2.10B). On the latter scale, normal intracranial soft tissues have a range of approxi-

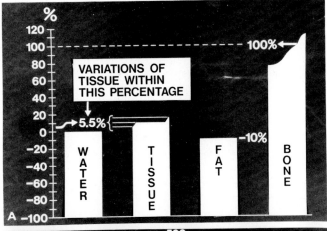

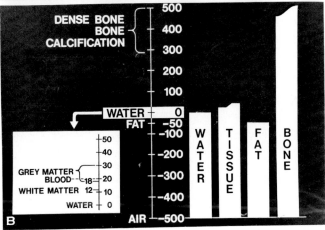

FIG. 2.10.

A. BASIC SCALE. The scale shown represents absorption coefficients of substances in percentages greater or lesser than water. With water representing 0, fat averages −10% and the majority of normal intracranial soft tissues lies in a 4% wide absorption band centered on approximately the 3% level. Dense bone has a mean value of about 100%, and calcifications range variably between a value somewhat higher than the densest soft tissues and somewhat less than bone, depending on their density of aggregation and size. On this scale, gas measures −100%. Equipment accuracy in determining absorption coefficients is approximately 0.5% on this scale.

B. WORKING SCALE. In practice, for working convenience, the above scale is expanded 5 times. As this scale uses the absorption of water as a reference (i.e., water = 0), to obtain the absolute absorption (attenuation) coefficient of any material for the 120 kV x-ray beam, 500 is added to the readings and the result is multiplied by a factor of 0.19/500. On this scale, equipment accuracy is approximately ±2.5 units (±½% standard deviation, measured on water). In practice, machine accuracy is frequently greater than this and may be as high as ±1 unit between 0 and +60 units.

mately 12 to approximately 30 units. However, it must be noted that the higher values in this range, occurring in the region of the peripheral cerebral cortex, are produced by an artifact. Note must be made of an important computational artifact that is identified in a broad zone internal to dense bone (or phantom material). This artifact results in the addition of 3–7 units to the correct absorption coefficients of materials lying in this zone (Fig. 4.1), and therefore this artifact affects the recorded absorption of cortex lying subjacent to the skull. Normal values of cerebral cortex in young adults lie in the range 19–22 units, but the above artifact produces values that range up to approximately 28–30 units in regions subjacent to the thicker and denser portions of the cranial vault. Absorption values in the cortical regions of the frontal and occipital areas may range several units higher, possibly due to the frequently thicker and denser bone in these regions. It has been noted that cortical grey matter in young children has an upper level less than that in the adult, and in infants, cortical grey matter may not be differentiated from subjacent white matter on the basis of higher absorption values. These findings may be due to the thinner and less dense calvaria in the younger age groups. The tendency for higher cortical values to be recorded in some elderly individuals may be the result of increased computational artifacts in regions beneath increasingly dense and thick portions of the cranial vault rather than to changes in the cortex itself.

Cerebral white matter normally lies in the range of 12–17 or 18 units. Central grey matter shows a mean absorption that is slightly greater than that of white matter and somewhat less than that of cortical grey matter, generally lying in the range of 15–20 units. There is a tendency for central grey matter to become denser in many elderly individuals, presumably due to the increased iron and calcium known to accumulate here with age. The head of the caudate nucleus is generally somewhat denser than the putamen, and the putamen is somewhat denser than the thalamus. It is at times possible to distinguish portions of the internal capsule by contrast with the slightly denser grey nuclei.

Our results have indicated the need for a modification of the absorption values provided with the equipment. Our measurements indicate that cerebrospinal fluid (CSF) is normally identified in the range of 0–11 units. The higher values (8–11) in this range represent CSF occupying less than the full thickness of the slice. The absorption coefficient (μ) is then averaged with the surrounding tissue in the block.

This feature of the method must be kept in mind when evaluating the absorption readings of all small tissue volumes (see Chapter 4, "Partial Volume Phenomenon").

Blood in the circulation was originally stated to have a value of 6 units, but our experimental results and clinical experience indicate much higher values (see Chapter 15).

The greater density of grey matter than white seems to be related to the markedly greater vascularity of grey matter and to the considerably greater lipid (myelin) content of white matter, although other factors probably are involved also. Fat, as seen in the orbit and in the lipoma of the corpus callosum, has values ranging down to −50. Lipid-containing lesions, such as craniopharyngiomatous cysts, have values that vary from negative values to levels of over +10, depending on the percentage of lipid (cholesterol) within the cyst fluid.

Pineal and glomus calcifications are regularly visible on scans, even when not visible on radiographs.

For further discussions of absorption values of normal tissues, see Chapter 5, and for discussions of absorption values of various pathological tissues, see appropriate chapters in Part Two.

SCAN PRINTOUT

Immediately after completion of absorption data processing of each scan section by the computer, printout of absorption values in that section in digital form can commence. Calculated numerical values according to the working scale of absorption (Fig. 2.10**B**) are printed for each matrix point of the 80 x 80 matrix (Fig. 2.11, **A** and **B**). Each value (in the range −500 to +500) represents the calculated absorption of a tissue block 3 x 3 x 13 (or 8) cubic mm. Printout time is 1 minute per slice. When the slice printout is complete, that slice can be viewed on the CRT display if the view control (C3) on the computer control panel is activated while the slice printout is in progress (see "Computer"). Printout of absorption data can be deferred or omitted if desired, with a saving of 2 minutes per scan pair (8 minutes for an examination of four scans). With the 160 matrix system, printout can be either on an 80 x 80 or a 160 x 160 matrix format.

Compared with the computer processing time of 4 minutes per section (8 minutes per scan sequence and 40 minutes per four-scan examination) required following scan completion with the 80 x 80 matrix system, the 160 x 160 matrix system requires less than ½ minute additional time for each pair of scan sections after the completion of scanning. With the new matrix, however, absorption data can be averaged and still printed out on an 80 x 80 matrix. Also, printout time remains 1 minute per slice. Guaranteed accuracy of absorption measurement is specified to be unchanged (± ½% standard deviation, measured on water), as compared with the 80 x 80 matrix system. However, our tests have indicated that the accuracy of resolution of absorption of cerebral

FIG. 2.11.

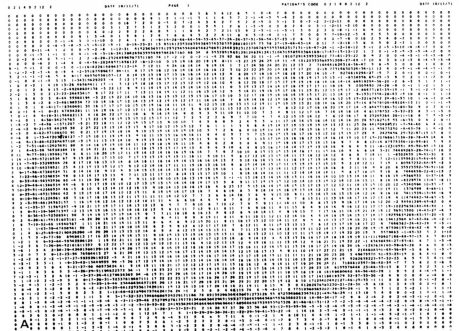

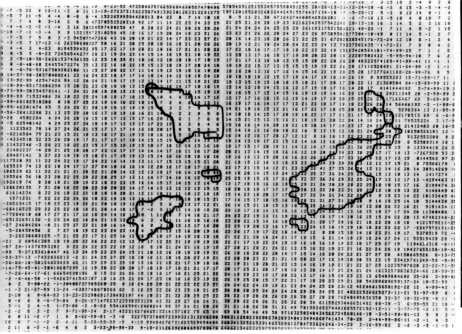

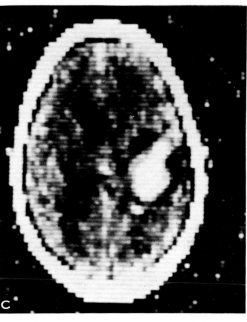

A. Digital paper printout at 8 lines per inch (lpi). The darker-appearing peripheral oval band represents the high absorption numbers of the bone of the skull vault. The light-appearing regions represent the low absorption values of the CSF-containing spaces (lateral and third ventricles, sylvian cisterns, and interfrontal longitudinal fissure). Intermediate values represent cerebral grey and white matter. Enlargement of CSF spaces represents diffuse cerebral atrophy. The oblique dark band tangent to the right side of the skull is due to false absorption values resulting from rotary head motion artifact. The low values just beneath the inner skull table, occupying a band 1 or 2 matrix points wide, is the result of computer "undershoot" (falsely low values in the zone of abrupt transition from high (bone) to low (CSF) readings). The geometric distortion of the scan is greater than in **B,** which shows a 6 lpi printout, with the 2 halves of the scan taped together.

B. Printout. This illustrates the use of the printout to identify certain anatomical features and an area of pathology. On the left side, the approximate configuration of a modestly dilated frontal horn and a somewhat dilated ventricular trigone are mapped out by drawing a line to include all figures consistent with partial or complete CSF volumes. In this example, the figures range from −1 to 10, with a single value of −2 within the trigone. In the center, the calcified pineal is represented by three values, 19, 19, and 44. All these values are less than would be the case if the calcification occupied the whole thickness of the slice. On the right side, a line is drawn around a zone to include values ranging from 25–38, inclusive. The major portion of this area represents a hematoma. A smaller irregular area extending anteriorly, enclosing values ranging from 25–30, probably includes portions of the frontal lobe cortex. The more posterior small separate zone encloses three values, 33, 37, and 41, representing partial volume values of calcification in the glomus of the choroid plexus.

C. Polaroid photograph taken from the CRT display with a window width of 20. The distribution of densities is not distorted by relative enlargement of the transverse axis as is the printout of the same data shown in **B. C** shows more clearly the anatomical and pathological features. In particular, it is much easier to appreciate the decreased absorption surrounding the hematoma and representing perifocal edema than on the printout. Also, a partial volume inclusion of the left occipital horn is much more readily identified in **C.**

soft tissues of approximately ±1.5 units with the original system has decreased to only slightly less than ±2.4 units with the 160 x 160 matrix system.

Printout Configuration

Owing to the construction of the printer (Tally), the configuration of the numerical printout has a reduced vertical dimension relative to the transverse (unlike the CRT display). Either a 6- or 8-lines per inch (lpi) format can be selected by means of a press-button printer control. At 6 lpi, the data for the right and left halves of the head are printed on separate paper sheets, one after the other. In addition to doubling the volume of paper used, time is required to match and tape the two halves of the printout together. On the other hand, the 8-lpi format, while printing all the data of a scan section on one paper sheet, results in further distortion of the axes of the scan and increases the difficulty in recognizing individual numbers and their correct spatial distribution. Since the actual numerical values in each tissue block are obtainable from the CRT display (by means of window width M setting and the window level control) in addition to a nondistorted pictorial representation, the CRT display is far superior to the printout in clinical investigations and in many experimental situations (Fig. 2.11, **B** and **C**).

CHAPTER 3

Patient Positioning

GENERAL CONSIDERATIONS

Except for the easing of constricting portions of clothing, particularly about the neck, for the purposes of comfort during scanning, no particular clothing requirements exist and the patient can be examined in street clothes.

PREPARATION OF THE PATIENT'S HEAD

No special preparations are obligatory but there are certain desiderata. A stockinette cap drawn over the head will compress the hair and reduce the amount of air trapped in this region (Figs. 2.8 and 3.1). An excessive amount of air between the scalp and the head bag may affect the quality of the scan adversely. For these reasons, it is desirable to avoid very bulky surgical dressings when scanning postoperative patients. All metal objects in the hair or in dressings should be removed to prevent artifacts in the subsequent scans.

If the patient has little or no hair, it is helpful to sprinkle the surface of the head bag with talcum power to prevent the rubber adhering to the scalp during patient insertion and cap adjustment.

MARKING OF REQUIRED LEVEL OF TOMOGRAPHIC SECTION

One method of identifying the surface level of the tomographic section is shown in Figure 3.2. In the example, the orbitomeatal line (OML) is used as the basic reference level and a tape band is applied firmly, perpendicular to the reference line. Alternatively, the anatomical (Reid's) base line may be used, and the band may be applied perpendicular to this line. Reference marks, as desired, are placed on the head band at desired levels above the reference line. It is helpful to draw the reference line on the skin surface and a second line below the reference line at the desired angle of the scan plane.

A second method is illustrated in Figure 3.3. In this illustration Reid's base line (RBL), extending from the inferior orbital margin to the superior portion of the external auditory meatus (EAM), is used as the reference plane. A line is drawn on the skin above RBL at the desired scan angle (e.g., 25°). As the zero (0) of the scale marked on the head cones and cylinders marks the upper edge of the upper slice (1B) scanned when the indicator is at 0 on the scanner reference scale, and the zero (0) of the cone or cylinder scale lies 5.1 cm from the surface of the base ring, when the line a–a' is brought into the plane of the surface of the base ring, the *upper edge* of the *low-*

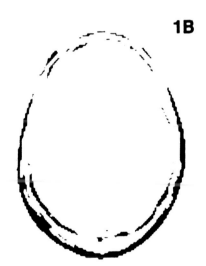

FIG. 3.1.
L −30   W M   160 x 160 matrix.
Photograph of a CRT scan display. At these viewer control settings, all substances in the scan with absorption values greater than −30 are white. Gas, being of very low density, is shown as black. The *outer black band* represents air trapped over the scalp beneath the head bag. The *inner narrow black zone* represents the remaining computer undershoot artifact of the abrupt and marked density change between bone and CSF. The latter artifact is less obtrusive with the 160 x 160 matrix system than with the 80 x 80 matrix system.

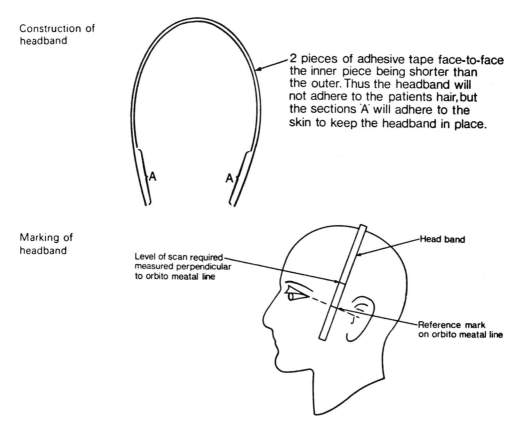

Construction of headband

2 pieces of adhesive tape face-to-face the inner piece being shorter than the outer. Thus the headband will not adhere to the patients hair, but the sections 'A' will adhere to the skin to keep the headband in place.

A   A'

Marking of headband

Level of scan required measured perpendicular to orbito meatal line

Head band

Reference mark on orbito meatal line

FIG. 3.2. Method of preparing and marking of headband for aid in positioning of the patient's head. In this example, the orbitomeatal line (OML) is used for reference. (Reprinted by permission of EMI Ltd.)

est slice (1A) will lie 3.8 cm above this line (A–A') and the plane of the tissue section will be parallel to this line. A second line (X–Y) is drawn on the skin of the face, 3.8 cm below and parallel to the first line. In final positioning of the patient for scanning, the line X–Y is related to the outer surface of the Tufnel base ring of the head cone or cylinder, which can be palpated immediately under the head bag at the rim of the portal of the scanner aperture. It X–Y is brought into the plane of the outer surface of the Tufnel base ring, *the upper edge of the initial section, 1A, will be in the plane of the external auditory meatus.* If X–Y is drawn 4.3 cm below the first line, the upper edge of the initial scan will be 0.5 cm below the plane of the EAM, etc.

The depth of the waterbox from the surface of the base ring of the cone or cylinder to the inner surface of the back wall of the plexiglas is approximately 18 cm. Initially, difficulty was experienced in obtaining sufficiently low scan sections for examination of the orbits and inferior portion of the posterior fossa, as the top of the adult head was prone to impinge upon the plastic overflow valve plate lying just inside the back wall of the waterbox. Removal of this valve plate permitted a few additional millimeters of head insertion, easing the problem of obtaining low cranial scans without causing difficulty in filling the box with water. However, the length of the waterbox still occasionally interferes with obtaining sufficiently low planes of scan when the patient's head is large in the vertical dimension. In positioning for low cranial scans, it is most important that contact between the head bag over the top of the head and the posterior surface of the waterbox is avoided. If contact is permitted, motion will be imparted to the head as the scanning gantry indexes, and this motion may cause degradation of scan quality.

The diameter of the portal of the waterbox is 22.0 cm. Occasionally, patients are encountered whose heads are too large to fit through this diameter. One such patient, an acromegalic, was encountered in our first 600 scans. Somewhat more frequently, the patient's maximum sagittal head diameter is too large to permit sufficiently deep insertion to permit low cranial scans. EMI Ltd. has been apprised of these problems and it is understood that a somewhat larger headbox will eventually be provided, or an alternative equilibrating substance may be used.

CHOICE OF HEAD CONE OR CYLINDER (FIG. 3.4)

Based on practice at Atkinson Morley's Hospital, we were originally advised that the head cone supplied should be used for routine scanning. It was found that

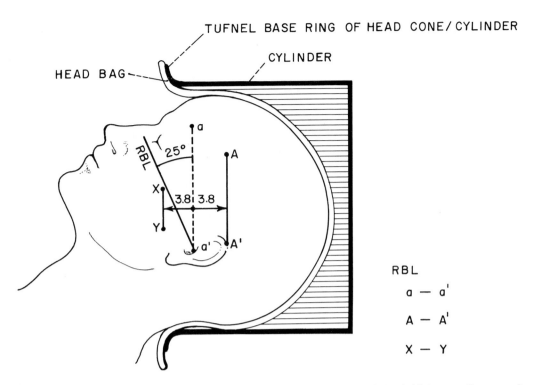

FIG. 3.3. Alternative method of marking for positioning the level and angle of the initial scan. See text for details. *RBL* = reference plane. Scan angle illustrated is 25°. With *X–Y* positioned in the plane of the outer margin of the base of the cone or cylinder waterbox insert, the *upper edge* of the lower scan section (1A) will lie at the level *a – a'*. If *a – a'* is in the plane of the outer margin of the insert base, the upper edge of section 1A will be at *A – A'*, 3.8 cm cephalad from *a – a'*.

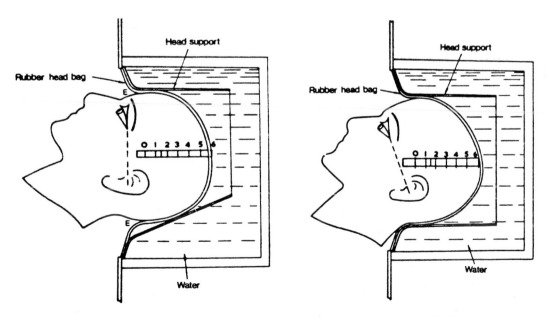

FIG. 3.4. Diagrammatic illustrations of patient positioning using a cone waterbox insert (*left*) and the cylinder insert (*right*). Deeper head insertion is possible with the cylinder, which is used when examination of the posterior fossa is required. The cylinder can also be used for general intracranial examinations. (Reprinted by permission of EMI Ltd.)

the extent to which the head could be inserted into the waterbox was relatively limited. When the cone was used, the base of the brain and the posterior fossa could not be examined routinely except in younger children. However, with the head cylinder insert in position, it was generally possible to obtain scans of the posterior fossa. Changing from cone to cylinder or vice versa requires as much as 10–15 minutes, since the waterbox must be emptied, the metal rim over the head cone removed, the insert changed, the head bag replaced, and the waterbox refilled. Refilling the waterbox requires a number of maneuvers to remove air bubbles adhering to the rubber bag, including repeated shaking of the bag and subsequent pumping out of the remaining air.

Since it was determined desirable to include the posterior fossa routinely in all patients examined, we elected to use the cylinder routinely, recognizing that the cylinder was not capable of providing support to the patient's head within the waterbox, a function that the head cone serves if the head is firmly impacted at the time of final positioning. Using the cylinder, the patient's head is given only the minimal support of the head bag and surrounding water. This undoubtedly increases the incidence of head motion during the scan as compared with the proper use of the head cone. This disadvantage was accepted for several months but spurred development of a dental fixation device (see below).

If it is elected to use the head cone (2 sizes of which are now provided), the level to which scanning can be accomplished in a caudal direction can be tested by placing the cone, or a duplicate, over the patient's head before insertion into the scanner. The beginning of the scale will indicate the *superior limit* of the 1B scan section obtainable in that patient (Fig. 3.4).

POSITIONING THE PATIENT IN THE SCANNING UNIT

With the patient lying on the table and the bar coupling the sliding tabletop to the waterbox assembly, the waterbox is withdrawn to within 0.5 cm of the maximum possible extension by means of the adjusting wheel on the table. A centimeter scale is provided on the side of the scanning gantry housing for reference when adjusting the levels of scan section. The head bag is expanded by operating the empty switch mounted on the scanning unit control panel until the bag is extended rearwards well into the cone.

After attaching the headband and marking it appropriately or drawing the appropriate reference lines on the face, the patient's head is eased into the rubber bag as far as possible while avoiding undue pressure on the nose. The rubber tabs of the head bag must not be trapped between the bag and the patient's head.

The table height is adjusted so that the chosen

reference line (OML or RBL) is at the chosen angle to the front ring of the scanner. The head should be carefully positioned so that the infraorbital or interpupillary line is exactly parallel to the face plate. Using the fill switch, the waterbox is filled so that the rubber cap collapses onto the patient's head and is eased caudally by pulling on the rubber tabs. Filling is stopped when the caudal portion of the rubber bag has extended as low as possible without pushing the head out of the waterbox by excessive water pressure. This initial positioning is to ensure that the head bag collapses evenly over the head. It is advisable to attach the canvas sling around the upper thighs and lower buttocks before completely filling the waterbox to avoid displacement outwards of the patient's head. The purpose of the sling is to oppose the water pressure, and therefore the elastic of the sling should be adjusted as tightly as the patient can accept comfortably.

If a cone is being used, one should check that the head is firmly seated in the cone by testing, using side to side motion of the patient's head, and observing flexing of the cone through the waterbox. If the head now requires deeper insertion into the waterbox, the empty switch can be operated for short periods and the patient can be eased further into the cone, with shoulder assistance if required. Final adjustment of the angle and position of the head is now made, and auxiliary head supports such as surgical tape, Velcro straps, or halters may be attached. Alternatively, and more satisfactorily, a dental holding device may be used (see below).

GENERAL CONSIDERATIONS IN PATIENT POSITIONING

With present equipment, CT scanning in planes approximating the horizontal (parallel to RBL) does not permit scanning of the bulk of the posterior fossa contents. Scanning at an angle of 30° to RBL generally provides the most satisfactory inclusion of the posterior fossa. This results in an anatomical presentation that is less than optimal for anatomical representation of posterior fossa structures and, in some respects, less than is optimal for representation of supratentorial structures. Logically, patients with suspected or known supratentorial pathology might be scanned in planes that are horizontal rather than angled. However, exigencies of machine operation and patient scheduling have dictated that an appropriate compromise angle for general intracranial examination is 25° to RBL. To ensure as complete as possible a coverage of the lower portions of the posterior fossa, an attempt is made to scan at an angle of 30° to RBL in patients with evidence of posterior fossa disease.

In the case of a normal-sized adult head, a series of four scan sequences (generating eight slices, each of

13 mm thickness) covers most of the intracranial anatomy (Fig. 5.1). If, after each scan sequence, the head position is moved 25 mm with respect to the scanning beam, a 1-mm overlap is provided between scan sequences (scan pairs). This will result in a total vertical scan coverage of the head of $(4 \times 10 \times 2) - 3 = 10.1$ cm.

Based on information supplied with the unit, this format had been in general use until it was announced by Hounsfield in April 1975 that section thicknesses actually obtained with the 13-min collimators were only 10 mm in thickness. Head position therefore must be moved 20 mm between scans, in order to avoid 5-mm tissue gaps between the section pairs of each scan sequence. It is indeed curious that many tens of thousands of studies have been obtained without realization that gaps of several millimeters existed between scan sequences. If no provision is made for overlap between sequences, a routine series of four scan pairs will cover a vertical dimension of 8 cm, and vertical coverage equivalent to previous routines will require five rather than four scan sequences.

If a routine scanning angle of 25° to Reid's base line is used and the upper edge of the lowest slice (1A) is placed at the level of the external auditory meatus (EAM) the upper surface of slice 1A will generally pass through the upper or mid-third of the orbit anteriorly and through the region of the foramen magnum or slightly above posteriorly. With a series of four scans, the upper surface of the highest tissue section, 4B, will lie a short distance below the vertex (superior parietal lobe area) (see Fig. 5.1).

Coverage of the brain by such a series of scans will be greater in dolichocephalic skulls with a relatively short vertical diameter and will be less in brachycephalic skulls with relatively larger vertical diameters. In heads with very large vertical dimensions, an additional scan sequence (5A, 5B) will be required to duplicate normal coverage. Heads of small vertical dimension (infants and very young children) will be covered satisfactorily by a series of three scans (six tissue sections of 13 mm thickness) or four scans (eight sections of 8 mm thickness).

DURATION OF EXAMINATION

The above represents a routine scanning format. Setup time for a cooperative patient is 5–10 minutes. Each scan sequence takes approximately 4½ minutes. Including the short time required to change cranial level after each scan sequence, a series of four scan sequences can be obtained in 25–30 minutes, assuming a cooperative patient. Also assuming that the patient is cooperative and remains still during each scan, the total examination can be completed in 35–40 minutes.

Using the iterative program supplied with the original 80 x 80 matrix, the computer requires an additional 4

minutes to process each slice. Computation of the first scan (initial two slices) cannot start until completion of this scan 4½ minutes after commencement of the scan, and computation of a series of four scans (eight slices) therefore requires 32 minutes (36½ minutes following the commencement of scanning). To this must be added the time required for digital printout of each slice, which is 1 minute per slice, or a total of 8 minutes. Printout can be omitted or deferred, but if it is elected to obtain each printout in routine sequence, the total time required for a four-scan examination is 36.5 + 8 or approximately 45 minutes from the beginning of the first scan to the end of processing of the last scan. Although computations will be proceeding during scanning, scans cannot be viewed on the CRT of the viewer during either actual scanning or computer processing of data. Thus, CRT data displays are not accessible unless the scanning or the computer processing is interrupted. As noted earlier, this limitation has caused considerable difficulty in patient scheduling and in efficient use of the radiologist's time.

If it is elected to perform only three scans (six slices) in routine examination, as for example by scanning only the supratentorial area or infratentorial region or by electing to exclude the equivalent of a 13-mm slice in the lower part of the posterior fossa and in the superior portion of the cerebrum, 25% of the total examination time (excluding patient setup time) will be saved, and a proportionate amount of time in later photographic recordings and analysis can also be saved. This will permit an increased number of patients to be scanned in a given session. However, this saving is accomplished only by accepting the risk of failing to include a pathological lesion lurking in the area not covered. A second metastatic neoplasm or a high parietal meningioma would be cases in point.

The optional new computer program and 160 x 160 matrix, with an increase in computer core *8K*, results in considerable decrease in computer processing (less than ½ minute for two slices after scan completion). This modification (which can be retrofitted to existing equipment in 1 day) therefore reduces the total scan procedure time to about 30 minutes (assuming a total scan time, which is unchanged with the new modification, of 25–30 minutes). With the modified system, processed scans can be viewed briefly on the CRT within ½ minute of the completion of each scan without significant delay in the examination.

This improvement permits decisions to be made regarding ongoing examinations, such as the technical adquacy of each scan, the presence or absence of obvious pathology, and the need or otherwise to supplement the examination with additional scans following intravenous injection of contrast material (contrast enhancement). Previously, such decisions could only be made by waiting approximately 15 minutes after completion of the actual scanning to view the scans. While the gross quality of the scan with respect to motion and the presence of quite gross lesions previously could be identified on the digital printout, the latter representation of scans is usually inadequate for making the aforementioned decisions, and it had proved most practical to scan a series of approximately eight patients without interruption for viewing, except for those cases in which the condition of the patient demanded very prompt diagnostic decisions. Such matters as technical adequacy of the scan with respect to motion and other factors, and decisions regarding the need to repeat scans with contrast enhancement, had generally been deferred until the scans were analyzed later in the day. Early reappointments were then required for patients in whom repeat study was considered necessary.

A further improvement in equipment is of high priority, that is, the availability of a separate viewing console, capable of operation remote from the scanner suite, with which tape or diskette scan records could be viewed and analyzed. The availability of such a remote viewer-analyzer would permit uninterrupted patient scanning during the day, whereas, with the single viewer, the scanner cannot be used during the time taken to make analyses and photographic records of completed scans. With complete study of the completed scans of 8–10 patients taking 2–3 hours, this represents a significant loss of patient examination time in a 9-hour day.

It is desirable that a radiologist review the patient's medical record and plain film skull examination in order to determine the best scan format for that patient. It is our practice to extract the salient features of the history, clinical findings, and results of previous studies and to enter these on a form (Fig. 3.5). This provides a convenient record at the time of interpretation of the CT scan and later review. This work takes only a fraction of the time required for a complete CT examination, and, unless the physician can use the intervening time profitably, considerable inefficiency results. The alternative is to give these responsibilities to the technologist, but this is considered to be an inappropriate delegation, even were it not the case that the technologist should be fully occupied in watching the patient during the scan (to monitor for movement and condition), observing the detector dials on the x-ray control unit, etc.

While the new program and matrix alleviate the problem to a degree, availability of a viewer capable of operation during scanning is still more advantageous (see Chapter 4).

CHOICE OF X-RAY FACTORS: KILOVOLTAGE (KV) AND CURRENT (MA)

The range of factors considered is as follows: 100 kV at 40 mA, 120 kV at 33 mA, and 140 kV at 28 mA.

Discrimination of atomic number falls significantly as kV 100 is increased to 140. The decrease in transmitted photons at the lower kV levels in this range does not greatly decrease the accuracy of measurement of absorption values, although there is some increase in standard deviation (32A). Although further investigation may result in a modification of our techniques, the present use of the factors is given here: routine adult examinations, 120 kV at 33 mA; adults with exceptionally thick and dense calvaria, 140 kV at 28 mA; primarily posterior fossa (adult) examinations, 140 kV at 28 mA; and infants, 100 kV at 40 mA.

CHOICE OF SCAN SECTION THICKNESS

In analyzing scans to detect specific anatomical features and variations in absorption indicative of pathology, two important elements must be kept constantly in mind: the possibility of artifacts created by a wide variety of factors, and the existence of the "Partial Volume Phenomenon" (see Chapter 4).

In evaluating these factors, the presence of coherent abnormalities of absorption pattern in more than a single section of scan is most helpful. For this reason, and for the additional reasons that a more adverse noise to signal ratio results from high x-ray photon absorption in the areas of denser bone in the region of the skull base and because of the smaller volume of the posterior fossa, it has appeared logical and advantageous to use 8-mm thick sections in posterior fossa scans.

POSTERIOR FOSSA ROUTINE

In order to scan as low as possible in the posterior fossa, an attempt is made to increase the angle of scan from the routine 25° to 30° to Reid's base line. Not all patients are able to sustain this degree of head and neck flexion comfortably, and this angle may be difficult to achieve in patients with short thick necks. For the reasons outlined above, the posterior fossa is usually scanned with a series of three scans with 8-mm sections (the 8-mm collimators replace the 13-mm collimators in the scanner). Following the initial scan, head level is changed by 15 mm (providing a 1-mm overlap between scan pairs). Following these three scans, the examination is completed with two further scans (four slices) using the 13-mm collimators. Thus, total of five scans (10 slices) is used, providing a total vertical cranial scan coverage of 9.5 cm (4.5 cm in the region of the posterior fossa and 5 cm superiorly). This is only 6 mm less than the routine coverage of 10.1 cm, using four slices with 13-mm thick sections. *Following Hounsfield's revised information (April 1975) concerning the actual thicknesses of the scanned sections with the 13-mm collimators, it is considered appropriate to regard the actual tissue sections obtained with the 8-mm collimators as*

C T SCAN

Clinical Information

Patient name

Hospital unit number
Age
Referring physician

Ward or Clinic

Clinical impression: a. pathology b. localization

Previous studies:	Results:	
	MGH	Outside
EEG		
SKULL study		
ISOTOPE scan		
CSF		
ANGIOGRAM(s)		
PNEUMOGRAM		
OTHER		

C T technique KV etc.

Reference plane (s)

No. of sections

Thickness

RESULT DIAGNOSIS FINAL DIAGNOSIS

Normal

Prob. normal

Prob. abnormal

Def. abnormal

FIG. 3.5. Form in use at the Massachusetts General Hospital for recording CT scan data. The reverse side is used for diagrams of abnormalities noted and for additional records of pathological absorption data at the time of scan analysis.

being 6 mm in thickness and to move the head 12 mm after each scan sequence using the 8-mm collimators.

It might be argued that the reduced number of photons per tissue block in the 8-mm section compared with the 13-mm section may produce less accurate absorption measurements and/or calculations. Thus far, we have felt that such loss has been more than offset by the availability of a greater number of sections through a given volume of tissue. An increased number of photons for measurements could be obtained by increasing the duration of scan above the standard 4½ minutes by means of the switch provided (6½, 8½, or 11½ minutes). Alternatively, higher photon transmission can be obtained by increasing kilovoltage from the standard 120 to 140 kV and accepting the somewhat reduced accuracy of the system in discrimination of tissue absorption that this entails. This has been part of our routine for posterior fossa scanning.

Similar considerations have applied to examination of the orbits (see Chapter 28) and to examination of selected areas of the brain (see Chapter 5) where maximum spatial discrimination is desired, even at the expense of some theoretical loss in discrimination of small absorption differences. This has been tested to an insufficient extent for final conclusions regarding applicability. One area in which this type of variation or supplementation of technique might be considered is examination for lacunar infarcts, in which fluid content apparently has an absorption characteristic similar to that of CSF. Lacunar infarcts should be readily discriminated from the density of surrounding brain, but their small size may result in obscuration, due to the averaging of the lower density of a small lesion with the higher density of a larger amount of brain tissue in the same slice (see Chapter 4, "Partial Volume Phenomenan"). Another area of possible use of the 8-mm section technique is in the region of the suprasellar cisterns and anterior third ventricle, where anatomical features are small and relatively crowded in a small volume. The capacity of the scanner to differentiate small lesions in such anatomical areas seems to be improved significantly by the selective use of the thinner sections.

Patient Immobilization

Movements of the patient's head during the 4½-minute scan period cause degradation of scan quality. Resolution of anatomical detail and accuracy of absorption measurements are both affected adversely. In certain areas, more or less serious artifacts are caused that may obliterate important details. In the first 600 CT examinations in our series (43, 46), it was found that 3% of the studies were technically unsatisfactory, most frequently due to excessive head motion (in some cases, unsatisfactory examinations resulted from intracranial gas, Pantopaque residues, or larger metal surgical devices such as shunt valves).

The problem was augmented by our decision not to use the cone-shaped insert. Although this insert provides support for the head, it restricts deep insertion of the adult head for basal region scanning compared with the cylindical insert.

Accuracy in measurement of photon absorption (attenuation) is markedly dependent upon the arranging of multiple measurements of the beam, which is projected from 180 different angles. If the individual tissue blocks do not remain in the same position throughout, false values will be calculated for individual blocks and spatial resolution will also be degraded. The adverse effects of motion and motion artifact production will be greater in areas where dense and irregular bone of the skull base produces sufficient beam attenuation to create an already adverse signal to noise ratio. The complex and dense bone configuration is such regions also makes for great difficulty in formulating computer program corrections to compensate for bone effects.

The use of various Velcro and surgical tape straps and halter arrangements meets with limited success, due to the mobility of soft tissues over bone. A dental plate and resin mold unit were therefore made and tested (Fig. 3.6). CT scans of 100 patients examined immediately before the introduction of the dental holder and a further 100 consecutive studies after institution of the holder were graded according to absence of motion artifact or presence and degree of such artifact on a scale of one to five (Fig. 3.7). Striking reduction in the incidence and degree of motion degradation resulted from the use of the device (Fig. 3.8). The incidence of moderate, severe, or gross motion was reduced from 43 to 9% (44).

The device has been well tolerated in general, but is unsuitable for very young children and semicomatose or comatose patients. It can be effective in edentulous individuals (in whom the use of double or triple layers of resin is helpful) and in those with well-fitting dentures. Subsequently, additional rigidity was introduced into the system by the installation of a duplicate post on the opposite side of the scanner ring.

A more generally applicable device using external pressure pads against the maxillae and upper lip is under construction.

Vigorous intercostal breathing with use of accessory muscles of respiration in obtunded or comatose patients can cause significant head motion.

PATIENT SCHEDULING

It can be understood readily from the foregoing sections that a large number of factors can affect the number of patients that may be scheduled in a given period. These may be summarized as follows.

a. Immutable factors.
   (1) Patient positioning, 5–10 minutes (may be much longer when patient condition requires intravenous equipment, vital function support and monitoring, orthopedic equipment, additional sedation, or general anesthesia).
   (2) Time per scan sequence (two sections), 4½–5 minutes.
   (3) Additional computer processing time, 8 minutes per scan sequence (80 x 80 matrix) or less than ½ minute per scan sequence following completion of scan (160 x 160 matrix).
   (4) Scan analysis and photography, 10 minutes minimum per case (requires cessation of patient scanning unless a remote console is available).

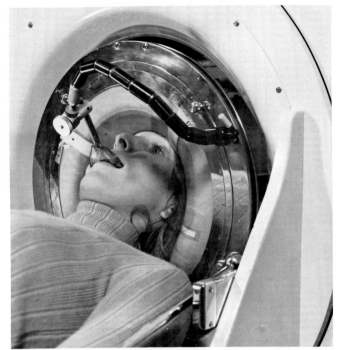

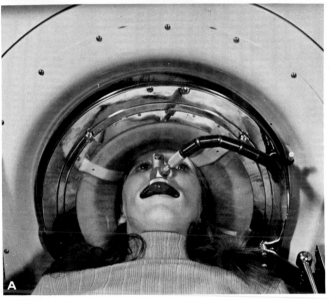

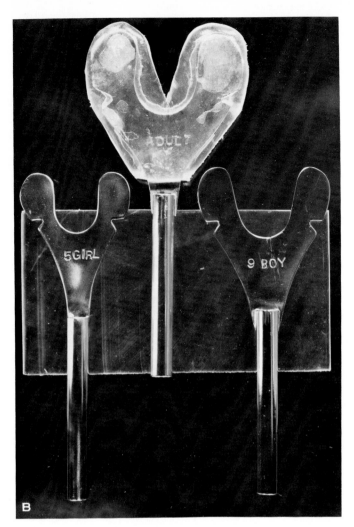

FIG. 3.6.

A. THE DENTAL HOLDER IN USE. The dental plate is supported by a jointed metal column (Model #657U Flex-O-Post Holder, Starrett Tool Company, Athol, Massachusetts), which consists of alternating cylindrical segments with concave ends and steel balls. A steel cable, ⅛ inch in diameter, passes through the spacers and balls and is attached to an adjustable collar and locknut (permitting adjustment for any stretching of the inner cable in use). Beyond the locknut is attached a thumbscrew lock and hole for the post of the dental plate. At the other end, the cable is attached to an internal cam, with an external lever permitting release and fixation of the joints of the post. The post is easily installed on the nonrotating portion of the ring of the EMI scanner by means of a base stud and a hole tapped in the ring. A point on the ring approximately 20° above the horizontal was chosen. Measuring inward from the outer edge ⁷⁄₁₆ inch along this radial, a punch hole starting center was made. Viewing the ring from the side, the EMI head was rotated until one of the notches of the rear rotating flange came opposite the hole starting center. This provided drill clearance and avoided damage to the thrust bearing of the EMI scanner. A hole was then drilled and tapped (½–20 UNC) in the

nonrotating ring only, and the Flex-O-Post Holder was attached, using both a flat and a lock washer. The position of the cam lever was adjusted so that it did not impinge upon the scanner ring when the cable was tightened to make the post rigid. The head collar, thread, and locknut must be adjusted periodically to allow for induced cable stretching. Materials that may act as lubricants must be kept out of the joints in the post or rigidity will be reduced. A second post has since been installed in a symmetrical position on the other side of the scanner ring to increase rigidity of the device still further.

B. STAINLESS STEEL DENTAL PLATES AND SUPPORTING RODS. ADULT SIZE AND TWO SMALLER SIZES FOR CHILDREN. Dental mold material is shown (nontoxic vinyl resin; STA-GUARD from Stalite, Inc., Hialeah, Florida). This material has been used principally as a protective mouthguard for athletes. The resin sheet is cut into squares. When softened in hot water, the material adheres about the dental plate. When cooled in cold water, the edges can be trimmed. Plastic is shown affixed to the adult plate, but the central tongue area has not been trimmed out fully by the scissors. In practice, it takes about 15 minutes to prepare five plates, which is done in advance. It is then only a matter of a few seconds to resoften the mold to take a dental impression, cool the mold under a tap, and reinsert it in the patient's mouth so that the teeth fit snugly into the appropriate impressions. The Flex-O-Post is then linked to the support rod and the patient's head is adjusted to final position before making the post rigid. When the water tank is filled, head position is rechecked. (Reprinted by permission from Radiology, 114: 474–476, 1975.)

31

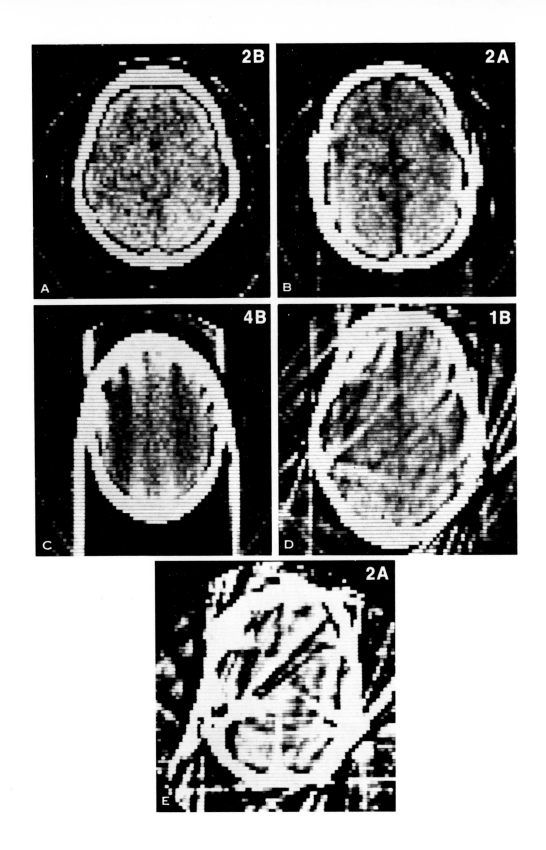

FIG. 3.7. GRADING OF SCANS FOR MOTION.

A. No detectable motion.

B. Minimal motion, indicated by the white lines extending through the water bath portion of the scan. Slight motion artifacts are visible as vertical white bands just internal to the right and left lateral portions of the skull in the temporal regions.

C. Moderate motion, indicated by the broad white bands extending through the water bath region. More obvious degradation of intracranial detail is expressed by broad white and dark bands extending vertically through the frontal and parietal regions.

D. Severe motion. Numerous vertical and oblique white bands are present in the water bath region and many oblique white and dark artifactual bands are shown in many areas of the cerebral scan.

E. Gross motion. Intracranial details are virtually completely obscured by artifacts.

(Reprinted by permission from Radiology, 114: 474–476, 1975.)

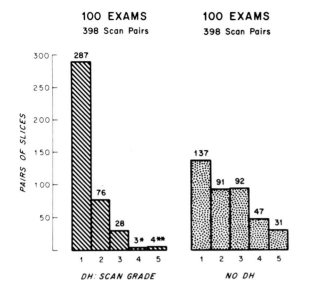

DH: SCAN GRADE   NO DH

FIG. 3.8. One hundred examinations obtained with the use of the dental holder (*DH*) and without the dental holder (*NO DH*) were analyzed for the absence or presence of motion and the degree of motion and were graded according to the classification shown in Figure 3.7. There were 398 scan pairs in each group (each scan sequence scans two slices of tissue simultaneously). Using the dental holder, 363 pairs of slices or 91% showed no motion or minimal motion and 35 pairs or 9% showed moderate, severe, or gross motion(**). The four scan pairs showing gross motion were all from a 16-year-old girl who had great difficulty swallowing with the dental plate in the mouth, due to omission of the trimming out of the central tongue area of the plastic (Fig. 3.6*B*)(*). Two of the three scan pairs showing severe motion were from examination of a female suffering from spasmodic torticollis with intermittent, involuntary twisting movements of the head. Of 398 pairs of slices scanned without the dental holder, 228 (57%) showed no motion or minimal motion, and 170 pairs (43%) showed moderate, severe, or gross motion. (Reprinted by permission from Radiology, 114: 474–476, 1975.)

  b. Optional Factors.
  (1) Routine examination consisting of three instead of four scans.
  (2) Omission of printout (saves 2 minutes per scan sequence).
  (3) More detailed scan analysis and photography (15–30 minutes per case).
  (4) Additional scans at new levels or following injection of contrast medium (up to doubling of examination time).

It is not surprising, therefore, that reported figures from different institutions vary from 6–16 patient examinations per 8–9 hour working day. It must also be appreciated that these figures are sustained only on days when equipment breakdowns do not occur (or are trivial and rapidly corrected). At the Massachusetts General Hospital, equipment "down time" during the first year was approximately 10% of working hours. Some recouping was achieved by extending the working day and by week end scheduling. With the 80 x 80 matrix system, it was found to be most efficient to scan patients sequentially during the morning and early afternoon, deferring all scan analysis and photography (except in emergency cases) until completion of computer processing. Assuming that a series of eight patients could be scanned in the session, processing of data and scan analysis by a neuroradiologist would be completed by late afternoon.

A second session was scheduled from 5:00 to 9:00 p.m., in which an additional three or four patients were scanned and a technologist made standardized photographic records. Further viewer analysis and photography were obtained the following day, as required, by the neuroradiologist on CT scan rotation that day.

Greater efficiency is possible with the 160 x 160 matrix system. Since scans can be viewed almost immediately after a scan is completed, decisions regarding the appropriate extent of a study can be made before the patient leaves the table. Some reduction in the number of scans per examination may be effected and decisions concerning the need for supplementary examinations with contrast medium may be made at that time. Thus, much of the rescheduling previously necessary is avoidable. On the other hand, it may be found advisable to take longer in the analysis of the new higher resolution scans than has been deemed necessary with the original system, and more frequent use of *supplemental* contrast enhancement studies is occurring.

SEDATION AND ANESTHESIA

The accuracy of CT scan data is very heavily dependent upon the absence of motion during the scan. Therefore, every effort must be made to ensure the least possible motion. There is generally no problem with the patient who can cooperate. With patients who are unable to cooperate, for such reasons as disease causing involuntary movements, depression of level of consciousness, or psychiatric disturbance and immaturity, sedation and occasionally general anesthesia will be required unless a more or less degraded scan quality is to be accepted. It is frequently the case that a trial scan will be made of a patient in fragile condition before more than minimal sedation is given. Depending upon the result and upon the type of lesion being sought, it may then be decided to give more sedation or general anesthesia. This very proper approach reduces the scanning time available for other patients. The long period of stillness required in CT scanning compared with that needed to produce a cranial radiograph or a series of angiograms or pneumoencephalograms represents a significant handicap, particularly in the examination of emergency patients. General anesthesia will often be necessary for a satisfactory CT scan in such patients when it would not be required for angiography. This problem is somewhat similar to that of radionuclide imaging but is of greater degree, in that the resolution of CT scanning is so much greater.

In neonates, satisfactory CT scans may be obtained with minor sedation and a steadying lead-gloved hand on the chin. The comatose infant can often be scanned in this way. Otherwise, general anesthesia will be necessary. For infants and older children, a sedative mixture of meperidine, promethazine and chlorpromazine given parenterally may prove satisfactory. Currently, anesthesia is regularly scheduled for infants and young children. Usually oxygen, nitrous oxide, and halothane are used up to 1 year of age. From 1 to approximately 6 years, Brevital has been favored (usually 8–10 mg per kg intramuscularly). This proves satisfactory in the majority; otherwise, nitrous oxide and halothane are used. For optimal scans in some adults under anesthesia, succinyl choline for muscular paralysis has been required.

In children over the age of 5–7 years who are cooperative, the pediatric size of the dental plate holder can be effective. Chloral hydrate has been found to be satisfactory for sedation of children by some. In our experience, Valium has generally been the most suitable drug for use in adults and has usually been given intramuscularly.

CHAPTER 4

Physical Considerations in Computed Tomography

The method under consideration represents a more or less detailed plot of x-ray absorption (attenuation) coefficients over a cross section of the body. The result is a quantitative transaxial tomograph.

The basic measurement obtained with the scanner is the x-ray absorption (attenuation) coefficient. For photon energies in this beam and for most biological materials of interest, the principal interaction is the Compton effect. The absorption values obtained vary according to a combination of atomic numbers of the elements in the scanned material and the physical density of the components of the structures. For the energy levels used (73 keV at 120 kVp), physical density contributes far more (over 90%) to the attenuation than does atomic number. X-ray attenuation through tissues (or other materials) is measured by means of photon detectors (sodium iodide crystals and photomultipliers) accurately aligned with the x-ray source. The degree of accuracy in measurement of attenuation at each point in the cross section is obtained by the use of multiple scans (180 transmissions) in each scan sequence. The fundamental concepts have been reviewed and considered in some detail by McCullough et al (38) recently, with particular reference to EMI scanning. These workers have also published results of experiments designed to evaluate the characteristics and accuracy of this scanner.

Following acquisition of attenuation data and before the reconstruction of scan can be attempted, the data must be preprocessed to convert exponential x-ray absorption to linearity.

MATHEMATICAL RECONSTRUCTION

It is possible to relate, by means of a set of linear equations, measured projections of a cross section to the density distribution of the section. Two principle methods of solving such a set of equations for cross-sec-

tional distribution of attenuation have been described. The first involves a solution of the equations directly by iterative (iterative-reiterative means) as described by Hounsfield, 1972; Gordon, Bender and Herman, 1970; and Herman, 1972. The second method utilizes Fourier transform (reciprocal space) methods as described by Crowther, DeRosier, and Klug, 1970; and Smith, Peters, and Bates, 1973.

Iterative Method

This method makes use of a series of assumptions regarding the absorption characteristics of a cross section and these are progressively modified as the attenuation results are recorded, with remodification following measurements from multiple subsequent scans until a "best fit" result is achieved. This is the method used in the 80 × 80 matrix system originally incorporated in the EMI scanner. One-hundred-and-sixty photon transmission measurements are made during each linear traverse. Following 180 traverses at 1° intervals, 28,800 (160 × 180) transmission measurements have been taken by each detector and are stored in a disc file for computer processing. A separate detector measures the intensity of the original x-ray beam, and these readings are used to calculate the absorption by the material along the beam path (absorption = original intensity/log-transmitted intensity). If the scanned material is partitioned into small volumes (blocks), each having a calculable value of absorption, then the sum of the absorption values of the blocks of material that are traversed by the x-ray beam will equal the total absorption of the beam. Each beam path therefore forms one of a series of 28,800 simultaneous equations in which there are 6,400 (80 × 80) variables. Provided that there are more equations than variables, the absorption values of each block can be solved. There must be more x-ray measurements than matrix points.

A numerical value is assigned to each point (block of material), indicating the absorption value of each block volume. The values derived are represented on a linear scale using water as the reference value 0. As the coefficient of absorption of water for the 120 kVp beam (effective energy, 73 keV) is in fact 0.19 cm^{-1}, the true coefficient of absorption for any material scanned is obtained by adding 500 to the scale reading and multiplying this by 0.19/500.

Fourier Transform

The purpose of this method is to break down a function into a number of sinusoidal components of varying frequency in such a way that, when these components are summed, the original function is restored. An algorithm ((from Arabic, al-Khuwarizmi (mathematician), a rule of procedure for solving a mathematical problem that frequently involves repetition of an operation)) developed by Cooley and Tukey (1965) has enabled extremely rapid evaluation of such transforms and has made processing by computer a realistic proposition. Using the Fourier transform approach, it has been found that algorithms based on this principle can be made to execute appreciably more rapidly than the alternative "direct" methods (53).

This reconstruction method makes use of an assumption that the Fourier transform of a one-dimensional projection of a cross section of an object is identical to the values on a line passing through the origin of the two-dimensional transform of the section. The Fourier transform of each of the projections for the various views of the section are computed and these are then interpolated on a grid to build up the two-dimensional transform of the section. For accurate build up of the entire Fourier transform plane of an image represented by N^2 points, approximately $N\pi/2$ different projections of the object must be viewed (Crowther et al, 1970). If the required resolution in the reconstruction is less than this, however, considerably fewer views are needed to obtain an adequate reconstruction. It has been shown that a simple linear interpolation scheme to assign values to the grid points of the two-dimensional Fourier transform allows a reconstruction that is virtually identical to that produced by more sophisticated schemes (Smith et al, 1973). A linear interpolation scheme permits much faster reconstruction times than do the alternative methods. An inverse two-dimensional transform then results in a numerical array, representing the reconstructed cross section.

A modification of the EMI system recently made available for this scanner provides a 160 x 160 matrix and an algorithm based on convolutional methods. The increased speed of data processing with the latter method has permitted a striking reduction in computation time required (two slices are now processed in less than ½ minute after scan completion, compared with the previous 8 minutes additional processing time required for two slices), in spite of the greatly increased number of calculations required for the finer matrix (240 measurements per linear sweep × 180 sweeps per scan = 43,200).

The new system provides a four-fold increase in the number of picture points, i.e., 25,600 (160 × 160) compared with 6,400 (80 × 80) in the CRT display, and each point represents absorption in a block 1.5 x 1.5 x 13 (or 8) cubic mm. It should be noted that the *thickness* of the block is unchanged and that there is *no change in the x-ray energy, x-ray dose, or scan time.* With both the old and the new systems, the diameter of the scanned circle of the waterbox is 23.4 cm. With the 80 × 80 matrix system, 160 measurements are taken during each traverse. Thus, the cross sections of the tissue blocks measured with this system are 1.47 mm square (although the information is presented on an 80 × 80 matrix, in which the blocks are 2.94 x 2.94 x 13 or 8 cubic mm). With the new system, the number of transmission measurements per sweep has been increased to 240 with the use of a finer graticule. The cross sections of the measured tissue blocks in this system are, therefore, 0.97 mm square (although the measurements are presented on a 160 × 160 matrix, in which the blocks have a cross section of 1.47 mm square). Therefore, the *ratio* of the number of photon being measured to the size of the measured blocks is unchanged. However, it is axiomatic that, all other factors remaining equal, the smaller the volume under consideration, the greater the quantum noise of the system. It is to be expected, therefore, that the new system will have a somewhat higher quantum noise level, and experience with the system is consonant (Fig. 4.3). With the new system, somewhat higher window widths are required to produce a coherent appearance of the image, as compared with the 80 × 80 matrix system. Additional phantom experiments are being made to quantitate these factors, but it is already clear that there is a greater spread of absorption values and that significantly more accurate measurements are possible with the 80 × 80 system than with the "high resolution" system.

The printout with the new system remains on an 80 × 80 matrix, with averaging of the four values for each block. However, it is not possible to switch from one system to another on the CRT display after the modification has been installed. This is hopefully correctable, as both the higher anatomical resolution and the higher absorption measurement accuracy are needed.

SPATIAL ORIENTATION OF ABSORPTION VALUES IN A MATRIX

Goitein (28) and Crowther et al (14) have discussed the accuracy and the number of scan passes at differing

CHARACTERISTICS OF X-RAY BEAM

For 120 kVp operation, the x-ray beam used in the EMI scanner has been shown to have an effective energy of 73 keV for the spectrum transmitted through water (the linear attenuation coefficient of the beam after traversing the waterbox has been measured for water to be 0.190 cm^{-1} for 120 kVp (52)). Phelps et al (54A) have analyzed the spectral distribution of the x-ray beam of the EMI scanner in the process of a major investigation into attenuation coefficients of various body tissues, fluids, and lesions, using a variety of radioactive sources. McCullough et al (38) have discussed the greater difficulties in computation of attenuation coefficients to the level of accuracy required in the case of a polychromatic beam, such as that used in an x-ray scanner, as compared with that of a monochromatic beam from a nuclear source. This is due to the hardening of the beam as it traverses the object scanned, introducing the possibility of undesirable spatial dependence on attenuation coefficient determinations. The possibility of simplifying computation and the mechanical complexity of a rotating scanning x-ray apparatus have led several investigators, including Hounsfield in the early stages of his work, to attempt development of a system using nuclear sources (30, 48, 62, 64). However, the specific activities of available nuclear sources are not adequate to provide the intensity of photons required for resolution of attenuation coefficients to an accuracy of 1% or better.

QUANTITATIVE ASPECTS

According to both Hounsfield and McCullough, satisfactory accuracy and interpretation of attenuation data require the scanning of the subject through an equilibrating waterbath of fixed length. The fixed waterbath length of the EMI scanner is 27 cm, and transmissions through the fixed path length are accomplished by rotating the water-filled box synchronously with the x-ray tube and detectors.

The contention of Hounsfield and McCullough, that scanning of objects in the absence of a surrounding homogeneous equilibrating substance of the density of water can introduce serious inaccuracies (such as non-linearity and spatial dependence), with difficulties in maintaining a consistent interpretation of incoming beam quality, seems to be borne out by the relatively poorer quality of CT brain scans thus far obtained by scanning through air.

The manufacturer claims an accuracy of ½ of 1% for the EMI scanner in determination of absorption (attenuation) coefficients. As the linear attenuation coefficient of the scanner beam after emergence from the waterbath has been measured to be 0.190 cm^{-1} for 120 kVp, indicating that the emerging beam has an effective energy of 73 keV, the accuracy and precision of the scanner can be determined from a comparison of the mass attenuation coefficient values for a variety of materials for a 73 keV beam and measured EMI values of those materials (EMI units + 500 × 0.190/500 = attenuation coefficient).

The results obtained by McCullough et al (38) in such comparisons indicate that there is agreement in most cases to better than ½ of 1%. Precision of scanner mean values of attenuation coefficients is greatest for materials (such as intracranial soft tissues) having absorption characteristics not markedly different from water.

We have found that EMI scan measurements are highly reproducible and appear to have a precision of ±1 unit in the range 0-60 units under optimal circumstances (MGH unit operating with the 80 × 80 system). However, this precision is affected readily and adversely by patient motion and in regions immediately adjacent to dense bone, metallic objects, and gas. In brain scans of good quality, it is possible to recognize large lesions (several centimeters in diameter) that differ in mean absorption value from surrounding brain by as little as 2-4 units. Discrimination (detectability of absorption differences between tissues) decreases with smaller lesions. In part, this is due to smaller lesions tending to occupy less than the full thickness of any single scanned section; but experimental findings, when partial volume phenomena are excluded, also reveal that there is a size factor that determines the minimum absorption difference that can be detected. Disappearance size for two materials differing in absorption values by 1% (5 EMI units) and 10% (50 EMI units) was found by McCullough et al (38) to be less than 6 mm (less than the width of two matrix blocks).

Inaccuracies of scan absorption measurements occur at interfaces between two substances of widely different absorption values. Inaccuracies have been shown to occur (38) in measurement of absorption in a 6.4-mm object (Lexan pin) having a true coefficient of 52.5 EMI units when scanned in water, whereas a correct measurement was obtained when the same object was scanned in Plexiglas. In the first instance the difference in coefficients was 10.5%; in the second instance the difference was 2%.

When the interface is between two objects having a coefficient difference of 60% or more, striking aberrations are seen within 6 mm of the interface in the case of the 80 × 80 matrix and iterative program ("undershoot" in the case of an interface between bone and CSF or brain, "overshoot" in the case of gas and adjacent tissue or CSF). These interface effects have been subdued some-

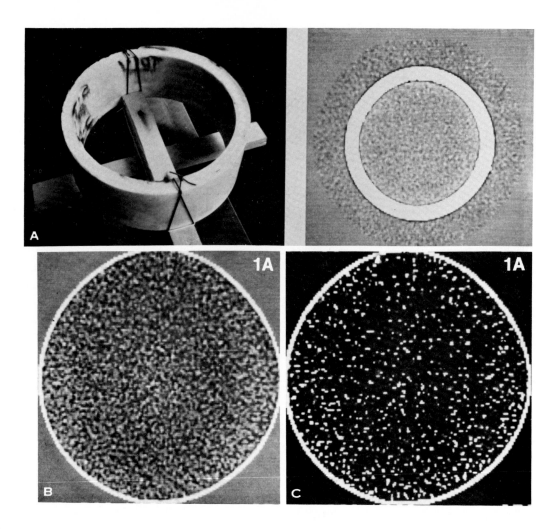

FIG. 4.1.

A. Photographs of a phantom representing dense skull (*left*) and of a CRT display of the CT scan of the phantom in water, obtained using the 160 x 160 matrix system (*right*). The scan was displayed with high contrast (sensitivity), which shows up the background noise. By suitable adjustments of the algorithm, the noise "grain" can be varied in area and amplitude *in inverse proportion*, and a suitable "grain" size may be chosen. In this scan display, the mean area of the noise "grain" is comparable with x-ray beam width, and Hounsfield considers the size chosen to be the best compromise for grain size. Objects that are greater in size than the noise amplitude stand out with better resolution. As the time of scanning is unchanged and the number of photons measured per reading is the same as in the 80 x 80 matrix system, the total information received is said to be the same. However, the form of noise represented by the geometric patterns and density edges of the coarse matrix has been removed. The "underswing" aberrations at the interface between the dense bone equivalent material and the water is much less than in the previous system. *Of note is the presence of factitious high values in the area equivalent to cerebral cortex* (values are increased 3–7 units in the zone internal to the dense phantom material). (Reprinted by permission of EMI Ltd.)

B and **C**. Waterbox scans using the 160 x 160 system.
B. L 0   W 20.
A circular band of factitiously increased absorption values for the water (an increase of 3–7 units) is visible extending inwards from the edge of the computed field for a distance of up to about 3.0 cm. The effect is less extensive in the upper part of the field than elsewhere.
C. L 3   W M.
The distribution of the elevated values peripherally is apparent. The *total* spread of values for water with this system was −10 to +10 in this test.

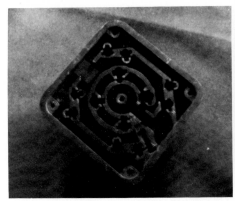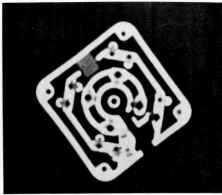

FIG. 4.2. Scan showing the high spatial resolution of a relatively dense object with the 160 x 160 matrix and new program. (Reprinted by permission of EMI Ltd.)

what in the case of the 160 × 160 matrix and the new program based upon convolutional methods (Fig. 4.1). The position of an object within the skull or phantom simulating a skull is otherwise said not to have an effect on the accuracy of absorption values produced (spatial independence), except for a zone adjacent to the internal surface (Fig. 4.1) where a 3–7 unit factitious increase in measurement is produced.

Spatial Resolution: 160 × 160 Matrix System

In the horizontal two dimensions of 160 × 160 matrix scans, with picture points of 1.5 square mm, quite sharp resolution of high-contrast margins is obtainable (Fig. 4.2). Spatial considerations with either matrix determine that resolution will be less with smaller objects (e.g., heads) than with large, in proportion to the number of matrix points included in the object.

Discrimination of Small Objects with Similar Absorption Values: 160 Matrix System

In phantoms, structures approximately 2.0 cm in diameter with absorption values 4 units different from the surrounding region can readily be discriminated with both the old and new systems. With objects smaller than 1.0 cm and of 3–4 units differential absorption value, discrimination is uncertain with the old system due to the "noise" of the coarse matrix pattern and is uncertain in the new system because of quantum noise. If scan time is increased to 11½ minutes, the increased photons available for measurement result in greatly reduced quantum noise and considerable increase in discrimination of small structures with very small differential absorptions (Fig. 4.3). Although x-ray dose will be increased, future development should clearly be directed towards increasing photon flux. Considerably greater x-ray dosage can be accepted if this results in a significantly increased detectability of lesions. A suitable

compromise with the need for shorter scan times must then be determined.

X-RAY DOSE

Studies of radiation dose have been reported by Perry and Bridges (52) and by McCullough et al (38).

Exposure at the surface of the filled waterbox, measured with a 240-cubic mm thimble ionization chamber at 120 kVp, was 2.2 mR per mA and, at 140 kVp, was 2.5 mR per mA for a single scan pass of the narrow beam (2.7 x 20 mm at 366 mm from anode). The measurements include scatter from the water-filled box. Measured half-value layers were 3.5 and 4 mm Al, respectively. Findings were consistent with a total filtration of 4 to 5 mm Al (52).

Head Phantom Measurements

Using a water-filled bladder within a Plexiglas cylinder of 152 mm diameter and a 240 cubic mm ionization chamber between the bladder and cylinder, the phantom was set into the scanner as a patient's head would be. Exposures for a complete scan sequence at 120 kVp and 27 mA were found to range from 1.9 R on the side of beam entry to 0.6 R on the side of beam emergence. A set of isodose curves was calculated from such measurements (Fig. 4.4A). From these data, it is calculated that a complete CT examination of three or four scans results in a cranial exposure of between 1 and 2.5 R, very similar to the dose resulting from a single radiograph of the skull. Male gonad dose was indicated to be considerably less than 0.1 mrad for each complete scan (52).

Measurements of exposure were made during scanning of an Alderson phantom containing thermoluminescent dosimetry powder (TLD-100). At 120 kVp, 32 mA, readings for one complete scan ranged from 0.6 to 1.5 R within the region of the scan section (38).

Radiation field measurements around the scanner

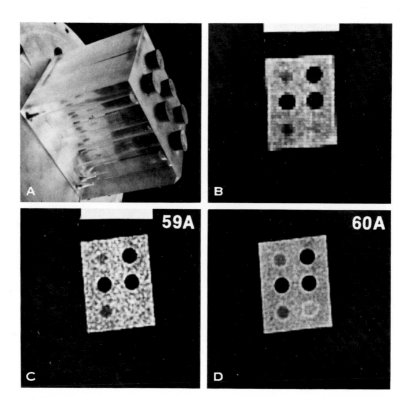

FIG. 4.3.

A–D. Test of discrimination using a phantom.

A. A Plexiglas block, in which six holes about 2 cm in diameter have been drilled and filled with water and various concentrations of copper sulphate, ready to be inserted into the waterbox for scanning.

B. Scan obtained with 80 x 80 matrix system; 4½-minute scan. The *numbers* shown above indicate the measured absorption values of the contents of the cavities *relative* to those of Plexiglas.

C. Scan obtained with the 160 x 160 matrix system; 4½-minute scan. Again, the figures indicate the absorption values of contents of the cavities relative to those of the Plexiglas.

Note: The cavities reading −50 contained water. The other values refer to different concentrations of copper sulphate. In the 3 hours that elapsed between scans **B** and **C**, there was a change in concentration of the copper sulphate solutions. A further change in the copper sulphate solutions had occurred on repeat scan on the 80 × 80 system.

D. 160 x 160 matrix; 11½-minute scan. Same absorption pattern as in **C**. Note the greatly smoothed images resulting from reduced quantum noise produced by the prolonged scan time (with proportionate increase in radiation dose). The *white bands* (circular denser zones) around the holes in the Plexiglas are probably due to diffusion of copper sulphate into the material.

This test, although incomplete, suggests that there is no significant loss of discriminatory capability with the 160 x 160 system compared with the 80 x 80 system in the case of larger objects and 13-mm sections and indicates the considerable improvement that could be obtained by increasing the scan duration were it not for the increased problem of patient motion. Increase in the patient dose would probably be acceptable for such an improvement in scan quality.

(Fig. 4.3, **A–D** reprinted by permission of EMI Ltd.)

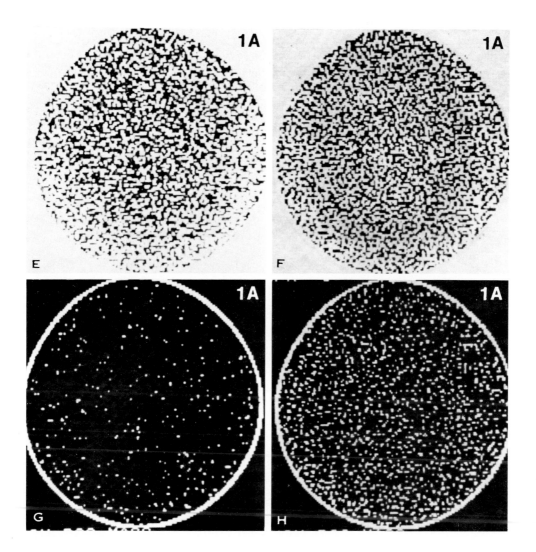

FIG. 4.3

E–H. Comparison of quantum noise levels in 13- and 8-mm scan sections with the 160 x 160 matrix system.

It has been noted that the quantum noise level is higher in the 160 matrix system than in the 80 matrix system. Accuracy of measurement of absorption differences is approximately one half that noted using the earlier system, although the accuracy is generally still somewhat better than the guaranteed $\pm \frac{1}{2}\%$ standard deviation. In the test illustrated here, the waterbath was scanned at 120 kV, first with the 13-mm collimators (**E** and **G**) and then with the 8-mm collimators (**F** and **H**). The scan results are displayed at L 0 W M (**E** and **F**) and at L 5 W M (**G** and **H**). The significantly increased noise when the thinner sections were scanned is clearly visible and reflects the reduced photons available for measurement. An obvious further increase in noise was found when specially constructed 4-mm collimators were used.

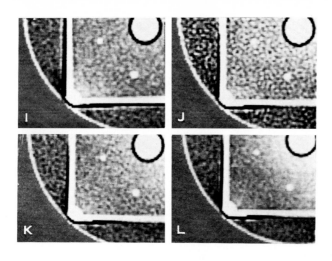

FIG. 4.3

I–L. Comparison of the effect of section thickness and scan duration on quantum noise.

Portions of scans of a phantom consisting of normal saline within a Plexiglas box containing plastic syringes filled with calcium chloride solution, one of which is visible as the large circle at the *top right* corner. Two nylon rods were included, one of 5 mm diameter, below the syringe, and one of 3 mm diameter to the left of the syringe. The scans were all obtained at 120 kV and the displays are all at L 0 W 40 control settings.

I. 13-mm scan section. The two small nylon rods are quite clearly visible against a background of noise.

J. 8-mm section. Noise is obviously greater than in the 13-mm section shown in I, and the rods are less distinctly visible.

K. 8-mm section. Duration of the scan sequence has been increased approximately 50%, by slowing the individual traverses (7 min, 30 sec). Noise is now very little different from that in the 5-min scan shown in I, and the nylon rods are again quite clearly discriminated.

L. 8-mm section. Scan time has been increased to 10 min, 20 sec. Noise is now less than in the 13-mm section scanned in 5 min, and the rods are relatively sharply defined against the more nearly homogeneous background of normal saline.

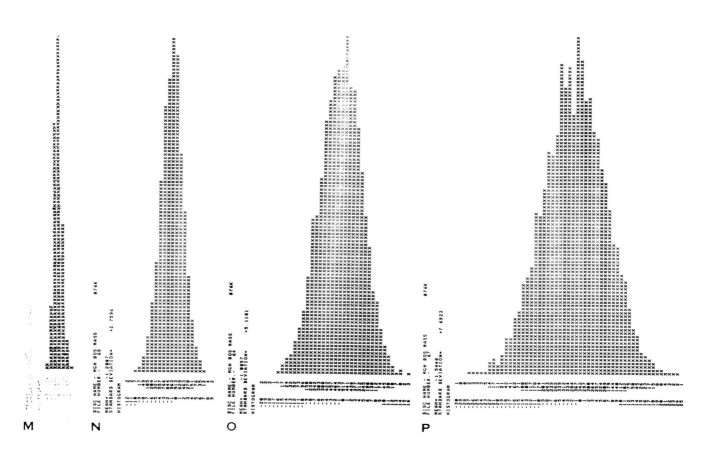

M   N   O   P

FIG. 4.3

M–P. Influence of matrix system and section thickness upon resolution of attenuation measurements and quantum noise. Histograms of attenuation measurements obtained with the 80 x 80 matrix system (**M**), 160 x 160 matrix system (**N**), obtained using the 13 mm collimators and 120 kV in each case. **O** and **P** are the histograms obtained with the 160 x 160 matrix system and 8-mm and 4-mm collimators, respectively, also using 120 kV. The scans are of water. The greater spread of values with the new matrix system compared with the old system and with the narrower sections is obvious. The mean attenuation measurements in each case are close to the true measurement of 0, but the standard deviation in **M** is approximately 1, in **N** is 2.7, in **O** is 5.1, and in **P** 7.7. Scans **N, O,** and **P** were obtained just before routine maintenance of the scanner and show slightly greater standard deviations than are obtained under optimum conditions. Under such conditions, the standard deviation of the new system, using the 13-mm collimators, is usually 2.3 to 2.4. The Conway remote console operated in the attenuation averaging mode reduces the noise characteristics of the scan shown in **N** to those shown in **M**, without significant alteration of the anatomical resolution.

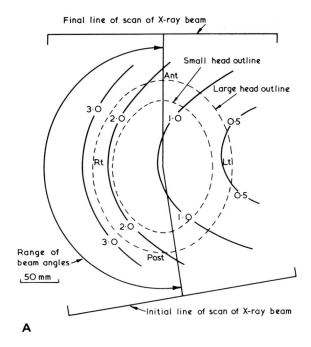

Final line of scan of X-ray beam

Small head outline

Ant

Large head outline

3·0   2·0   1·0   0·5

Rt

Ltl

0·5

1·0

2·0

3·0

Post

Range of beam angles

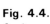
50 mm

Initial line of scan of X-ray beam

A

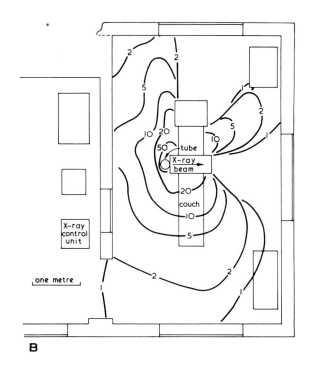

B

Fig. 4.4.

A. Isoexposure curves in a water phantom for a single complete scan, 120 kVp at 32 mA. Exposure in Roentgens. Total scan time, 5.3 minutes. The exposure to the head is relatively uniform and represents that to a slice of tissue between 20 and 40 mm thick for any one complete scan. No attempt is made here to allow for the effect of skull attenuation and, therefore, these calculations represent an overestimate of the dose received at the center of the head of the order of 30%. In practice, a narrow zone of tissue at the overlap between successive scan sections will receive up to double these doses.

B. Radiation field in x-ray room from stationary, horizontal x-ray beam, showing tube leakage and beam scatter, 120 kVp at 32 mA. Figures are mR per hour. The water-filled box is fully into the tube gantry. If the figures on the isodose curves are divided by 10, they will represent the approximate exposure in mR from one complete scan.

(Fig. 4.4, **A** and **B** is reprinted courtesy of Mr. B. J. Perry (52) and by permission of the Editors, British Journal of Radiology 46: December, 1973.)

were made and isodose curves were plotted for the different x-ray tube loadings used clinically, but without a patient in position. One such plot is illustrated in figure 4.4B. The x-ray tube manufacturers claim a maximum leakage from the present tube housing of less than 10 R per hour at 140 kVp in any direction from the tube (52).

Studies of exposures at 140 kVp, 27 mA, 1 meter from the scanner indicated values less than 3 mR per hour except opposite the high-voltage cable tube terminals, where maximum exposure rates of 12 and 25 mR per hour were found for 120 and 140 kVp operation (38).

SCAN ARTIFACTS

Partial Volume Phenomena

These are features of the method that must be kept constantly in mind when interpreting CT scans. Accuracy of measurement of absorption values of substances of which the equipment is capable cannot be achieved unless the substance being measured occupies at least the full thickness of the scan section. If the substance occupies less than the full thickness of the scan section (13 or 8 mm), the absorption value obtained will be an average of that of the substance under consideration and that of the surrounding material, according to the proportions of each in the scan section. If the absorption value of a given type of material (tissue or other) is only slightly different from the surrounding material, so that it would just be visible (discriminated) under conditions in which it occupied the entire thickness of the scan section, complete loss of discrimination would occur readily if it occupied only a fraction of the slice thickness. On the other hand, if the material under consideration had a much higher or lower absorption value than did the ambient material, discrimination would tend to be preserved under partial volume conditions. Knowledge of the true absorption values of the material and of the surrounding substance will permit calculation of the approximate amount of the material that must be present in the scan section for discrimination to be possible.

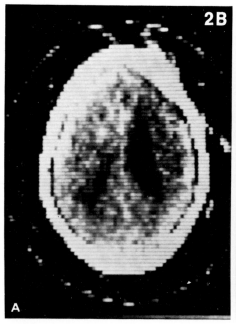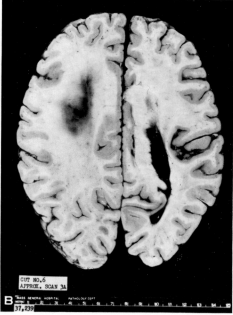

FIG. 4.5. PARTIAL VOLUME REPRESENTATION OF AN INTRACEREBRAL HEMATOMA

A. L 16　　W 20.

The more inferior sections of this patient's examination revealed a typical large dense intracerebral hematoma (Fig. 16.2). At the scan level shown, the superior extremity of the hematoma extends to occupy portions of the scan section. Averaging of absorption values with surrounding brain results in falsely low values for the hematoma in this section, although portions of the hematoma encroaching upon the section remain quite readily visible against the absorption of adjacent brain and some edema. It is probable that CSF in the anterior portion of the compressed left lateral ventricle contributes to the lowering of absorption measurement of the blood.

B. Brain slice approximately corresponding to the scan section shown in **A**. Although the brain section is slightly higher than the scan, the extension of the upper portion of the hemorrhage into this slice is visible in the left frontal lobe.

An exceedingly dense object such as a metal clip will be identifiable even though it is surrounded by a low absorber such as CSF or edema fluid, although its true absorption value will not be obtained. Small particles of bone or densely aggregated calcium will also tend to remain visible, even though they may occupy only a very small percentage of the slice thickness. Hematomas, considerably denser than white matter, and cavities containing low absorption fluids can often be discriminated although they occupy only a portion of the scan section thickness. In considering intracranial lesions in general, if they are of sufficiently large size to occupy at least the full thickness of one section, they will commonly be traceable into adjacent sections on careful analysis, although they might occupy only a portion of the adjacent sections (Fig. 4.5). A greater problem is the lesion that is too small to occupy the full thickness of any section and has an absorption not greatly different from that of surrounding normal issues. Under these conditions, a lesion that would otherwise be readily identified may be overlooked. For example, a small dense nodule of metastatic adenocarcinoma, occupying only a portion of the section thickness, may not be discriminated when its density is averaged with the low absorption of surrounding edema. The likelihood of discrimination of such small lesions may be increased by intravenous injection of a large volume of contrast medium. The density of a small vascular lesion (vascular tumor nodule or small aneurysm) may be sufficiently increased by these means to permit identification that would otherwise be impossible. Small lesions may fortuitously occupy contiguous portions of two slices or be entirely included in one slice. Clearly, the former situation is the more adverse. Assuming equally accurate absorption measurements in 8- and 13-mm sections, use of the former will tend to increase the possibility of discriminating small lesions.

Another aspect of the partial volume phenomenon involves the measurement averaging that occurs when a small object extends to occupy only a portion of an adjacent matrix point. The absorption value of the material encroaching partially upon an adjacent matrix point will be averaged with the material occupying the remainder of the matrix point, resulting in a form of

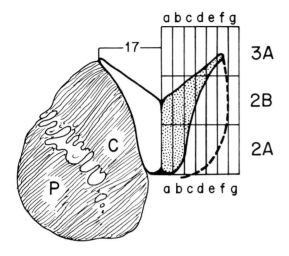

FIG. 4.6. DIAGRAMMATIC REPRESENTATION OF THE PARTIAL VOLUME PHENOMENON AS IT AFFECTS SMALL LATERAL VENTRICLES. The lateral ventricular contours were traced from a pneumoencephalogram of an 8-year-old girl, and the matrix blocks of 13-mm scan sections (80 x 80 matrix) were drawn to scale and are superimposed upon the anterior portion of the left lateral ventricle. On the *left* side are drawn representations of the caudate nucleus (*C*) and putamen (*P*). Although there are innumerable alternative possible relationships between the scan sections and matrix blocks and the lateral ventricle, those shown serve to illustrate the varying degree of inclusion of the ventricular cavity in various matrix blocks. Ventricular CSF occupies 100% of block *a, 2A*. The ventricular cavity occupies less than 100% of all of the other matrix blocks in each of the scan sections shown. The ventricle occupies approximately 30% of block *d, 2B*, and only some 15% of block *e, 3A*. About 5% of block *f, 3A*, is occupied by ventricle. Assuming that the mean absorption of CSF is 4 and that of the surrounding brain tissue is approximately 18 (white and grey matter above and central grey matter below), and assuming that loss of discrimination is likely when differential attenuation is less than 3 units, CT discrimination of the lateral ventricle will be lost lateral to block *d, 2B*. Therefore, the ventricular span will appear to be only 11 mm on the CT scan, rather than the actual span of 17 mm. When the ventricles are even smaller than in this example, the factitious reduction in size will be greater and microventricles may not be visible at all. If 8-mm sections are scanned, the partial volume effect will be less and the artifactual reduction in lateral ventricular size will also be less.

"smearing" in the transverse plane of the section. This feature is of considerably lesser importance in the 160 × 160 matrix system, in which the matrix point is only 1.5 mm square.

False Representation of Ventricular Size

It has been observed that the dimensions of small lateral ventricles are regularly represented as smaller than reality on CT scans. This is explained by partial

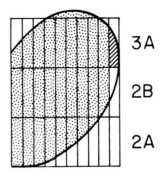

FIG. 4.7. DIAGRAMMATIC REPRESENTATION IN THE CASE OF A DILATED LATERAL VENTRICLE. The rounded configuration occurring laterally makes significant partial volume effects unlikely, and ventricular size is depicted much more accurately. The *heavily shaded zone* occupies over 50% of the tissue block in this example, and discrimination will occur. Ventricular span will therefore be demonstrated accurately.

volume averaging (Fig. 4.6). As the thinner lateral portions of the lateral ventricles are not discriminated, the ventricles of many young individuals and those of patients who have been effectively shunted appear much smaller than they actually are. Under some conditions of placement of the scan sections in relation to the lateral ventricles, very small ventricles may appear minute. Portions of the third ventricle and the entire fourth ventricle may be difficult or impossible to identify under such conditions. On the other hand, the greater the dilatation of the ventricular system, the more likely it is that the ventricular dimensions will be accurately represented (Fig. 4.7).

Overshadowing by Bone of Cerebral Anatomy in the Superior Convexity and Parasagittal Regions

Owing to the increasing obliquity of these anatomical structures relative to the scan sections, bone is included in the scan sections in the superior scans (Fig. 4.8). Thus, the absorption readings at the periphery are incorrect and window width and level will often require increasing for visualization of the cerebral surface structures at these higher levels.

MEASUREMENT OF LESION SIZE

To obtain the "true"* dimensions of an object or lesion from a Polaroid record of the CRT display, the diameter of the water bath field display on the photograph is checked. This should be perfectly circular (or the viewer requires adjustment). Since the actual diameter of the circle is 21.8 cm in the 160 × 160 matrix system, the

---

*In measuring on Polaroid records, due allowance must be made for partial volume phenomena.

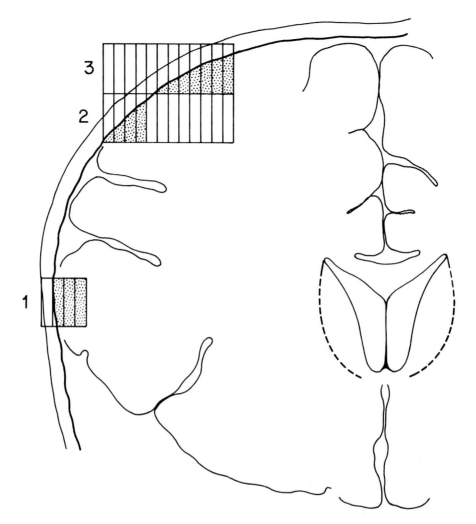

FIG. 4.8. Inclusion of bone in superior cerebral scan volumes. The increasing inclusion of bone in the matrix blocks of more superior sections is demonstrated (*2* and *3*). More inferiorly, the relatively vertically oriented bone encroaches only slightly (*1*). The abrupt change from high absorption of bone to low absorption of CSF and brain causes a degree of computer error (undershoot) just beneath the inner table in the lower scan sections. The gradual change that occurs in the more superior sections results in an absence of the undershoot phenomenon in these sections.

minification factor is:

$$\frac{\text{Diameter of field on Polaroid } (D)}{21.8}$$

and the "true" size of a lesion is obtained by:

$$\text{Measured size of lesion on Polaroid} \times 21.8/D$$

At present, on the MGH system, D = 6.6 cm and the correction factor is therefore 3.3.

MOTION ARTIFACTS

If any form of head motion occurs during the period of scanning, individual structures will lie in different positions during different portions of the scan sequence and a wide variety of false absorption readings can be produced. At scan levels above the basal bone structures, slight head movements during scanning produce only a relatively subtle degradation of the quality of the intracranial scan. The appearance of rather obvious streaks in the surrounding water bath represents a useful general indication of the amount of movement that has occurred under such conditions. More striking artifacts are produced in the more basal cranial scans, even when cranial motion is relatively slight. Such motion artifacts are most serious when the motion is in the axis perpendicular to that of the x-ray beam (in and out movements of the head). Such movements can result in the inclusion of bone in the scan section during part of the scan sequence and absence of bone during other portions of the scan sequence. The attenuation measurements obtained, therefore, vary very widely for the same matrix region at different times during the scan, and, following processing, these changes are represented by alternating white and black bands on each side of the area of bone involved. The sign of the artifact changes across the region of bone involved. If the latter is part of the cranial periphery, the white and black bands external to the head are aligned with black and white bands within the cranium, respectively (Fig. 4.9A). If the region of bone is intracranial, for example, the petrous pyramid, the alternating black and white artifactual bands that are always vertically oriented in the processed scan, will be on either side of the petrous pyramid (Fig. 4.9B).

Movement of the head from side to side rather than in and out of the water bath (and shifting of air trapped in the temporal hollows under the head bag) produces vertically oriented white and black bands in the water bath and lateral portions of the cranial cavity. Rotary movement of the head during scanning produces similar bands that are tangent to the calvaria and run obliquely. With considerable movement of the patient, both of the latter types of motion artifact tend to be seen together in the processed scans (Fig. 4.9C).

In and out head movements or shifting fluid within the frontal sinus may cause different transmission readings in different points in the scan, due to the presence or

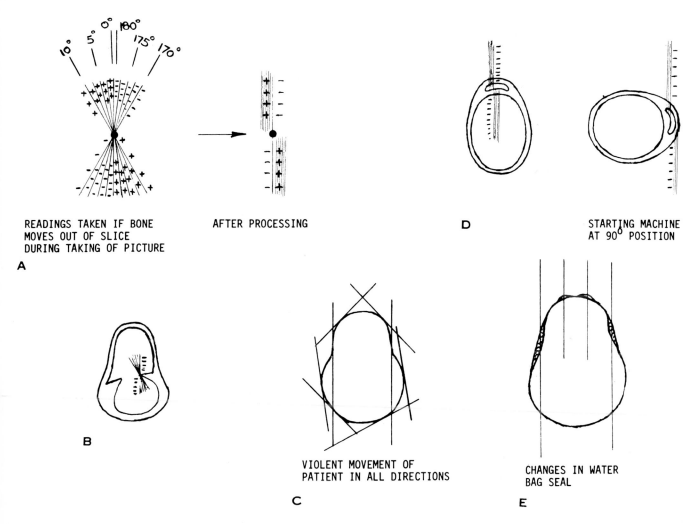

A — READINGS TAKEN IF BONE MOVES OUT OF SLICE DURING TAKING OF PICTURE

AFTER PROCESSING

D — STARTING MACHINE AT 90° POSITION

B

C — VIOLENT MOVEMENT OF PATIENT IN ALL DIRECTIONS

E — CHANGES IN WATER BAG SEAL

FIG. 4.9. DIAGRAMMATIC REPRESENTATION OF THE PRODUCTION AND FINAL APPEARANCE ON PROCESSED SCANS OF VARIOUS FORMS OF MOTION ARTIFACT. When there is a change in position of a very high- or very low-density structure during the course of the 180° scan sequence, there is a conflict in the measurement related to the region in which movement has caused a change in structure position. The end result is a number of white and black alternating bands proximal and distal to the region that has moved. If such artifactual bands extend into the cranial cavity, as many will under conditions of motion, more or less serious obscuration of anatomical and pathological details will occur. Motion during scanning is anathema to CT scanning, and every reasonable effort must be made to prevent motion or to reduce it to an acceptable minimum. To achieve this end, comfortable patient positioning, tolerable fixation devices, sedation, and general anesthesia must all be used appropriately. (Reprinted by permission of EMI Ltd).

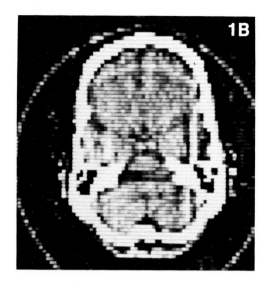

1B

FIG. 4.10. SCAN ARTIFACT IN THE REGION OF THE PONS

L 10   W 30.

This very commonly occurring artifact between the anterior portions of the petrous pyramids has a typical horizontal geometrical appearance of factitiously low absorption. The cause of the artifact is not readily explained. Anatomical considerations exclude partial volume inclusion of the interpeduncular cistern. A possible explanation that has been put forward is that this represents an artifact secondary to a deficiency in computer programming. The program supplied with the 80 x 80 matrix provides a total of 16,000 numbers as a maximum for any horizontal scan matrix line. If the total of absorption values in each matrix point of the line exceeds this figure, other matrix points in the line will be assigned factitiously low absorption values. The absorption values through both dense petrous bones is likely to exhaust the assigned numerical total, so that the intervening region, extending across the pons, would show abnormally low values.

absence of very dense bone and very low-density air in the sinus. The processed scan section at the involved level will show vertical alternating bands of white and black, with a change in sign between the exterior and interior of the skull (Fig. 4.9D). If this type of artifact is a problem in a particular case, repeating the scan at this level by commencing the scan at the 90° position (utilizing the scanner over-ride switch) may solve the problem by causing the artifactual bands to pass exterior to the intracranial cavity.

A patient movement correction (PMC) capability has been made available in the EMI scanner system. Use of this option requires an extension of the scan sequence time to 6 minutes, ±15 seconds, to provide a 225° scan. When some motion of the patient's head has been observed during the initial 180° scan, use of the above extension, with subsequent automatic rejection of the least valid absorption data acquired during individual traverses at any angle up to a total of 45 different angles, may result in appreciable improvement of the total scan sequence quality (Fig. 4.16).

If a greater than usual amount of air is trapped in the temporal hollows beneath the rubber cap, changes in distribution of this gas during the period of scanning may cause similar, vertically oriented alternating white and black artifactual lines extending through the temporal fossa regions (Fig. 4.9E).

Computer overswing and underswing artifacts that result from an abrupt and marked density difference and that generally involve one or two matrix squares adjacent to the discontinuity are generally registered as a reading of approximately 3% of the absorption difference at the discontinuity. The 160×160 matrix and new program combine to reduce the prominence of such artifacts. Various forms of CT artifact are additionally described and illustrated in other portions of this book.

MISCELLANEOUS ARTIFACTS

The artifacts that may be produced by the presence of extremely low or high absorption substances are illustrated in Figs. 4.10, 4.11, 4.12, and 4.13.

AUXILIARY VIEWING UNITS

The rapid development of auxiliary viewing units capable of operating completely independently of the scanner system itself was inevitable. Such units can be relatively small and made to provide complete viewing and analytical facilities at various remote stations, using scan records transferred to magnetic tape or small flexible discs. A variety of modifications of data display on television monitors of different sizes can be tested. Larger displays suitable for conferences, with small slave monitors for photographic recording, are desirable. It should be possible to provide selection of an 80×80 matrix display of averaged values for more accurate measurement of absorption coefficients and a 160×160 display for the greater anatomical resolution provided by that system. Simultaneous presentation of both forms of display would be even more convenient. These options are presently being explored by us.

An interesting remote display modification has been developed by C. J. Thompson, Computing Systems Engineer at the Montreal Neurological Institute. His method uses taped records produced by the EMI scanner. These are read into a Fortran program on a PDP-12 computer. A grey scale image is produced on the storage

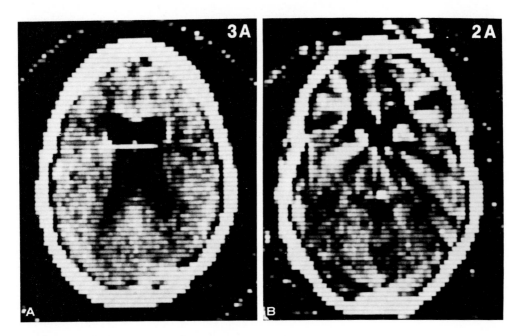

Fig. 4.11. ARTIFACTS CAUSED BY INTRAVENTRICULAR GAS.

A. L 16   W 20.

Gas is present in the frontal horns, from recent pneumoencephalography. At the air fluid level, a 1 matrix-wide horizontal band of factitiously high readings is present and, less clearly seen, a similar narrow band of incorrect high readings extends about most of the perimeter of each frontal horn.

B. L 17   W 20.

The gas in the frontal horns has produced very extensive and striking fan-shaped alternating white and black zones of factitious absorption readings, probably due to associated motion of the head during the scan. Extensive portions of the scan are degraded below diagnostic levels.

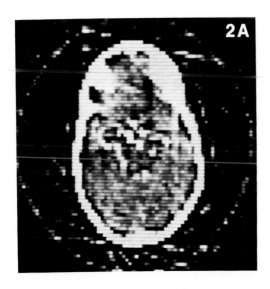

FIG. 4.12. An occasional droplet of Pantopaque retained within the cranium from previous intracranial or intrathecal instillation of Pantopaque does not create significant problems of artifact. However, if Pantopaque residues are very extensive, and especially if the Pantopaque drops are large, the underswing artifacts adjacent to the high-density droplets will tend to obscure details. The same is true of intracranial surgical clips. An occasional small clip provides no appreciable problem in analysis of absorption values of adjacent regions and can be of great help in defining the extent of the surgical procedure. However, a close grouping of multiple clips, particularly of larger size, can produce significant adjacent artifacts when the 80 x 80 matrix system is used. The program used with the 160 x 160 matrix handles such metallic aggregations without producing quite such severe artifacts, since computation of the absorption of dense metal is cut off at a little above the level of dense bone (approximately 800 units).

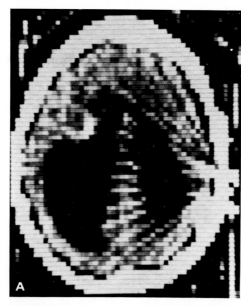

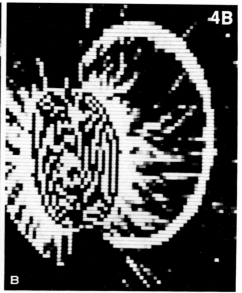

FIG. 4.13. ARTIFACTS PRODUCED BY DENSE METALLIC OBJECTS OF MORE THAN MINUTE SIZE

A. The scan of this patient, who suffered from severe obstructive hydrocephalus treated by ventriculoatrial shunting, shows lateral ventricles that are still greatly dilated and exhibits the alternating radiating black and white artifactual streaks extending into the head from the site of the metal casing of the valve on the right side. The artifacts produced in this particular scan are not as striking as are commonly seen under such circumstances, because the valve is included in only a portion of the scan section (partial volume averag-

ing). One manufacturer of ventricular shunt valves has produced a modification using a plastic casing to replace the original metal. Testing of the modified valves reveals that no intracranial artifacts are produced thereby.

B. This scan was obtained in a patient who had received a large tantulum plate following extensive craniectomy. The very extensive artifacts produced on the 80 x 80 matrix system obscured much of the intracranial anatomical detail. The degree to which the 160 matrix program can compensate for this type of situation is at present unknown.

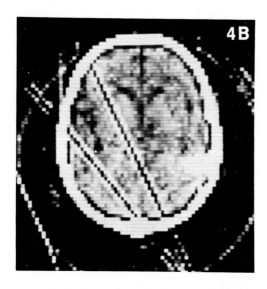

FIG. 4.14. This artifact is seen rarely. The radiating lightning-like streaks of white with an intervening black band are the result of brief loss of power during the scan, so that no reading is received from the detectors during these portions of the scan. A major dip in main voltage or a loose detector connection could produce such artifacts. Faulty indexing of the scanner causes a "herring bone" pattern of alternating light and dark bands at 2° *intervals*.

screen of a Tektronix terminal. The window level and width for the images are adjusted in a manner similar to the viewer controls of the EMI scanner. On this image, an "area of interest" may be defined (selected) by the operator. The matrix points within the defined area can either be printed out numerically, together with their mean and standard deviations, or can be viewed from any of four angles as an isometric display (Fig. 4.15, *A* and *B*). To form an isometric display viewed from the anterior left corner of the region of interest, points from right to left are laid out along the horizontal axis of the screen, the rows of points from anterior or posterior are projected onto the screen (away from the observer), and the relative density of each point is drawn vertically. Lines are drawn between the points along all rows and along all columns. If a line would be hidden behind one that had already been drawn when seen from the point of view of the observer, it is not drawn. This is done simply by drawing the lines nearest the observer first and keeping track of the horizontal and vertical coordinates up until that time. The resulting picture is such that, if the lesion is of relatively constant density (e.g., a hematoma), the height above the base line indicates the extent of the lesion in that scan section. Three slices on a smaller scale can also be drawn.

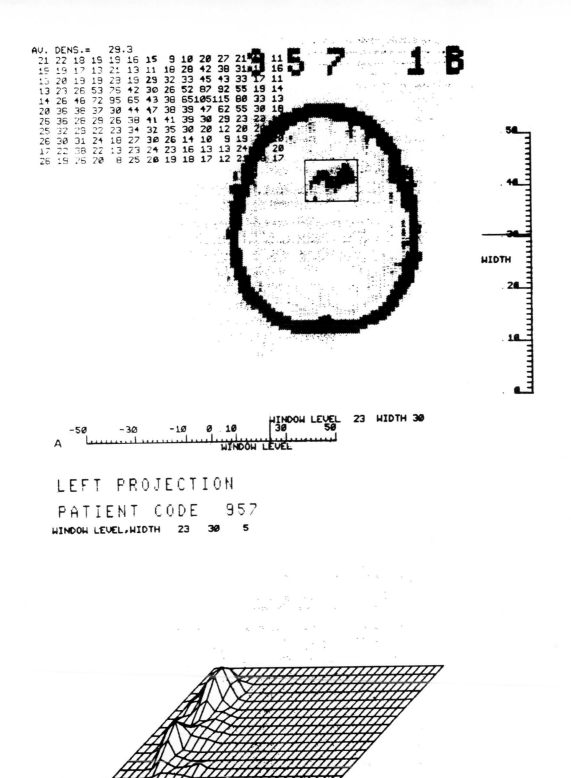

AV. DENS.= 29.3
```
21 22 18 19 19 16 15  9 10 20 27 21   9 11
19 19 17 13 21 13 11 18 20 42 38 31   1 16
13 20 19 19 23 19 29 32 33 45 43 33 17 11
13 23 26 53 75 42 30 26 52 87 92 55 19 14
14 26 48 72 95 65 43 38 65105115 80 33 13
20 36 38 37 30 44 47 38 39 47 62 55 30 18
25 36 28 29 26 38 41 41 39 30 29 23 23
25 32 23 22 23 34 32 35 30 20 12 20 20
26 30 31 24 18 27 30 26 14 10  9 19
17 22 38 22 13 23 24 23 16 13 13 24   20
26 19 26 20  8 25 20 19 18 17 12 23   17
```

WIDTH

-50   -30   -10   0 10   WINDOW LEVEL   23 WIDTH 30
                              30   50
A   WINDOW LEVEL

LEFT PROJECTION

PATIENT CODE   957

WINDOW LEVEL,WIDTH   23   30   5

B   18

FIG. 4.15.

A. Photocopy of a scan section display on the storage screen of a Tektronix terminal. The patient scan code number and slice level displayed are shown at the *top* in large letters. Cursors can be moved along the vertical and horizontal scales to select an area of particular interest and numerical printout can be obtained of that area only. The area selected is shown within the *rectangle* in the frontal region. The associated absorption values have been printed out in the *top left* portion of the display and indicate the presence of small areas of calcification and a larger area of blood clot. The average absorption (*AV. DENS.*) of a selected area is also given.

B. Isometric display from a Tektronix terminal, viewed from the left anterior corner of region of interest. The selected window level and width are printed *above*. The regions of relative increase in absorption at these viewer settings are shown projecting upwards to a height proportionate to the values at each matrix point.

(Illustrations by courtesy of Mr. Christopher Thompson, Montreal Neurological Institute.)

Diagnostic Display Console (DDC) (EMI)

This auxiliary console enables processed pictures to be recorded from the EMI scanner system onto a floppy disc, the capacity of which is 8 pictures. The write and read check time is less than 45 seconds. For recording on the floppy discs, the console must be connected with the computer with a maximum cable length of 8 meters. The recorded pictures are displayed on a 12-inch black-and-white television monitor, and the unit has window width and level controls similar to those of the primary viewing unit. Following recording on the floppy disc, the pictures on the disc can be viewed and analyzed on a second display console operating completely independently at any remote site. Once the initial information transfer has taken place, the primary console also becomes independent of any input from the main system. Therefore, scan records on this unit can be studied whether or not the scanner is engaged in scanning, processing, or transferring data to tape, etc. Whether linked to the scanner or used as a completely remote system, the console may be connected with other television monitors, allowing multistation viewing of scan records. Polaroid records can be obtained by any display, using a camera attached to a small slave television monitor.

Video Display Processor (VDP) (Elscint)

Another off-line static display system has been described by Shields et al (60). Scan data are stored on tape cassettes (38 image capacity) and may be displayed on a television monitor in eight shades of grey or in eight colors. The colors are used quantitatively to display an adjustable band of available data. Scan sections can be analyzed and viewed by superimposition or by subtraction.

Modular Magnetic Tape Viewer

This viewer was designed and built by Melvin E. Conway, Ph.D., under contract to the Massachusetts General Hospital. It consists of two cable-connected electronic units and one or more black-and-white television monitors. A typical configuration with one television monitor can be placed on a standard office desk with room left over for working surface.

The tape unit accepts magnetic tapes written by the magnetic tape option that EMI offers. All viewing controls are on a movable control unit. The control unit allows the operator to peruse the directory written at the front of the tape, to search for a particular image, and to view that image. The viewing controls include the conventional continuous level control and a discrete window width selection control. An averaging switch permits choice of two different image presentations. In addition to the 160×160 matrix picture produced by the scanner, a presentation is available in which each picture element is an average of four neighboring elements. This choice permits a reduction of the noise accompanying absorption values, with no apparent loss of spatial resolution. A 15-inch monitor provides images of full anatomical size. Film records on 90-mm roll film appear to be convenient and economical.

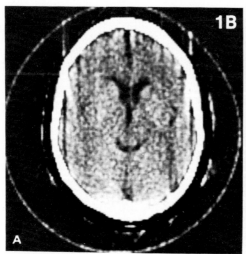 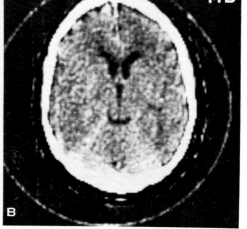

FIG. 4.16. PATIENT MOVEMENT CORRECTION (PMC) SYSTEM

A. During this scan, the patient's head moved sufficiently to cause disturbing artifacts in both temporal areas and to a lesser extent in the anterior frontal region. Other scan levels showed similar motion artifacts.

B. Following injection of intravenous contrast medium, the scan series was repeated, using the PMC program. Although patient motion was similar to that in the initial series, use of the PMC resulted in significantly less interference with intracranial anatomical detail.

THIN SECTION SCANNING AND DEVELOPMENT OF CORONAL AND SAGITTAL SECTIONS FROM CONVENTIONAL TRANSVERSE DATA

Present x-ray tube output places limitations upon the capability of scanning thinner cranial sections (less than 6–8 mm in thickness), due to unacceptably high noise-to-signal ratios produced when using acceptably short scan times (Fig. 4.3). Dr. William Glenn, during his residency in Radiology at the Massachusetts General Hospital, conceived an ingenious solution to the current problem. His approach involves repeated scanning in standard planes using the EMI 8-mm collimators with standard scan times. Following each scan sequence, succeeding scans are obtained after movement of the section plane by a fraction of the slice thickness. The movement could be, for example, 1, 2, or 4 mm. The scan data acquired by such a series of overlapping scans are sufficient for reconstruction of scan sections of 1, 2, or 4 mm in thickness, respectively.

Following a study of step function on Plexiglas phantoms, Glenn and his coworkers at the University of Missouri's Image Analysis Laboratory were able to deconvolve the data acquired by such multiple overlapping scans and to reconstruct, by means of a suitable algorithm programmed on a small computer, highly detailed thin scan sections in not only the original scan plane but also in coronal and sagittal planes. In the coronal and sagittal reconstructions, sections can be reconstructed to the thickness of the matrix elements (1.47 mm) or in multiples of this thickness. In the original scan plane, sections can be reconstructed according to the thickness of the original overlap or in multiples thereof, to give somewhat thicker sections. The method was tested on cadavers and demonstrated a most satisfactory degree of anatomical and pathological detail in both the original scan plane and the coronal and sagittal planes (27A).

Of particular interest is the effectiveness of the reconstructed scans in showing anatomical details that cannot be appreciated in the original thickness and plane of scan. In particular, the cross-sectional configuration of the temporal horns and the lateral and third ventricles in the coronal sections and the configuration of the aqueduct, fourth ventricle, and median cisterns in the sagittal sections were noteworthy.

The computer algorithm, which has been programmed in Fortran on a standard small computer system (Digital Equipment Corporation PDP 11/20), is an interpolation procedure based on the experimentally determined photon flux across the collimated 8-mm beam. Processing time required for the reconstruction of coronal and sagittal images is long in comparison to the 5–10 minutes that will be required when computer programs have been optimized for speed and applied only to local volumes of interest, e.g., an orbit or the perisellar region.

While the prolonged examination time required by this technique will limit its application to relatively narrow zones within the orbit and cranium until faster scan systems become available, the method should be applicable shortly to patient examinations in the planes of the orbit, the supra- and parasellar regions, and the cerebellopontine angles. Although only a limited number of patient studies has been obtained thus far, satisfactory signal-to-noise ratios are present on the reconstructed scans, and the method appears capable of development *pari passu* with general improvements in CT scanning technology.

CHAPTER 5

Anatomical Correlations

INTRODUCTION

The present technique of computed tomography entails a distinct reorientation of thought in evaluating intracranial anatomy. Radiologists have been accustomed to thinking of this anatomy largely in the direction of construction of 3-dimensional concepts from lateral and sagittal projections as obtained particularly from angiographic and pneumographic studies. Oblique, axial, and subaxial projections have played a distinctly subsidiary role.

Computed tomography at present displays cranial and intracranial anatomy in a transaxial or subaxial manner. While this anatomical orientation is more familiar to neuropathologists, brain cutting has been dominated in the past by coronal sections in the supratentorial regions. In the future, in cases in which CT scans have been obtained in life, it is likely that there will be a steady trend towards transaxial brain cutting, with the aim of reproducing the angle of the scan and the scan section thicknesses as accurately as possible. This has become a common practice in such cases at the Massachusetts General Hospital.

The *Atlas of the Human Brain in Section* by Roberts and Hanaway is of particular value in the study of anatomy as presented by CT scans, as it includes a chapter illustrating horizontal sections, serially sliced at 4-mm intervals and well annotated. However, the illustrated horizontal sections are limited to the region of anatomy between the following planes: inferiorly, the medial orbital gyri of the frontal lobe anteriorly, the optic chiasm and midbrain centrally, and the superior cerebellar vermis and occipital lobes posteriorly; and superiorly, a plane at the level of the most superior portion of the corpus callosum and the superior limit of the caudate nucleus. These planes of section lie at approximately 5° to Reid's anatomical base line. In order to supplement the Roberts and Hanaway *Atlas* and to provide an anatomical reference more

readily correlated with the angled transverse sections commonly used in CT scanning, a series of brain sections made at an angle of approximately 30° to Reid's base line (corresponding to an angle of approximately 20° to the orbitomeatal line) is illustrated in this chapter. Naturally, the wide individual anatomical variations that exist make it impossible to derive anatomical illustrations that are more than rather generally representative.

An attempt has not been made to annotate the illustrated brain sections fully. Emphasis has been placed upon those structures that are more or less frequently recognizable on CT scans and certain other structures that form useful landmarks that can be located approximately on the scans.

Individual differences in anatomical configuration of the skull and brain result in variations in effective inclinations and levels of CT scan sections, even if positioning is accomplished precisely according to external landmarks. Such variations can be minimized by using a true lateral skull radiograph of known magnification as a preliminary reference for standarizing scan angles and levels.

The brain specimen sections illustrated in this chapter are each 7 mm in thickness and are consecutive from below upwards. The slices were photographed from their superior aspects with one exception. Instead of reproducing the superior aspect of the brain slice next superior to that in Figure 5.7, the immediately superjacent inferior aspect of the succeeding slice is represented in Figure 5.14, in order to display the optic chiasm and other structures adjacent to the anterior portion of the third ventricle. The approximate level of each slice is indicated in Figure 5.3.

In the section following each brain slice illustrated, approximately corresponding Polaroid photographs taken from the CRT display are presented for correlation. The CT scans shown do not necessarily correlate precisely with the levels of the anatomical sections, for reasons stated above. Thus, it has been necessary to include a representative range of scans at *similar* anatomical levels.* All of the CT scans illustrated are of 13-mm thick sections unless otherwise stated. The majority of the examples of CT scans obtained using the new 160 x 160 matrix and program included in this chapter were made available through the courtesy of Dr. James Ambrose, Consultant Radiologist at Atkinson Morley's Hospital, and his kind cooperation is gratefully acknowledged.

Anatomical diagrams in the form of acetate overlays are provided as aids to orientation of scan sections with respect to various gross anatomical features. These diagrams can be used singly or in various combinations when interpreting CT scans and when comparing scan findings with those of angiography and pneumoencephalography.

---

* Nil thickness for the surface of anatomic sections versus 8 or 13 mm thickness integrated for CT scans also precludes exact correspondence between anatomic sections and CT scans.

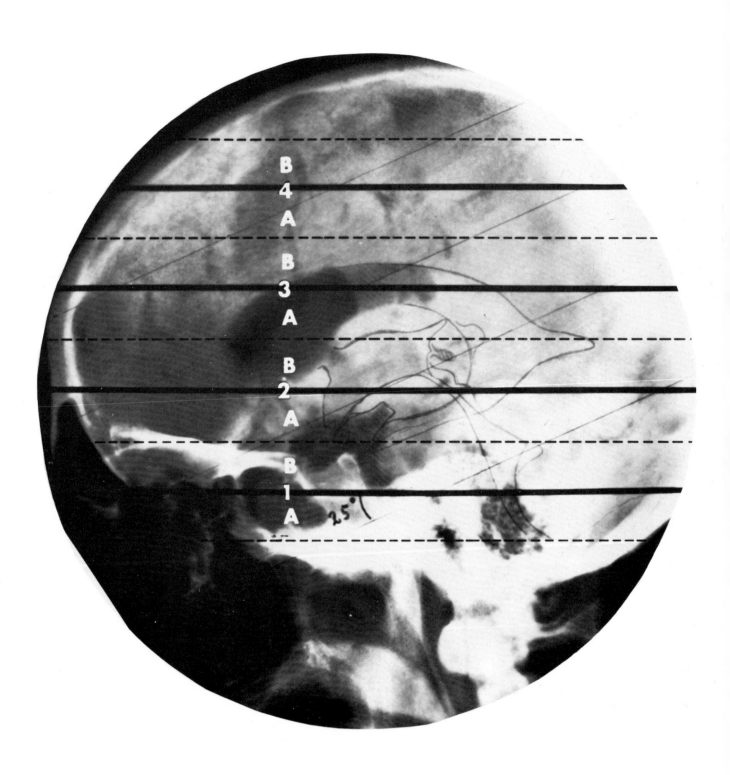

FIG 5.1. Skull, PEG with grid. Standard technique with 13-mm sections and 25° angle coverage. The reference levels for a set of four scans are superimposed on a lateral brow up film taken at pneumoencephalography. The heavy *solid black lines* represent the midplanes of the contiguous pairs of scan sections obtained in each scan sequence. The *interrupted lines* indicate the limits of each scanned tissue section (1.3 cm thick in this example). The scan angle is 25° to Reid's base line (RBL) and the section thicknesses have been adjusted to compensate for the radiographic magnification of the pneumogram. The midplane between the lowest two scan sections was placed 1 cm above the external auditory meatus (EAM). With this placement and scan angle, *in this individual anatomical configuration*, the lowest scan section includes the midorbits anteriorly, the base of the middle fossae, and the posterior fossa a few millimeters above the foramen magnum. A series of four scan sequences (eight sections) encompasses most of the intracranial volume in the adult, and the highest scan (4B) includes the superior parietal region and a small portion of the upper posterior part of the frontal lobes. The *light continuous lines* indicate planes parallel to RBL. Note that scans parallel to RBL will not include much of the lower posterior fossa and will include more of the frontal lobes than parietal lobes superiorly. Scans parallel to RBL will also produce less "distorted" representations of the anatomy of certain structures, including those in the upper part of the posterior fossa, the ambient cisterns, third ventricle, optic chiasm, temporal lobes, and temporal horns. Ideally, scan angle (and section thickness) should be selected for optimum display of anatomical regions suspected to be involved in pathology, but reduced angles involve sacrifice of the extent of coverage of the caudal regions with the present EMI waterbox configuration. Alternatively, the number of patients that can be examined is reduced if it is elected to add additional scans with modified angles and/or thicknesses and levels to the basic routine.

The above-described relationship of section thicknesses to intracranial anatomy represents the concept followed by all workers in the field until the announcement by G. N. Hounsfield in April 1975 that the individual tissue section thicknesses obtained with the 13-mm collimators were actually 10 mm. Thus, the previously established routines of moving the position of the patient's head 25 mm between scan pairs left 5-mm tissue gaps between each scan pair. For uninterrupted coverage, therefore, a shift of 2 cm between scan pairs is required. With the use of 8-mm collimators, a shift of 12 mm rather than 15 mm is required for complete coverage.

It is interesting to reflect that many tens of thousands of patients had been studied without the discrepancy being noted. **The grid overlay supplied with this volume is scaled to reflect individual scan sections of 13 mm. We are continuing to move the head 2.5 cm between "13-mm" scans and 1.5 cm between "8-mm" scans.**

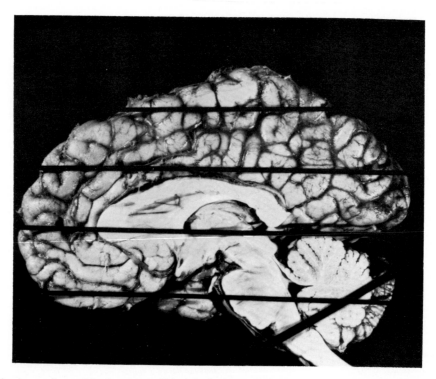

FIG. 5.2. Midsagittal brain section, with placement of *black tape strips* to indicate the general orientation of anatomical features that will be produced by scans at approximately 25° to RBL. There has been some postmortem deformation of the brain. A *thicker tape* has been placed across the cerebellum and medulla to indicate a plane parallel to Reid's anatomic base line, a plane more suitable for displaying the anatomy of posterior fossa structures. Such a plane of section cannot be obtained with the EMI scanner in its present form. A deeper waterbox could allow such scan planes only with special provision for patient respiration. Even then, air in the maxillary antra and pharynx would tend to affect adversely the quality of such scans.

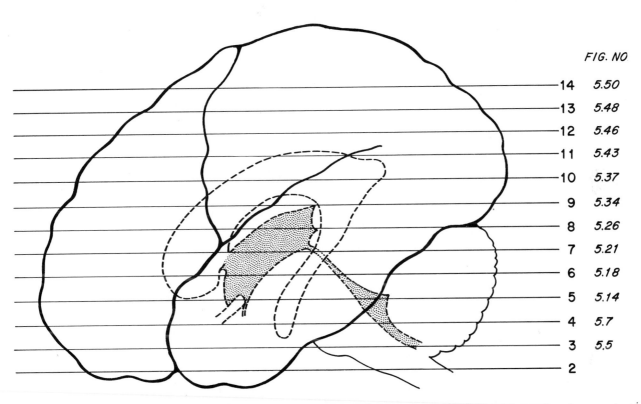

	FIG. NO
14	5.50
13	5.48
12	5.46
11	5.43
10	5.37
9	5.34
8	5.26
7	5.21
6	5.18
5	5.14
4	5.7
3	5.5
2	

FIG. 5.3. Diagrammatic representation of the angle (approximately 30° to RBL) and the levels of the series of anatomical brain sections illustrated in this chapter. Anatomical sections corresponding to the lowest two levels are not included in the series.

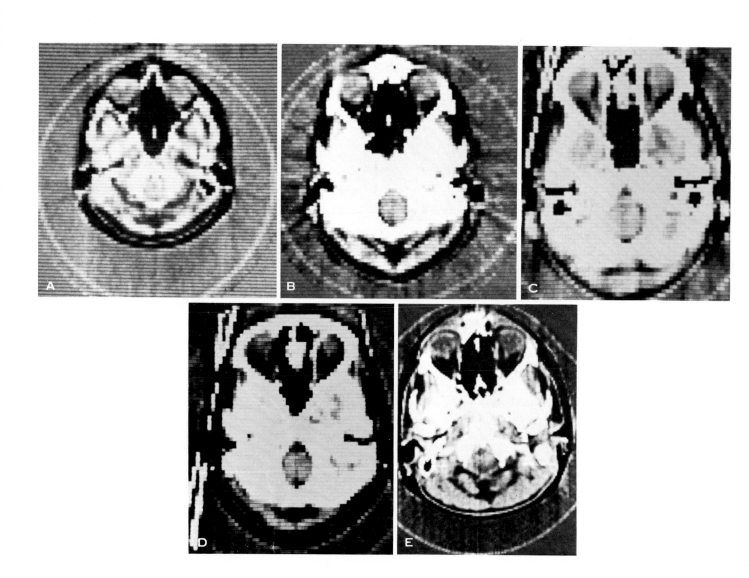

FIG. 5.4. A–D. SCAN SECTIONS THROUGH THE ORBIT AND BASAL SKULL REGIONS.
A. L −2   W 75.
This scan section extends through the middle third of the orbit anteriorly and the foramen magnum posteriorly. The wide window width and negative window level commonly provide the best display of intraorbital structures and basal cerebral and skull detail, but the control positions will need to be modified depending upon the anatomical area of maximum interest and the precise scan angle and plane. This scan demonstrates the globes. The lens can be identified on each side, more clearly on the left. The globes are sharply demarcated by contrast with the low density (−40 to −50) of the orbital fat, and there is some discrimination of the higher density of the walls of the globes and the lower density vitreous. The muscles of mastication below inferior portions of the middle fossae are shown. The scan plane passes through the inferior portions of the petrous bones (oblique white areas) and the mastoids (bilateral rounded black areas representing gas in the mastoid air cells, surrounded by narrow white zones representing mastoid cortex). The large diamond-shaped black zone centrally in the anterior and middle thirds of the scan represents the combined air spaces of the ethmoid and sphenoid sinuses. A portion of a septum of sphenoid sinus is present posteriorly. Scan angle is approximately 30° and the scan extends posteriorly to include the foramen magnum and the subjacent occipital condyles; circular light grey area representing the medulla, surrounded by a white area representing the posterior margin of foramen magnum, the lateral foraminal margins and occipital condyles together bilaterally, and the lower portion of the clivus anteriorly. The control settings are less than optimal for discrimination of the foramen magnum and medulla (see below). Owing to the obliquity of the scan, there is partial inclusion in the scan section of more posterior and superior segments of the occipital bone at the posterior margin of the scan.
B. The scan level is slightly higher than that shown in **A**. Window width was decreased to provide higher contrast and optimum display of the medulla within the foramen magnum. Many of the features demonstrated in **A** are again visible. The black zone surrounding the head in **A** and **B** represents a layer of air between the head bag and scalp.
C. L −3   W 75.
These control settings were optimal for display of the globes and of the optic nerves; both contrasted with the low density of orbital fat. The black zones anteriorly and in the central portion of the scan represent the inferior extremities of the frontal sinuses, ethmoidal sinuses, and large sphenoid sinus. The scan passes through the inferior portions of the middle fossae and the region of foramen magnum posteriorly, but the temporal lobes and medulla are not well displayed by these control settings. Air in the external auditory canals, mastoid air cells, and possibly middle ear cavities is indicated by the black rectangular zones in the petrous temporal regions. The slightly oblique white band adjacent to the left side of the head is an expression of minor movement of the head during the scan.
D. L 14   W 20.
These control settings provided optimum demonstration of the medulla within the foramen magnum in another case in which the scan angle and level were very similar to those shown in **C**. Note that there is a much less satisfactory display of the globes and optic nerves with these settings. The intraorbital structures were displayed well by control settings similar to those used in **C**. Due to the angle of the section, there is again a "stepped" appearance in the posterior occipital region, due to partial inclusion of a more posterosuperior segment of the occipital squama. In this region, the dark zone of CSF representing cisterna magna is visible.
E. L 15   W 50   160 x 160 matrix system.
Scan section similar to that in **A**, showing the improved anatomical resolution of the new system. The section is slightly inferior to **A** and shows the occipital condyles, then passes above the laminae of the first cervical vertebra. The suboccipital musculature is outlined by fat.

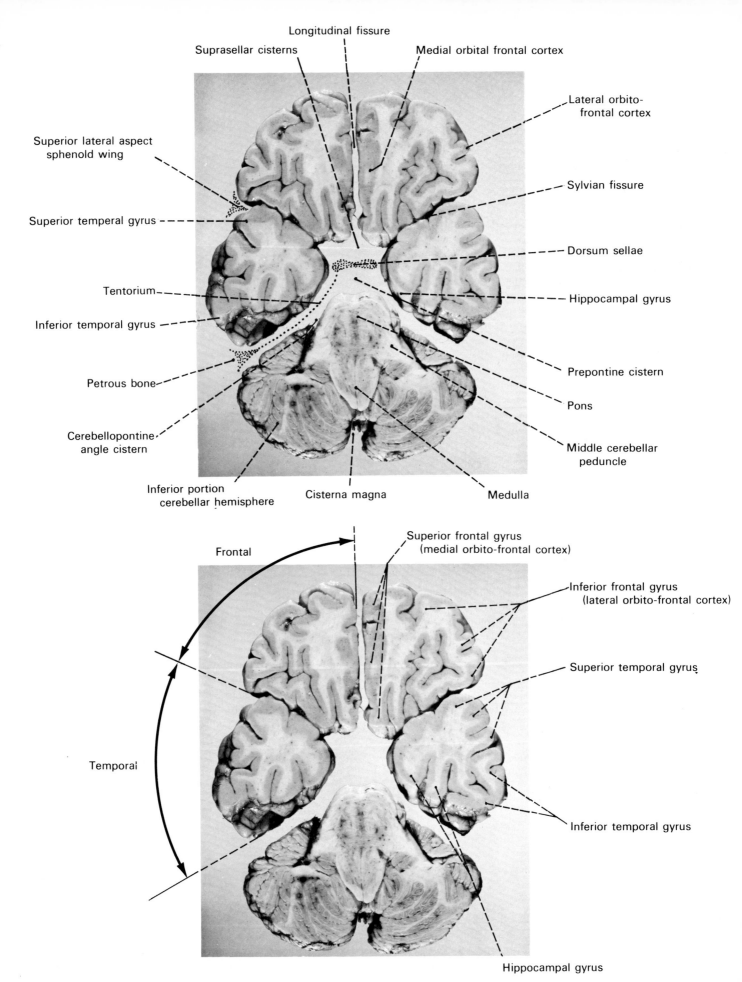

Longitudinal fissure

Suprasellar cisterns

Medial orbital frontal cortex

Lateral orbito-frontal cortex

Superior lateral aspect sphenold wing

Superior temperal gyrus

Sylvian fissure

Dorsum sellae

Tentorium

Inferior temporal gyrus

Hippocampal gyrus

Petrous bone

Prepontine cistern

Pons

Cerebellopontine angle cistern

Middle cerebellar peduncle

Inferior portion cerebellar hemisphere

Cisterna magna

Medulla

Frontal

Superior frontal gyrus (medial orbito-frontal cortex)

Inferior frontal gyrus (lateral orbito-frontal cortex)

Superior temporal gyrus

Temporal

Inferior temporal gyrus

Hippocampal gyrus

FIG. 5.5

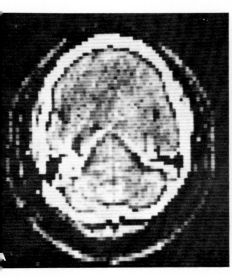 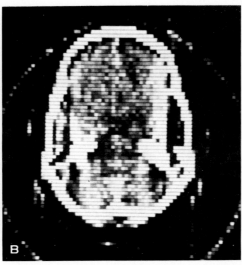 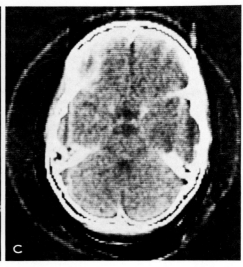

FIG. 5.6.

A. L 15   W 20.

Scan angle approximately 35° to Reid's base line. Anteriorly, the scan passes through the inferior portions of the frontal lobes. Posteriorly, the scan includes the petrous pyramids, upper portion of the pontine cistern at the level of the dorsum sellae, cerebellopontine angles, pons, and inferior portion of the cerebellum. The steep scan angle results in representation of the superior portion of the pons anteriorly and the middle to inferior portion of the pons posteriorly. The inferior extremity of the fourth ventricle is just visible (irregular light grey midline area). Just behind the fourth ventricle is a broad area of much greater density (white) representing the inferior cerebellar vermis. On each side, the grey matter of the cerebellar hemispheres is discriminated as arching zones, denser (whiter) than the cerebellar white matter and the intermediate density of the pons. On each side, within the dense (white) petrous bones are irregular black areas, representing the petromastoid air cell complexes. The narrow, almost black, zone adjacent to the posterior surfaces of the petrous pyramids represents the cerebellopontine angle cisterns, merging with the upper pontine cistern anteriorly. The portion of this dark zone immediately adjacent to the petrous may be due to computer undershoot, which occurs at an abrupt change from very high density (bone) to a much lower density (CSF or brain substance). This undershoot phenomenon is seen more regularly between the inner table of the skull and the external surfaces of the cerebrum and cerebellum and is restricted to a zone 1–2 matrix squares wide. This computer artifact obscures the subarachnoid spaces unless these are considerably widened. The small dark areas in each anterior temporal region represent the anterior inferior portions of the sylvian cisterns.

B. L 14   W 20.

The inferior vermis is represented by a moderate-sized white area posteriorly. The vermis frequently exhibits very dense characteristics and the appearance must not be mistaken for a dense midline cerebellar lesion. There was only slight side-to-side head movement during this scan, indicated by the vertical white streaks in the waterbath adjacent to the head, but striking scan artifacts are present in the lateral portion of each temporal region and lateral cerebellar hemisphere areas. These are characterized by vertically oriented alternating white and black bands of varying width. These typical and frequently appearing artifacts interfere with evaluation of absorption characteristics where they occur and in proportion to their prominence. Another form of frequently occurring artifact is prominent also in this scan. This is in the area of the pons, between the anterior portions of the petrous pyramids. In typical form, these artifacts show rectangular configurations of black or dark grey and are commonly arranged primarily in a transverse direction across the area of the pons. These may cause serious difficulties in evaluation of the pons. The upper pontine and suprasellar cisterns are visible in this scan as black areas. Viewer controls were not set for optimum demonstration of these cisterns.

C. L 16   W 40   160 x 160 matrix.

This scan reveals the smoothing effect on anatomical contours resulting from the finer matrix (four-fold increase in number of matrix points compared with the 80 x 80 matrix). The scan angle was considerably less (approximately 15°) than in **A**. The plane of section passes through the inferior portions of the frontal lobes, just above the orbital roofs (lateral portion of left orbital roof partially included), through the upper portions of the petrous pyramids and the fourth ventricle. The dark grey rectangular central area represents the suprasellar cistern, bounded on each side in this scan by the anterior clinoid processes (bilateral light grey areas) and posteriorly by a slightly dumbbell-like transverse band of light grey. The latter represents partial inclusion of the upper portion of the dorsum sellae and posterior clinoid processes in the scan section. The recorded density of these bone structures will be less than anticipated, as their absorption characteristics are averaged with the very low absorption of superjacent cisternal CSF. Under such circumstances, the measured absorption value may be similar to that of soft tissue, and these structures should not be mistaken for representations of the optic chiasm. Immediately behind the dorsum is a dark grey zone representing the upper portion of the pontine cistern. Alternating vertical white and dark bands in the lateral temporal regions represent minor manifestations of the commonly occurring form of artifact described in **B**. Anteriorly, a narrow dark grey zone in the midline represents the inferior portion of the interfrontal segment of the longitudinal fissure, leading up to the internal frontal crest. The internal occipital crest can be seen posteriorly, just behind a light grey zone representing the vallecula. The higher window width setting (40) of this scan display renders appreciably less contrast than do the settings shown in **A** and **B** (W 20).

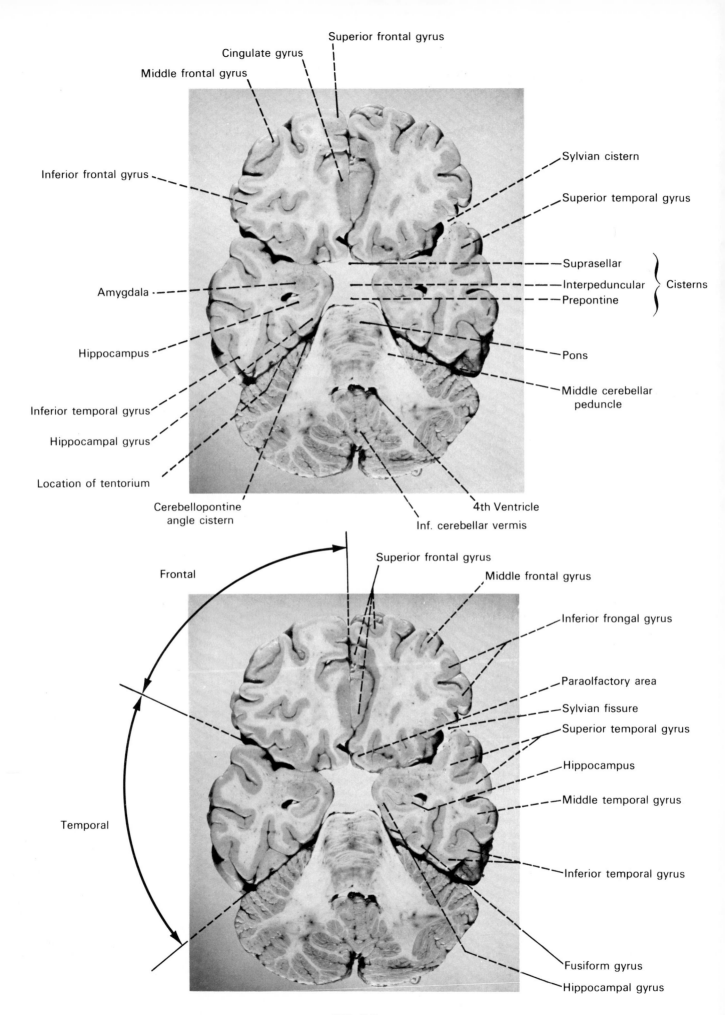

Middle frontal gyrus

Cingulate gyrus

Superior frontal gyrus

Inferior frontal gyrus

Sylvian cistern

Superior temporal gyrus

Suprasellar

Interpeduncular — Cisterns

Prepontine

Amygdala

Hippocampus

Pons

Middle cerebellar peduncle

Inferior temporal gyrus

Hippocampal gyrus

Location of tentorium

Cerebellopontine angle cistern

4th Ventricle

Inf. cerebellar vermis

Frontal

Superior frontal gyrus

Middle frontal gyrus

Inferior frongal gyrus

Paraolfactory area

Sylvian fissure

Superior temporal gyrus

Hippocampus

Middle temporal gyrus

Temporal

Inferior temporal gyrus

Fusiform gyrus

Hippocampal gyrus

FIG. 5.7

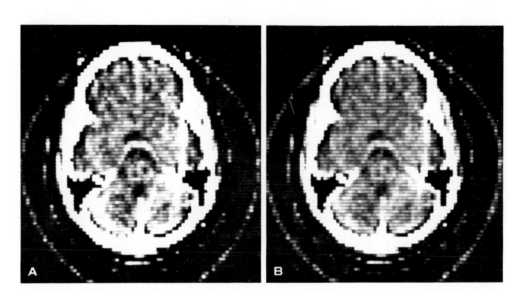

FIG. 5.8.
A. L 17   W 20.
Large petromastoid air cell complexes are shown as irregular black triangles on each side. Anteriorly, the section passes through the inferior portions of the frontal lobes and, posteriorly, through the upper pons, pontine cistern, and middle to lower portion of the fourth ventricle. The dorsum sellae and petroclinoid ligaments are shown as a whitish arch centrally in the scan. Just anterior to the dorsum sellae, the most inferior portion of the suprasellar cistern is visible as a dark area. The cerebellopontine angle cisterns are small and quite inconspicuous in this case. The white peripheral contour of high-density bone is visible. Anteriorly, on each side, a triangular inward projection of bone marks the region of the pterion and superolateral extremity of the sphenoid ridge.
B. L 17   W 30.
This is the same scan as is shown in **A.** The lesser contrast of the higher window setting is apparent. The vertical white bands shown in the right temporal region and in the region of the cerebellar vermis represent scan artifacts. These are partially suppressed by the higher window setting. The greater density of the cerebellar grey matter compared with white matter is visible. This is better seen on the left side than on the right and **A**, where the lower window setting favors differentiation.

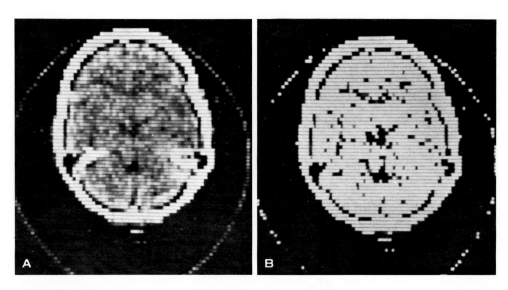

FIG. 5.9.

A. L 15   W 20.

The scan level is slightly higher than in the preceding figure. The dorsum sellae is not included and the section is nearer to the petrous ridges. Anteriorly, the cortex of the frontal lobes, being denser than the subjacent white matter, is shown as a very light grey area differentiated from the darker grey of the white matter. In the central area, the dark zone represents suprasellar cistern. Within this are smaller denser zones, contrasted with the CSF of the cistern. Structures that may contribute to such densities in the cistern include the portions of the chiasm, hypophyseal stalk, and cisternal segments of the internal carotid arteries. These structures generally cannot be differentiated satisfactorily. Further posteriorly, in the midline area, the dark zone of the inferior portion of the fourth ventricle is shown and, arching to the left is the left lateral recess of the fourth ventricle, which is rarely shown clearly in CT scans. On the right side, the lateral recess of the fourth ventricle is not visible, presumably due to slight head tilting or anatomical asymmetry.

B. L 13   WM

These viewer control settings provide maximum contrast between the CSF-containing spaces (fourth ventricle, suprasellar cistern, and small segments of the sylvian cisterns). At this window level, scattered areas of relatively low absorption are visible in the white matter of the frontal lobes. Relatively low white matter densities are commonly found in the frontal lobes adjacent to the frontal horns, particularly in children and young adults. These must be differentiated from decreased absorption resulting from pathological changes. The denser appearance of the cerebellar grey matter compared with white matter is visible in **A** but is obscured at the window level selected for **B**. With window width of M, a higher window level setting would be required for discrimination of grey matter and white matter. In normal individuals, the cerebellar vermis frequently presents a distinctly denser appearance than does the grey matter of the cerebellar hemispheres. This must be kept in mind when evaluating scans for possible pathology in the cerebellar vermis.

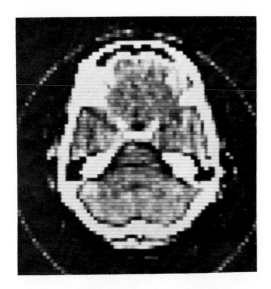

FIG. 5.10. Eight-mm section. Anteriorly are shown the broad frontal sinuses (black) and much of the left orbital roof (white). On the right, the section passed slightly higher and only a small segment of the orbital roof is included with the frontal lobe. Centrally, the anterior clinoids, dorsum sellae, and lower suprasellar cistern are visible. Due to the slight head asymmetry or tilt, the left lesser wing of sphenoid is seen faintly in its medial portion, while the right wing is not visible. Posteriorly, the pontine cistern, large cerebellopontine angle cisterns, and the inferior portion of the fourth ventricle are visible. The difference in density of the cerebellar grey and white matter is inconspicuous. Note the transverse dark band extending across the density of the pons. This is a commonly recurring artifact, that is frequently more obtrusive than in this scan. This particular artifact occurs between the dense bone of the anterior portions of the petrous pyramids.

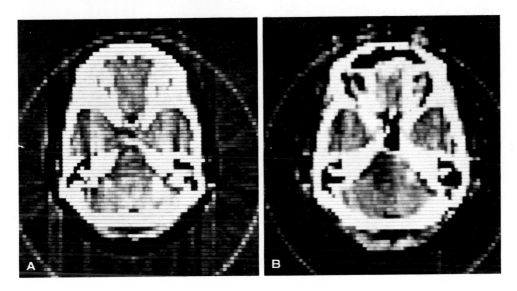

FIG. 5.11.
A. L 10   W 50.
Anteriorly, the section includes the orbital roofs laterally and the medial orbital and recti of the inferior medial portions of the frontal lobes centrally. The sphenoid wings, anterior clinoid processes, region of the diaphragma sellae, and uppermost portion of the dorsum sellae are included. Posteriorly, the pons and the lower cerebellum are included. The fourth ventricle is not visible. The vertical white and dark bands in each temporal area represent commonly occurring artifacts. Dark horizontal bands across the pons are also artifacts. There is a "stepped" appearance of the squamous occiput due to the shelving contour of the inferior portion of the occiput. The latter type of artifact is very pronounced in **B**.
B. Eight-mm section through large frontal sinuses, upper orbits, sphenoid wings, petrous pyramids, and lower cerebellum. The low density of air in the frontal sinus, sphenoid sinus (rectangular area in the center of the scan), and petromastoid air cells is shown as black, as is fat in the orbits. The vertical artifacts in the lateral regions (black) are not as pronounced as in **A**. The "stepped" appearance of the shelving contour of the inferior occipital squama is pronounced. The black zone in this region represents a large cisterna magna. The approximately 9 mm white area in the region of the right cerebellopontine angle represents partial inclusion of the upper segment of the jugular eminence in the scan section. The density of the bone in this region is averaged with overlying soft tissues so that its apparent absorption value is reduced to 50 in this section. This phenomenon (partial volume inclusion of bone, with downward averaging of density) must be differentiated from nodular lesions, such as tumors in the cerebellopontine angle. The low density in the left pons is probably artifactual: this type of asymmetry in pontine density is fairly common and may interfere with accurate diagnosis of pontine pathology.

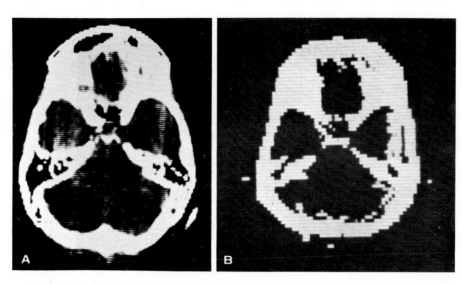

FIG. 5.12.   A. 160 x 160 matrix.   **B.** 80 x 80 matrix.

These sections, obtained in two different cases, are similar in orientation to those in the preceding figure.

A. Note the greatly improved bone detail, which shows the orbital roofs, inferior medial portion of the anterior fossa, including the inferior medial segments of the frontal lobes, lesser wings of sphenoid, anterior clinoids, limbus sphenoidale, dorsum sellae, and petroclinoid ligaments. A fringe of bone (dural ossification) at the posterior margin of the upper dorsum sellae is visible. A bone bar is shown extending between the left anterior and posterior clinoid processes. Some internal structure is visible in the petromastoid air cell complexes and the right internal auditory meatus is just recognizable. The prominence of the torcula is visible posteriorly. A high window level setting accentuates the display of bone and practically no details of brain are shown.

B. L 32   W M.

The rectangular steps of the 3-mm picture points of the 80 x 80 matrix interfere with recognition of bone details. The anterior clinoid processes and dorsum sellae are visible and an interclinoid bar is visible on the *left*. There is also some representation of the limbus sphenoidale and there is even a suggestion of the left internal auditory meatus. The latter is extremely rarely indicated on scans with the 80 x 80 matrix. The broad white vertical band in the lateral portion of the right middle fossa represents a characteristic artifact of this region. At this window level a small amount of cerebellar grey matter is still visible (*white*).

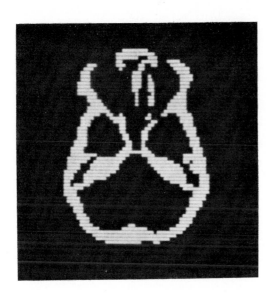

FIG. 5.13.
L 50   W M.
Section taken through the upper orbits, ethmoid sinuses, sphenoid sinus, and petrous pyramids. Viewer controls were set to display bone only (*white*), with all other tissues being invisible (*black*). The lateral and posterior walls of the sphenoid sinus are visible, but the anterior wall of this sinus and the lateral wall of the left ethmoid sinus are too thin and irregular to be displayed at this window level. (The right tegmen tympani of the petrous bone is also too thin to be visualized at this setting.) The densities of the walls were averaged with adjacent soft tissues and air. They became visible as the window level was reduced.

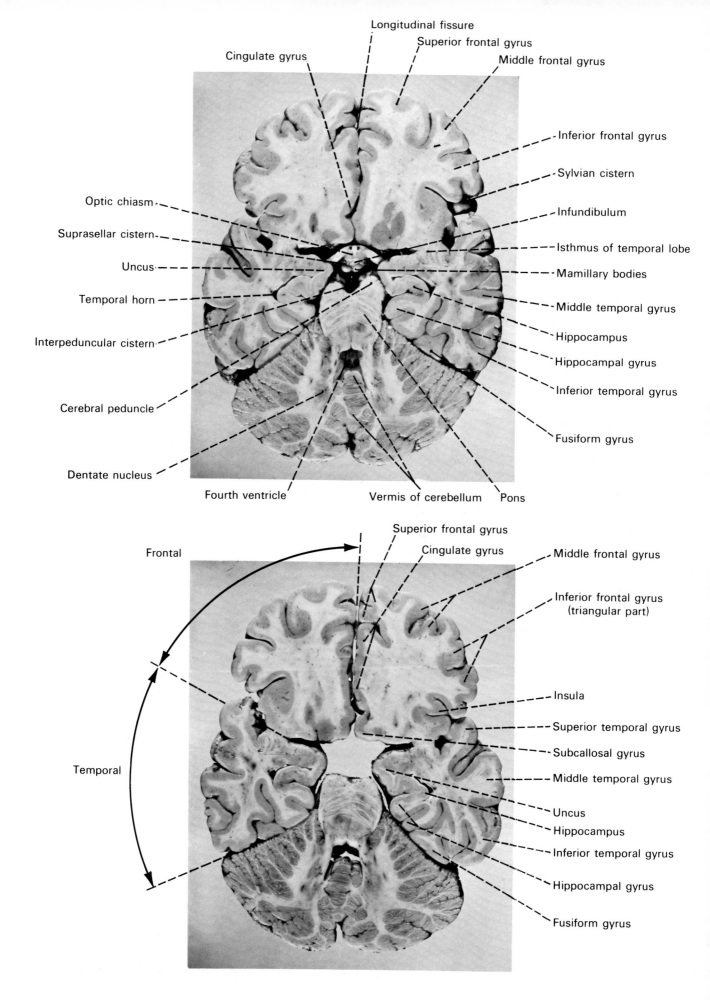

Longitudinal fissure
Cingulate gyrus
Superior frontal gyrus
Middle frontal gyrus
Inferior frontal gyrus
Sylvian cistern
Optic chiasm
Infundibulum
Suprasellar cistern
Isthmus of temporal lobe
Uncus
Mamillary bodies
Temporal horn
Middle temporal gyrus
Hippocampus
Interpeduncular cistern
Hippocampal gyrus
Inferior temporal gyrus
Cerebral peduncle
Fusiform gyrus
Dentate nucleus
Fourth ventricle
Vermis of cerebellum
Pons

Superior frontal gyrus
Cingulate gyrus
Middle frontal gyrus
Frontal
Inferior frontal gyrus
(triangular part)
Insula
Superior temporal gyrus
Subcallosal gyrus
Temporal
Middle temporal gyrus
Uncus
Hippocampus
Inferior temporal gyrus
Hippocampal gyrus
Fusiform gyrus

FIG. 5.14

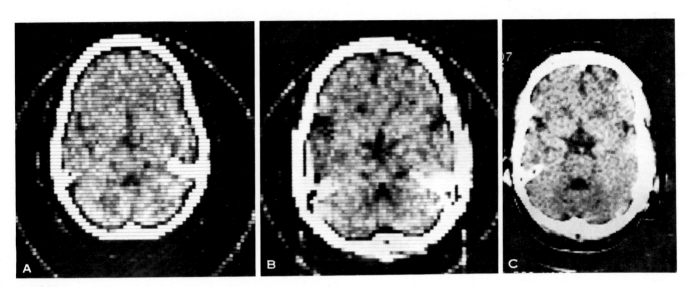

FIG. 5.15.
A. L 15   W 20.
This section corresponds well with the anatomical slice (Fig. 5.14) posteriorly but passes slightly higher than the latter anteriorly, where the upper part of the interpeduncular cistern and anterior third ventricle are visible. What is probably the posterior inferior portion of frontal longitudinal fissure appears to merge with the anterior third ventricle. The left sylvian cistern is visible, but not the right. More of the right petrous bone is included in the section than the left, indicating anatomical asymmetry of the petrous bones or slight upward tilting of the head. Review of sagittal skull films will allow differentiation. The anterior part of the longitudinal fissure is just visible. The left temporal horn is barely visible. The fourth ventricle is well shown and is probably in the region of the upper limit of normal in size. Small fourth ventricles are often difficult or impossible to identify. The lower density of cerebellar white matter is quite clearly differentiated from the higher density grey matter. Rarely, the dentate nuclei, being very slightly denser than the white matter, may be very incompletely and imperfectly differentiated.
B. L 15   W 20.
This section, which corresponds well with the anatomical slice (Fig. 5.14), was obtained in a patient who had modest cerebral atrophy. The interfrontal portion of the longitudinal fissure and the anterior portions of the sylvian fissures are enlarged. The suprasellar cisterns are generous in size. The appearance of the cerebellum and fourth ventricle is normal. Note that the posterosuperior recesses of the fourth ventricle can be distinguished, as can the median portion of a small cisterna magna.
C. L 15   W 30   160 x 160 matrix system.
Sections similar to those in **A** and **B**. The new system improves detail in the suprasellar cistern. Its pentagonal shape is well shown here, as are the ventral surface of the pons, basilar artery, and small paired densities in the anterior part of the cistern. The latter probably represent the anterior optic chiasm, although medially arching internal carotid arteries may be responsible.

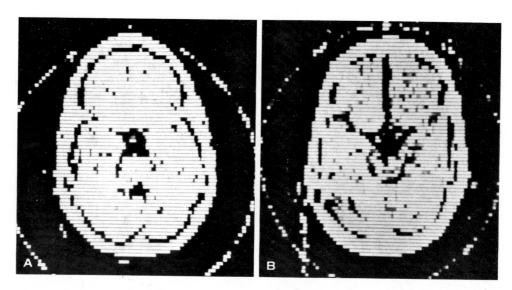

FIG. 5.16.

A. L 12   W M.

These viewer control settings generally provide the best discrimination of CSF-containing spaces (including as much as possible of their partial volume representations) from brain substance. Small zones in white matter tend to appear black also at the level setting of 12. Most of the black rim directly under the inner skull table represents a computer undershoot artifact rather than actual subarachnoid space, and much of the black rim remains black when window level settings are reduced to the −5 to −10 range. True CSF spaces occupying full section thickness will change from black to white at, or very close to, a window level setting of 0. The computer undershoot artifact involves a region only 1–2 picture points in width (3–6 mm on the 80 x 80 matrix; 1.5–3 mm on the 160 x 160 matrix). When the subarachnoid spaces are considerably widened, as in very severe cortical atrophy, they can be identified extending more than 2 matrix points internal to the inner table. The computer undershoot phenomenon interferes with evaluation of the narrow peripheral zone underneath the inner table, but this feature is much less obtrusive in the case of the new computer program and 160 x 160 matrix. The general configuration of the suprasellar cisterns is shown, with part of the connections with the sylvian cisterns anteriorly and with the ambient cisterns posteriorly. These connections are shown better in **B**. The 6-mm white zone in the center of the suprasellar cistern probably represents part of the optic chiasm and/or hypophyseal stalk. The fourth ventricle, including its superolateral recesses, is visible.

B. L 11   W 5.

The latitude of the display is slightly greater here than in **A** and therefore more black areas are visible in white matter, but the general effect is similar. The suprasellar cisterns are clearly visible, with their sylvian and ambient cisternal connections. The slightly higher level of this slice compared with that in **A** results in a more complete demonstration of the ambient cisterns. The bilateral, small (3–6 mm) white spots on either side of the suprasellar cistern are probably the internal carotid arteries in the "carotid cisterns". The carotid arteries (and the vertebral and basilar arteries) are far more likely to be recognized when calcified. Such structures and the optic chiasm are rarely identifiable with the 80 x 80 matrix, but are likely to be seen more frequently with the higher resolution system. Care must be taken to avoid mistaking a partial volume representation of the upper dorsum sellae for the optic chiasm by careful comparison with the subjacent scan section. The vertical black band in the median frontal region is partly artifact and partly representative of the longitudinal fissure.

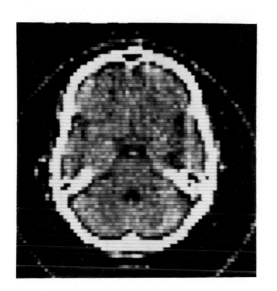

FIG. 5.17. This is an 8-mm section, showing somewhat enlarged sylvian cisterns, a probably normal interpeduncular cistern and a normal fourth ventricle. In the interpeduncular cistern, a dense 6-mm white spot just anterior to the brain stem may represent the basilar artery (containing calcification) in this 60-year-old male, who also appeared to have calcification in the left vertebral artery in a lower section. Computer undershoot is responsible for the narrow black zone immediately subjacent to the inner table and is seen well here in the posterior fossa. A similar phenomenon probably contributes to the narrow black zone immediately posterior to the petrous pyramids, but, in the latter regions, a narrow black zone is less constantly seen than around the external surfaces of the cerebrum and cerebellum. Nevertheless, the possible presence of such an artifact makes for difficulties in assessment of the subarachnoid spaces in the region of the cerebellopontine angle cisterns.

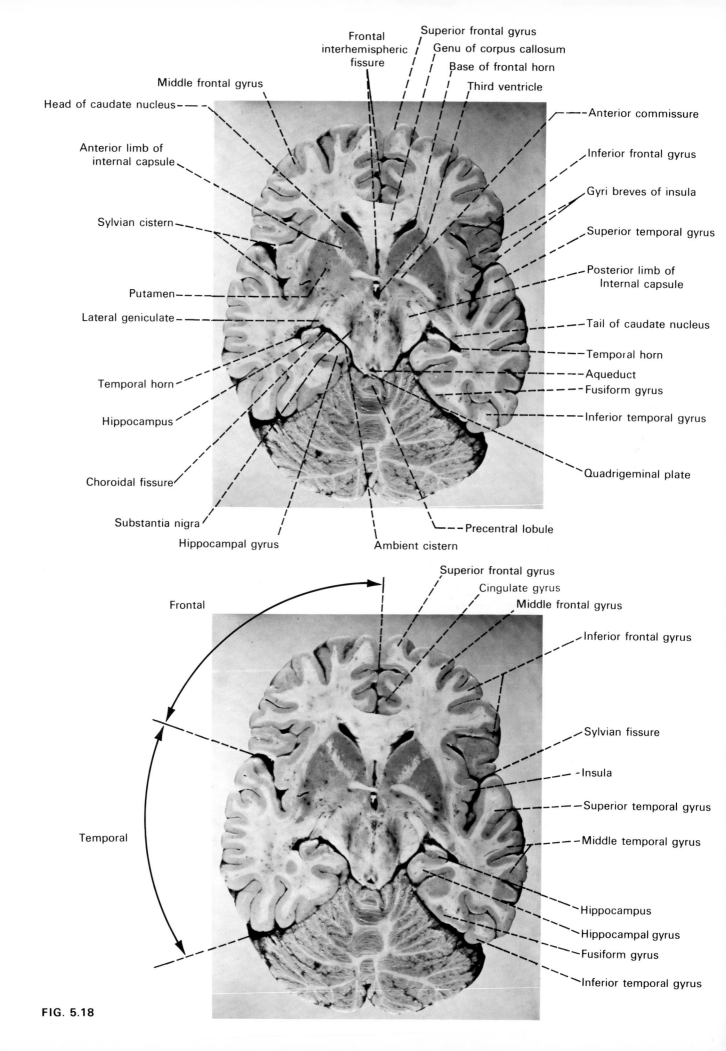

Middle frontal gyrus

Head of caudate nucleus

Anterior limb of internal capsule

Frontal interhemispheric fissure

Superior frontal gyrus

Genu of corpus callosum

Base of frontal horn

Third ventricle

Anterior commissure

Inferior frontal gyrus

Gyri breves of insula

Superior temporal gyrus

Sylvian cistern

Putamen

Lateral geniculate

Temporal horn

Hippocampus

Posterior limb of Internal capsule

Tail of caudate nucleus

Temporal horn

Aqueduct

Fusiform gyrus

Inferior temporal gyrus

Quadrigeminal plate

Choroidal fissure

Substantia nigra

Hippocampal gyrus

Ambient cistern

Precentral lobule

Frontal

Temporal

Superior frontal gyrus

Cingulate gyrus

Middle frontal gyrus

Inferior frontal gyrus

Sylvian fissure

Insula

Superior temporal gyrus

Middle temporal gyrus

Hippocampus

Hippocampal gyrus

Fusiform gyrus

Inferior temporal gyrus

FIG. 5.18

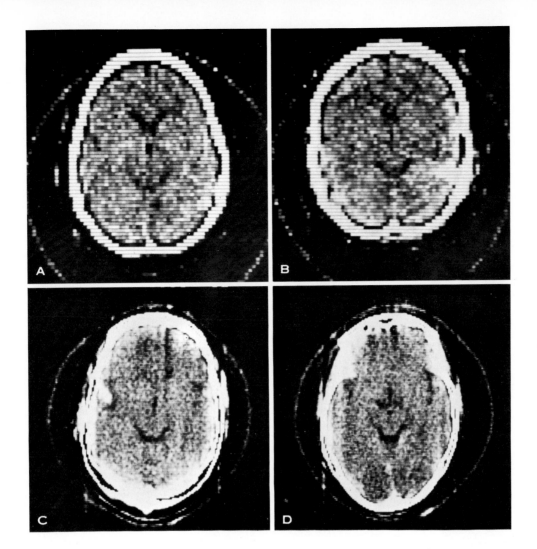

FIG. 5.19.
A. L 14 W 20. **B.** L 15 W 20.

These sections pass through the inferior portions of the frontal lobes, frontal horns, anterior portion of the third ventricle, and the quadrigeminal plate. A very slight change in scan angle can greatly alter visibility and apparent size of the inferior portions of normal-sized frontal horns by varying the amount of frontal lobe substance included with the frontal horns in the particular section. The normal anterior third ventricle, the axis of which is inclined to the scan plane, tends to be obscured by averaging with adjacent brain and/or the optic chiasm. (A scan obtained parallel to Reid's base line would favor the demonstration of the anterior third ventricle and the optic chiasm, compared with one angled at 25 or 30°. The use of 8-mm sections would also improve visibility of the anterior third ventricle and optic chiasm.) Slight changes in scan level will readily affect the view of the anterior third ventricle and optic chiasm and also the view of the midbrain and ambient cisterns. The latter structures are frequently demonstrated more completely (expecially in a single section) by scans parallel to Reid's base line or at small angles to the base line (Fig. 5.20). In **A**, the anterior third ventricle is approximately 2 picture points wide (6 mm) and in **B**, it is visible as a vertical black line 3 mm wide. Smaller frontal horns are difficult to see in scans at this level. A hint of the greater density of the head of the caudate nuclei and putamina relative to white matter is present, but this is generally better seen at the next superior scan level. The contours of the midbrain are visible posteriorly and laterally by virtue of the low density of the dorsal segments of the ambient cisterns and of the quadrigeminal cistern. The choroidal fissure is not commonly visible unless dilated. The normal aqueduct is not visible and becomes visible only rarely when markedly dilated. Owing to the presence of less dense and more regularly distributed bone, artifacts are less obvious and less frequent at this level and above than in more caudal sections. The lower absorption of the white matter of the frontal lobes in the areas adjacent to the frontal horns and anterior to the frontal horns compared with white matter elsewhere tends to be more obvious at this level and on the next superior section compared with more inferior scans. The temporal horns are rarely distinguishable on this or adjacent scan sections unless dilated, although hints of their presence may be obtained at times. Due to the angle of scan, the temporal horns are sectioned more coronally than axially.

C and **D.** 160 × 160 matrix.

C. Scan at approximately 15° to RBL, just including the inferior extremities of the frontal horns (barely visible). The third ventricle is visible centrally and the ambient and quadrigeminal cisterns allow the configuration of the quadrigeminal plate to be seen. The right and left colliculi can be identified. Even with this degree of resolution, the aqueduct is not discriminated. A scan at or near right angles to the aqueduct would minimize the partial volume effect and favor demonstration of a wide aqueduct.

D. The superior portion of the interpeduncular cistern, including its coronal extensions, is included with the posterior inferior portion of the third ventricle. The more caudal portions of the ambient cisterns are visible compared with **C**, and most of the outline of the midbrain is shown. Portions of the sylvian cisterns are visible in **C** and **D**.

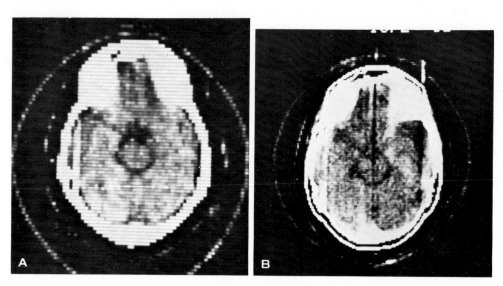

FIG. 5.20.
A. 80 × 80 matrix.   **B.** 160 × 160 matrix.
Both scans at approximately 10° to RBL. The shallower scan angle results in a complete demonstration of the ambient cisterns in the single section. The contour of the midbrain is shown well. The scan in **A** includes more of the interpeduncular cistern than that in **B**. The crural segments of this cistern are visible in both bases. The cisterns are enlarged in **A** (69-year-old female).

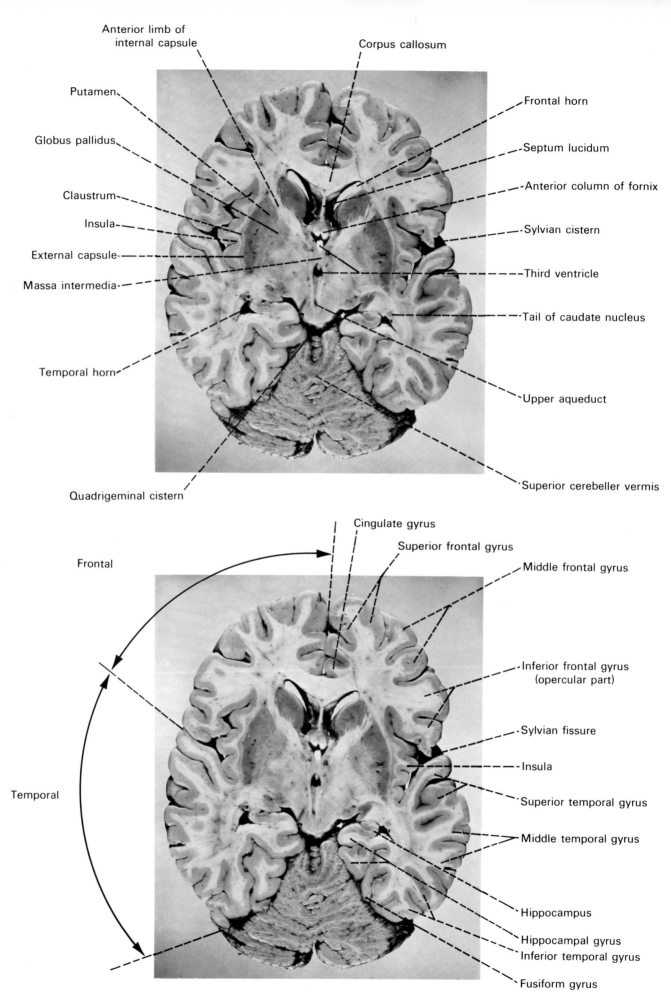

Anterior limb of internal capsule

Corpus callosum

Putamen

Globus pallidus

Claustrum

Insula

External capsule

Massa intermedia

Temporal horn

Quadrigeminal cistern

Frontal horn

Septum lucidum

Anterior column of fornix

Sylvian cistern

Third ventricle

Tail of caudate nucleus

Upper aqueduct

Superior cerebeller vermis

Cingulate gyrus

Superior frontal gyrus

Frontal

Middle frontal gyrus

Inferior frontal gyrus (opercular part)

Sylvian fissure

Insula

Temporal

Superior temporal gyrus

Middle temporal gyrus

Hippocampus

Hippocampal gyrus

Inferior temporal gyrus

Fusiform gyrus

FIG. 5.21

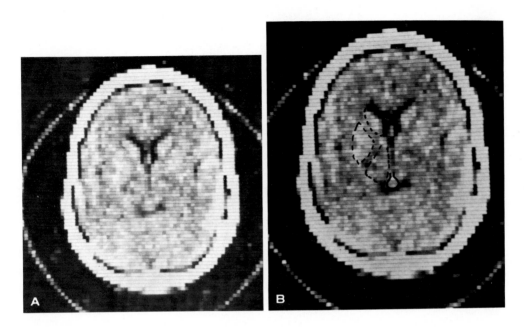

FIG. 5.22.
A. L   14   W   20.
At this level is represented the bulk of the frontal horns. The septum lucidum is regularly visible. Although narrower than a single matrix square, it occupies a full or nearly full section thickness, is dense enough to contrast well with the surrounding low density of CSF, and is seen as a whitish band one matrix square wide if the window level is not set too high. Just posterior to the septum lucidum, the broader and denser (whiter) anterior columns of the fornix are commonly seen. Immediately posterior to the fornix, the dark area of the third ventricle is visible, normally one or two squares wide on the 80 × 80 matrix. Angling posteromedially from the frontal horns to the third ventricle, the foramina of Monro are often seen, at least in part. A variable extent of the middle and posterior segments of the third ventricle is seen at this level, depending on the precise anatomical inclination of the ventricle, scan angle, and scan level. The massa intermedia can be seen occasionally. As with the septum lucidum and other smaller structures surrounded by CSF, the massa intermedia is best discriminated by the maximum contrast window setting M and a window level in the region of 12. Barely visible in this figure, the massa intermedia is clearly visible in Fig. 5.23C. Posteriorly, the inferior portion of noncalcified pineal is visible by contrast with adjacent cisternal CSF. Although generally less dense than cerebral cortex, the grey matter of the corpus striatum is commonly sufficiently denser than white matter to be identified in a general manner. The head of the caudate nucleus, putamen, and thalamus are generally in that order of decreasing density. Under favorable conditions, the internal capsule, having the density of white matter, can just be distinguished in whole or in part, with careful manipulation of the viewer controls. Most of the internal capsule is just distinguishable in this illustration.
B. This is a photographic copy of the original Polaroid shown in **A,** with the outlines of the left head of caudate nucleus, lenticular nucleus, and thalamus drawn in *interrupted lines*. The pineal is outlined by *continuous line*.

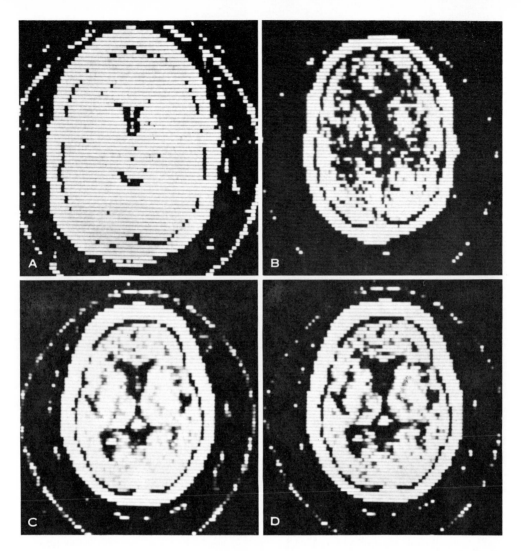

FIG. 5.23.

A. L   8   W M.

Although hardly visible on the routine display at L   13, W   20, the septum lucidum is clearly visible in this case with the maximum contrast provided by the M setting, at level 8.

B. L   17   W M.

A different case, in which the left internal capsule is quite well differentiated from the denser (white) putamen laterally and caudate nucleus anteromedially at these settings. Because of the lower density of portions of the left thalamus, the posterior limb of the internal capsule is not as well discriminated. As white matter generally lies in the absorption range 12–17 or 18, and the central grey matter lies in the very approximate range 15–22, the best discrimination of the two is to be expected at window levels 17 or 18. Cortical grey matter has an absorption range extending upwards from 17 or 18 (usually to 28–32 in adults and occasionally as high as 36–38). Thus, all of the cortex, including that of the insula, is shown as *white* in this illustration. For unknown reasons, the contours of the right internal capsule are much less clear in this scan. Appreciable asymmetry of apparent contours and densities of grey and white matter may be caused by even slight tilting of the head (canting). The density range of white matter appears the same in infants and young children as in young adults, but the density range of cerebral cortex in early life appears to be less and the density appears to be lower than in older individuals. In adults, the cortex in the anterior frontal region and in the occipital region frequently appears denser than elsewhere. These apparent differences in cortex at different ages have not yet been investigated fully. The differences in thickness and density of the skull at different ages and in different regions produce artifacts in computation of the absorption of cortex that may explain the observed variations (see Chapter 4, page 38).

C. L   13   W   10.

D. L   13   W   5.

In another case, the massa intermedia was clearly shown at these high contrast settings. The posterior limbs of both internal capsules and the anterior limb of the right internal capsule were visible at these settings but were better displayed at the higher contrast of W 5 shown in **D** (same scan as in **C**). The appearance of the foramina of Monro should be noted in **C** and **D**. The scan shown in these illustrations extended posteriorly at a higher level than is illustrated by the brain slice in Fig. 5.21 and included the retrothalamic cisterns, pineal, and left trigone. Somewhat enlarged sylvian cisterns are demonstrated.

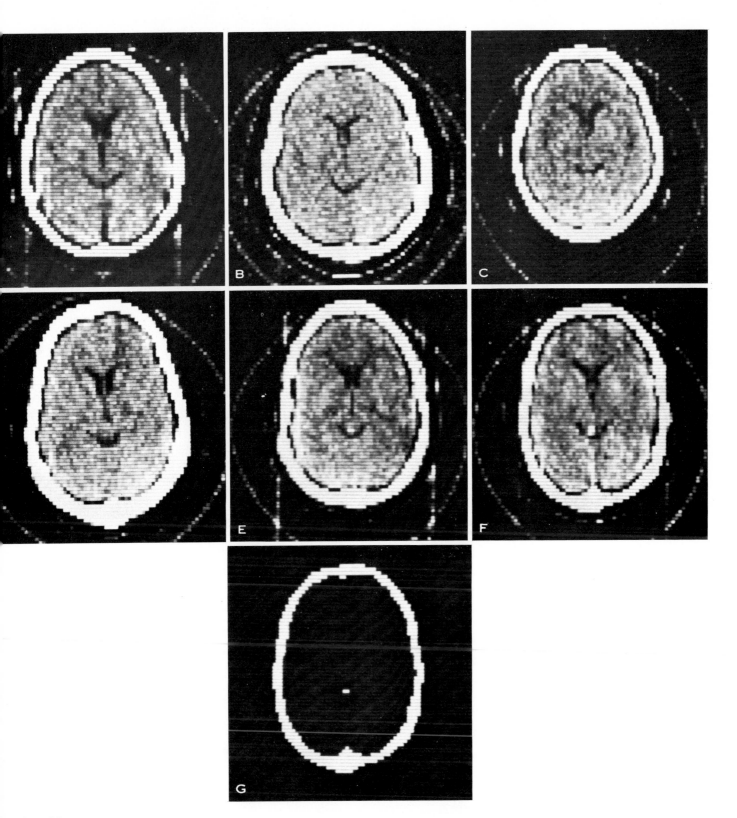

FIG. 5.24.

A–F. All scans photographed at W 20 and L 15 or 16. These scans of six different patients illustrate the individual variability in appearance of normal scans, due to minor individual anatomical differences and slight differences in scan angles and levels. Note that pineal calcification has been partially included in the section shown in **E** and more completely included in that shown in **F**. In **F**, the torcula and posterior portion of the straight sinus (and/or falx) are visible.

G. Same scan as **F**, but displayed at L 55 and W M. At this window level, only calvarial bone and pineal calcification are visible (*white*). Because some of the pineal calcification are was less densely aggregated, or as a result of averaging of the calcification with adjacent tissue and/or CSF, much of the calcification was recorded as having a lower absorption (down to 25), and, like all soft tissues in this slice, is shown as homogeneous black (compare apparent size of pineal calcification in F). The pineal calcification therefore appears smaller in **G** than in **F**, which was displayed at L 15.

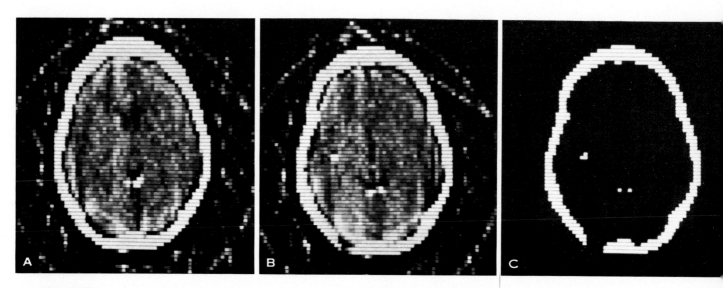

FIG. 5.25.
A. L 14   W 30.

Calcification (ossification) in the posterior tentorial margin. No calcification is evident in the pineal, but quite dense calcification or ossification is shown just behind the quadrigeminal cistern. **B.** This is the section immediately inferior to that shown in **A** and reveals calcification in the region of the left temporal horn, probably in the choroid plexus. This section also includes some of the tentorial ossification.

C. L 70   W M.

A different display of the section shown in **B**. The peak absorption value of the tentorial ossification was 70 (since it occupied only a portion of the scan section) and that in the tentorial horn showed a peak absorption value of 140 (calcification also occupying only a portion of the section). Note the craniotomy defect in the left occipital area.

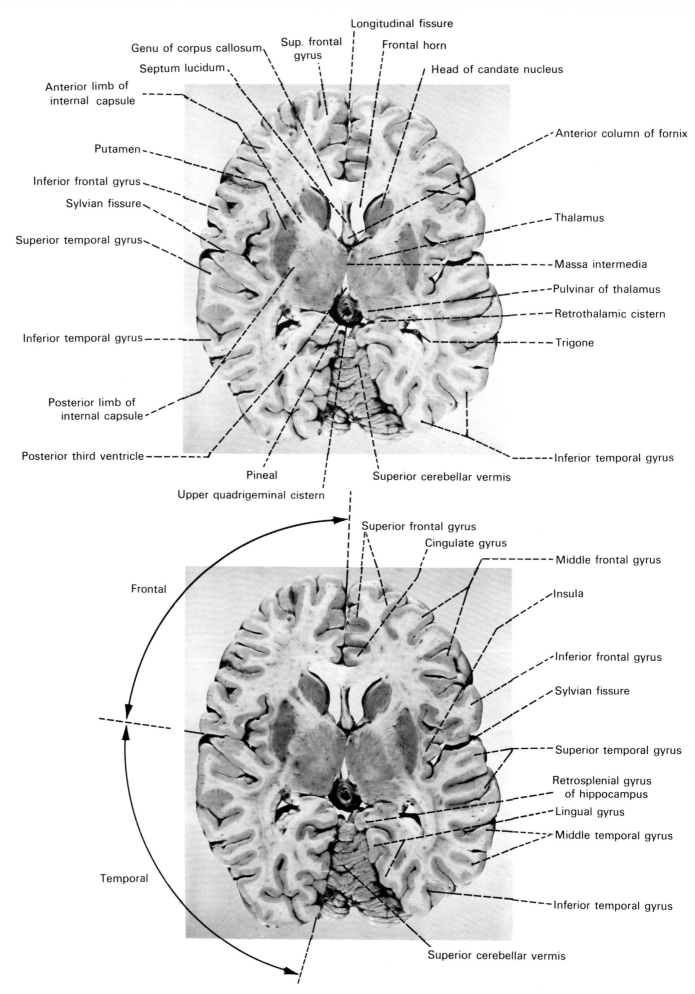

Genu of corpus callosum
Septum lucidum
Sup. frontal gyrus
Longitudinal fissure
Frontal horn
Head of candate nucleus

Anterior limb of internal capsule
Putamen
Inferior frontal gyrus
Sylvian fissure
Superior temporal gyrus

Anterior column of fornix
Thalamus
Massa intermedia
Pulvinar of thalamus
Retrothalamic cistern
Trigone

Inferior temporal gyrus

Posterior limb of internal capsule

Posterior third ventricle
Pineal
Upper quadrigeminal cistern
Superior cerebellar vermis
Inferior temporal gyrus

Frontal

Superior frontal gyrus
Cingulate gyrus
Middle frontal gyrus
Insula
Inferior frontal gyrus
Sylvian fissure

Superior temporal gyrus

Retrosplenial gyrus of hippocampus
Lingual gyrus
Middle temporal gyrus

Temporal

Inferior temporal gyrus

Superior cerebellar vermis

FIG. 5.26

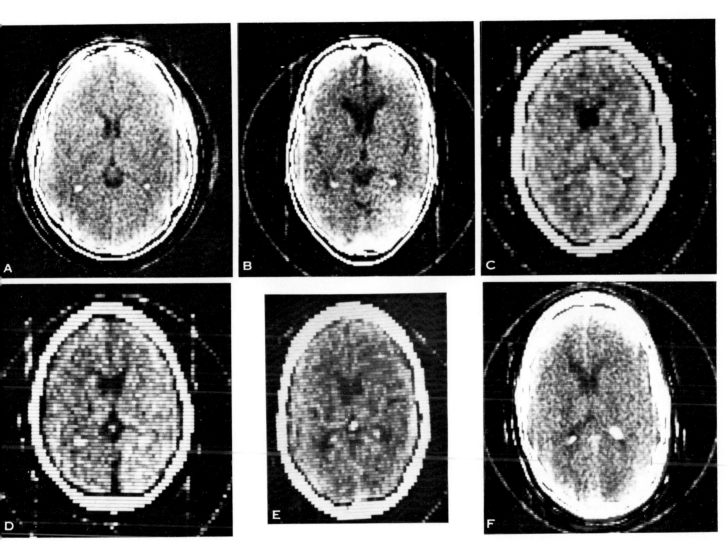

(Legend for FIG. 5.27 on page 86)

FIG. 5.27.

A. L 16   W 40   160 × 160 matrix.
Improved anatomical resolution compared with the 80 × 80 matrix (**C, D,** and **E**) is apparent. Picture points represent 1.5- × 1.5-mm squares of anatomy, rather than 3 × 3-mm (giving a four-fold increase in horizontal resolution), and the soft tissue display no longer has a geometrical appearance. "Steps" are still visible in the bone display, but bone edges are much smoother in appearance. Vertical "resolution" remains 13 (or 8) mm. Since the number of photons available for measuring and averaging absorption in each tissue block of 3 × 3 × 13 cubic mm remains the same as with the 80 × 80 matrix, and is therefore 1/4 the number available per computation compared with the 80 × 80 matrix, "noise" has somewhat increased. This accounts for a rather "wormy" appearance of the soft tissue display at lower window settings and the somewhat wider minimum window setting generally required for the "best" picture display on the CRT, as compared with the previous matrix (W 30 or 40 versus W 20 to 30). The alternating white and black vertical streaks in the right temporal area are typical artifacts secondary to air trapping over the scalp in the slightly concave frontotemporal area and have been pointed out in scans at lower cranial levels. In sections at this level, the frontal horns and septum lucidum are again visible. The posterior portion of the third ventricle tends to be seen more clearly than the midportion. The massa intermedia is sometimes identifiable. The noncalcified or calcified pineal is visible, contrasted with the adjacent CSF. In this scan, the pineal appears noncalcified. A flake of calcification (single matrix point, white spot) at the junction of the third ventricle and pineal probably represents calcification related to habenular commissure. The heads of the caudate nuclei can be distinguished, but there is only a hint of a minimally greater differential density of each putamen. The normal sylvian cisterns can just be detected on each side. They are often not visible or are barely detectable unless enlarged. The greater density of the cerebral cortex can be seen. Because of the irregular convolutional configuration of the cortex and the varying amounts of white matter within the gyri included with the cortex in the scan section, highly variable cortical density readings are obtained in different areas, and the inner cortical contours are generally not well defined. Artifacts secondary to the presence of dense overlying bone also cause some aberration in the apparent density of cerebral cortex and cerebellar grey matter. At this level, the scan section passes below the lateral ventricular bodies and through the thalami, reentering the lateral ventricles at the trigones. In the case of small lateral ventricles, the trigones may barely be detectable (especially if they are quite incompletely included in the section, as in this illustration and in **C** and **D**). However, calcification in the glomi of the choroid plexuses in the trigones is commonly obvious (**A–F**). Slight anatomical asymmetry or head tilting may cause a false appearance of asymmetry in size and density of glomus calcifications, and only one glomus may appear in the slice. Also of course, the glomi may be asymmetrically calcified (**F**). A portion of the frontal segment of the longitudinal fissure may be visible as in **A,** but this feature is often inconspicuous or invisible unless the fissure is widened as it is in **B**. The falx may be visible (**A** and **F**) anteriorly and/or posteriorly, and occasionally the vein of Galen and/or the anterior portion of the straight sinus (**F**) is visible. The lozenge-shaped light grey area between the glomus calcifications probably represents the vein of Galen in this scan. The falx and the larger vascular structures are seen more frequently and are denser in scans obtained after intravenous (or intra-arterial) injections of contrast medium. A small portion of the cerebellum is included at this scan level. The superior vermis is shown in **B,** contrasted with CSF in the upper portion of the quadrigeminal cistern anteriorly and part of the superior cerebellar cistern posteriorly (U-shaped dark region). The upper quadrigeminal cistern (retrothalamic cistern) outlines the pulvinar of each thalamus (**A, B,** and **D**).

B. 160 × 160 matrix.
This scan reveals slight enlargement of the frontal horns and probably minimal widening of the interfrontal portion of the longitudinal fissure. All these features would probably be considered to be within normal limits for an individual of 60 years of age or older.

C. The upper quadrigeminal and superior cerebellar cisterns are larger than average, although probably within normal anatomical limits.

C, D, and **E.** Representative scans on 80 × 80 matrix.

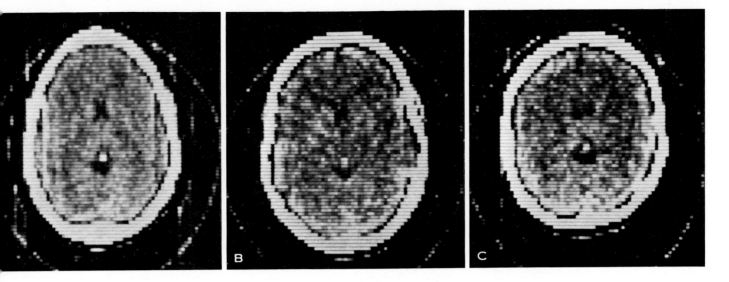

FIG. 5.28.

A–C. The normal frontal horns in these three young patients (14-year-old-male, 32-year-old-male, and 23-year-old-female, respectively) appear smaller than they actually are, due to the partial volume effect. This effect results in upward averaging of the absorption values of the small lateral portions of the frontal horns with those of surrounding brain substance (corpus callosum above and caudate nuclei below). This results in loss of discrimination of the upper lateral portions of the frontal horns, and the apparent total transverse ventricular span at the coronal plane of the foramina of Monro appears to be only 12 mm (4 matrix squares × 3 mm per square) in this scan. The third ventricle is very narrow and is barely detectable in **A** and **B**. It is not discriminated in **C**, probably because it is even narrower than usual. The measured absorption of pineal calcification is highly variable, due to variable density of aggregation, variable size of the area calcified, and varying degrees of inclusion of the pineal calcification in the section. Measured absorption of this calcification commonly ranges between 25 and 80 units rather than in the hundreds of units.

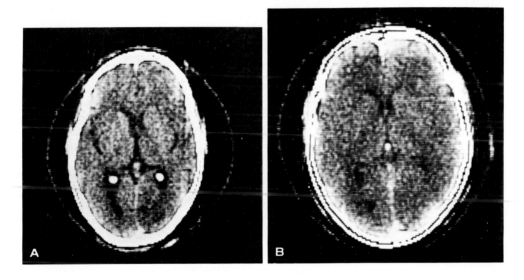

FIG. 5.29.

A. L 14   W 30   160 × 160 matrix.

This scan section of a 61-year-old female reveals a normal appearance of the frontal horns, a generous width of the third ventricle, and an appearance of slight enlargement of the trigones. The retrothalamic cisterns are well demonstrated bilaterally. On the left side, there is a large occipital horn. The sylvian cisterns are slightly widened and there was a little widening of a number of cerebral sulci at higher scan levels. The scan was obtained following intravenous injection of Conray 60. Just posterior to the third ventricle and density of the pineal is an area less dense and smaller than the pineal that is also surrounded by the darker zone of CSF in the quadrigeminal cistern. This density represents the great vein of Galen. A narrow, light grey, vertically oriented band extends posteriorly, with gentle curving to the right in the region of the torcula. This density represents the straight sinus, although the falx may contribute to the density.

B. L 16   W 40   160 × 160 matrix.

This scan, in another case, was also obtained following intravenous injection of Conray 60. The medium light grey, vertically oriented band extending from the posterior part of the upper quadrigeminal cistern and inclining very slightly to the right as it approaches the torcular region appears to represent the great vein of Galen and the straight sinus. The internal frontal crest is visible in both **A** and **B**. The frontal horns and narrow third ventricle are normal in appearance. The small trigones are faintly represented as slightly darker areas on each side, with faintly visible choroid plexus glomi. The sylvian cisterns are not visible in this scan.

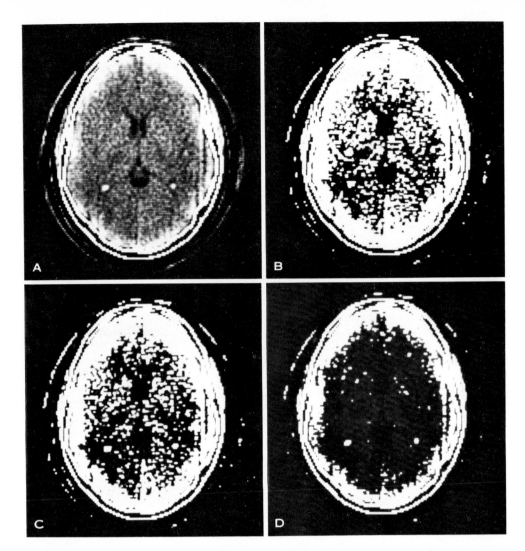

FIG. 5.30. A–D.   A series of photographs of the same scan with different viewer control settings.
A. L   18   W   30.
There is visible differential absorption of cerebral cortex and white matter. The corpus striatum is partially and faintly discriminated at these control settings. Alternating vertical light and dark bands in the lateral temporal region on the right side of the scan represent common artifactual aberrations in absorption calculations.
B. L   16   W   M.
These control settings provided the most complete demonstration of the corpus striatum in this scan. The right head of caudate nucleus is partly separated from the putamen by an incomplete visualization of the lower density anterior limb of the internal capsule. There is better separation of the densities of the right putamen and thalamus by the posterior limb of the internal capsule. The components of the left corpus striatum are less well differentiated. Such an asymmetry in discrimination of the elements of the corpus striatum is a common normal finding. Much of the cerebral white matter appears black at this window level and, of course, ventricular CSF is also shown black at this level setting.
C. L   18   W   M.
Raising the level setting 2 units reveals the maximum amount of white matter as black, while providing the best discrimination between white matter, cerebral cortex, and central grey matter in this typical normal case. In other normal cases, and at other levels of scan, the level of best discrimination of grey and white matter may be at slightly higher or lower window level settings.
D. L   22   W   M.
These settings provide a clear differentiation of the higher density cortex (*white*) and the lower absorption level white matter (*black*). However, some of the cortical densities exhibited at lower window level settings have become black. These areas were less dense, due to the downward averaging effect on the inner portions of the cortical convolutions caused by white matter contained in the scanned volumes. The central grey matter, being intermediate in absorption levels between white matter and cerebral cortex, is shown as progressively decreasing white areas as the window level is raised from 18 to 22. Only a few small scattered areas in the caudate nuclei and putamina remain white at L   22. These remaining white zones in the central grey matter dropped out (changed to black) between levels 22 and 23, indicating peak absorption values in the central grey matter of 22 in this case. Other small scattered white areas between the peripheral cortical zone and central grey matter probably represent portions of the inner cortical convolutions at the depths of the sulci where there is irregular and highly variable averaging with different amounts of white matter in the scanned volumes. Larger arteries and veins probably contribute. Occasional computational errors due to program imperfections and statistical fluctuations may also contribute. The vertical artifacts in the right lateral temporal region are still partly visible. The glomus calcifications stand out clearly at this window level.

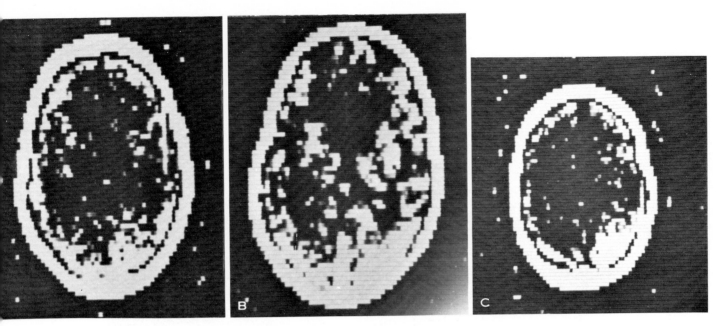

FIG. 5.31.   CORTICAL AND CENTRAL GREY MATTER REPRESENTATIONS

A. L   21   W   M.

Section from a normal CT scan of a 19-year-old female, obtained without intravenous contrast medium injection (plain scan). These window settings provide high contrast between the denser cerebral cortex (*white*) and white matter (*black*). Some areas in the putamina are of higher density than 21 and are still shown white. In addition, small areas of insular cortex are visible on each side and pineal calcification is visible centrally. The vertical white band in the lateral right temporal region represents common artifact. The asymmetrical configuration and extent of grey matter in the occipital regions is a frequently noted normal feature, believed to represent slight asymmetry of anatomy or positioning. The greater extent of the occipital cortical density on the right side probably represents scanning through the cortex of the inferior surface of the occipital lobe. Superior cerebellar grey matter may be included. This feature is quite commonly seen in normal scans. When asymmetrical, as in this scan, the reason is probably that the occipital portion of the scan was slightly lower on the side of the most extensive cortical representation (see **C**). As the window level is raised gradually from 18, the inner portions of the cortical convolutions drop out (change from black to white) earlier than do the more superficial portions of the cortex, due to the downward averaging of cortical values in the inner portions of the convolutions resulting from included adjacent white matter in these convolutions. Similarly, as the window level is gradually raised, the central grey matter, being less dense than cerebral cortex, changes from white to black at lower levels than does most of the peripheral portion of the cerebral cortex. The level at which all of the central grey matter changes from white to black indicates the peak absorption values in these structures.

B. L   22   W   M.

Scan obtained in an 84-year-old male with severe atherosclerosis, and following intravenous injection of 45 ml of Hypaque 60 M. It has been observed that the absorption values of cerebral cortex increased by several units following intravenous contrast injection, compared with the values obtained on a preceding plain CT scan. Some increase in absorption values of central grey matter has also been observed, generally a lesser increase than is observed in the cerebral cortex. No increase in absorption has been identified thus far in white matter following intravenous (or interarterial) contrast injection up to volumes of 50 ml of contrast medium. Density of the central grey matter was increased following intravenous contrast injection in the case illustrated here. The density of the thalami (generally less dense than the caudate nuclei and putamina in plain scans) is shown exceptionally clearly in this scan with contrast enhancement. The lateral ventricles were moderately enlarged in this patient. The gaps in cortical representation in both frontal regions were caused by pathological changes, thought to represent encephalomalacia resulting from ischemia. Increasing the density of the central grey matter by contrast medium injection has the effect of providing clearer discrimination of the internal capsule. In older patients, the density of the basal ganglia is not infrequently greater than in younger individuals, no doubt as a result of the known frequently occurring increase in deposition of calcium and iron in these structures.

C. L   20   W   M.

Plain CT scan section. Striking asymmetry in the extent of cortical density is shown in the parietal and occipital regions. The great extent of the cortical density on the right side is believed to be due to the scan section passing through the inferior cortical surface of this cerebral hemisphere. On the left side, the scan section has evidently passed through the parietal and occipital lobes at a slightly higher level so that the inferior cortex is not included. This effect is believed to be due to slight anatomical asymmetries in the cerebral hemispheres or to slight canting of the head (i.e., right parieto-occipital region slightly higher than on the left side in this scan).

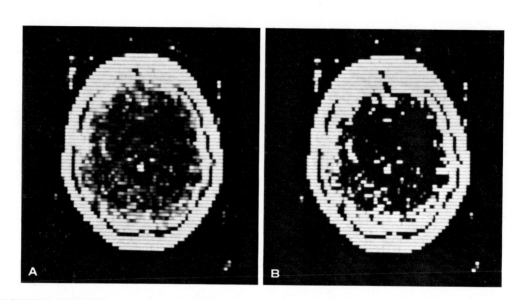

FIG. 5.32. INSULAR CORTEX. A. and **B.** While small portions of the cortex of the insula are commonly seen, rarely is it possible to identify the insula clearly. This is probably the result of downward averaging of the absorption values of insular cortex with the low absorption of adjacent CSF in the sylvian cisterns and with the intermediate absorption of adjacent white matter.
A. L 21 W 10.
At these settings, the pineal calcification and cerebral cortex are displayed as white or very light grey. Tissues having absorption values ranging from 16 (21 − ¹⁰⁄₂) to 26 (21 + ¹⁰⁄₂) are displayed in this window and so some of the denser areas of white matter are shown as grey rather than black. Normal white matter absorption range is 12 to 17 or 18. The cortex of the insula is shown as a grey-white curved strip on the left side. Rarely is the insula as clearly shown as on the left side in this scan. It is not known if this represents a pathological change in this individual.
B. L 21 W M.
The maximum contrast of the M window setting permits maximum differentiation between cortex and white matter in this case, and the left insula stands out very clearly on the left side. The cortical density of the medial portions of the superior frontal gyri are shown and partial representation of the cortex of the medial surface of the left occipital lobe in the region of the retrosplenial and lingual gyri is depicted. An asymmetrical appearance of cerebral cortex may be marked in individual cases (as here) and may be due to anatomical cerebral asymmetry or head tilting. Slight variations in symmetry of planes on the two sides can result in markedly different cortical configurations in anatomical brain sections and in CT scans.

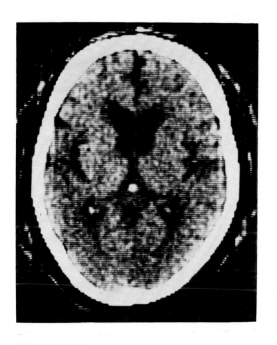

FIG. 5.33. 160 × 160 matrix. An example of cerebral atrophy. There is moderate widening of the sylvian cisterns and of the frontal horns bilaterally. The third ventricle and the trigones are slightly enlarged. Upper quadrigeminal, retro-thalamic, and superior cerebellar cisterns are continuous, and they appear to merge with third ventricle from which there is only a membranous separation. In addition, widening of the interfrontal portion of the longitudinal fissure and of several sulci is evident, including the cingulate sulci, the sulcus of the left superior frontal gyrus, the sulci between the right and left superior and middle frontal gyri, and the sulci between the right and left middle and inferior frontal gyri. In addition to the sylvian cisterns, portions of the widened sylvian fissures are demonstrated. Although visible, the septum lucidum is demonstrated poorly on this photograph. It was clearly visible at lower window level settings, but, at lower settings, the cisterns and sulci were depicted less well.

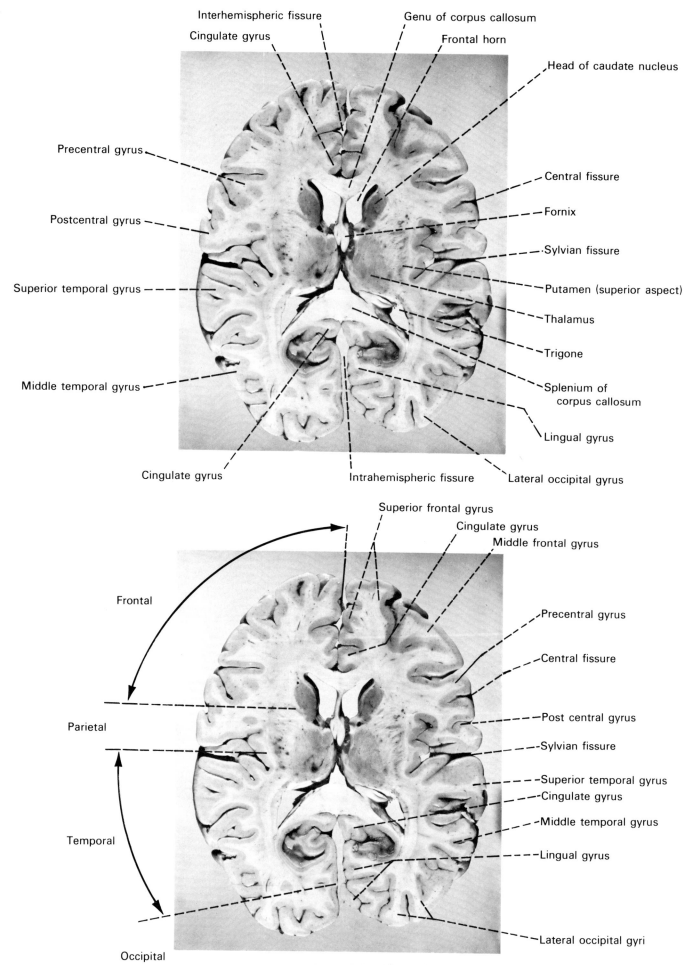

Interhemispheric fissure

Cingulate gyrus

Genu of corpus callosum

Frontal horn

Head of caudate nucleus

Precentral gyrus

Postcentral gyrus

Superior temporal gyrus

Middle temporal gyrus

Central fissure

Fornix

Sylvian fissure

Putamen (superior aspect)

Thalamus

Trigone

Splenium of corpus callosum

Lingual gyrus

Cingulate gyrus

Intrahemispheric fissure

Lateral occipital gyrus

Superior frontal gyrus

Cingulate gyrus

Middle frontal gyrus

Frontal

Precentral gyrus

Central fissure

Parietal

Post central gyrus

Sylvian fissure

Superior temporal gyrus

Cingulate gyrus

Temporal

Middle temporal gyrus

Lingual gyrus

Occipital

Lateral occipital gyri

FIG. 5.34

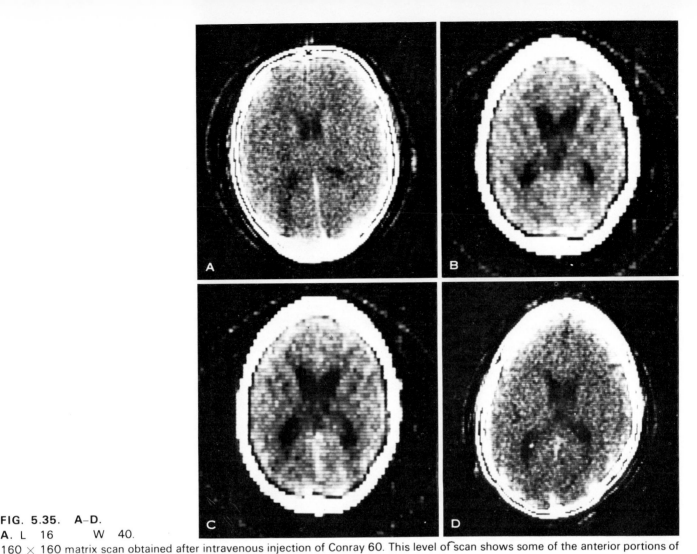

FIG. 5.35. A–D.
A. L 16   W 40.

160 × 160 matrix scan obtained after intravenous injection of Conray 60. This level of scan shows some of the anterior portions of the bodies of the lateral ventricles but may still include no recognizable portion of the posterior segments of the bodies of these ventricles. If the section includes superiorly only a narrow segment of the lower portions of these segments of the lateral ventricles, averaging of the CSF values and those of the subjacent thalami will tend to render the ventricles inconspicuous or unrecognizable in this region. It should be noted that the result of such averaging will cause lower than correct absorption values in the upper thalamic regions. As the ventricular bodies are traced posteriorly from the frontal horns, the apparent density gradually increases as progressively less of the ventricles are included in the section. Thus, the lateral ventricles appear to "fade away" posteriorly. Very slight angular and/or level changes in the scan plane and slight differences in individual curvature of the ventricular floor will produce variations in the appearance of the thalamic and posterior ventricular body regions. As more of the ventricular bodies are included in the section, the absorption level of these regions decreases, the lateral boundaries of the bodies of the ventricles become more visible, and segments of the choroid plexuses may be shown. A thalamic "hump" appearance may occur as the density of the ventricular bodies is locally increased by the intrusion of the superior convexities of the thalami (**B, C,** and **D**). In the latter scans, the choroid plexuses can just be distinguished as arching bands about 6 mm wide, in addition to the more diffuse thalamic densities. The noncalcified segments of the choroid plexuses can be differentiated from surrounding CSF and adjacent brain in many plain CT scans but tend to be recognizably denser following injection of contrast medium intravenously or intra-arterially (Fig. 5.41). The same is true of the falx cerebri, the tentorium, and occasionally the falx cerebelli. The vertical dimensions of the falx cause this structure generally to occupy full scan sections. However, while denser than the noncalcified choroid plexus, the falx is usually surrounded by such narrow and irregular subarachnoid spaces that it tends to be obscured by immediately adjacent high-density cerebral cortex. It is markedly increased in density by intravascular contrast medium injection (an effect that is frequently visible at angiography, on the far less sensitive recording medium of radiographic film).

B. L 16   W 20   80 × 80 matrix.

Plain CT scan. Irregular areas of greater density representing the upper portions of the thalami and choroid plexuses encroach upon the partially included bodies of the lateral ventricles. The lateral ventricles are slightly enlarged.

C. L 16   W 20   80 × 80 matrix.

Scan following intravenous injection of 50 ml of Hypaque 60 M. Scan from the same patient as in **B**, at a closely similar, although not identical, plane of section. Following intravenous injection of Hypaque, there has been no definite change in density of the choroid plexuses, but the vein of Galen and the anterior two-thirds of the straight sinus are now visible. The difference in *precise* duplication of scan angle and level prior to and after injection of contrast medium makes for significant uncertainties in evaluating such changes in scan appearance.

D. L 16   W 40   160 × 160 matrix.

Scan following intravenous injection of Conray 60. A scan of a different patient. The lozenge-shaped area of considerable density between the trigones represents the vein of Galen. The choroid plexuses are visible, arching over the floors of the lateral ventricular bodies from the trigones. A small spot of calcification is visible in the glomus of the left choroid plexus.

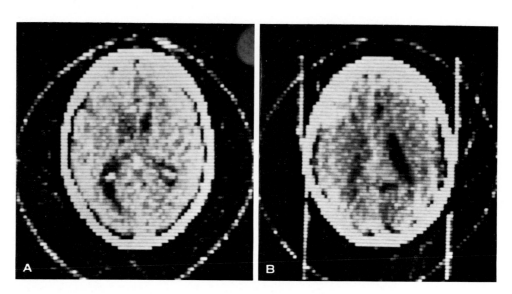

FIG. 5.36.
A. L 12   W 20.
There is inclusion of the lower portions of the lateral ventricular bodies in the section. Densities included in these regions represent the superior portions of the thalami and the choroid plexuses. As the right side of the head is tilted up slightly compared with the left, there is inclusion of more of the thalamus on the right side. Normal anatomical asymmetry can produce such appearances, which should not be mistaken for intraventricular masses or extensions of masses into the ventricle from the side or from below. The tilt of the head was identified by the appearance of lower and higher scan sections (see below).
B. L 12   W 20.
This is the next scan section superior to that shown in **A.** Upward tilt of the head on the right results in more complete inclusion of the right lateral ventricle than of the left in this section. This leads to a false appearance of asymmetry in the ventricular size. Review of plain skull film examination is necessary to differentiate between developmental asymmetries of the skull and brain in a vertical direction from a canted positioning of the patient's head during CT scanning. As the lateral ventricles become larger with disease, such apparent asymmetries and simulations of encroaching masses are less likely to be troublesome with given degrees of head canting or anatomical asymmetry.

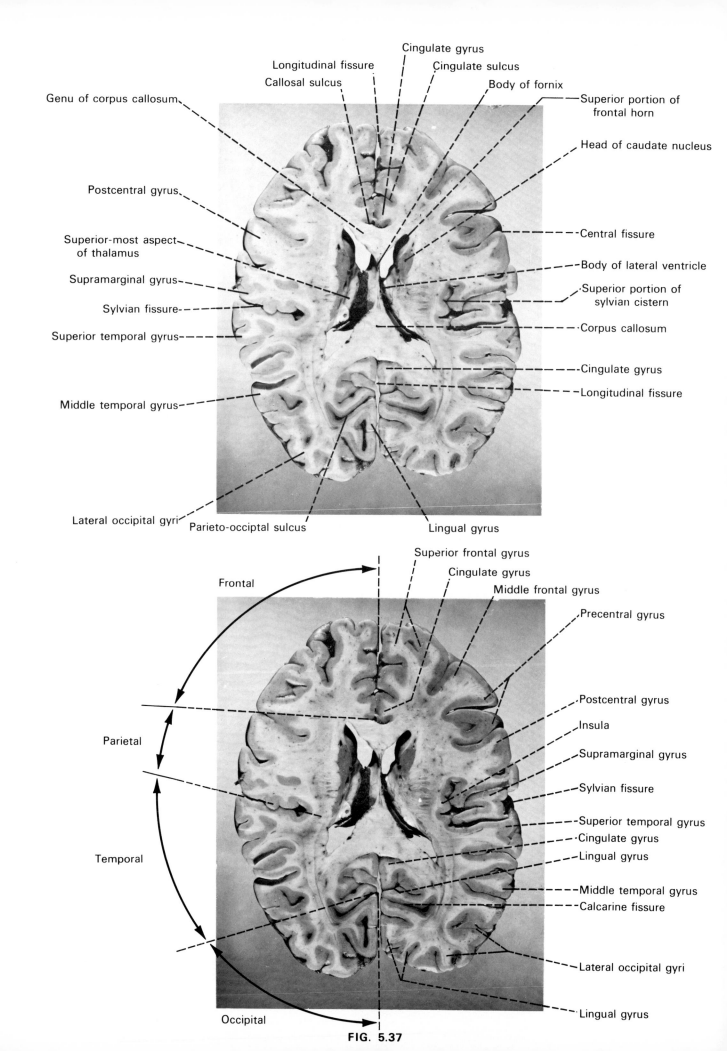

Longitudinal fissure
Cingulate gyrus
Callosal sulcus
Cingulate sulcus
Body of fornix

Genu of corpus callosum

Superior portion of frontal horn

Head of caudate nucleus

Postcentral gyrus

Superior-most aspect of thalamus

Central fissure

Body of lateral ventricle

Supramarginal gyrus

Superior portion of sylvian cistern

Sylvian fissure

Corpus callosum

Superior temporal gyrus

Cingulate gyrus

Longitudinal fissure

Middle temporal gyrus

Lateral occipital gyri
Parieto-occiptal sulcus
Lingual gyrus

Superior frontal gyrus
Cingulate gyrus
Middle frontal gyrus

Frontal

Precentral gyrus

Parietal

Postcentral gyrus

Insula

Supramarginal gyrus

Temporal

Sylvian fissure

Superior temporal gyrus

Cingulate gyrus

Lingual gyrus

Middle temporal gyrus

Calcarine fissure

Lateral occipital gyri

Occipital

Lingual gyrus

FIG. 5.37

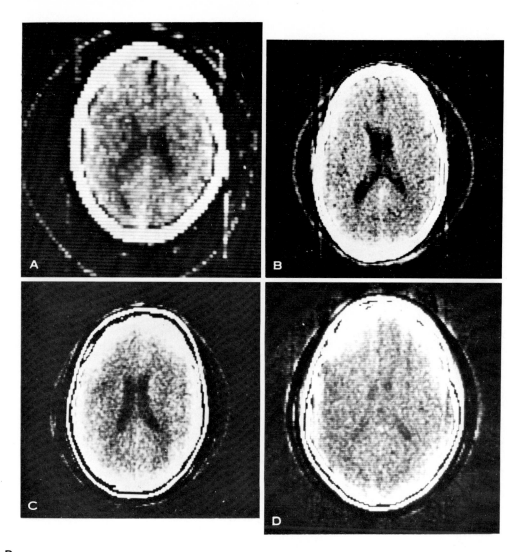

FIG. 5.38. A–D.
A. L   19   W   20.   **B.** L   14   W   30   160 x 160 matrix.
C. L   14   W   30   160 x 160 matrix.   **D.** L   14   W   40   160 x 160 matrix.
At this level of section, the bodies of the lateral ventricles are seen most completely. Frequently, the occipital horns are visible, especially if they are larger than usual. A long narrow occipital horn is visible on the left in **A**. The plane includes the upper portions of the trigones. The body of the fornix is visible between the ventricular bodies. Depending on the precise angle and level of the scan, part of the septum lucidum may be visible anteriorly, as in **C**. The anterior and posterior portions of the corpus callosum are sectioned. The plane includes little or no putamen, but the superior portion of the caudate nucleus is included and appears to be visible as a narrow whitish zone adjacent to and paralleling the lateral walls of the anterior portions of the bodies of the lateral ventricles in **B** and **C**. Narrow dense zones at the lateral ventricular margins are produced by intravenous contrast medium injection, when the subependymal convergence of veins of white matter seems to be responsible. The upper convexities of the thalami may be visible, jutting into the ventricular bodies posteriorly (thalamic "humps"), as in **B,** and the choroid plexuses contribute to these densities, even if they are not separately distinguishable. A high-thrusting great vein of Galen may be included in the section and may be represented by the small whitish area in the midline between the trigones in **B**. Very little or nothing is seen of the uppermost sylvian cisterns, unless they are greatly enlarged.

D. In the case of small lateral ventricles (as in children and young adults) and especially when the lateral ventricles are reduced in size by diffuse cerebral swelling, as may be seen in benign intracranial hypertension, it may be difficult to recognize their contours. Difficulty in recognition of the lateral ventricles will be most likely if the scan section also includes them incompletely. High contrast of the M setting of window width can increase discrimination usefully under these circumstances.

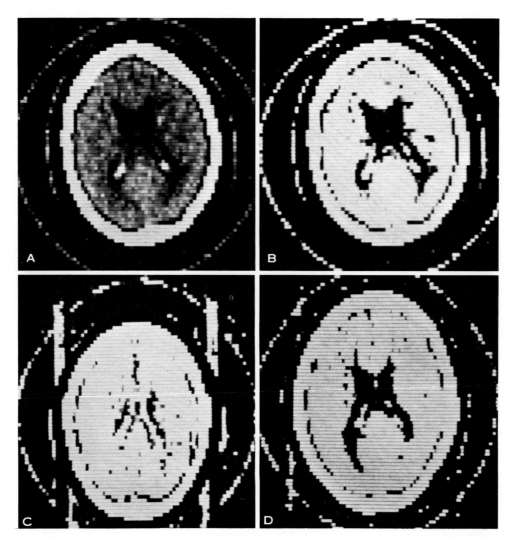

FIG. 5.39. A–D. A series of scans showing the choroid plexuses of the lateral ventricles. The noncalcified extensions of the choroid plexuses into the bodies of the lateral ventricles tend to be more frequently and more clearly visible when the lateral ventricles are a little enlarged than when normal or smaller than normal in size.
A. L 20   W 20.
The lateral ventricles are modestly enlarged in this scan of a 64-year-old female. The calcifications in the glomi are quite large. Extending anteriorly and slightly medially from these calcifications, the noncalcified portions of the choroid plexuses are visible.
B. L 12   W M.
This is the same scan as is represented in **A**. These viewer control settings provide maximum contrast of the ventricular cavities and of the choroid plexuses.
C. L 11   W M.
The choroid plexuses of the lateral ventricles are seen more extensively than usual in this example and are also wider than usual. A very slightly widened interfrontal segment of the longitudinal fissure is visible.
D. L 11   W M.
Scan of a patient who had evidence of mild cerebral atrophy. The choroid plexuses are visible, with more complete demonstration on the left side. A prominent left occipital horn is shown.

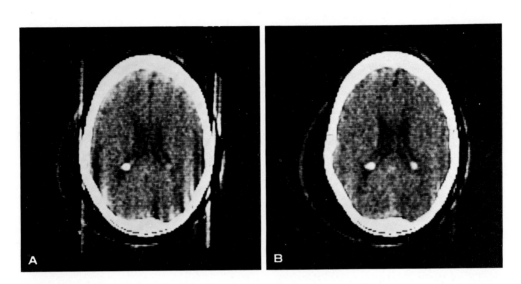

FIG. 5.40. A and **B.**   160 x 160 matrix.

A. Plain CT scan. Bilateral glomus calcifications are visible. That on the left is much denser than on the right, owing to slight anatomical asymmetry or head tilting, which resulted in incomplete inclusion of the right glomus calcification in the scan section. A falsely low absorption level was therefore calculated for right glomus. The soft tissue portions of the choroid plexuses are shown extending anteromedially into the posterior portions of the bodies of the lateral ventricles. There was a little movement of the head from side to side during the period of the scan, resulting in the white vertical bands in the region of the waterbath and causing alternating white and dark vertical bands within the cranium. These movement artifacts are more striking on the right side in this case.

B. Same patient as illustrated in **A,** but scanned following intravenous injection of Conray 60. A slight difference in scan level is present, indicated by the greater calculated absorption of the right glomus calcification, which has been more completely included in this scan section than in **A.** Viewer control settings are the same as in **A.** There was barely appreciable motion during this scan. There appears to be a slight increase in density of the noncalcified portions of the choroid plexuses compared with **A.** However, the slight change in scan level makes evaluation unreliable. This underscores the difficulty in obtaining precise comparative measurements on different scans in the same patient.

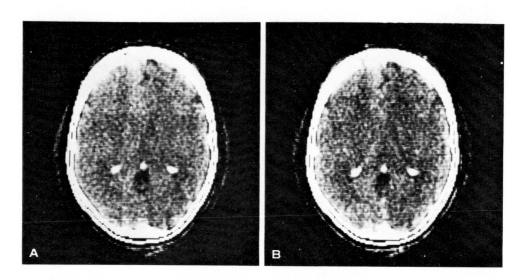

FIG. 5.41. A and **B.** 160 x 160 matrix. Same viewer control settings in each scan.
A. Plain CT scan. Bilateral glomus calcifications are shown, in addition to pineal calcification. Virtually nothing is visible of the noncalcified segments of the choroid plexuses and the small lateral ventricles are quite incompletely discriminated.
B. Same patient. Scan repeated following intravenous injection of Conray 60. The scan angle and plane appear to be practically identical to those in the scan in **A.** The noncalcified portions of the choroid plexus in each ventricle are now distinctly visible, passing anteromedially through the ventricles from the trigones. There is reason to believe that the noncalcified portions of the choroid plexuses have been increased in density as a result of circulation through them of blood that has been rendered more dense as a result of the injection of contrast medium. More recent use of high-dose contrast enhancement confirms that increased choroid plexus density is produced.

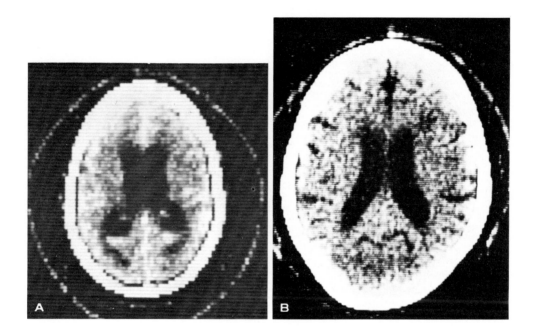

FIG. 5.42.
A. L 19   W 20.
Scan of a patient with communicating obstructive hydrocephalus, examined 1 day after acute subarachnoid hemorrhage. The lateral ventricles show moderate generalized enlargement. The glomi of the choroid plexuses are visible. Bilateral soft tissue prominences project into the prominent occipital horns from their medial aspects. These seem to represent very prominent and asymmetrical expressions of the calcar avis (elevation in the occipital horns at the depth of the anterior portions of the calcarine fissures).
B. Scan in a patient with cerebral atrophy, demonstrating modest enlargement of the lateral ventricles, moderate enlargement of the interfrontal portion of the longitudinal fissure, and minor to moderate widening of many sulci of the frontal and parietal lobes. The calcarine fissures were widened and are visible behind the trigones and posterior portion of the corpus callosum.

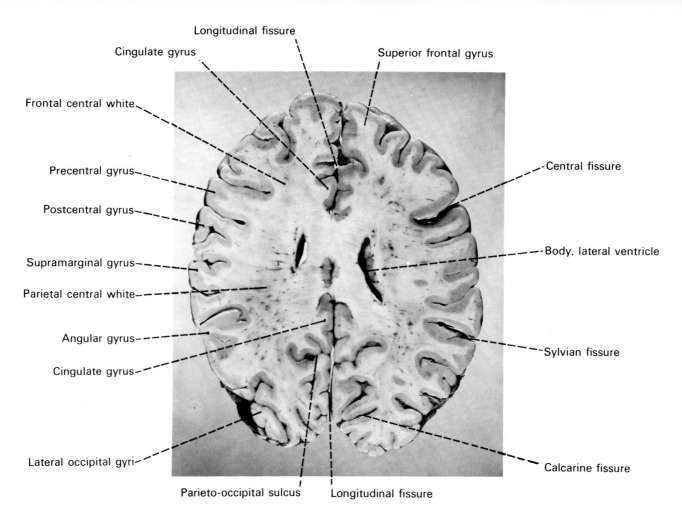

Longitudinal fissure

Cingulate gyrus

Superior frontal gyrus

Frontal central white

Precentral gyrus

Central fissure

Postcentral gyrus

Supramarginal gyrus

Body, lateral ventricle

Parietal central white

Angular gyrus

Cingulate gyrus

Sylvian fissure

Lateral occipital gyri

Calcarine fissure

Parieto-occipital sulcus

Longitudinal fissure

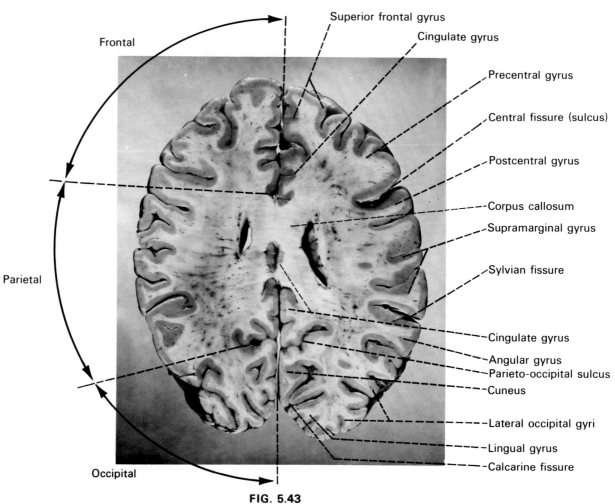

Superior frontal gyrus

Cingulate gyrus

Frontal

Precentral gyrus

Central fissure (sulcus)

Postcentral gyrus

Corpus callosum

Supramarginal gyrus

Sylvian fissure

Parietal

Cingulate gyrus

Angular gyrus

Parieto-occipital sulcus

Cuneus

Lateral occipital gyri

Lingual gyrus

Occipital

Calcarine fissure

FIG. 5.43

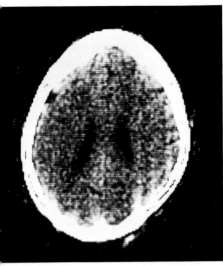 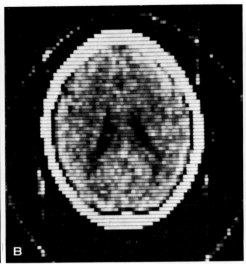 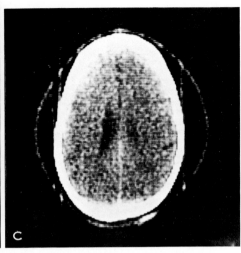

FIG. 5.44. A–C. At this level of scan, only the uppermost portions of the lateral ventricles are included. Depending on the precise angle and level of scan, the included portions of the lateral ventricles will be the superior portions of the bodies of the ventricles, but the relative extents of the anterior and/or posterior portions of the ventricular bodies will vary. With shallower angles, proportionately more of the anterior portions of the bodies will be included and, with steeper angles, more of the posterior portions of the bodies. Very steep angles will tend to include the superior portions of the trigones. With change in scan angle, the position of the central point of the portions of the lateral ventricles shown will tend to move anteriorly or posteriorly but the positions of the anterior and posterior arcs of the cranial vault will tend to move in the same direction, so that the anteroposterior position of the venticular segments will not alter greatly. However, the position of visualized cerebral sulci will be altered in relationship to the anterior or posterior portions of the cranial vault by angular changes. For example, a steeper scan angle will cause the central sulcus to lie nearer the anterior margin of the skull vault and further from the posterior skull vault, as compared with shallower scan angles. The higher the level of the scan plane, the more marked is the change in position of the sulcus relative to the skull vault with change in scan angle. The individual shape of the scanned cranial vault and brain will further influence the positions of the sulci and gyri relative to the bone contours in the scan. For this reason, reconstruction of the anatomical relationships likely to be present, using a suitable graticle and a lateral skull film, is highly desirable when attempting to localize the relative positions of anatomical features and lesions. The angle of the individual scan can be reconstructed quite accurately from osseous, cisternal, ventricular, and pineal landmarks obtained at multiple levels in an individual examination, provided that there has not been a change in angle due to patient movement between scans.

A. L 16　　W 40　　　　160 x 160 matrix.

An irregular band of greater density representing the cortex is evident peripherally. Beneath this is a large and broadly crescentic zone of relatively homogeneous density representing the centrum semiovale. The more posterior portions of the bodies of the lateral ventricles and adjacent superior portions of the trigones are demonstrated. While reasonably sharply defined in this case, the contours of the included segments of the lateral ventricles may appear relatively indistinct when less of the ventricle is included in the scan section. The superior portion of the corpus callosum is present between the ventricular cavities. If a portion of the cortex of the cingulate gyrus is included, there may be visible local modification upwards of the absorption values in the region of the central portion of the corpus callosum. On this scan, a minute portion of the interfrontal segment of the longitudinal fissure is visible, and there is an appearance of minimal widening of sulci.

B. L 15　　W 20　　　　80 x 80 matrix.

Scan at a closely similar plane and level to that shown in **A**. The peripheral cortical density and subjacent extensive lesser density of white matter is visible. In both **A** and **B,** larger volumes of the lateral ventricles are included than in the anatomical slice in Figure 5.43. No sulci are identified with certainty in this scan, although a small amount of the subarachnoid space of the anterior portion of the longitudinal fissure appears to be visible.

C. L 15　　W 20　　　　160 x 160 matrix.

In this scan, less of the superior portion of the body of the right lateral ventricle has been included than of the left, giving a spurious appearance of asymmetrical ventricular size. This scan was obtained following intravenous injection of contrast material, and the posterior portion of the falx is relatively dense. Small sections of the subarachnoid space of the anterior portion of the longitudinal fissure are visible, and there appears to be minimal enlargement of one sulcus in the right parietal region.

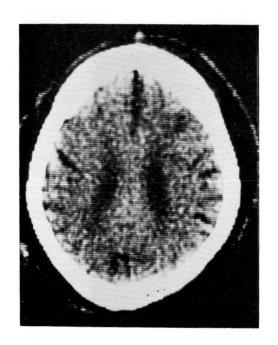

FIG. 5.45. 160 x 160 matrix scan. The lateral ventricles were slightly enlarged due to cerebral atrophy. The frontal portion of the longitudinal fissure is markedly widened, and numerous slightly and moderately widened sulci are demonstrated laterally in the frontal, parietal, and occipital regions. These include the precentral, central, and postcentral sulci on each side and possibly portions of the depths of the superior frontal sulci anterior to the bodies of the lateral ventricles. Individual variations and bilateral asymmetries in sulcal pattern in different individuals make identification of specific sulci and gyri difficult or impossible. Variations in sulcal position relative to bone contours are readily produced by differing scan angles and levels. When there is widespread sulcal dilatation, the major sulci may be identified with reasonable assurance after close study of the scan orientation and the series of higher scan sections.

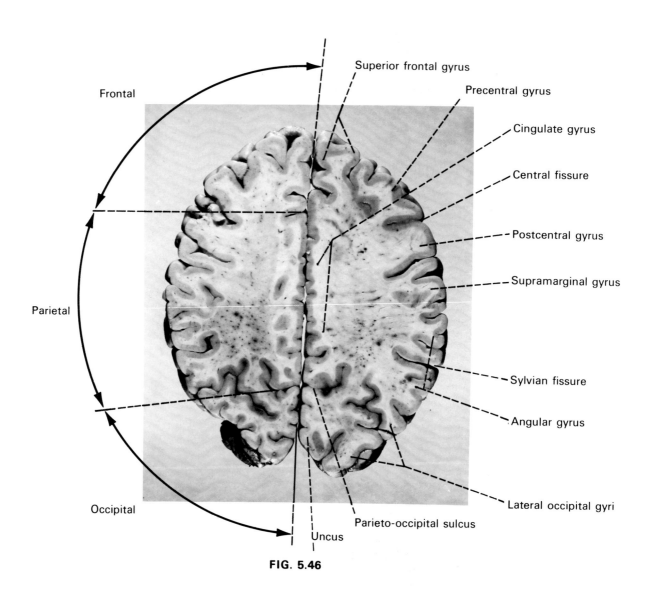

Frontal

Superior frontal gyrus

Precentral gyrus

Cingulate gyrus

Central fissure

Postcentral gyrus

Supramarginal gyrus

Parietal

Sylvian fissure

Angular gyrus

Occipital

Lateral occipital gyri

Uncus

Parieto-occipital sulcus

FIG. 5.46

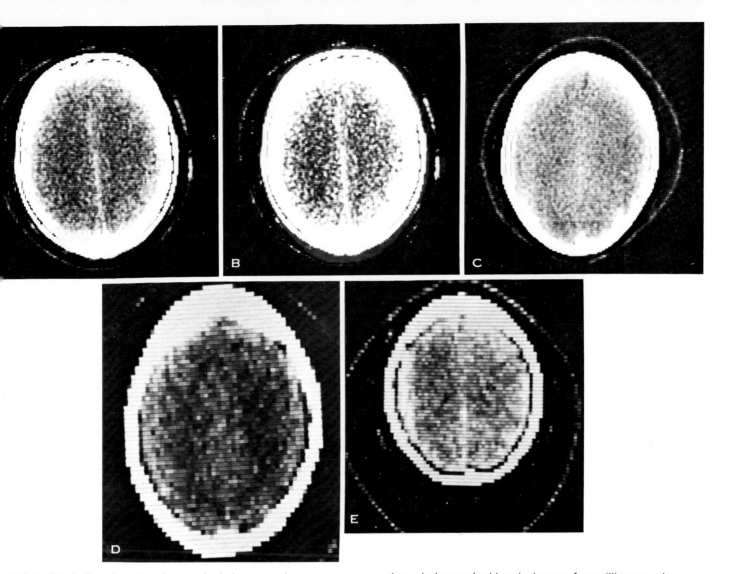

FIG. 5.47. A–E. A series of scans depicting normal scan appearances through the cerebral hemispheres a few millimeters above the lateral ventricles. In the normal case, scans at this level are relatively featureless. The peripheral denser zone of cerebral cortex is visible. This generally appears denser than the cortex of the mesial aspects of the cerebral hemispheres due to computer artifact. The relatively homogeneous and less dense white matter of the centrum semiovale is extensive and again has a broad crescentic configuration. Portions of the falx may be identified. In normal children and young adults, cerebral sulci are not visible or are extremely inconspicuous.

A. L 16   W 40.   **B.** L 16   W 20.

These two illustrations are of the same scan, obtained with the 160 x 160 matrix and following intravenous injection of Conray. **B** illustrates an effect routinely seen with either matrix at superior levels of cerebral scan section. The most peripheral portions of the cerebral hemispheres are "overshadowed" to a varying degree by the inward shelving of the cranial vault superiorly. This results in a varying degree of inclusion of some bone in the peripheral portion of the scan section of the brain; thus, the peripheral portion of the brain slice is recorded as having a falsely high absorption and is incompletely seen on the CRT display at standard viewer control settings. The peripheral anatomy is better demonstrated under these circumstances when the window width is increased, as was done in **A.** The cerebral surface area was even more completely visualized when the window width was increased to 60, but this resulted in an extremely low contrast in the more central portions of the cerebral scan. The injection of contrast medium has resulted in a denser and more clearly visible falx cerebri.

C. L 18   W 40   160 x 160 matrix.   **D.** L 16   W 20.

The difference in density of the cerebral cortex and white matter is more clearly visible with the higher contrast of the settings in **D,** as compared with **C.** In **D,** much of the centrum semiovale on the right side exhibits lower absorption values than that on the left, although the configuration is quite symmetrical in the two cerebral hemispheres. These asymmetries of absorption of centrum semiovale (amounting to a difference of several units) are quite common at higher levels of scan and may be due to even minor anatomical asymmetries or canting of the head. Care must be taken to avoid erroneous diagnosis of pathology on the basis of this asymmetry. In most such instances, the general crescentic configuration of the white matter is maintained as the region is observed with the M setting, and the window level is gradually altered through the appropriate range, in spite of the difference in density levels in the two hemispheres.

E. L 14   W 20.

In this case, the shelving effect of the cranial vault is not apparent except in the frontal region, where the slope of the cranial vault at this level is greater than elsewhere. The computer overswing artifact causing a narrow black band subjacent to the inner table is not visible in the frontal region, since the shelving configuration here avoids the abrupt and marked change in absorption between the cranial vault and the cerebral cortex.

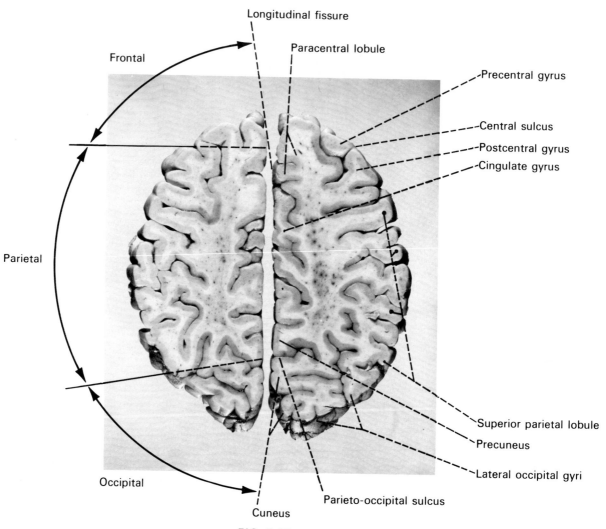

Longitudinal fissure

Paracentral lobule

Frontal

Precentral gyrus

Central sulcus

Postcentral gyrus

Cingulate gyrus

Parietal

Superior parietal lobule

Precuneus

Occipital

Lateral occipital gyri

Cuneus

Parieto-occipital sulcus

FIG. 5.48

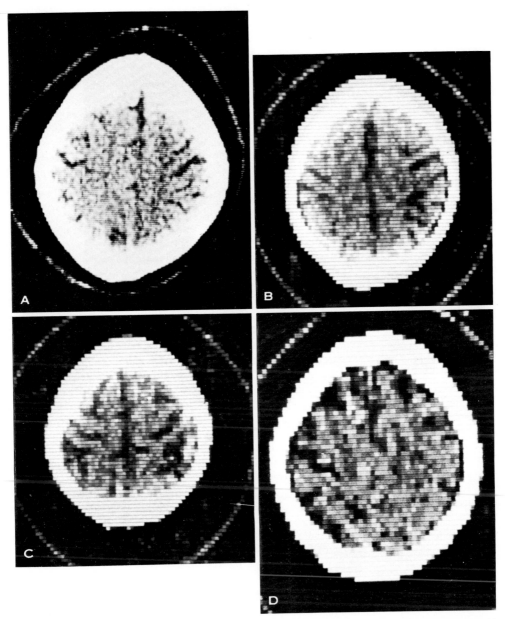

(Legend for FIG. 5.49 on page 110)

FIG. 5.49. A–D. The position of gyri and sulci within the contour of the cranial vault is very markedly dependent upon the precise angle and level of the scan plane in these superior sections. At an angle to Reid's base line of 30°, as in the anatomical brain slices, the central sulcus lies almost at the anterior extremity of the CT scan and will appear to move anteriorly, the higher the scan level. Individual variations in skull and brain contour will also affect the position of cerebral anatomy relative to the bone contours. The series of CT scans shown here were obtained at angles of approximately 10 to 20° to Reid's base line and the central sulci appear to be more posteriorly situated with respect to the cranial contour. It may be quite tedious and occasionally impossible to identify some individual sulci with any certainty, even when there is quite extensive and obvious sulcal enlargement.

A. 160 × 160 matrix.

Slight widening of the longitudinal fissure is present, particularly anteriorly. There is mild but apparently widespread enlargement of sulci. On the left side, the sulcus lying just anterior to the midsection of the scan may be the central sulcus. On the right side, the widest sulcus, lying slightly posterior to that on the left, also may be the central sulcus, with a somewhat less wide precentral sulcus just anteriorly. There is less certainty regarding the anatomy of the slightly widened appearing sulci visible elsewhere.

B. 80 × 80 matrix.

The two modestly widened sulci laterally in the midportion of the left cerebral hemisphere appear to represent the central sulcus and postcentral sulcus. The latter appears to be just traceable upwards and posteriorly into the interparietal sulcus. On the right side, there appears to be a moderately widened central sulcus, slightly anterior to its fellow on the left, with less widened precentral and postcentral sulci. There is considerable widening of the longitudinal fissure, especially anteriorly.

C. 80 × 80 matrix.

The three moderately severely widened sulci extending medially and somewhat posteriorly from the lateral surface appear to represent the precentral, central, and postcentral sulci, and the sulcus arching anteriorly and medially from the presumed precentral sulcus may represent the superior frontal sulcus. More severe widening of the right central and postcentral sulci is indicated. There is moderate widening of the longitudinal fissure and an appearance of "pooling" of CSF over the parietal lobe, in and behind the area of the presumed postcentral sulcus.

D. 80 × 80 matrix.

On the left side, the considerably widened sulcus, which can be followed for the greatest distance, running posteriorly and medially from a point just anterior to the midsegment of the scan, is presumed to represent the postcentral sulcus. It appears to be traceable posteriorly and medially into the interparietal sulcus. Just anterior to the presumed postcentral sulcus is an area of CSF pooling that may represent the area of the central sulcus and an even larger area of CSF pooling immediately anterior to the latter that may represent the area of the precentral sulcus. There is also a cluster of CSF pools in the left parietal region behind the postcentral sulcus.

At these high levels of cerebral scan, there is a greater area of cortex and a lesser area of white matter than in the subjacent sections.

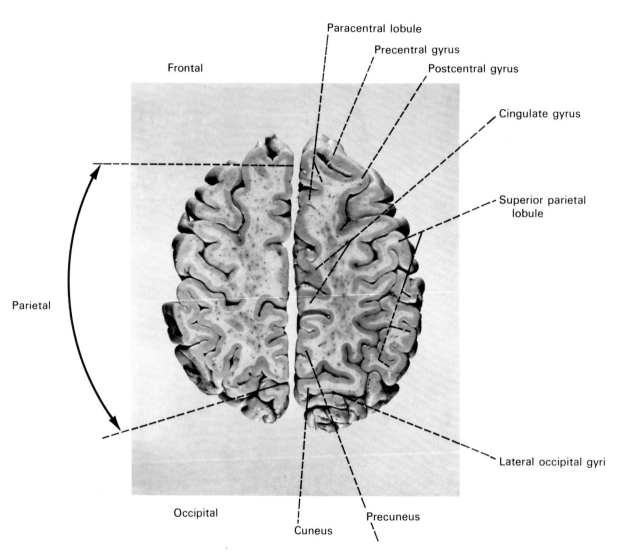

Paracentral lobule

Precentral gyrus

Postcentral gyrus

Frontal

Cingulate gyrus

Superior parietal lobule

Parietal

Lateral occipital gyri

Occipital

Precuneus

Cuneus

FIG. 5.50

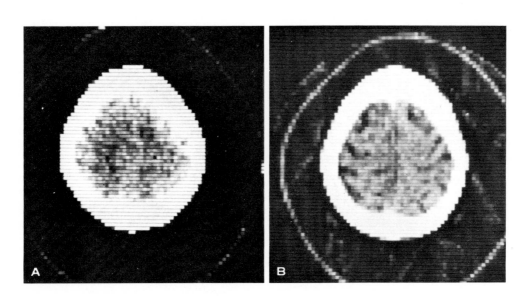

FIG. 5.51. A and **B.**   80 x 80 matrix.
A. L   18   W   20.
Normal scan. There is no evidence of sulcal enlargement. Very little white matter is present at this level, as compared with the widespread distribution of cortex. The shelving bone of the superior portion of the skull vault is included with the cortex. In the absence of an abrupt change from very high bone values to much lower cortical values, the computer undershoot phenomenon of a narrow black zone beneath the inner table is not present. An additional effect is that the anatomical contours of the periphery of the brain are not observed at the standard window width. Widening of the window increases visibility of the cerebral surfaces (see **B**).
B. L   18   W   30.
The wider window reduces the obscuring effect of partial volume inclusion of shelving bone in the peripheral cerebral volumes. Some increase in window level also decreases obscuration, but may result in an unsatisfactory display of lower density regions more centrally. In this case, moderately severe and widespread cerebral atrophy was present. The two wide sulci extending posteromedially in the midportion of the right cerebral hemisphere appear to represent the central and postcentral sulci. The angle of the scan is approximately 15 to 20° to Reid's base line, rather than 30° as in the case of the anatomical brain slice (Figure 5.50). A marked difference in the relative positions of the central sulci and bone contours is therefore to be expected, compared with that illustrated by the anatomical brain slice.

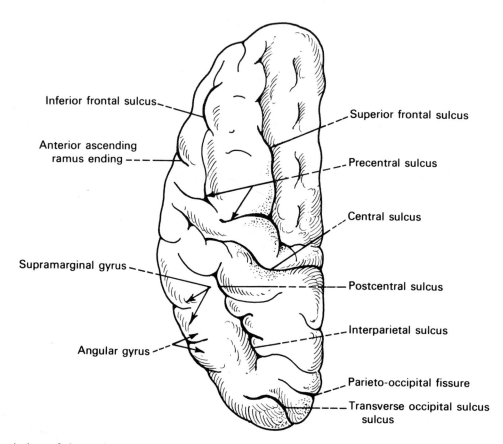

Inferior frontal sulcus

Anterior ascending
ramus ending

Supramarginal gyrus

Angular gyrus

Superior frontal sulcus

Precentral sulcus

Central sulcus

Postcentral sulcus

Interparietal sulcus

Parieto-occipital fissure

Transverse occipital sulcus
sulcus

FIG. 5.52 General view of the entire left cerebral hemisphere from above. There is no angulation involved. Note the spatial reorientation produced by the angled sections illustrated in the anatomical photographs and equivalent CT sections.

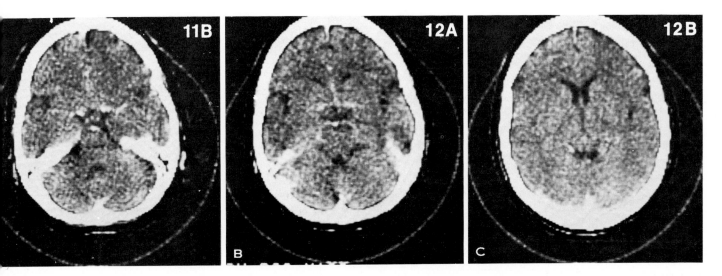

FIG. 5.53. Visualization of intracranial vessels following intravenous drip infusion of 300 ml of 30% meglumine diatrizoate. Contiguous 8-mm scan sections.
L 15   W 30   160 x 160 matrix system.
A. This scan section is through the suprasellar and interpeduncular cisterns and shows the distal segments of the internal carotid arteries. On each side, the proximal portions of the middle cerebral arteries are visible extending into the sylvian fissures (the right is denser, being more completely included in the scan section). In the midline just anterior to the petrous apices, the superior portion of the basilar artery is visible immediately anterior to the upper pons. Further posteriorly, the fourth ventricle is visible, with more of the left posterosuperior recess visible than the right. Immediately to the left of the midline, midway between the internal carotid arteries and the internal frontal crest, a segment of the pericallosal arteries is visible as a single irregular white spot. This arterial segment is a little more clearly visible in **B**.

B. Section immediately above that in **A**. The anterior cerebral arteries are visible extending almost transversely to the midline, and the pericallosal arteries are shown extending anteriorly from the region of the anterior communicating artery, with an inclination slightly to the left. At the coronal plane of the most inferior portions of the frontal horns, the pericallosal arteries move out of the section, but become visible again a few millimeters further anteriorly, where they pass vertically through the slice. Near the posterior portion of the interpeduncular cistern, the upper extremity of the basilar artery is again visible, with the posterior cerebral arteries arching around the anterior half of the midbrain. The section extends through the inferior colliculi and posterior portions of the ambient cisterns.

C. This section clearly shows the frontal horns and also extends through the superior colliculi. Irregular high absorption areas in the superior portions of the ambient cisterns are visible on each side, presumably representing portions of the posterior cerebral arteries and the basal veins.

Part TWO

Introduction

In the second portion of this work are presented the CT scan findings in different varieties of intracranial disease. Apparently typical and atypical CT scan representations in different pathological conditions are included. A chapter is also devoted to anatomical correlations in orbital scanning, with examples of orbital pathology as demonstrated by CT scans.

Clinical histories, the results of neurological examinations, pertinent laboratory data, and the results of examination by other radiological methods, including radionuclide brain scanning, are included as summaries where possible. In order to include a wider spectrum of CT scan representations of pathological conditions, the number of actual illustrations of traditional studies has been kept small. Those included have been selected to illustrate certain fundamental differences in capability of the various modalities.

In several chapters, the results of comparative studies of the accuracy of CT scanning, radionuclide brain scanning, cerebral angiography, and cerebral pneumography have been included. Such data have not yet been analyzed for all pathological conditions represented here, although this work is in progress.

As radionuclide scans may show increased activity secondary to the effects of surgery for prolonged periods after operation, the diagnosis of recurrence of tumor, other pathological processes, or postsurgical complications by this means may be extremely difficult or impossible. Postoperative CT scans are often more difficult to interpret than are preoperative scans, but the method is far less subject to the above disadvantage, in that absorption characteristics of tissue changes offer the possibility of specific evaluation.

Where comparative data regarding relative accuracy is given, the individual traditional radiological examinations have been interpreted by highly qualified individuals in the respective fields. The diagnoses made on the basis of each modality were arrived at with knowledge of the clinical and laboratory data. In some cases, the diagnoses made from CT scans, radionuclide brain scans, cerebral angiography, and pneumoencephalography were arrived at with some knowledge of the results of studies by one or more of the alternative examinations. To the degree that this occurred, the scientific validity of the comparative studies was impaired, but every effort was made to ensure an unbiased assessment of the diagnostic value of each form of study independently.

Five institutions, including the Massachusetts General Hospital, are cooperating in a study to evaluate the use of computed tomography in the diagnosis of brain tumors. This study is sponsored by the National Cancer Institute, National Institutes of Health, and is expected, in due course, to provide definitive answers to many questions that can only be addressed tentatively in the chapters on intracranial neoplasms to follow.

In order to achieve high fidelity, the large majority of the illustrations of CT scans was made directly from the original Polaroid records.

ATLAS OF PATHOLOGY:

Including consideration of the comparative value of computed tomography and traditional radiological studies.

CHAPTER 6

Gliomas

INTRODUCTION

Of the initial 600 CT scan examinations performed at the Massachusetts General Hospital (MGH), gliomas comprised 7%. The cases illustrated in this chapter were selected from a total of approximately 2400 CT scan examinations as illustrative of the various scan appearances that may be encountered in this class of tumor. As would be expected from the gross pathology of gliomas, the CT scan patterns are highly variable, not only from case to case, but in different portions of the same tumors when these are relatively large.

The typical appearance of a low or intermediate grade astrocytoma is an area of reduced absorption relative to white matter, the margin of which is irregular, showing an ameboid or frond-like configuration. Absorption values generally lie in the range of 6–16 or 18, with small regions of the tumor extending slightly outside of this range. Typically, the absorption is nonhomogeneous, with patchy areas of greater and lesser absorption being intermingled through the lesion. Glioblastomas may have a similar appearance to astrocytoma Grades I and II but commonly show a more heterogeneous pattern of absorption values, in which ill-defined patches of greater density than normal brain are distributed through the lesion or occur in one area of it. These regions of higher density generally represent areas of minor local hemorrhagic extravasation or areas of more densely compacted cells. The latter pattern can mimic quite closely that of hemorrhagic infarction, although, as with lower grade astrocytomas, the margins of the tumor tend to be more markedly irregular than in infarction. In a small minority of cases, there may be difficulty on the initial CT scan in differentiation of glioma from infarction. If the clinical presentation is equivocal, differentiation should readily be made by repeating the CT scan after an interval of 2–3 weeks, at which time the edema accompanying an acute infraction will have subsided to some degree, whereas the neoplasm will generally appear unchanged or larger. Cystic changes in gliomas are usually shown clearly by virtue of generally low absorption values, in the range 0–14, of the contained fluid. Occasionally, cystic areas in a glioma may contain sufficiently proteinaceous fluid that the absorption of the cystic region will not be discriminated from surrounding tumor tissue. It is not to be expected that microcystic changes will be identifiable on CT scans, although in areas where such changes are marked, the overall absorption of the region will probably be reduced further. Areas of cystic necrosis in a malignant glioma tend to be less regular and less sharply defined than the cysts of low-grade astrocytomas.

Mass effects upon the ventricular contour and displacement of midline structures are generally obvious, although in the more infiltrating forms of glioma these changes may be very slight. Mass effects are generally greater in the case of glioma than in ischemic infarcts of equal volume.

Any calcific foci present in gliomas are much more readily identifiable on CT scans than on plain film examination, due to the far greater sensitivity of the former system. However, the exact morphological pattern of calcification is not shown on CT scan, as a consequence both of the increased sensitivity and the lower resolution of the system. *This is one of the many reasons that plain film cranial examination must be regarded as a necessary complement to CT scanning.* Preferably, the two examinations should be interpreted together. In some gliomas, absorption characteristics may be very similar to those of adjacent brain, either throughout the lesion or in certain areas. Presumably, such gliomas, or portions of gliomas, have less fluid content than in the typical case. It is extremely difficult at times to identify the margin of the tumor, due to the imperceptible mixture of tumor cells and normal brain. At other times, edema peripheral to the tumor creates conditions that make differentiation of the actual tumor margin impossible. These limitations notwithstanding, the extent of a glioma is usually far more clearly identifiable on CT scans than on radionuclide scans (even when these are clearly positive) and as compared with angiography. Generally, the less vascular the tumor, the more accurate is the CT scan in demonstrating its extent, as compared with angiography. Generally, extension of glioma into the ventricular system is more readily identified on CT scans than on angiograms. This type of extension, however, is generally most accurately revealed by pneumoencephalography. The greater the vascularity of a glioma, the more likely it is that angiography will provide important additional evidence regarding the nature of the lesion and its extent. Pneumoencephalography remains supreme in the identification of small tumors involving the optic chiasm, third ventricle, temporal horn, aqueduct, fourth ventricle, and the region of the lower cisterna magna and foramen magnum. The present resolution of the CT scan renders a negative study quite unreliable in the diagnosis of such tumors. While the 160 x 160 matrix system will no doubt increase the sensitivity of CT scanning in such cases, the thickness of the tissue section militates against high effectiveness in such situations, even if an 8-mm scan series is obtained. Partial volume effects further impair the accuracy under such circumstances.

Supplementary CT scanning following intravenous injection of contrast medium was originally used relatively infrequently by us in the study of gliomas, partly due to exigencies of scheduling and partly due to the evidence that most *symptomatic* gliomas are identifiable on plain CT scans. It is now clear that the overall accuracy of diagnosis and differential diagnosis is increased by more frequent use of supplementary scans following contrast injection, and this will probably be used more and more frequently in the future, since the almost immediate availability of scan viewing with the new matrix system will ease scheduling pressures somewhat and will permit such decisions to be made before the patient leaves the table. It has been demonstrated that the sensitivity of CT scan examination can be enhanced by the use of intravenous contrast medium in some cases to the point that a previously unrecognized small lesion is clearly recognizable. In other cases, it has been shown that the extent of the lesion can be identified with greater reliability following contrast injection. In cases of significant doubt, when clinical features are appropriate, repeating scans at one or more levels a few minutes after intravenous injection of 40 or 50 ml of standard contrast material may improve the differential contrast in absorption values to the point that a definite diagnosis can be made. As in the case of angiography, CT scans following intravenous injection of contrast medium in the order of 50 ml will generally not produce visible increase in absorption values of astrocytoma Grades I and II, whereas an increase in absorption is usually identified in some areas of glioblastomas or throughout

TABLE 6.1
GLIOMAS: 35 CASES

	CT* scans (35)	RN scans (24)	Angiograms (22)	PEGs (12)
Positive	32†	21	≫ 10‡ > 6	≫ 1 > 5
Negative	1 + ? 1§	3	= 5 ≪ 1	= 2 < 2 ≪ 1 + ? 1§
Technically unsatisfactory	1 (motion)	0	0	0

* CT, computed tomographic; RN, radionuclide.

† Interpretation error regarding nature of tumor in two cases; diagnosed as metastases.

‡ ≫, CT very much superior to angiography or pneumoencephalography; >, CT distinctly superior to angiography or pneumoencephalography; =, CT approximately equal to angiography or pneumoencephalography; ≪, CT very much inferior to angiography or pneumoencephalography.

§ Suspected optic chiasmal glioma (unproved).

these tumors. Larger intravenous doses have not been tested fully in this regard as yet by us (see Chapter 27).

COMPARATIVE DIAGNOSTIC EFFECTIVENESS OF CT SCANS IN GLIOMA (TABLE 6.1).

Of the 35 cases of glioma scanned in the initial 600 consecutive CT scans, only 1 false negative diagnosis is known. This is the case of temporal glioma illustrated by Figure 6.9. In another case, pneumoencephalography indicated either perichiasmatic arachnoid adhesions or a very small optic chiasm glioma. The case is not finally proved but is retained here because it is clear that very small tumors in the region of the optic chiasm and hypothalamus are unlikely to be diagnosable on CT scans. Two cases were falsely diagnosed as glioma, but these were examples of metastatic malignant neoplasms seen early in the series. With greater experience, we would expect to diagnose both correctly. In general, therefore, CT scanning proved highly accurate in the diagnosis of *symptomatic* glioma. Of the 35 cases, 24 had radionuclide (RN) scans, of which 21 were positive and 3 were negative. CT scans were very much superior in diagnosis of the extent and type of lesion. Angiography was performed in 22 cases. CT scans were considered to be very much superior in the diagnosis of glioma and its extent in 10 cases, distinctly superior in six cases, and approximately equal in five cases. One case of glioma diagnosed by angiography had a technically unsatisfactory CT scan due to motion. Twelve cases had pneumoencephalograms. CT scans were considered to be very much superior in one case, distinctly better in five cases, equal in two cases, somewhat less informative in two cases, and very much less informative in one case. The one CT scan that was negative in a case of suspected small optic chiasmal glioma is also shown in Table 6.1.

POSTOPERATIVE CT SCANS IN GLIOMA CASES

Although much useful information can be obtained following surgery in these cases, particularly information concerning the presence or absence of mass effects, the extent of surgical excision, evidence of obstructive hydrocephalus, and the presence of extensive residual tumor or further tumor growth, interpretation of postoperative CT scans tends to be more difficult than in preoperative cases, owing to problems in differentiating tissue changes consequent upon surgery from residual tumor. Postoperative complications, such as intracerebral or extracerebral hemorrhage, are generally readily recognized, and the effects of ventricular decompression are readily evaluated. Postoperative cerebral angiography and pneumography are notoriously difficult to evaluate, and, in general, the CT scanning can be expected to provide more useful information, particularly if intravenous contrast enhancement is also used.

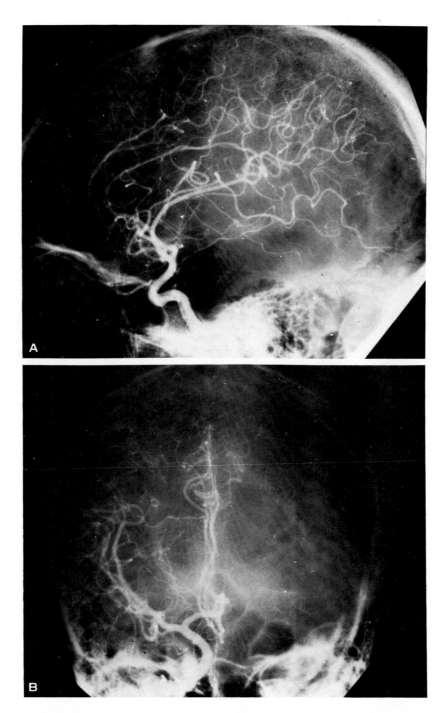

FIG. 6.1. ASTROCYTOMA OF TEMPORAL LOBE GRADE II-III

Clinical Features. A 33 y.o. male who presented with temporal lobe epilepsy, with his first seizure 4 years previously.

Neurological Examination. Within normal limits.

EEG. Suggested a right temporal focus.

Skull Examination. Normal.

RN Scan. Tcp, normal.

CSF Protein. 30 mg%.

Angio. Bilateral carotid, abnormal (Fig. 6.1, A and B).

CT Scan. Abnormal (Fig. 6.1, C and D).

Operation. 6.5 cm of the temporal lobe was resected (Dr. Michael Scott). There was obvious tumor extending deeply from the resection margin. The tumor was firm and avascular, containing a few microcysts.

Histology. Grade II-III astrocytoma.

Postoperative CT Scan. (Fig. 6.1, E and F).

A, lateral, and **B,** frontal arterial phase films of the right carotid angiogram, showing a large, completely avascular holotemporal mass. The degree of medial displacement of the lenticulostriate arteries is consistent with centrosylvian extension of the mass. Very slight dislocation of midline vessels to the left.

C. L   16   W   20.

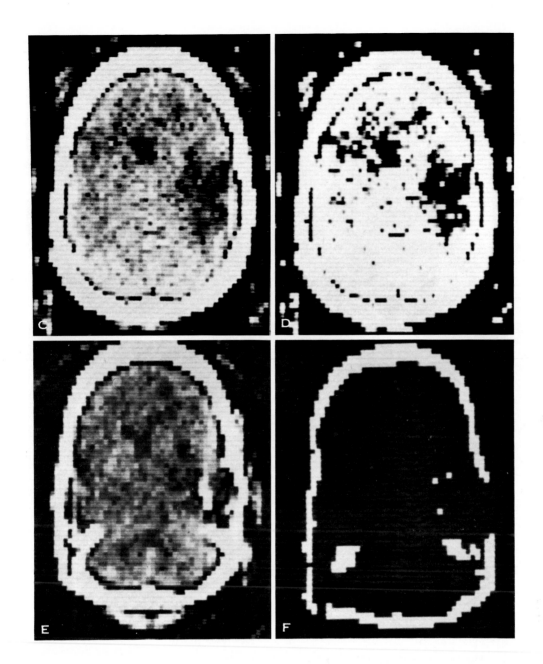

One section showing a large, highly irregularly marginated zone of decreased absorption (average 8–10) involving the entire right temporal lobe and extending in a frond-like manner into the frontal and parietal lobes and centrally almost to the midline. There is obvious displacement of the frontal horns to the left and compression of the right frontal horn. The heterogeneous absorption results in a patchy appearance of the area of pathology. (Reprinted by permission from Radiology, 110: 109–123, 1974.)

D. L 15   W M.

Same section as in **C**, with maximum contrast between the tumor and surrounding brain. At this window level, some of the white matter in the anterior portions of both frontal lobes is black, which is not necessarily abnormal in these areas in younger individuals. However, on the right side just anterior to the frontal horn, the appearance is very suggestive of additional tumor extension.

E. Postoperative CT scan a few days after surgery. The very low absorption in the right temporal area represents the resection bed, bounded medially by the density of silver clips. Deep to the latter, irregular areas of abnormally low absorption indicate the residual deep portions of the tumor. Displacement of the frontal horns to the left is somewhat greater than before surgery, due to postoperative edema. The extent of surgery and postoperative status is more completely revealed by this technique than would be possible by any other method. The postoperative examination is very helpful in the planning of radiotherapy.

F. L 50   W M.

At these control settings, all soft tissues appear black and only bone and 3 silver clips are shown white. The craniectomy defect is obvious.

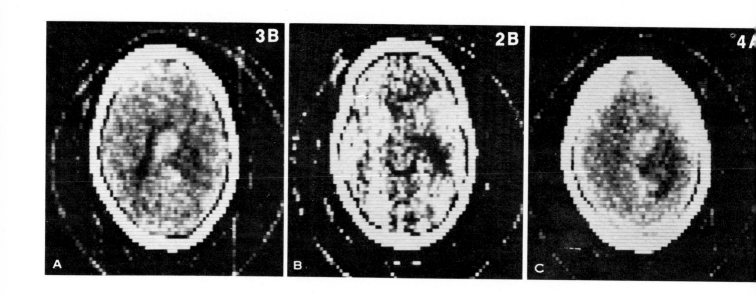

FIG. 6.2. GLIOBLASTOMA

Clinical Features. A 44 y.o. woman with multiple progressive neurological symptoms involving the left side of her body. Sensory seizures started 4 months previously. These initially involved the left lower extremity and then extended to the left upper extremity and to the face. She started to note twitching of the left leg and left side of the jaw. Headaches, dizziness, and unsteadiness for $1\frac{1}{2}$ months. Recent left hemiparesis.

Neurological Examination. Revealed a typical right parietal sensory deficit.

EEG. Normal on two occasions.

Skull Examination. Normal 3 weeks earlier.

RN Scan. Tcp, showed increased uptake in right superior and midparietal convexity regions 3 weeks before CT.

Angio. Bilateral carotid, obtained elsewhere 3 weeks earlier, interpreted as negative. On review, minimal abnormality indicative of a very poorly localized avascular right frontoparietal mass. Repeat angio at MGH just before CT revealed increased, poorly localized, right cerebral hemisphere mass effect with a few small scattered areas of pathological vascularity.

CT Scan. Abnormalities involving most of right cerebral hemisphere and extending across the midline (Fig. 6.2, A–C). Patient advised to undergo radiotherapy, but returned to home state and underwent biopsy. She died the following day. Autopsy revealed glioblastoma involving most of the right cerebral hemisphere.

CT brain scan revealed irregularly distributed areas of abnormal absorption involving all lobes of the right cerebral hemisphere. Large regions of decreased absorption (9–16) with focal areas of greater (20–26) and lesser (4–12) absorption.

A. L 16 　 W 20.

Section at the level of the bodies and trigones of the lateral ventricles. An irregularly rounded area of increased density, 20–26, measuring some 2.5 cm in diameter, is shown within the region of the body of the right lateral ventricle and extending into the medial portion of the body of the left lateral ventricle. A similar but smaller area of increased absorption is present posterior to the trigone of the right lateral ventricle, near the midline. Widespread, nonhomogeneous abnormality of absorption, mainly in the range 9–16, extends through a large portion of the right cerebral hemisphere. The denser areas of the tumor probably contain some extravasated blood.

B. L 16 　 W 10.

Section 2.5 cm below **A.** In the deep temporal and posterior centrosylvian regions is a large ovoid zone of very low absorption (4–12), consistent with a large area of cystic degeneration in the tumor. Irregular patchy areas of decreased absorption are shown extending through the right frontal, temporal, parietal, and occipital lobes. The right frontal horn is grossly compressed.

C. L 16 　 W 20.

Section immediately above **A.**

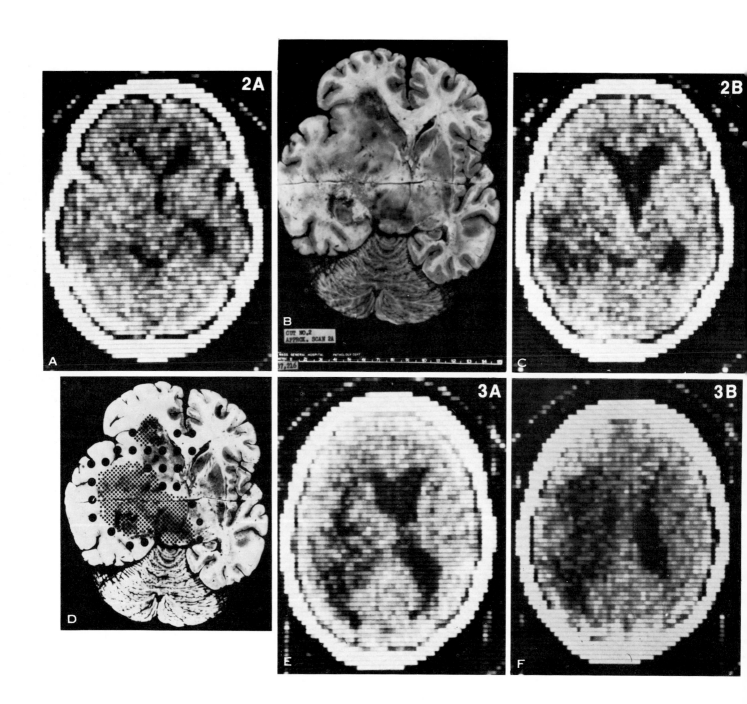

FIG. 6.3. EXTENSIVE GLIOBLASTOMA ORIGINATING IN THE REGION OF THE LEFT THALAMUS

Clinical Features. A 39 y.o. male. A diagnosis of vascular thalamic glioma was made by angiography 7 months earlier. He received radiation therapy. Deterioration again became progressive.

Skull Examination. Pineal displaced 4 mm to right.

RN Scan. As[74], 7 months earlier, showed an abnormal left central cerebral uptake. Repeat scan 3 months later showed essentially no change.

CT Scan. Widespread abnormality consistent with glioblastoma.

Angio. Carotid angiography within 3 days of CT revealed a huge mass in thalamic and temporal regions, with a marked malignant neovascularization and ventricular compression.

Successive 13-mm slices extending superiorly. L 14–16 W 20.

A. Obvious compression of the left frontal horn and several mm displacement of the septum pellucidum and anterior third ventricle to the right. A subtle widespread abnormality of absorption pattern is present through most of the frontal and temporal lobe areas and throughout the area of the left corpus striatum. In the frontal and temporal lobes, there is a patchy, slight decrease in absorption compared with normal white matter. In the area of the corpus striatum, there is also a patchy abnormality of absorption with numerous areas of increased absorption and some zones of decreased absorption compared with normal. There is modest enlargement of the right temporal horn and slight enlargement of the inferior portion of the right frontal horn. The superior portion of the left ambient cistern is wider than on the right. (Reprinted by permission from Radiology 114: January 1975.)

B. Autopsy brain slice similar in angle and level to the CT section in **A**. Widespread glioblastoma was demonstrated in the abnormal areas referred to in **A**, and tumor extended laterally from the wall of the frontal horn and of the third ventricle. A boundary zone anterolaterally, laterally, and posterolaterally was found to consist primarily of reactive gliosis and edema, with possibly a few malignant cells distributed through the zone. Absorption values on the CT scan did not permit differentiation between this boundary zone and the area of gross tumor, but the general correspondence between the scan and the pathological findings was remarkably good. (Reprinted by permission from Radiology 114: January 1975.)

C. A large, irregularly marginated region of variably decreased absorption is present in the temporal lobe and extending into the lateral portion of the corpus striatum. Compression of the left frontal horn is obvious. There is marked compression and displacement to the right of the posterior portion of the third ventricle and modest enlargement of the frontal horn and trigone of the right lateral ventricle. A subtle nonhomogeneous increase in absorption is present in the more anterior and medial portions of the corpus striatum. (Reprinted by permission from Radiology 114: January 1975.)

D. Same brain slice as in **B**. *Small dots* show the area of gross glioblastoma and the *large dots* show the region consisting primarily of reactive gliosis and edema, with some tumor cells probably distributed through the zone. Interval between CT scan and autopsy was 23 days. (Reprinted by permission from Neurology 25(3): 201–209, 1975.)

E. Widespread mottled decrease in absorption is present in the temporal and parietal lobes and in the lateral portion of the corpus striatum. Denser tumor areas are present in the region of the thalamus, a portion of the lenticular nucleus, and the head of the caudate nucleus. Encroachment by the tumor upon the ventricular system medially is evident.

F. At this level, a very widespread decrease in absorption represents the tumor and edema extending through a broad confluent region of the frontal, parietal, and temporal lobes and causing compression of the body of the left lateral ventricle. (Reprinted by permission from Radiology 114: January 1975.)

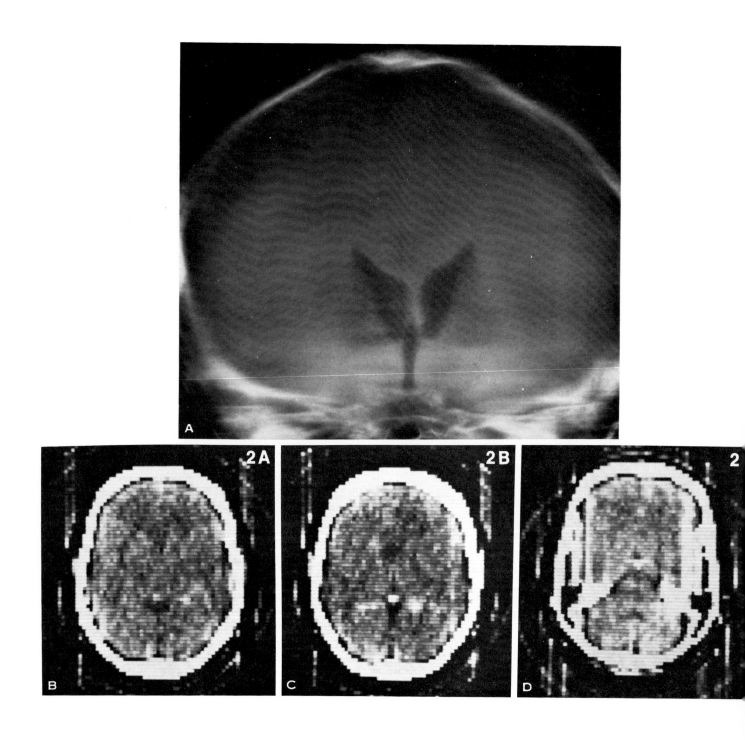

FIG. 6.4. GLIOMA: WIDESPREAD BIFRONTAL AND CORPUS CALLOSUM INVOLVEMENT

Clinical Features. A 54 y.o. female with a history of episodic emotional instability and depression for several years. Progressive deterioration of memory, particularly of recent memory. Weight loss of 40 lbs. Normal neurological examination.

EEG. Frequent intermittent right temporal slowing.

RN Scan. Tcp, normal 5 days before second CT scan. Clinically, question of early Alzheimer's disease.

Skull Examination. Increased density right frontal bone, involving inner table.

CT Scan. First CT scan revealed abnormally low absorption in the right frontal lobe, but there was considerable motion artifact on this study. Repeat CT scan 4 days later, between 1 and 2 hours after angiography with injection of 94 ml Conray-60. Widespread bifrontal abnormality (Fig. 6.4, **B–D**).

Angio. Bilateral transfemoral carotid angiograms, including right selective external carotid injection and left vertebrobasilar angiogram. An extensive but poorly localized mass lesion was identified in the right frontal lobe, with modest displacement of pericallosal branches to the left and subfalcial herniation. Minimal indication of hypervascularity on subtraction films. Evidence of deep extension revealed by lateral displacement of insular branches. Internal cerebral vein in midline. *No indication of left hemispheric lesion.* Normal appearance of vertebral angiogram.

Diagnosis. Extensive avascular anterior right frontal mass, with primary or secondary neoplasm being the most likely.

PEG. Abnormal (Fig. 6.4A).

Patient referred for radiotherapy without biopsy. No histological verification to date.

The second CT scan is illustrated. Widespread diminution of absorption is visible in the anterior portions of both frontal lobes and in the region of the anterior portion of the corpus callosum. Absorption values range between 10 and 19, with the average

values being somewhat lower in the right frontal lobe compared with the left. The vertical extent of the pathology appears greater in the medial anterior portion of the right frontal lobe than elsewhere. Comparing the absorption values on the two scans, no definite increase in absorption was produced by the circulating contrast medium in the second examination, indicating an avascular lesion and relatively intact blood-brain barrier.

A. PEG. AP brow-up film, one of a laminagraphic series. This study demonstrated a moderate mass effect in the region of the corpus callosum, separating and indenting the roofs of the lateral ventricles. The mass effect is slightly greater to the right of the midline and extended from the frontal horns posteriorly to involve the bodies of the ventricles. The examination indicated a mass in the corpus callosum but did not indicate the wide extent of the tumor in both frontal lobes.

B, C, and **D. B** and **C** are from the second CT scan, and **D** is from the first. Widespread diminution of absorption is visible in the anterior portions of both frontal lobes and in the region of the anterior portion of the corpus callosum. Absorption values range between 9 and 19, with the average values being somewhat lower in the right frontal lobe as compared with the left. The vertical extent of the pathology also appears greater in the medial anterior portion of the right frontal lobe than elsewhere (**C**). Much of the lesion on both sides of the midline lies in the absorption range 9–13. Although the absorption of the lesion is only very slightly different from surrounding brain, demarcation from surrounding brain is fairly easily defined.

B and **C** are contiguous sections. **D**, an inferior frontal section from the first CT scan, is below the level shown in **B**. Comparing the absorption values on the two CT scans, no definite increase in absorption was caused by the circulating contrast medium in the second examination.

Diagnosis: Extensive low-grade bifrontal and corpus callosum glioma (no histological verification to date).

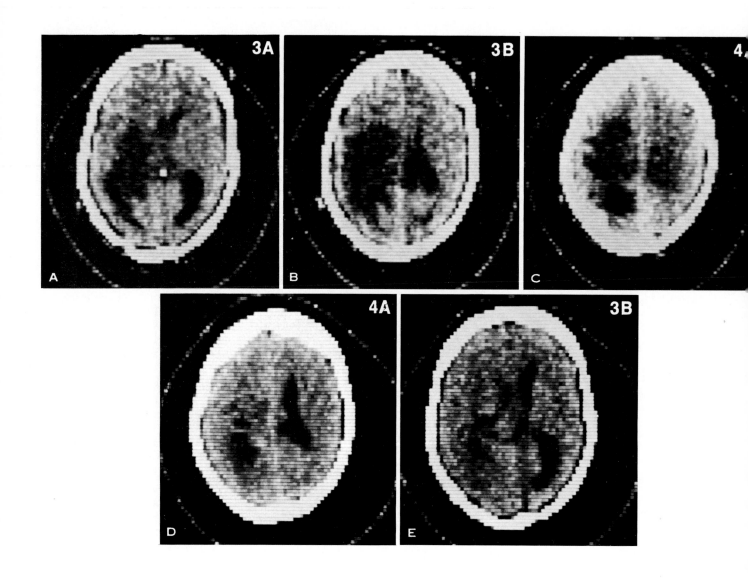

FIG. 6.5. GLIOBLASTOMA: EXTENSIVE, PARTLY CYSTIC, TUMOR

Clinical Features. A 51 y.o. male, who presented with symptoms of a depressive illness. Elevation of CSF protein led to further investigation.

CT Scan. Initial CT scan revealed a cystic mass in the posterior portion of the corpus callosum, with deformity of both lateral ventricles. Equipment failure prevented completion of the scan.

PEG. Obtained elsewhere before admission; showed no filling of the posterior portion of the left lateral ventricle and a large tumor mass near the midline in the medial parietal area.

Operation. Left parieto-occipital craniotomy, with a very limited resection of tumor in this region, revealed a cystic glioblastoma (Dr. Robert G. Ojemann).

First postoperative CT Scan. Approximately one month later; widespread abnormality (Fig. 6.5, **A**–**C**).

Second CT Scan. Six months after postoperative radiation therapy (4600 R). Striking reduction in abnormality (Fig. 6.5, **D** and **E**).

Histology. Glioblastoma, mixed with fibrosarcoma.

The very wide extent of the tumor is now shown.

A. A large region of diminished absorption, mostly in the range 5–13, with irregular margins, is shown extending widely through the central portions of the frontal, temporal, and parietal lobes. The septum pellucidum and pineal are displaced markedly to the right, and the left lateral ventricle is compressed. The right lateral ventricle is enlarged, particulary in the region of the trigone and occipital horn. The abnormal reduction in tissue absorption extends to the displaced midline, and there is evidence of extension to the medial portion of the *right* thalamus.

B. Next superior section. The area of diminished tissue absorption is more extensive at this level and is clearly seen to involve most of the left cerebral hemisphere from the plane of the central sulcus posteriorly. There is more striking evidence of extension of the lesion to the right of the midline in the region of the posterior portion of the corpus callosum (black area immediately medial to the right trigone).

C. Next contiguous superior section. The left cerebral hemisphere is again shown to be widely involved at this level, and there is an extensive area of reduced absorption in the right parietal lobe, indicating considerable extension across the midline. The rounded area in the left parieto-occipital region has a lower absorption than does the remainder of the lesion (4–10) and represents partly the original cystic region of the tumor and partly the region of surgical excision.

CT Diagnosis. Extensive cerebral glioblastoma, partly cystic.

D and **E**. Scans obtained 6 months after radiotherapy. The patient had been much improved and had resumed strenuous athletic activities. For 1 week before the scan, he had noted marked weakness of the right extremities and unsteady gait.

D. Scan level similar to that in **B** and **E**, level similar to that in **A**. There is much less extensive reduction in absorption but extensive tumor (with absorption very close to that of normal brain) is visible growing into the lateral ventricles from left to right (tumor absorption 12–16 in **D** and 13–21 in **E**). The septum lucidum is thickened and displaced to the right.

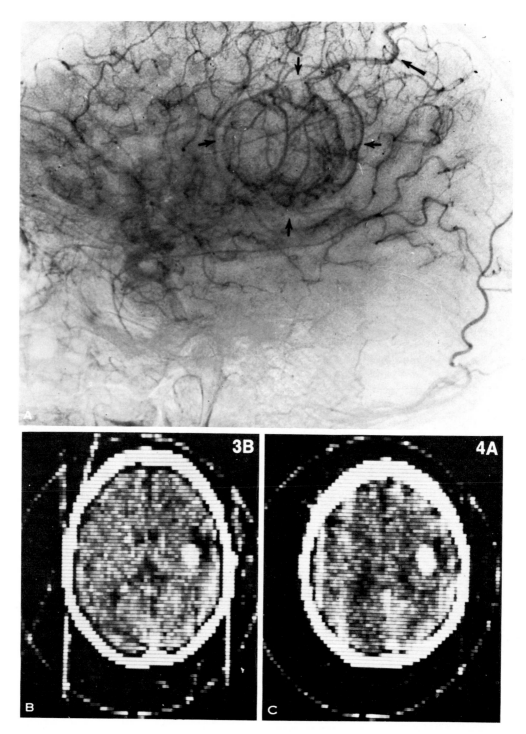

FIG. 6.6. GLIOBLASTOMA, WITH NECROSIS AND BLOOD CLOT

Clinical Features. A 56 y.o. hypertensive male, with a 2–3 year history of episodic numbness of the left hand. For several months he had noted occasional cramping in the muscles of the left hand and occasional pins and needles paresthesias in the entire hand. Over the previous few days he had noted twitching in his upper lip followed by twitching of the left side of the face and shaking of both hands and feet, without loss of consciousness. Neurological examination was normal.

EEG. Normal.

Skull Examination. Normal.

CSF Protein. 58 mg%.

RN Scan. Tcp, abnormal, with an area of increased uptake in the area of right parietal lobe in the region of the Sylvian fissure. This extended out to the inner table.

CT Scan. Abnormal, with evidence of hematoma, but atypical of simple intracerebral hemorrhage (Fig. 6.6, **B** and **C**).

Angio. Right carotid angiography demonstrated a moderate-sized, smoothly rounded mass with a peripheral zone of considerably increased vascularity above the posterior two-thirds of the depressed Sylvian triangle. There was rapid filling of an ascending parietal vein from the tumor circulation (Fig. 6.6A).

Operation. Partial excisional biopsy of a cystic tumor through a small corticetomy (Dr. Robert Crowell). A sphere of old blood clot was present in the deeper portions of the mass, partly surrounded on the lateral and anterolateral aspects by a space containing 10 ml of xanthochromic and viscid fluid, and multiple small grey areas of gritty tissue containing thrombosed veins at the outer rim.

Histology. Glioblastoma.

A. Right carotid angiogram, lateral projection, late arterial

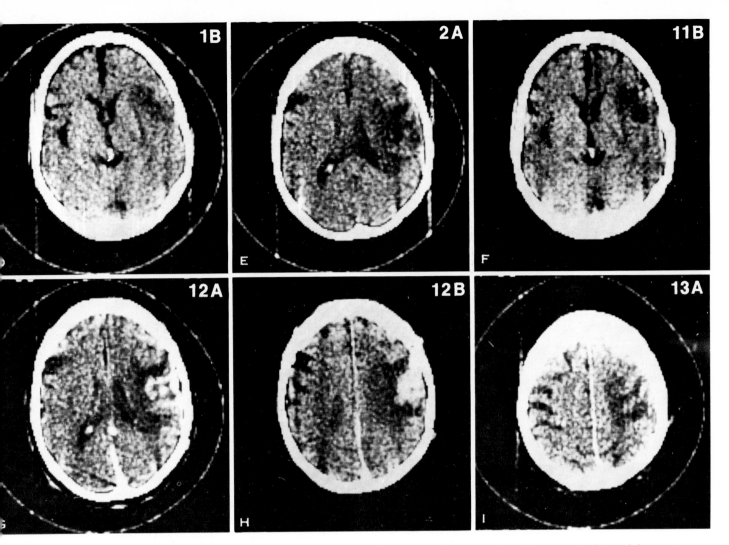

phase. The ovoid mass, with a well-vascularized periphery, is shown immediately above the depressed posterior two-thirds of the Sylvian triangle (*small arrows*). There is rapid filling of a superficial parietal vein by shunting through the tumor vessels.
B and **C**. Two adjacent 13-mm CT sections.
B. Section at the level of the frontal horns and trigones. A rounded area of high absorption (20–38) is shown in the region of the insula, extending to the lateral superior region of the putamen. Immediately lateral and anteriolateral to this is an irregular region of abnormally low density (5–14). It was tempting to diagnose this as a hematoma with associated edema, particularly in view of the history of hypertension. However, there is no suggestion of abnormally low absorption adjacent to the medial and posteromedial aspects of the hematoma. This suggested the possibility of hemorrhage into a metastatic tumor. The septum pellucidum and third ventricle are slightly displaced to the left, and there is some compression of the right ventricular trigone.
C. In this succeeding section just above **B**, the blood clot shows a larger and oval configuration. The low absorption abnormality laterally is still visible and again extends to the subcortical level. The two components have the same absorption values as in the section shown in **B**. Just medial to the blood clot is an area of lesser absorption representing a portion of the right lateral ventricle. A definitive CT scan diagnosis was not reached before the angiogram was obtained very shortly after. The combined CT scan and angiographic findings strongly suggested the diagnosis of hemorrhage into a neoplasm, and metastatic melanoma was thought to be the most likely diagnosis at this point. This unusual case serves to illustrate

an important advantage of angiography in determining anatomical localization. It was clear from angiography that the mass lay in an expanded portion of the frontoparietal operculum, depressing the Sylvian triangle. This particular feature could not be identified from the CT scan.
D–I. 160 x 160 matrix system. CT scan obtained 9 months following surgery and subsequent radiation therapy. The patient had recently experienced twitching of the left upper lip and some malaise.
D and **E**. Sections at levels similar to those in **B** and **C** before injection of contrast medium. A quite extensive area of diminished absorption (8–18) is shown in the lateral portion of the right frontal lobe, extending into the parietal lobe. There is a suggestion of nodularity in the lateral portion of the lesion in **B**. There is slight mass effect, evidenced by sharpening of the right frontal horn and minimal displacement of the septum lucidum and third ventricle to the left.
F–I. Sequential sections from below superiorly following injection of 300 ml of 30% meglumine diatrizoate. A very irregular nodular lesion has become densely enhanced (18–48). Irregular areas of lesser absorption are distributed within the main nodular mass and irregular smaller nodules are visible adjacent to the main mass. A large, irregularly marginated zone of decreased absorption extends medially to the lateral wall of the right lateral ventricle. This zone is evidently edematous, but probably contains foci of nodular and infiltrating tumor. *Although this patient had been operated upon and had received radiation therapy, the CT pattern exhibited is one form of characteristic pattern seen in glioblastomas ab initio.*

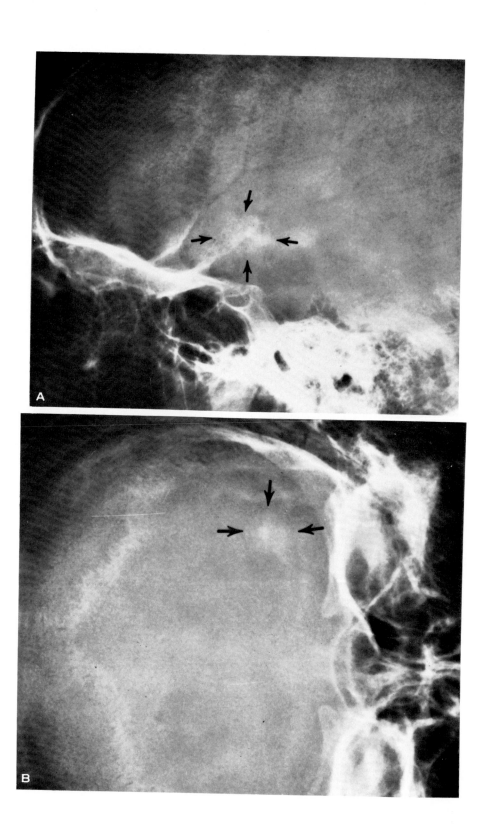

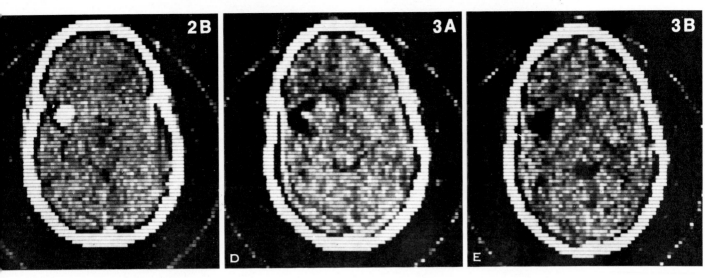

FIG. 6.7. ASTROCYTOMA, GRADE I

Clinical Features. A 14 y.o. male with recurrent psychomotor seizures for 4 years, starting with an abnormal taste in the mouth, followed by a tonic phase, involving twisting of the right side of the face. He heard everything said during attacks but could not respond. The attacks lasted ½ to 2 minutes and had been rather poorly controlled by medication.

Neurological Examination. Normal.

EEG. Bilateral temporal sharp waves, greater on the left side.

Skull Examination. Granular and nodular amorphous calcification in an ovoid region, measuring approximately 1.8 x 1.5 x 1.5 cm in the area of the left insula (Fig. 6.7, **A** and **B**).

RN Scan. Tcp, 1 year earlier, normal. Tcd scan within 1 week of CT showed no definite abnormality, although there was questionable, borderline increased activity in the temporal area, seen only in the left lateral view.

CT Scan. Abnormal, with obvious left anterior insular area lesion containing calcification (Fig. 6.7, **C–E**).

Angio. Left carotid angiography with internal and external injections revealed a small rounded, somewhat vascularized, mass lying in and just deep to the insula in the region of the corpus striatum. The insular vessels were displaced slightly laterally and the lenticulostriate vessels slightly medially. The latter vessels appeared irregular and very slightly enlarged. The Sylvian triangle was slightly elevated and there was spreading apart of anterior insular branches. There was an early draining vein that appeared to be an uncal vein draining to the region of the cavernous sinus. The midline was not dislocated and ventricular size appeared normal. There was no contribution from the external carotid circulation.

Diagnosis. Probable low-grade glioma.

Operation. (Dr. Paul Chapman). An incision was made in the superior temporal gyrus and a dense mass in the insula and lateral putamen was excised, with the area of calcification. *No cyst was identified.* The tumor extended medially from the resection margin for a distance that could not be determined at surgery.

Histology. Astrocytoma, Grade I.

A and **B.** Lateral and frontal skull films. The high resolution and relative insensitivity of absorption recording of the standard skull radiograph brings out details of texture in calcifications that are extremely useful in diagnosis (*arrows*). Conversely, the sensitivity and rather poor resolution of the CT scan causes the calcification to appear completely homogeneous, which obviates any attempt to derive a more specific diagnosis from the appearance of this feature. While the radiographic appearance of the calcification does not by any means exclude other possibilities, it suggests the probability of a low-grade glioma.

Markedly diminished absorption, similar to that of CSF (0–12), consistent with a cystic fluid-filled space that may represent a locally dilated portion of the Sylvian cistern or a cystic component of the mass (**D** and **E**). There is no visible compression or displacement of the lateral ventricles. The third ventricle is hardly visible but does not appear displaced.

CT Scan, C, D, and E. An approximately 2-cm, roughly spherical mass with absorption characteristics indicative of calcification (peak value, 230) was demonstrated immediately adjacent to and above the left sphenoid ridge (**C**). Around the calcific mass, especially superiorly, is a crescentic broad zone of **C**. Maximum dimension of the calcification in the anterior insular region is shown in this section, which is just below the frontal horns. A narrow vertical dark band is present posterior to the calcification, probably representing a minimally enlarged left temporal horn.

D. A 13-mm section immediately above that in **C**. Only the apex of the calcification is visible, and the low absorption space is much larger at this level. The absorption range of this space is too low, and it is too sharply marginated for it to be accepted as edema. There are some irregular areas of suspiciously high absorption immediately posterior to the frontal horn, between it and the nodular calcification.

E. The section immediately above that in **D** is above the nodular calcification and shows the large cystic-appearing space very clearly. Just medial to its anterior portion are some small islands of somewhat greater density than expected in normal corpus striatum.

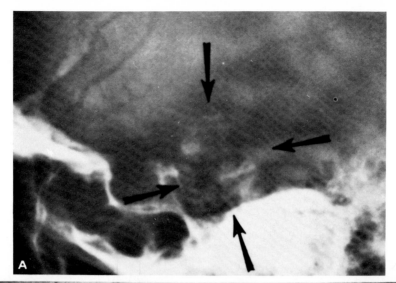

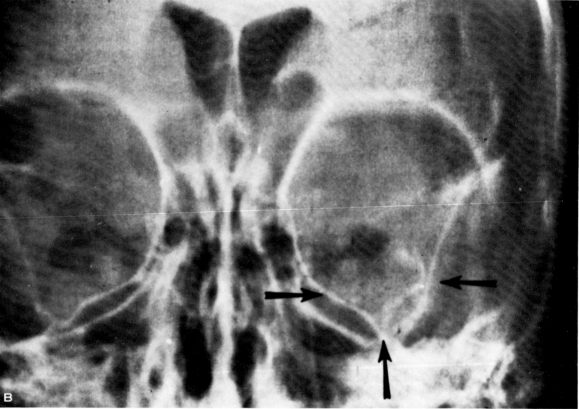

FIG. 6.8. Astrocytoma.

Clinical Features. A 22 y.o. female with a 7 year history of temporal lobe seizures, recently with grand mal seizures associated with unpleasant smell. Recent increase in seizure frequency and poor seizure control by medication.

Skull Examination. Linear and amorphous low-density calcification in a 2-cm area of the temporal lobe, extending to a point approximately 4.5 cm behind the anterior wall of the middle fossa, was demonstrated in 1968. By 1974, there had been a slight but distinct increase in extent of the calcification (Fig. 6.8A).

Angio. A left carotid angiogram in 1968 showed no definite abnormality, but there was a slight appearance of stretching of the anterior choroidal artery and a somewhat higher than usual inferior aspect of the Sylvian triangle, suggesting a temporal lobe mass effect.

PEG. In 1968, there was no general mass effect, but a few mm medial and very slight superior displacement of the temporal horn was demonstrated, with calcification extending to the surface of the temporal horn laterally and inferiorly (Fig. 6.8B).

CT Scan. In 1974, obvious temporal lobe lesion, containing calcification (Fig. 6.8, C–F).

Operation. (Dr. William H. Sweet) Through a cortical incision in the middle temporal gyrus extending to 5 cm behind the temporal tip, a grey and soft, deep-reddish obvious neoplasm was found extending well beyond the granular calcification, which was readily identified. A reddish soft nodule of tumor extending posterior to the limit of the cortical incision was seen through the operative microscope, and it was suspected that malignant glioma extended beyond the boundary of the excision. Exploration extended to the posterior portion of the floor of the middle fossa and the adjacent portion of the tentorium. There was suspicion of medial extension of the tumor beyond the limits of excision.

Histology. Microscopy indicated astrocytoma Grade II, but at surgery it was suspected that areas beyond the excision were more malignant.

A. Lateral skull projection. Amorphous and nodular calcification is shown in the temporal lobe (*arrows*). The appearance is strongly suggestive of a glioma.

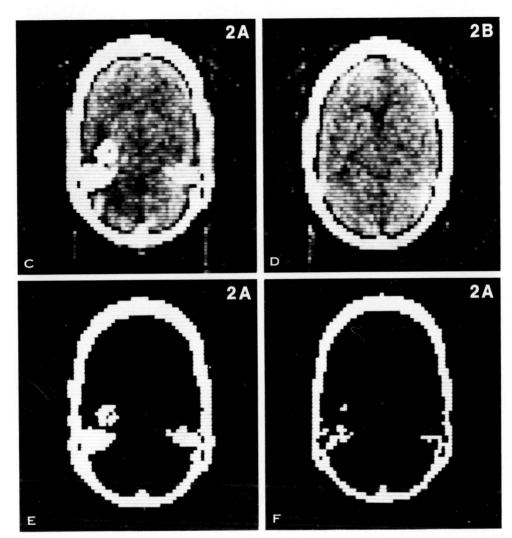

B. Pneumoencephalogram, obtained 6 years before operation, shows the relationship of the area of temporal lobe calcification (*arrows*) to the deformed and displaced temporal horn. The texture of the calcification is informative, suggesting a glioma, whereas the higher sensitivity of the CT scan in detecting calcification results in almost homogeneous and virtually featureless representation of the region containing calcification.
C and **D.** L 15   W 20.
The rounded homogeneous appearance of the calcification, which measures 7 matrix squares in diameter ($7 \times 3 = 21$ mm), is shown. There is a narrow rim of abnormally low density bounding the lateral aspect of region of calcification, and a broad vertical zone of reduced density extends anteriorly in the temporal lobe. The region of calcification shows a peak absorption of 165. The adjacent low absorption region measured in the range 4–16, consistent with tumor tissue. It should be noted that the absorption values measured in the region immediately adjacent to high absorption calcification are almost certainly factitiously low, due to the high absorption gradient between this zone and the calcification.

D. A 13-mm section immediately superior to that in **C.** A very small partial volume of the calcification is barely detectable. Small irregular areas of abnormally low absorption are shown extending for a distance of approximately 16 mm deeply from the subjacent calcification and a few millimeters posteriorly. This could be due to edema peripheral to the tumor, but the irregular configuration strongly suggests that this represents medial and posterior infiltration of neoplasm. In the case of an avascular neoplasm such as this, angiography is inadequate to reveal such important details.
E. L 40   W M.
These viewer control settings provided demonstration of the maximum extent of the region of calcification.
F. L 160   W M.
This setting is close to the upper limit of the absorption of the densest portion of the calcification, which is shown as a small white area slightly anterior to the density of the petrous pyramid.

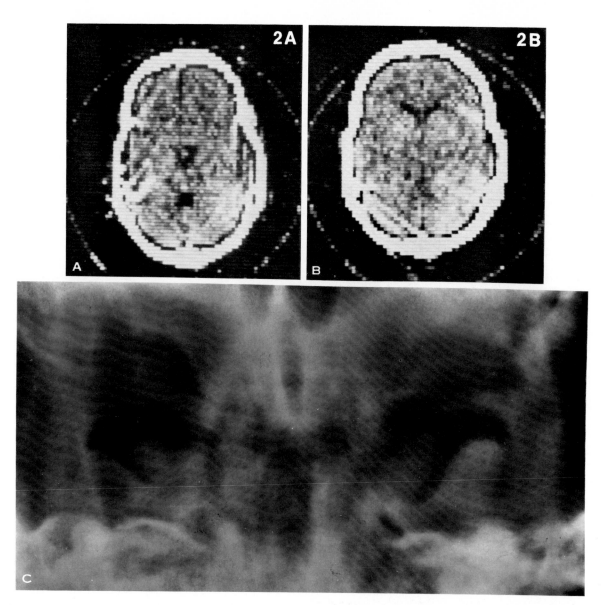

FIG. 6.9. Glioma.

Clinical Features. A 45 y.o. man with a 3 year history of temporal lobe seizures.

Skull Examination. Normal.

RN Scan. Tcp, normal.

CT Scan. Two examinations at an interval of 5 months revealed no convincing evidence of abnormality (Fig 6.9, **A** and **B**).

Angio. Left carotid angiogram, interpreted as probably normal.

PEG. An exceptional prominence of the collateral eminence on the left side, associated with a stretched, elongated appearance of the anterior portion of the temporal horn and additional subtle appearances of distortion of the temporal horn, were interpreted as probably representative of a temporal lobe mass, in spite of the fact that there was no change in the findings on repeat PEG 5 months later (Fig.6.9C).

Operation. Dr. William H. Sweet. An en bloc medial temporal lobectomy was carried out.

Histology. No histological abnormality was identified in the portion of the resected specimen subjected to neuropathological examination by light microscopy. However, tissue culture from an adjacent portion of the specimen resulted in growth of cells, 41% of which were multinucleated and which, on electron microscopy, continued many 90–100 Ångström glial-type fibrils. The cells have continued to grow in a rapid and vigorous fashion, more compatible with tumor than with normal brain (Dr. Paul L. Kornblith).

A and **B.** Two contiguous 13-mm sections. No good evidence of abnormal absorption values is detected in the region of the left temporal lobe. Artifacts are present in both temporal areas in **A**, more prominently on the right side. One could question the configuration of the suprasellar cisterns in **A**. There may be a slight encroachment on the left side, but this was not considered to be adequate evidence of abnormality. The area of density in the central portion of the suprasellar cisterns is believed to represent the hypophyseal stalk and possibly a portion of the optic chiasm. *It is possible that CT scans following intravenous injection of contrast medium would have provided evidence of neoplasm.*

C. A brow-up pneumoencephalogram, showing a configuration of the left temporal horn, which, together with additional minor deformities of the temporal horn shown on polytomography, was interpreted as indicating a temporal lobe mass lesion.

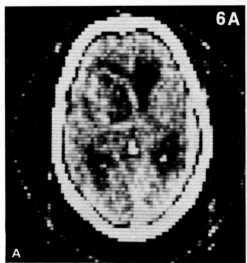
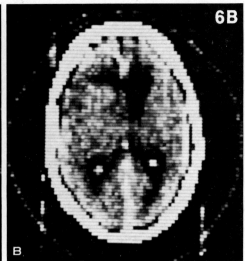

Fig. 6.10. Glioma of mixed cell type; features of astrocytoma and oligodendroglioma, Grade II–III.

Clinical Features. A 45 y.o. male with a 1 month history of personality changes and more recent slowing of gait, movements, and speech, with marked memory impairment; known to have hypertension for the past 5 years, well controlled on medication. Malignant tumor of bladder resected 5 years ago.

Neurological Examination. Moderately disoriented; thinking and speech slow and hesitant. Inappropriate affect and gross memory impairment. Bilateral papilledema with some hemorrhages. Apart from a suggestion of slight weakness of right upper extremity, motor system normal. Sensory examination normal. Cerebellar tests normal except for slight dysmetria on finger to nose testing. Provisional clinical diagnosis, anterior midline tumor with increased intracranial pressure.

Skull Examination. Normal.

RN Scan. Obtained at another center; showed large area of increased activity in the suprasellar region.

CT Scan. Striking abnormality (Fig. 6.10).

Angio. Bilateral carotid study showed a markedly vascular lesion in the deep left frontal region, involving the basal ganglia and anterior thalamus, with premature venous filling. The tumor vessels were fed principally from the lenticulostriate arteries and it was noted that peripheral vascularity was considerably more than the central, raising suspicion of a cystic lesion. Ventricular dilatation and 5-mm dislocation of the internal cerebral vein to the right were noted. Conclusion: probable glioblastoma.

Operation. (Dr. Robert Ojemann.) Left frontal craniotomy, with subtotal removal of malignant glioma. Large hemorrhage found in the deep portion of the tumor, extending into the deep portions of the corpus striatum. Anteromedial left frontal lobectomy performed.

Histology. Moderately soft homogeneous focally ecchymotic

tumor fragments; glioma of mixed cell type, with features of astrocytoma and oligodendroglioma, Grade II–III.

A and B. CT scans following intravenous injection of 50 ml of Hypaque 60, showing a large oval mass extending from the compressed left frontal horn, posteriorly to the region of the thalamus and measuring approximately 5.5 × 5.0 cm.

A. L 16   W 20.

The mass shows a 6- to 9-mm rim of greater density (19–30) than much of the central region (10–16). The peripheral denser rim was visible on the plain CT scan, but there was a significant increase in density following contrast injection, consistent with a moderate degree of vascularity. The more central absorption values showed no apparent increase following contrast injection. The lateral portions of the central areas of the mass showed heterogeneous intermediate absorption values.

B. Scan section immediately superior to that in **A**, showing moderate ventricular dilatation due to obstruction in the region of the foramina of Munro and/or anterior third ventricle. The section includes the superior pole of the central mass, indicated as an area of moderately increased density in the area of the head of the caudate nucleus and anterior portion of corpus striatum. This represents the superior segment of the more vascular tumor periphery, and a zone of diminished absorption situated lateral to this may represent edema rather than tumor. CT diagnosis was neoplasm, with glioblastoma more probable than a very large metastatic neoplasm. Absorption values suggest areas of necrosis centrally, without gross cyst formation. No obvious cystic formation was noted at surgery. The scan does not show gross hemorrhage, although some of the higher absorption values within the lateral portion of the denser rim may represent areas of hemorrhagic extravasation. Presumably the major hemorrhage noted in the tumor at surgery had occurred in the 2-day interval between scan and operation.

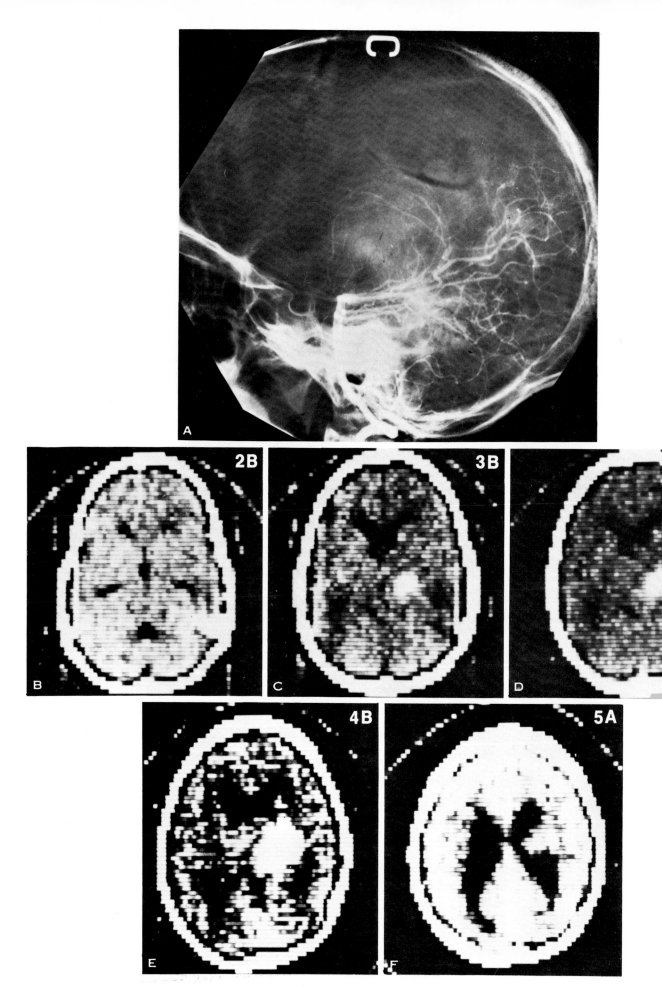

FIG. 6.11. Glioma (not histologically verified).
Clinical Features. A 7 y.o. boy, with a 2 months history of lethargy, 1 month of progressive left hemiparesis, and bilateral chronic ear infection, with drainage from the right ear.
Skull Examination. Normal except for lack of aeration of the right mastoid, without bone destruction.
RN Scan. Tcp, dynamic and static; equivocal. Suspicion of increased uptake right temporoparietal, seen only in right lateral view.
CT Scan. With contrast enhancement only (20 ml Hypaque 60); obvious abnormality (Fig. 6.11, **B–F**).
Angio. Transfemoral selective right internal carotid and vertebral study. Internal cerebral vein displaced 0.5 cm to left, with midline anterior cerebral artery branches. Anterior choroidal artery displaced inferiorly in the posterior part of its course. Similar displacement of basal vein of Rosenthal. Posterior and lateral displacement of the posterior choroidal vessels, which were hypertrophied. Thalamoperforating and posterior choroidal arteries large and stretched and distorted by mass. No definite tumor circulation identified. Findings consistent with a deep-seated right thalamic space-occupying lesion, most likely a tumor (Fig. 6.11A).
A. Vertebral angiogram, right lateral projection in the early arterial phase. Depression and flattening of the posterior cerebral arteries. Stretching and disorganization of the thalamoperforating branches and of the medial and lateral posterior choroidal branches by a thalamic area mass without definite tumor circulation. (Courtesy of Dr. Roy Strand, Children's Hospital Medical Center, Boston, Massachusetts).

B–F. A series of 8-mm thick CT sections obtained following intravenous injection of 20 ml of Hypaque.
B. L 10   W 20.
This section is below the level of the lesion and is virtually normal.
C. L 16   W 20.   D. L 18   W 20.
These contiguous sections reveal a rounded area of high density (13–30) occupying the region of the right thalamus and adjacent structures. The more posterior portions of the third ventricle are compressed.
E. L 15   W 5.
This section is immediately above the level shown in **D** and shows the maximum horizontal dimensions of the lesion that extends to the region of the caudate nucleus anteriorly, to the trigone posteriorly, and slightly across the midline at the level of the suprapineal recess medially. Absorption values at this level were also 13–30.
F. L 11   W 10.
This section demonstrates considerable encroachment by the vascular mass upon the posterior potion of the body of the right lateral ventricle. *Information obtainable regarding the nature of the mass from the CT scan alone is limited by the absence of a plain CT scan. Under these circumstances it is not possible to differentiate between a bascularized lesion and one consisting largely of extravasated blood.* In other anatomical sites, the possibility of a mass containing diffuse psammomatous calcification would also have to be considered.

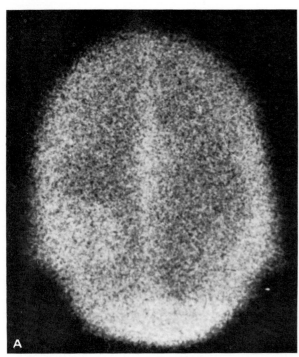

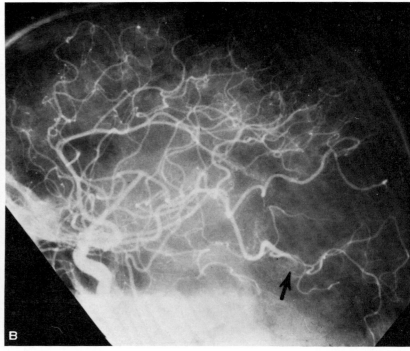

FIG. 6.12. Glioblastoma.

Clinical Features. A 67 y.o. female with a two months history of progressive difficulty with word finding and memory. Neurological examination revealed moderate posterior type of dysphasia, with dyscalculia and dyslexia. No definite visual field defect. Carcinoma of the breast was diagnosed in 1954 and treated by radical mastectomy and radiotherapy, without evidence of recurrence.

EEG. Intermittent left temporal slowing.

Skull Examination. Essentially normal.

RN Scan. Tcp; large area of increased activity in left parietal region, suggesting malignant glioma (Fig. 6.12**A**).

Angio. Left percutaneous carotid study. Abnormalities suggesting either infarct or neoplasm in retrosylvian area (Fig. 6.12**B**).

PEG. Multiple abnormalities, suggesting cavitating neoplasm or infarction (Fig. 6.12**C**).

Operation. (Dr. William H. Sweet.) Biopsy of what appeared to be an area of hemorrhage and infarction from the region just above the higher of two large angular branches of the middle cerebral artery (Fig. 6.12**F**).

Histology. No evidence of neoplasm; hemorrhagic white matter, probably representing infarction.

Tissue Culture. Growth of multinucleate large cells, characteristic of malignant glioma. Review of biopsy specimen; confirmed diagnosis of malignant glioma. RN and CT scans, angio, and PEG were all performed within an 8-day period.

A. Tcp static scan, vertex view. There is a large circumscribed rounded area of considerably increased activity superiorly in the left parieto-occipital region.

B. Left carotid angiogram, lateral view in arterial phase. Separation and distortion of the angular and posterior temporal branches of the middle cerebral artery, indicating a mass lesion in the retrosylvian area. Moderately severe stenosis is present

distally in the posterior temporal artery (*arrow*). Initially, the findings were thought to favor the diagnosis of infarction rather than neoplasm.

C. PEG; lateral erect film. Slight diffuse mass effect in left parietal lobe area, with a few mm displacement of midline structures to the right. Cavities in the posterior superior frontal and in the parietal areas, lying superficially and filling with gas from the subarachnoid spaces, are shown (*1 and 2, arrow and arrowheads*). In the parietal cavity, a smooth convex nodule of tissue projects into the cavity from the posterior aspect (*arrowheads*). The findings suggested cavitating neoplasm or infarction.

D. L 22   W M.

This was the fifth clinical CT scan in the MGH series. Obvious large area of abnormality in the left parieto-occipital region. CT scan at 25° to RBL. A 13-mm section through the level of the pineal (central white rectangle that does not appear laterally displaced). Suspiciously high absorption values are noted in the region of the left thalamus and retrosplenial gyrus of the hippocampus.

E. L 16   W 20.

Third section above that shown in **D.** A relatively poorly marginated region of high absorption is shown extending to the cortical surface in the left parietal lobe in the region of the angular gyrus (*arrow*); absorption 18–32, consistent with hemorrhage. Extending anteriorly and medially from the dense area is an irregular zone of diminished density, approximately 8–18. A low absorption region on the left side anteriorly extends forward from the region of the precentral gyrus and corresponds with the area of cavitation, 1, shown in the PEG. Absorption values here were largely those of CSF. Diagnosis on the CT findings was infiltrating malignant glioma containing an area of hemorrhage and was made prior to angiography and PEG.

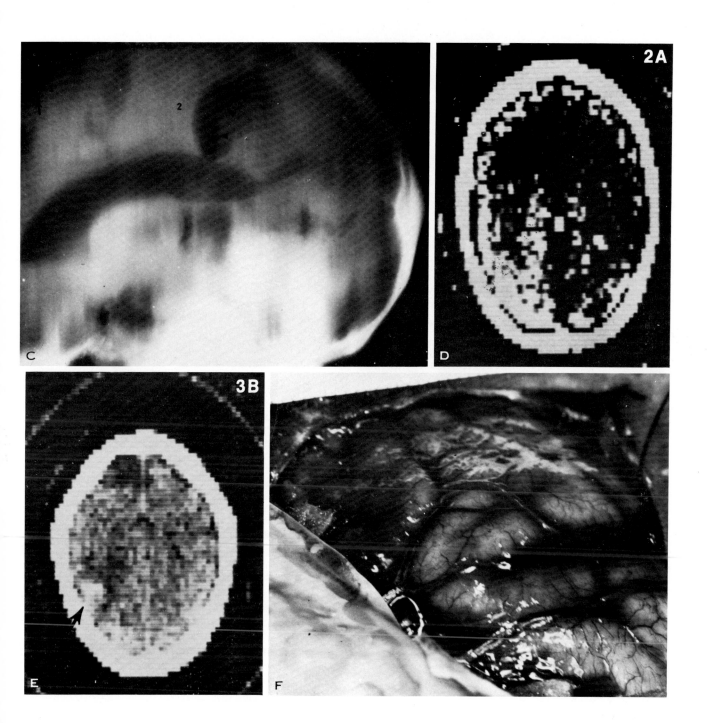

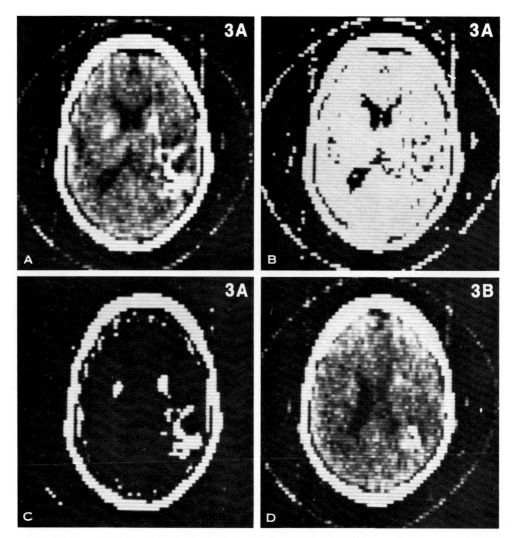

FIG. 6.13. Oligodendroglioma and idiopathic calcification of basal ganglia (not histologically verified).

Clinical Features. A 61 y.o. male. First grand mal seizure 17 years previously. Good seizure control with phenobarbital. Three year history of attacks of tingling and burning paresthesias in the left hand, extending up the arm to the left side and then to the left leg and foot.

Skull Examination. Increasing extent of serpiginous calcification in the right temporoparietal area over many years.

RN Scan. Mercury scan, normal.

CT Scan. Striking abnormalities (Fig. 6.13, **A**–**D**).

Angio. Right carotid study showed an avascular mass in the temporoparietal region.

No histological verification.

A. CT scan: L 15   W 20.

Extensive irregular calcification is present in the temporal and parietal lobes, with abnormally low absorption regions intermingled and extending well beyond the calcific zones. Immediately adjacent to the very dense calcification, the soft tissue readings were factitiously low, due to computer undershoot. Elsewhere, abnormal soft tissue readings ranged between 9 and 16. These abnormal readings extended to the region adjacent to the right frontal horn, which showed minor compression. There was more marked compression of the

region of the body and trigone of the right lateral ventricle. There was several mm displacement of the septum lucidum to the left, better shown in **B**. Dense islands of calcification were present in the caudate nuclei and putamina bilaterally, far more readily identified than on plain skull examination.

B. Same section as in **A**. L   12   W   M.

Small portions of the soft tissue components of the tumor are shown as black areas in the temporal and posterior corpus striatum regions. Compression of the right lateral ventricle and midline dislocation to the left are better demonstrated with these control settings.

C. L   24   W   M.

At these settings, the basal ganglionic calcification and irregular calcification in the tumor are shown white. A little of the denser cortex also remains white.

D. Section immediately above that in **A,** at the level of the bodies of the lateral ventricles. Further irregular calcification is present in the posterior parietal region. The superior extremity of the right caudate nucleus calcification is visible anteriorly adjacent to the lateral ventricle, which is generally slightly compressed. Quite extensive, poorly marginated, abnormally low absorption readings are shown between the lateral to these two calcific regions. Diagnosis is extensive oligodendroglioma and idiopathic calcification of basal ganglia.

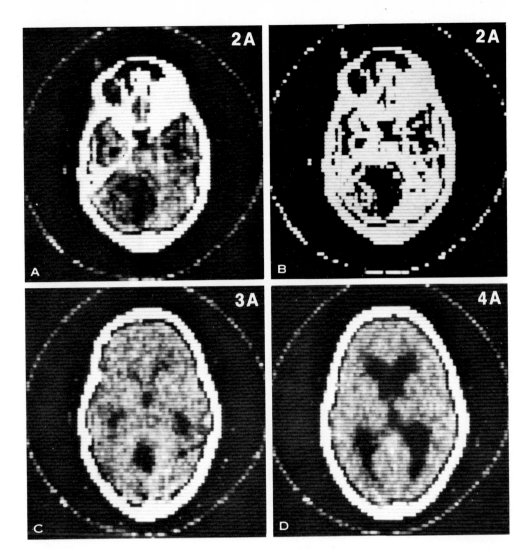

FIG. 6.14. Astrocytoma; cystic cerebellar, Grade I.

Clinical Features. A 7 y.o. girl, complaining of generalized headaches for 3 weeks and double vision for 1 week.

Neurological examination. Bilateral papilledema with punctate hemorrhages, bilateral sixth cranial nerve palsies, mild left facial weakness, generalized hypotonia, truncal ataxia, and instability of gait, with falling to the left.

RN Scan. Tcp; increased uptake in the anterior superior portion of posterior fossa, left side.

CT Scan. Extensive and striking abnormalities (Fig. 6.14, A–D).

Angio. Transfemoral left vertebral study. Evidence of a large avascular left cerebellar hemisphere mass, with stretching of hemispheric arterial branches and contralateral displacement of the vermian arteries. Considerable herniation of the tonsillar-hemispheric branches of the pica below the foramen magnum. Precentral vein displaced anteriorly. Diagnosis: a large avascular left cerebellar hemisphere mass with severe tonsillar herniation. Probable large tumor, likely cystic.

Operation. (Dr. Robert Crowell.) Following ventricular decompression by lateral ventricular catheter, radical and hopefully complete excision of a very large cystic tumor was performed. A large volume of yellowish viscid fluid, which did not clot on standing, was obtained from the cyst. On the left side, a nodular tumor mass projected into the cyst. Tumor tissue was noted peripherally around the cyst, which extended superiorly close to the superior aspect of the cerebellar hemisphere and tentorial margin.

Histology. Astrocytoma, Grade I.

A. CT scan. L   16   W 20.

The plane of scan extends from the region of the orbital roofs through the region near the top of the left petrous ridge. The head was canted slightly upwards on the left side. A large rounded area of diminished absorption (4–11) occupies almost all of the area of the left cerebellar hemisphere and bulges 12–15 mm to the right of the midline. The anteroposterior diameter of the cyst measures 4.8 cm (16 matrix squares). A large nodule projects into the cyst cavity from the left side (11–14). (Reprinted by permission from Radiology, 114: January 1975.)

B. Same section as in **A.** L   13   W M.

High contrast settings to show the cyst contours and nodule. (Reprinted by permission from Radiology, 114: January 1975.)

C. Section 15 mm above **A** (sections 8 mm in thickness). L   15   W   20.

The section shows the inferior portions of the frontal horns, a widened anterior third ventricle, moderately dilated temporal horns, and the superior portion of the cerebellar cyst. Surrounding the cyst at this level is a broad zone of slightly increased tissue absorption that may represent compressed cerebral tissue rather than tumor. A repeat scan after intravenous injection of contrast medium would probably have differentiated, but it was not done. In both **A** and **C,** but more clearly visible in **A,** a 6- to 9-mm arcuate band of decreased absorption is shown adjacent to the anteromesial aspect of the cyst and is consistent with tumor tissue.

D. 13-mm section 8 mm above **C,** showing markedly dilated lateral and third ventricles. Trigone asymmetry is due to slight head tilting.

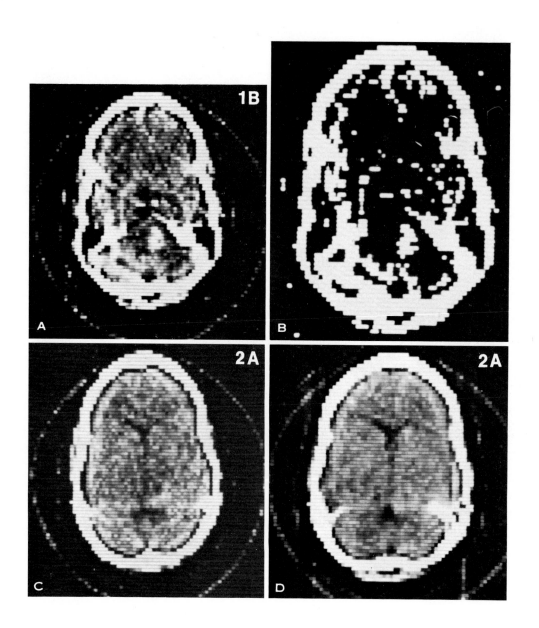

FIG. 6.15. Glioma of brain stem. No histological verification.
Clinical Features. A 35 y.o. female with a 2 months history of a progressive brain stem syndrome, including decreased hearing. Question of brain stem tumor versus multiple sclerosis.
Skull Examination. Normal.
RN Scan. Tcp; no evidence of posterior fossa mass.
CT Scan. Obvious abnormalities (Fig. 6.15, **A–C**).
Angio. Transfemoral vertebral study; findings equivocal, but somewhat suggestive of an avascular pontine mass.
PEG. There was very little enlargement of the anteroposterior diameter of the pons, but marked enlargement of its transverse diameter, indicating the presence of a neoplasm. The fourth ventricle was displaced posteriorly and to the left, with marked compression and indentation. Linear tomography used.
No histological verification. Patient treated with radiation and chemotherapy, with marked improvement.
Second CT Scan. Five months after the first; showed a reduction in size of both the increased and decreased absorption portions of the lesion, with some lowering of the remaining absorption values in the pons. There was an irregular nodule approximately 1 cm in diameter in the right paramedian pontine tegmentum and dorsal basis pontis, indenting the fourth ventricle slightly (Fig. 6.15**D**).
A. CT scan. L   16   W   20.
An oval area of increased absorption, 20–30, approximately

2.5 cm in maximum diameter, is shown in the pons, extending to the right from the midline. Surrounding this region is a poorly demarcated zone of lowered absorption (10–17). The fourth ventricle was not clearly identified, but there was a suggestion that it was compressed and displaced posteriorly and to the left. All scans in the supratentorial regions were normal in appearance.
B. L 22   W M.
Same section as in **A**. The dense area of the pontine lesion is more clearly shown. Densely compacted tissue with some hemorrhage is suggested by the absorption values. The surrounding absorption values are more consistent with tumor tissue than with edema.
C. Section immediately superior to that in **A**. The zone of decreased absorption (10–16), extending bilaterally across the pons, is seen more clearly (part of this is the fourth ventricle). The normal-sized ventricles are seen anteriorly.
D. Section from CT scan obtained 5 months later, following radiation and chemotherapy. Comparison with scans at all levels showed that the lateral and third ventricles were slightly larger than before, but still within normal limits. The fourth ventricle is now clearly identified and appears very slightly indented on the right side, and displaced slightly to the left. Both the high- and low-density components of the lesion are smaller in extent, particularly the high-density component.

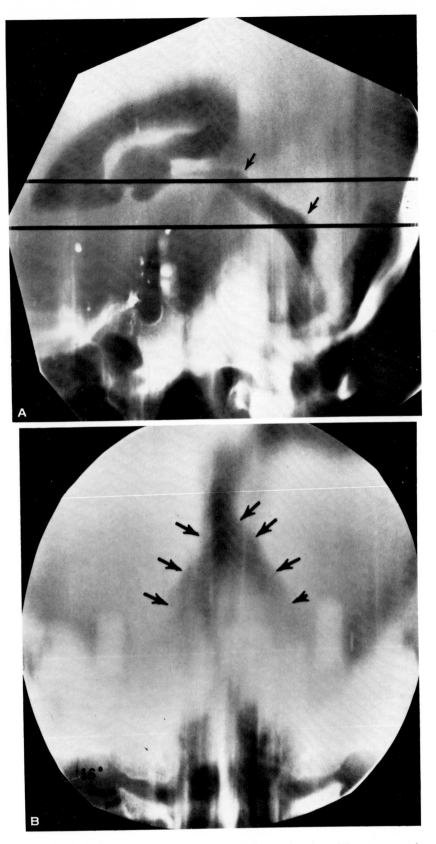

FIG. 6.16. Pontine glioma, histologically verified.

Clinical Features. A 7 y.o. girl in whom a pontine glioma was diagnosed 2 years previously. Following radiation therapy with 4500 rads she improved, then again deteriorated and was treated with an additional 1500 rads and methyltrexate, with improvement again.

Neurological Examination. Right sixth nerve paresis and paresis of right arm and leg.

Skull Examination. Considerable scattered Pantopaque in the subarachnoid spaces.

CT Scan. A series of 4 scans was abnormal (Fig. 6.16, **C–F**).

PEG. Obtained 3 days after the fourth CT scan. Evidence of an extensive brain stem mass that had extended to the cerebellar vermis (Fig. 6.16, **A** and **B**).

Operation. (Dr. William H. Sweet.) Following ventriculoatrial shunting, suboccipital craniectomy, with aspiration of a tiny cyst in the floor of the fourth ventricle and biopsy of solid tumor in the pons; decompression using pericranial graft in dura. Little indication of tumor in the cerebellum was noted at surgery. A suspicious-appearing area under the operative microscope in

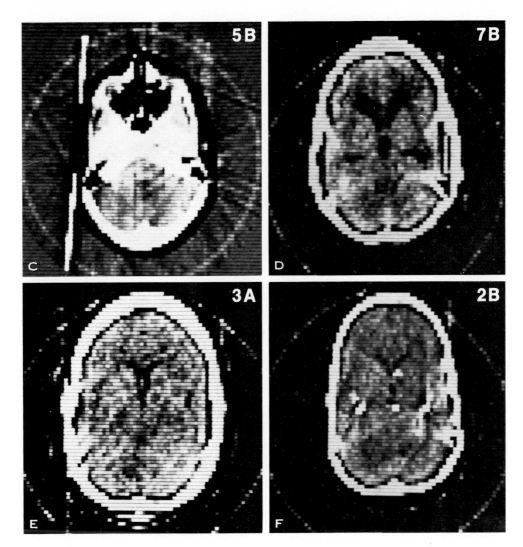

the medial aspect of the left cerebellar hemisphere at the upper end of the vallecula was biopsied, but this was reported as showing no neoplasm on histological examination.

Histological Diagnosis. Tissue culture of the biopsy of solid tumor in the floor of the fourth ventricle resulted in growth of a modest number of multinucleated giant cells, characteristic of astrocytic malignant tumor. The majority of the cells in the culture appeared to be relatively normal-appearing astrocytes. This picture was considered to be compatible with astrocytoma of intermediate grade (Dr. Paul Kornblith).

A and B. Lateral and frontal PEG laminographic projections obtained 3 days after the last CT scan, which is shown in **F.** The two *horizontal lines* in **A** show the upper and lower boundaries of the CT section illustrated in **E.** There is stretching and posterosuperior displacement of the aqueduct and fourth ventricle by a mass extending from the midbrain caudally to include the medulla. The greatly elongated fourth ventricle is indented posteriorly (between the *arrows*), indicating extension of tumor to the superior vermis. Pontine cistern is markedly compressed. There are Pantopaque residues in suprasellar region and temporal horn. **B** shows stretching of the fourth ventricle transversely, with slight displacement to the left (*arrows*).

C. Initial CT scan at approximately 0° to RBL, showing an appearance of compression of the pontine and CT angle cisterns. Irregular areas of greater and lesser density than normal are distributed through the area of the pons. The fourth ventricle is difficult to see and appears compressed and displaced posteriorly.

D. Approximately 1 month later. Higher scan section than in

C. Considerable ventricular dilatation had developed in the interval. Decreased absorption values were distributed through the brain stem and there was suspicion of a slight decrease in absorption in the central portions of the left cerebellar hemisphere.

E. Further CT scan at a similar level to that in **D** following ventricular shunting. The lateral and third ventricles are now close to normal in size for the age, but there is clear indication of pathologically reduced absorption values through the brain stem, left cerebellar hemisphere, and region of the vermis.

F. Scan at a similar level to that in **E** 6 months after the scan shown in **C** and 3 days before the PEG shown in **A** and **B.** The lateral and third ventricles are normal in size. The small area of marked density in the region of the right frontal horn represents the tip of a ventricular shunt tube. Densities in the left temporal region are due to Pantopaque droplets. There is now a widespread zone of abnormally low absorption (8–14) involving the brain stem, much of the left cerebellar hemisphere, vermis, and medial portion of the right cerebellar hemisphere. The full intracerebellar extent of the tumor is more clearly revealed than in the PEG. The latter shows evidence of extension of the tumor to the superior vermis (indentation in roof of fourth ventricle between the two *arrows* in **A**). CT studies in brain stem gliomas are frequently very difficult to interpret, mainly due to the artifacts that commonly obscure details and render difficult reliable absorption measurements here. *Additional scans after high-dose intravenous contrast medium injection may be very useful in differentiating tumor extension and reactive edema.*

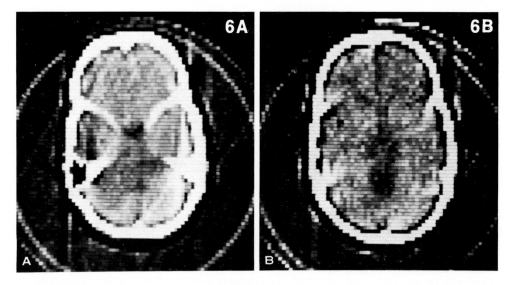

FIG. 6.17

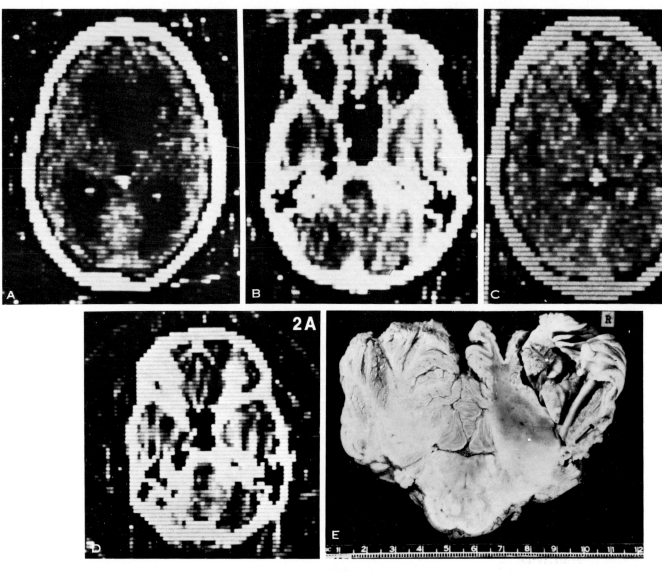

FIG. 6.18

FIG. 6.17. Glioma, extensively involving the brain stem and extending to the thalami.
Clinical Features. An 8 y.o. boy with complaints of loss of balance and diplopia for 6 months.
CT Scan. Abnormal (Fig. 6.17, **A** and **B**).
PEG. Marked enlargement of the brain stem, with greatly indented and posterosuperiorly displaced fourth ventricle. The fourth ventricle was also slightly displaced to the right.
Histology. Not obtained to date.
A and **B**. Eight-mm CT sections.
A. W 40.   **B.** W 20.
The CP angle, pontine, and interpeduncular cisterns are obviously compressed. In **A**, a small fourth ventricle is shown to be displaced posteriorly and to the right. Extending anteriorly and to the left from the fourth ventricle is a fairly homogeneous, very widespread zone of diminished absorption (8–11), involving the anterior half of the left cerebellar hemisphere and the entire region of the pons. CSF in the anterior portion of the suprasellar cisterns is shown between the anterior clinoid processes. The midbrain evidently bulges anteriorly to obliterate the interpeduncular cistern.
B. Eight-mm section immediately above that in **A**. A patchy zone of diminished absorption (8–11) is shown extending upwards from the region of the midbrain into the inferior portion of each thalamus.

FIG. 6.18. Glioblastoma, widely involving both cerebellar hemispheres and extending to the brain stem.
Clinical Features. A 77 y.o. female who had become progressively and severely depressed since her husband's death 6 months earlier. She developed unsteadiness of gait, tending to fall backwards. Two months earlier, she slipped and fractued her left hip. She had recently been partially disoriented and withdrawn. Her handwriting deteriorated, her affect flat, and her speech barely audible. She had episodic urinary incontinence.
Neurologic Examination. Examination was difficult. Snout and grasp reflexes were present. Speech was slow. General motor and sensory examinations were within normal limits. The provisional clinical diagnosis was probable normal pressure hydrocephalus, but with some question concerning senile dementia.
EEG. Generalized slowing, more prominent anteriorly than posteriorly.
Skull Examination. Normal.
RN Scan. Tcp, normal.
CT Scan. Abnormal (Fig. 6.18, **A–D**).
Lumbar Puncture. Opening pressure ?250/closing pressure 70; 0 cells, protein 38 mgm%, sugar 75 mgm%, cytology negative. Katzman infusion test was terminated after 20 minutes as the pressure exceeded 600, indicating a CSF absorption defect, consistent with normal pressure hydrocephalus.
Angio. Transfemoral carotid and left vertebral angiograms revealed marked lateral ventricular enlargement and were suggestive of an avascular posterior fossa mass.
In spite of the findings on two CT scans at a short interval, it was believed that the clinical features and other tests were so strongly indicative of nontumorous normal or near normal pressure hydrocephalus that a PEG should be avoided in this fragile elderly lady.
Operation. (Dr. William H. Sweet.) Right ventriculoatrial shunt. Three days postshunt personality improvement was noted, and, after 5 days, she was more alert with fluent speech. She was able to walk alone and writing improved. She expired two months later.

Histology. Autopsy revealed extensive glioblastoma involving both cerebellar hemispheres. A 3.5 x 3.0 cm area of cystic necrosis was present in the right cerebellar hemisphere. Infiltrating tumor extended widely, including involvement of the brain stem. Meningeal seeding was noted over the pons.
A and **B.** CT scans obtained before ventricular shunting.
A. Marked generalized enlargement of the lateral and third ventricles is shown. No focal abnormalities of absorption were demonstrated in the supratentorial portions of the brain.
B. Representative section through the posterior fossa. In spite of the marked enlargement of the lateral and third ventricles, the fourth ventricle *could not be identified*. A very widespread, irregularly marginated, low absorption lesion (8–15) was shown in the left cerebellar hemisphere, extending into the medial portion of the right cerebellar hemisphere.
These CT scan findings were interpreted as indicating an extensive cerebellar tumor, with obstructive hydrocephalus.
C and **D.** CT scans obtained shortly after ventriculoartrial shunting.
C. The high absorption region in the right frontal horn represents the tip of the shunt tube. This scan section is very similar in level and angle to that in **A**. Marked ventricular decompression has been achieved. The sylvian cisterns are now gaping.
D. The fourth ventricle was again not identified. A large area of markedly diminished absorption (approximately 3–10) is shown extending through the right cerebellar hemisphere from its posterior surface to the CP angle. Patchy areas of diminished absorption are shown in the region of the vermis. The findings were again indicative of an extensive neoplasm involving the cerebellum, but extensive artifacts are also apparent.
E. Autopsy section through the pons and cerebellum. The right cerebellar hemisphere is to the right in the photograph. The extensive involement of both cerebellar hemispheres by glioblastoma is shown. There is a large area of cystic necrosis involving much of the right cerebellar hemisphere and there is extension of tumor into the pons.

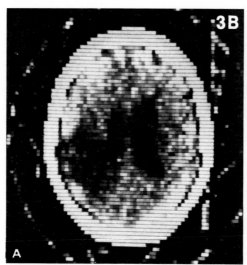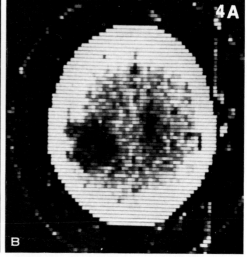

FIG. 6.19. Glioblastoma (not histologically verified).
Clinical Features. A 50 y.o. female. Four months before CT scan, a Tcp scan had revealed a large rounded area of increased activity with a "cold" central area in the left superior parietal region. Carotid angiography on the same day as the RN scan demonstrated a typical appearance of a very large and very vascular parieto-occipital malignant glioma. The patient was given radiotherapy (4000 rads to the whole brain and an additional 1500 rads tumor boost) without biopsy. CCNU chemotherapy was started approximately 10 weeks prior to CT scan.
A and **B**. L 14   W   20.
A large (9 cm diameter) irregularly rounded area of markedly

diminished absorption is shown in the parietal and temporal lobes, with extension into the occipital lobe on the left side. Absorption values through most of the region ranged from 2–12 in **A**, at the level of the bodies of the lateral ventricles, and 2–14 in **B**, the next section superiorly. Scattered small islands of density within the lesion measured approximately 23 laterally (in the abnormal cortical region) and 7–13 medially (in the abnormal centrum semiovale). There was little displacement of midline structures to the right, in spite of the massive size of the lesion. This feature and the very low absorption values through most of the lesion are consistent with considerable necrosis within the tumor, presumably induced by the combined therapy.

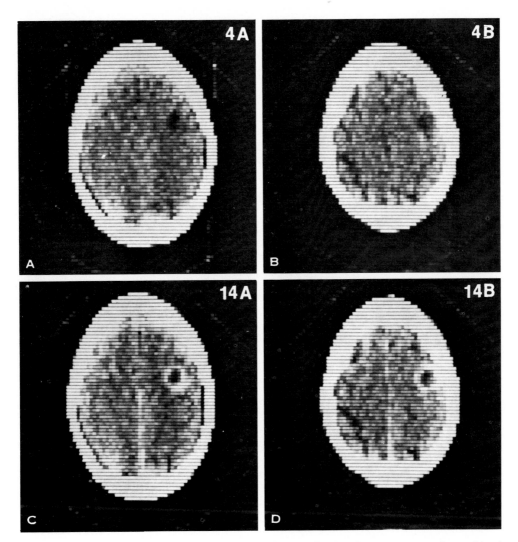

FIG. 6.20. Malignant glioma.

Clinical Features. A 52 y.o. man with focal motor seizures of 2 years duration involving the left corner of the mouth and the left hand.

Neurological Examination. Normal.

Skull Examination. Normal.

RN Scan. Normal.

Angio. Right carotid study 1½ years previously was normal, except for questionable slightly early filling of a parietal vein. Recent right carotid study showed subtle evidence of an avascular mass in the superior frontoparietal region without early venous filling.

PEG. Negative, 1½ years previously.

CT Scan. Abnormal (Fig. 6.20).

Operation. (Dr. J. Golden.) Resection of a right anterior superior parietal and posterior frontal tumor, containing cystic necrosis centrally.

Histology. Malignant glioma.

A and **B.** L 17   W 20.

Plain scan, showing a rounded 2.5-cm diameter zone of diminished absorption (7–14) in the anterior superior portion of the right parietal lobe. Lower sections (not shown) revealed a normal-appearing ventricular system with no midline dislocation.

C and **D.** Sections corresponding with those in **A** and **B** following intravenous infusion of 300 ml of Hypaque 30. A ring of increased absorption (16–31) is now present in the peripheral region of the previously entirely low-absorption abnormality. The center of the lesion remains of low density, consistent with central necrosis.

Peripheral venous blood samples obtained before and immediately after contrast infusion in this patient revealed an increase in blood absorption of 25 units (27 before injection and 52 after injection). As illustrated by this case, some neoplasms will increase markedly in absorption, even though they appear totally avascular on angiography. Although increased absorption following contrast injection may be identified on CT scans as a result of *intravascular* contrast medium when no opacification is visible on angiography, due to the greater sensitivity of CT, a marked increase in absorption on CT, with no visible tumor opacification on subtraction angiography, suggests that there has been *extravascular* diffusion of contrast medium into the neoplasm (see Chapter 27). The regularity of the ring of increased absorption in this case is somewhat unusual for glioma and is more suggestive of a metastasis with central necrosis or an abscess with a thick capsule (see Fig. 21.3).

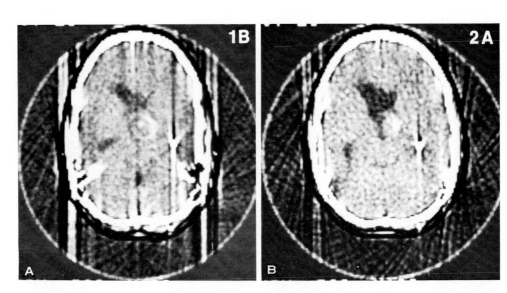

FIG. 6.21. Neoplasm of basal ganglia, probable glioma.
Clinical Features. A 14 y.o. girl with a history of headaches and vomiting of 15 days duration.
Neurological Examination. Severe bilateral papilledema was present. There were no localizing neurological signs.
EEG. Diffuse slow waves posteriorly.
Ventriculography and Pneumoencephalography. Asymmetrical dilatation of the lateral ventricles, left larger than right. Dilatation of the anterior portion of the third ventricle, the right wall of which was markedly indented by a mass that also bulged upwards into the right lateral ventricle at the level of the foramen of Munro. (Dr. Roy Strand, Children's Hospital Medical Center, Boston, Massachusetts.)
CT Scan. Abnormal (Fig. 6.21).
She was subsequently treated with radiation (5500 rads) to the area of tumor, in her home state.

Contiguous CT sections. 160 x 160 matrix system. Contrast enhancement with 40 ml of Hypaque 60 M only.
A. The lower section shows a 2.7-cm rounded mass that has a peripheral zone of increased absorption (23–37) that is broader laterally than medially. Within this peripheral zone is a region of absorption indistinguishable from that of white matter. A small, more central zone of increased absorption, similar to the peripheral zone, is visible.
A and **B.** The mass indents the lateral wall of the third ventricle, which is displaced to the left, and bulges into the right lateral ventricle in the region of the foramen of Munro. The right lateral ventricle had been decompressed (high absorption consistent with metal in the posterior portion of the right temporal horn, with accompanying vertical band artifacts). This study was obtained two weeks after the pneumogram.

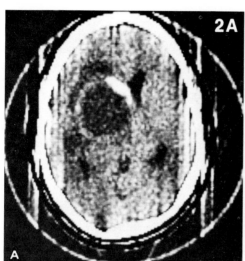 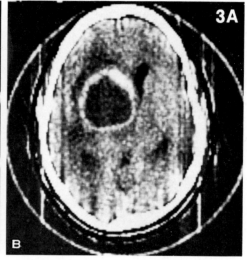

FIG. 6.22. Cystic astrocytoma, Grade III–IV. (Case contributed by Dr. Jeffrey Gawler, National Hospital, Queen Square, London, England.)

Clinical Features. A 44 y.o. male with a 3 month history of somnolence. He had a head injury 6 days before admission and there was a 3 day history of headache, vomiting, and right-sided weakness.

Neurological Examination. Bilateral papilledema, dysphasia, and right hemiparesis.

CT Scan. Abnormal (Fig. 6.22).

Angio. A left carotid study revealed a large deep left frontal mass lesion, with a very narrow but moderately intense capillary blush that outlined a large, apparently cystic, mass lesion.

Operation. A large cystic malignant astrocytoma was identified. There was an entrapped hematoma in the left frontal horn.

A. Plain scan. **B.** Scan following intravenous injection of 40 ml of Conray 60. L 13   W   30   160 x 160 matrix system.

A. The wall of the cystic mass is visible as a faint ring, with average density of 15 units, 4–6 mm in thickness and 5.3 cm in diameter. Absorption within the ring is quite homogeneous and a few units higher than that of CSF. A peripheral zone of diminished absorption consistent with edema is visible. The midline structures are displaced markedly to the right. The high absorption (peak 42) in the region of the compressed left frontal horn was found to be entrapped hematoma at operation.

B. The tumor capsule has increased some 5 or 6 units following contrast injection, while the cyst content and surrounding edema are unchanged in absorption.

(Illustrations courtesy of J. Gawler, M. D.)

CHAPTER 7

Meningiomas

Meningiomas are frequently, although not invariably, moderately dense, with absorption values ranging from the 20's to the 40's. These values are not remarkably different from those seen in intracerebral hematomas, and a possibility of confusion exists if the site of the lesion is atypical. However, even in these cases, the clinical context should serve to distinguish between the two. Subsequent scanning following intravenous injection of contrast medium should also differentiate meningiomas from hematomas, as there will generally be an obvious increase in density of meningiomas of the lower and medium density ranges and no increase in the density of hematomas will occur. In other cases, the plain CT scan density is only a little above that of white matter. In general, when the initial density of meningioma is relatively low, the density is markedly increased by intravenous contrast injection, as a function both of the vascularity of the tumor and of extravascular diffusion of contrast medium. A feature of some larger acoustic neuromas, i.e., increase in density following intravenous contrast injection in the form of a broad peripheral zone with a less dense center, representing less vascularity or actual necrotic changes centrally, is not common in meninigioma, although it is occasionally seen. Various portions of meningioma may show varying degrees of increase in density with intravenous contrast injection, but the lack of a distinct ring-shaped contour can serve to differentiate the two conditions. In this context, it should be remembered that, at angiography, a meningioma may show only a peripheral zone of vascularity when the internal carotid circulation only is opacified, while the central region of the tumor is opacified when the contrast medium is injected into the external carotid artery.

In many cases, the plain CT density of meningioma is very high, ranging up to as much as 90 units or more, due to psammomatous calcification. In such cases, the regions calcified show little or no further increase in density following intravenous contrast injection. The presence of calcification can be diagnosed on the CT scan when absorption values extend above 60 and may be identified when none is visible on plain film skull examination. With less extensive psammomatous calcification or with partial volume representations, the density may be less than 60 units.

Whether initially of lesser or greater density, meningiomas generally show a relatively homogeneous absorption, although large lobulated tumors may have different densities in different lobules. Occasionally, foci of dense amorphous calcification can be identified in the meningioma. The absence of evidence of central necrotic change aids in differentiation from dense malignant tumors. Not infrequently, resolution of the CT scan is sufficient to reveal associated hyperostosis.

Twenty-one consecutive cases of meningioma were diagnosed correctly, with one exception, which was a case seen early in the series (Fig. 7.3). In this case, inexperience led to a diagnosis of glioblastoma, an error not likely to be repeated now that the dramatic appearance of surrounding edema in some cases of large meningioma has been appreciated.

The accuracy of CT scan diagnosis of meningioma should approach 100%, provided that intravenous (or postangiographic) contrast enhancement is used appropriately and provided that the region of the tumor is appropriately covered by the scan sections. The latter caveat applies particularly to meningiomas in the lower portion of the posterior fossa and in the high parasagittal regions. A potential source of error exists when a thick region of bone is scanned obliquely on the highest sections and may appear nodular.

In the initial consecutive series of 600 CT examinations there were 11 cases of meningioma. The accuracy of CT scan diagnosis is compared with that of other radiological methods in Table 7.1.

TABLE 7.1
Meningiomas: 11 Cases

	CT Scans (11)	RN Scans (11)	Angiograms* (9)	PEGs (1)
Positive	11†	9	≫3 =3 <2	? Arnold-Chiari malformation
Negative	0	2‡	≪1	

* ≫, CT very much superior to angiography or pneumoencephalography; =, CT approximately equal to angiography or pneumoencephalography; <, CT distinctly inferior to angiography or pneumoencephalography; ≪, CT very much inferior to angiography or pneumoencephalography.

† Specific diagnosis in 10 cases.

‡ One postoperative recurrence.

Of 11 cases of meningioma in this series, there were no false negative or false positive CT diagnoses. In 10 cases, a specific diagnosis was made. RN scans were obtained in each case, with nine positive results and two negative scans. Angiography was obtained in nine of the 11 cases. CT scans were very much superior to angiography in diagnostic information in three cases, approximately equal to angiography in three cases, distinctly inferior to angiography in two cases, and very much inferior to angiography in one case. PEG was obtained in only one of the cases and suggested the diagnosis of Arnold-Chiari malformation.

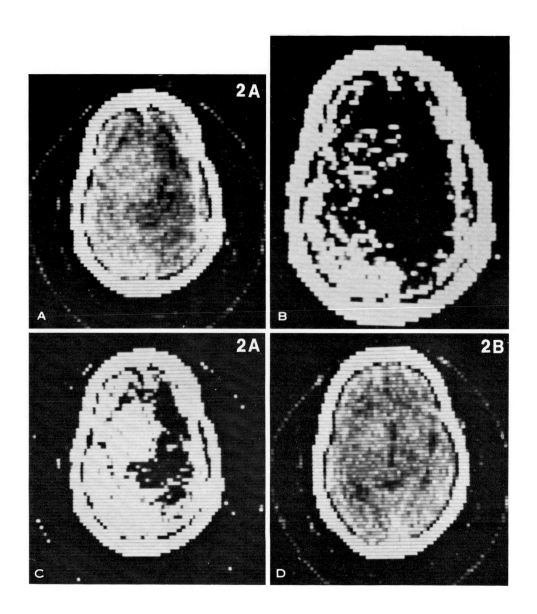

FIG. 7.1. SPHENOID WING AND TUBERCULUM SELLAE MENINGIOMA, LARGE AND HIGHLY VASCULAR.

Clinical Features. A 62 y.o. female with a history of radical mastectomy for breast carcinoma 6 years earlier. Had suffered transient attacks of loss of vision on the left eye for 5 years, with permanent loss of vision in that eye for the past 4 years. She had complained of left frontal headaches and temporal visual field loss in the right eye during the past year.

EEG. Slowing in the left temporal area.

Skull Examination. Including polytomography. Sclerosis and "blistering" of planum sphenoidale. Hyperostosis of the greater and lesser wings of sphenoid.

RN Scan. Tcp; showed increased uptake in the left frontal area.

CT Scan. Abnormal (Fig. 7.1).

Angio. Transfemoral bilateral internal carotid and left common carotid studies revealed a 6-cm diameter ovoid, highly vascularized, smoothly rounded mass arising from the planum sphenoidale and left sphenoid wings, supplied by many small branches from the left ophthalmic artery and anterior cerebral arteries. The mass was shown to extend 1.5 cm to the right of the midline beneath markedly elevated anterior cerebral arteries. The intrinsic tumor vasculature had a typical regular radiating pattern of miningioma.

Operation. (Dr. Michael Scott.) Left frontotemporal craniotomy, with gross but subtotal excision of a massive meningioma attached to the sphenoid ridge and planum sphenoidale. The tumor was highly vascular but relatively firm in consistency. It encased the left optic nerve and compressed and displaced the right optic nerve and chiasm.

Histology. Meningioma.

Plain CT Scan.

A. L 16   W 20.

A 6-cm rounded area of increased absorption (18–30) is visible in this section, which is just above the level of the sphenoid ridge. The area of abnormal density extends from the lateral temporal region anteriorly into the inferior frontal region and approximately 15 mm to the right of the midline. Posteriorly, the margin of the lesion extends to the region above the petrous apex. The increased absorption is relatively homogeneous throughout.

B. L 22   W M.

Same section as in **A**. The portions of the mass with higher absorption than 22 units are shown as white.

C. L 18   W M.

Same section as **A** and **B**. At these control settings, the entire mass is shown as white and its contours merge with the high absorption of cortex laterally and posterolaterally.

D. L 16   W 20.

Section immediately above that in **A**. The upper pole of the mass is just visible as a poorly defined area of increased density immediately lateral to a vertical dark band representing the third ventricle, which is displaced several millimeters to the right but not markedly compressed at this level. The quadrigeminal cistern is visible behind the third ventricle. There is minimal indication of lowered absorption of edema around this very large mass.

As angiography was obviously required, additional scans following intravenous contrast injection were not obtained and the patient was not rescanned following angiography. The highly vascular appearance of the meningioma at angiography indicated that the mass would have been very much denser with contrast enhancement.

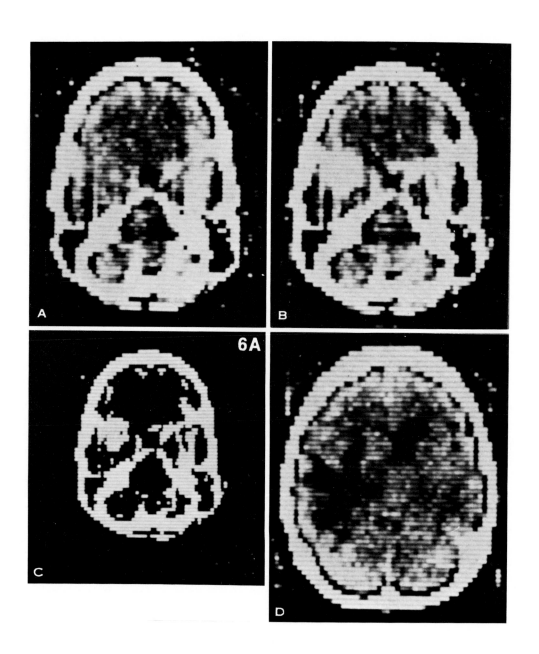

6A

FIG. 7.2. MENINGIOMA, HIGHLY VASCULARIZED.

Clinical Features. A 39 y.o. female with a history of headaches of increasing severity for several months, with intermittent diplopia and vague dizziness. Diminishing vision for several weeks and one episode of numbness of the left arm and left side of the face.

Neurological Examination. Bilateral papilledema, greater on the left side, and mild decrease in left visual acuity. Examination otherwise normal.

Skull Examination. No specific abnormalities.

RN Scan. Tcp; considerably increased activity was noted in the left frontotemporal region, suggesting a meningioma.

CT Scan. Abnormal (Fig. 7.2).

Angio. A 3-cm highly vascularized mass was shown in the anterior portion of the left middle fossa, associated with a disproportionately severe mass effect throughout the temporal lobe area. The combination of findings caused difficulty in differentiating between a meningioma and a temporal lobe glioma (study performed at another hospital and reviewed).

Operation. (Dr. Robert G. Ojemann.) Frontotemporal craniotomy, with total removal of sphenoid wing meningioma.

Histology. Meningioma.

Plain CT scan and scan following contrast enhancement with 50 ml of intravenous Hypaque.

A. L   15   W   20.

Plain CT scan section immediately above the left sphenoid wing. In the central area, the densities of the anterior clinoids and dorsum sellae are evident. In the left temporal region, a rather heterogeneous area of increased absorption (19–27) is evident, with a more dense portion, approximately 12 mm in diameter, lying just lateral to the sella.

B. After contrast enhancement, a very dense (23–39) rounded lesion, 3-cm in diameter, is shown extending posteriorly from the plane of the sphenoid ridge and medially to the parasellar region.

(Fig. 7.2, **A** and **B** reprinted by permission from Radiology, 114: 75–87, 1975.)

C. L   29   W   M.

Same section as **B**. The dense lesion is shown extending laterally to the region of the pterion and medially to within approximately 6 mm of the sella.

D. L   15   W   20.

Section above that shown in **A**. A large, irregularly lobulated region of markedly diminished absorption (7–15) is shown extending through the temporal lobe and centrally to the region adjacent to the markedly compressed left frontal horn and almost to the midline adjacent to the third ventricle, which is not shown in this section. Displacement of the frontal horns to the right is visible. The large area of diminished absorption is indicative of extensive edema associated with the 3-cm, very vascular meningioma. Absorption values in these regions did not change following contrast enhancement.

This case illustrates the very extensive volume of edema that may accompany meningioma. It also illustrates the need for contrast enhancement for clear delineation of the extent of some tumors. A CT scan may be very helpful in evaluation of such secondary changes, particularly when angiographic findings are equivocal.

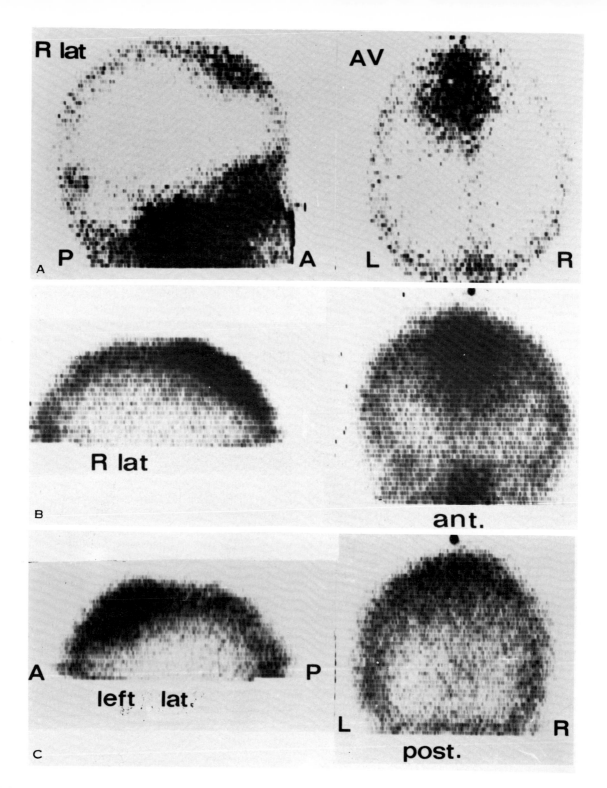

FIG. 7.3. MENINGIOMA, LARGE AND WELL VASCULARIZED, INVOLVING THE FRONTAL FALX AND PARASAGITTAL REGION.

Clinical Features. A 72 y.o. female with progressive slowing of mentation for 1 to 2 months, with recent urinary incontinence.

Neurological Examination. Alert, but slow in responses, without other neurological findings. The syndrome of abulia and incontinence raised suspicion of normal pressure hydrocephalus or bifrontal glioma.

EEG. Bifrontal and right temporal slowing and high voltage delta activity.

Skull Examination. Normal.

RN Scans. Tcp brain scan revealed an area of markedly increased activity of large size in the midline superior frontal area, but extending more to the left side than the right (Fig. 7.3A). Tcd scan revealed a striking area of increased activity of large size in the superior and anterior portions of the frontal bone, also extending further to the left than to the right (Fig. 7.3B and C).

CT Scan. Extensive and marked abnormalities (Fig. 7.3, D–G).

Angio. Transfemoral bilateral carotid studies revealed a large vascular mass in the region of the frontal portion of the falx, extending more to the left than to the right. The mass was supplied by dural and cerebral arterial branches, developed a homogeneous vascular stain, and was shown be drained by quite large cerebral veins extending deeply in the frontal area to connect with the deep venous system. The intrinsic tumor vessels, the arterial supply, and the drainage pattern raised

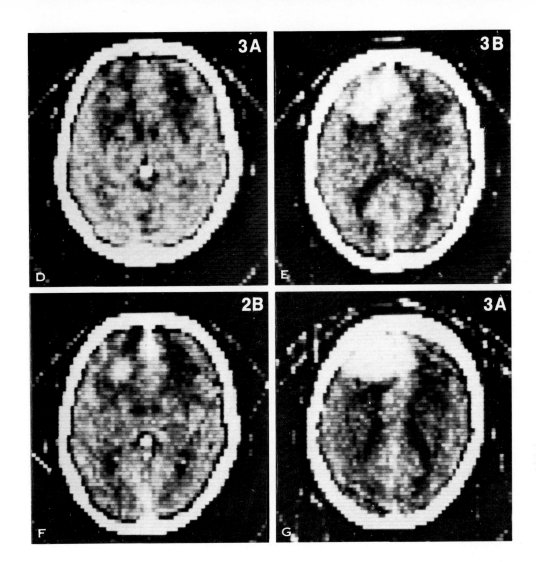

suspicion of a malignant lesion, although the primary diagnosis was a falx meningioma.

Operation. (Dr. James Wepsic.) A very large, reddish, firm tumor arising from the frontal portion of the falx and adjacent parasagittal dura was completely excised.

Histology. Meningioma with atypical cells. The presence of some very large hyperchromatic nuclei were considered to be possibly, but not necessarily, indicative of malignant characteristics.

A–C. Radionuclide rectilinear scans.

A. Tcp brain scan. Right lateral and vertex views, showing a large area of markedly increased activity in the superior frontal region, extending more to the left than to the right of the midline.

B and C. Tcd scans, showing a very large area of markedly increased activity in the anterior and superior portions of the frontal bone, extending further to the left than to the right of the midline. Radionuclide scans are strongly indicative of frontal meningioma with bone involvement. Although skull examination was normal, some erosive bone thinning, without apparent invasion by tumor, was noted in the frontal area at surgery.

D–G. CT scans before and after intravenous contrast enhancement with 45 ml of Hypaque 60.

D anu E: Contiguous 13-mm sections, without contrast enhancement, showing a fusiform area of density in the frontal midline area with compression of the frontal horns from the anterior-superior aspect. The mass extends much further to the left of the midline than to the right, and the absorption range

was 22–28. Extensive areas of diminished absorption are shown around the mass in both frontal lobes (6–14).

F and G. Contrast-enhanced scan sections very similar in levels to those shown in **D** and **E**. There has been considerable increase in absorption values through the irregularly lobulated lesion, which now measures 24–35. The much greater extent to the left of the midline is now more striking. No change in absorption was evident in the low density areas, which represent large volumes of edema in both frontal lobes.

(Fig. 7.3, **E–G** reprinted by permission from Radiology, 114: 75–87, 1975.)

This case, seen early in the series, before it was appreciated that large *irregular* volumes of edema may be seen around meningiomas, was originally misinterpreted as indicating an extensive bifrontal malignant glioma. The more homogeneous appearance of the lesion after intravenous contrast injection is of interest because the carotid angiograms did not result in obvious opacification of much of the mass extending far laterally in the left anterior frontal region. We have seen a number of other examples of tumors that appeared largely as totally avascular in angiography and that increased markedly in density on CT scans after intravenous contrast. *This indicates that diffusion of medium through the impaired blood-brain barriers can be an important factor.* The density of the mass in the left medial parasagittal region on plain scan **(E)** is consistent with diffuse psammomatous calcification in this portion of the tumor. Postoperative scans showed resolving frontal lobe edema.

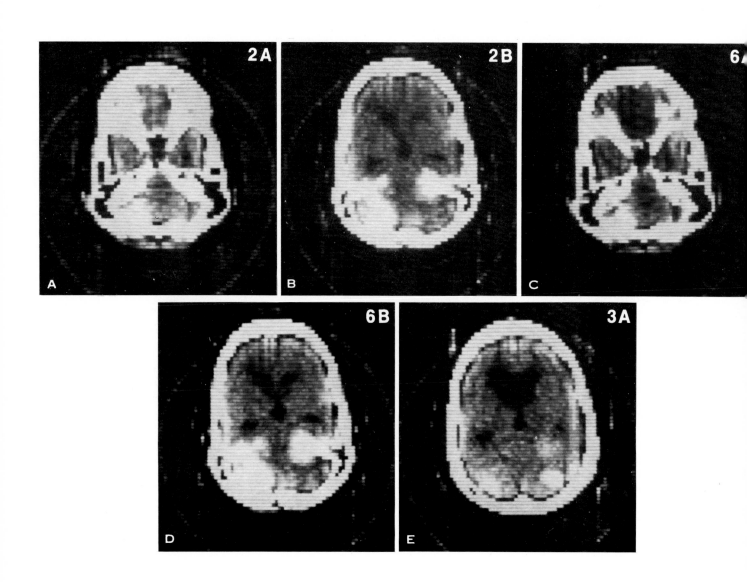

FIG. 7.4. MULTIPLE POSTERIOR FOSSA MENINGIO-MAS.

Clinical Features. A 57 y.o. female with a history of 3 years of progressive hearing loss, 2 years of unsteady gait, tinnitus, and 1 episode of diplopia. Six years earlier, she had been treated with INH, PAS, and streptomycin for pulmonary tuberculosis.

Neurological Examination. Blurring of the right optic disc and a left sixth nerve palsy were noted. She also had right lateral gaze weakness, hyperactive reflexes, a broad-based gait, and poor coordination of her extremities.

Skull Examination. Sellar enlargement and erosive changes consistent with chronic increase in intracranial pressure.

RN Scan. An area of increased activity was evident in the region of the right cerebellopontine angle and a larger diffuse area of increased activity was present in the left cerebellar region.

Angio. Transfemoral carotid and vertebrobasilar studies revealed a moderately large avascular mass in the region of the right CP angle, probably extra-axial. A diffuse and extensive mass, also avascular, was evident in the region of the left cerebellar hemisphere, appearing to be intra-axial. Tonsillar herniation and considerable hydrocephalus were also identified. These studies raised suspicion of metastatic malignancy or multiple tuberculomas.

PEG. No ventricular filling was obtained. Herniation of the cerebellar tonsils was noted. The study failed to localize the position and nature of the major mass effect.

CT Scan. This study was obtained after angio and PEG, for clarification (Fig. 7.4, **A–E**).

Operation. (Dr. Robert G. Ojemann.) Suboccipital craniectomy. A 6-cm, hard, encapsulated tumor with necrotic central area was excised from the left side. Area of dural involvement.

Histology. Meningioma.

A–E. CT scans obtained before and after contrast enhancement with 50 ml of Hypaque 60.

A and **B.** Plain scans. **C** and **D.** Scans at similar levels following intravenous contrast injection.

L 20–23   W 30–50.

The dense, rounded mass extending posteriorly from the right petrous pyramid measured 25–75 on plain scan and 26–85 after injection. The very large, dense mass occupying much of the left side of the posterior fossa measured 39–170 before and 40–170 after injection. This mass showed slight lobulation.

E. A third mass, smaller than the other two, not recognized by RN scanning or angiography, was shown projecting from the region of the left side of the tentorium. This measured approximately 15 x 18 mm and measured 32–110. The considerable obstructive hydrocephalus is visible. The upper pole of the mass in the right CP angle is partially included in this section as a less dense area anterior to the third lesion.

(Fig. 7.4, **D** and **E** reprinted by permission from Radiology, 114: 75–87, 1974.)

The homogeneous appearance of these three lesions and the high absorption range, indicative of considerable psammomatous calcification, strongly indicated the diagnosis of multiple meningiomas. Negligible increase in density after intravenous injection is consistent.

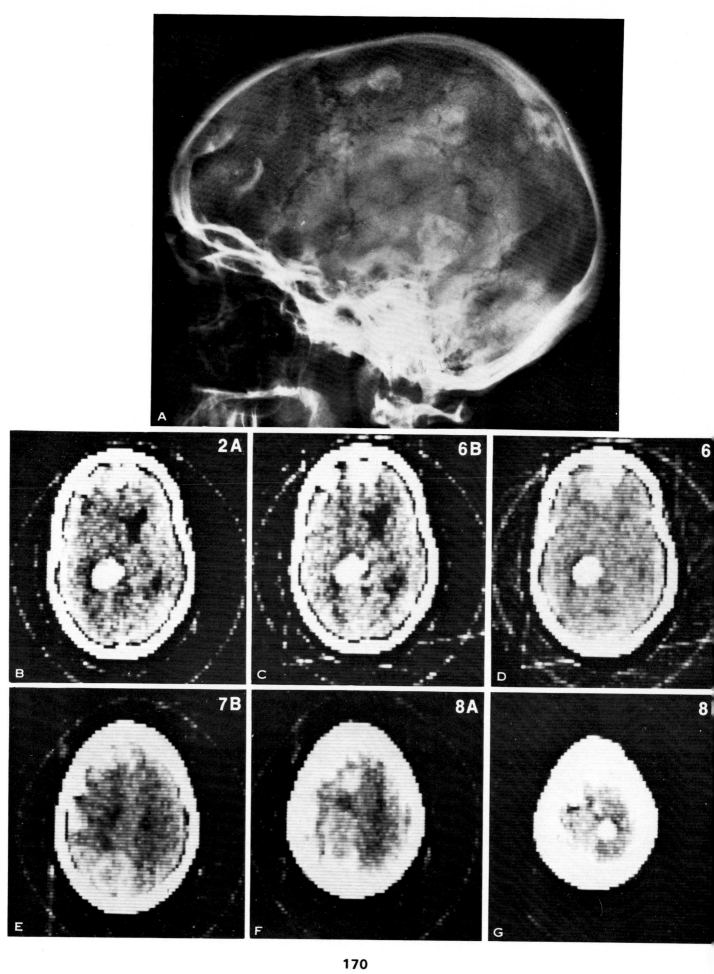

FIG. 7.5. MENINGIOMATOSIS.

Clinical Features. A 50 y.o. woman with chronic anxiety, depression, and numerous cyclic symptoms for several years, including recurrent weakness, abdominal pain, and headaches.

Neurological Examination. Question slight weakness of right arm, otherwise essentially normal.

Skull Examination. Numerous calcific lesions varying from a few millimeters up to approximately 2.5 cm, widely distributed throughout the cranial cavity, and having both nodular and irregular amorphous characteristics in different areas. Prominent meningeal arterial channels (Fig. 7.5A).

RN Scan. Tcp. Very numerous areas of increased activity were noted in the frontal and parietal regions, particularly superiorly, with one area of activity in the region of the left choroid plexus.

Angio. Left direct carotid study at another hospital revealed moderate dislocation of midline structures to the right, widespread local mass effects in the areas of calcification, and enlargement of meningeal arterial branches extending to supply several convexity meningiomas.

CT Scan. This study was obtained to confirm the diagnosis and to provide further information regarding intracranial anatomy, with particular reference to the possibility of a markedly dilated, obstructed left temporal horn (Fig. 7.5, **B–G**). Plain and contrast-enhanced scans were obtained. At least 10 nodular masses were identified over the convexities of the cerebral hemispheres. Absorption ranges varied widely, from as low as 22–28 to as high as 360. There is a widely variable increase in absorption values in many of the masses. The high absorption values of many of the lesions were clearly indicative of variable amounts of contained calcification. One tumor was demonstrated in the left trigone, and measured approximately 3.6 cm in diameter. This lesion measured 33–195, with the peak value increasing to 285 after contrast injection. There was no important obstructive dilatation of the left temporal horn. There was marked compression of the left lateral ventricle and dislocation of midline to the right (**B** and **C**).

B and **C.** Scans at the same level obtained before and after injection, showing the left atrial tumor and adjacent tumors in the frontal midline region and left frontal area.

D. Section immediately below that in **C**, again showing multiple frontal tumors and the left atrial mass.

E–G. Successive 13-mm thick sections superiorly from the section in **C**. Numerous rounded masses of varying size, from a few millimeters to several centimeters in diameter, are shown, predominantly over the left cerebral hemisphere. The obliquely curving vault is included in the high sections (**F** and **G**), tending to obscure the laterally situated masses.

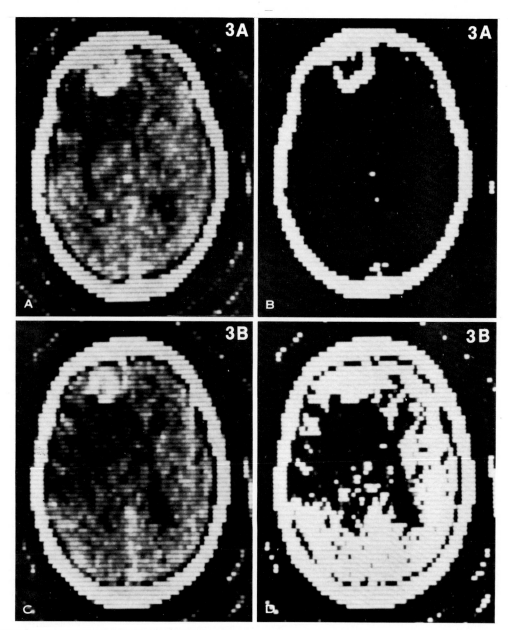

FIG. 7.6. MENINGIOMA, WELL VASCULARIZED AND CONTAINING AMORPHOUS CALCIFICATION.

Clinical Features. A 72 y.o. female with increasing memory difficulty for several years and now disoriented.

Neurological Examination. Mild right hemiparesis.

Skull Examination. Amorphous dense calcifications in the area of the left frontal pole.

RN Scan. Tcp; dynamic and static studies. These revealed increased dynamic activity in the left anterior inferior frontal region, and an area of increased activity in the same region on static scans.

Angio. Left carotid study revealed a very vascular tumor in the anterior inferior region, adjacent to the falx, and supplied by branches of the ophthalmic artery and by the anterior falx artery. Tumor vessels and homogeneous stain were considered characteristic of meningioma. The surrounding avascular region, showing a mass effect, was indicative of considerable associated cerebral edema.

CT Scan. Abnormal (Fig. 7.6, **A–D**).

CT scan without contrast enhancement.

A. Section extending through the lower portions of the frontal lobes and pineal and showing a circumscribed dense mass

(30–60) immediately adjacent to the skull vault. Surrounding this mass elsewhere is a very large zone of decreased absorption (6–14), typical of edema. Behind this is visible a somewhat enlarged left temporal horn. Minor patchy decrease in density in the central portion of the right frontal lobe presumably represents a small amount of edema in this lobe also.

B. L 60 W M.

These control settings reveal considerable hyperostosis in the frontal bone adjacent to the midline and the mass. The broad white crescent beneath this represents a thick calcific rim in the mass (70–85 units).

C. Section immediately above that in **A** and **B**. The superior portion of the meningioma is shown and there is a more extensive zone of edema involving the frontal lobe, extending through the corpus striatum and into the temporal lobe. Compression of the left lateral ventricle is evident, with marked displacement of the midline. Lowered absorption values in the right frontal region represent a small amount of edema and a slightly enlarged and dislocated right frontal horn.

D. L 14 W M.

These control settings accentuate the very large volume of edema in the left cerebral hemisphere, which, towards the right, merges with the compressed and displaced ventricular system.

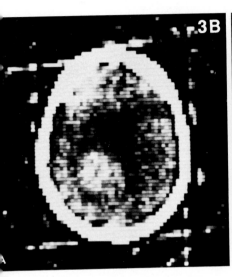 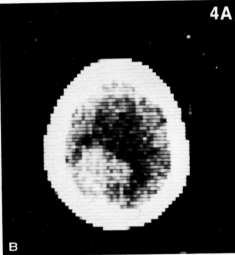 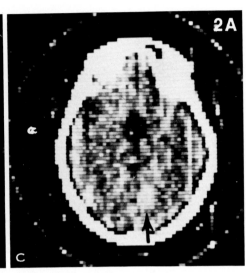

FIG. 7.7. MENINGIOMA, MILDLY VASCULAR.

Clinical Features. A 71 y.o. female who complained of general lack of energy and mild but increasing difficulty with walking. She had also noted a recent decrease in powers of concentration and some difficulty with memory.

Neurological Examination. Apart from impaired coordination of right lower extremity and very mild right hemiparesis, the neurological examination was normal.

Skull Examination. Apart from some prominence of vascular channels in the frontal and parietal regions, no indication of abnormality was detected.

RN Scan. Tcp; revealed increased uptake in the parasagittal region, suggesting a 4.5-cm meningioma.

CT Scan. Abnormal (Fig. 7.7).

Angio. Retrograde femoral carotid study revealed a large "deep" parasagittal mass in the frontoparietal region, supplied by the right pericallosal and left middle meningeal arteries and both occipital arteries. A faint stain appeared in the late arterial phase and persisted through the venous phases. Diagnosis was meningioma, approximately 5.5 x 4.5 cm in diameter.

Operation. (Dr. Robert G. Ojemann.) Excision of a parietal falx meningioma, with much greater extension to the left than to the right. It was noted that the tumor was not visible from the surface, as it projected approximately 2 cm below the upper margin of the falx and bulged into the medial portions of the parietal lobes.

Histology. Meningioma.

CT scan without contrast enhancement.

A and **B.** Contiguous scans through the middle and superior portions of the parietal lobes. A rounded mass, 19–30, with a maximum transverse diameter of 5.5 and AP diameter of 4.5 cm, is demonstrated. A zone of decreased absorption (7–14), 1 to 2 cm in width, represents parietal lobe edema around the mass. The tumor can be seen extending approximately 12 mm to the right of the midline in **B.** If the more superior section had not been included, the full dimensions of the mass would not have been demonstrated.

C. Section at the level of the tentorium. A 2-cm diameter region of density, measuring 20–23 units, is shown and presumably represents a small second meningioma arising from the tentorium. This lesion has not been confirmed.

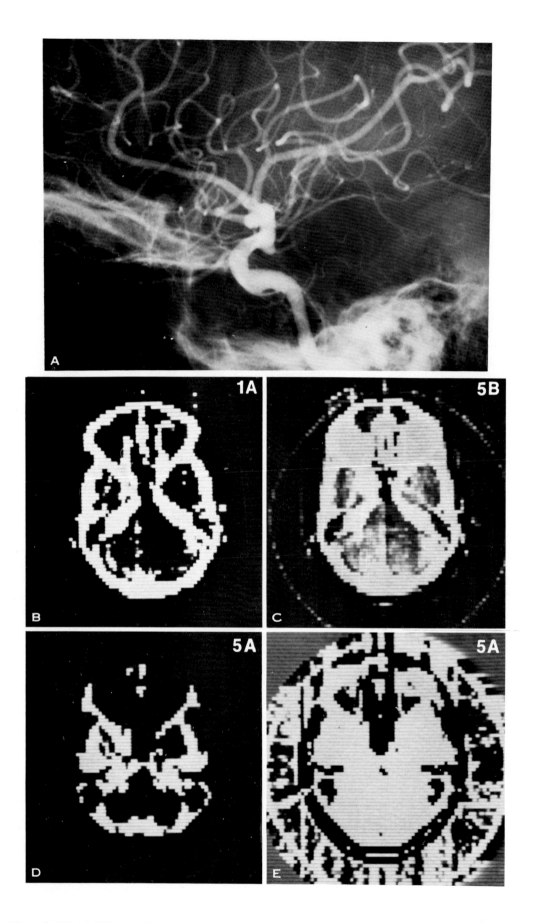

FIG. 7.8. MENINGIOMA, PARASELLAR.

Clinical Features. A 44 y.o. female who had noted mild headaches of 2 to 3 years duration in the left frontal region and gradual onset of blurred vision in the left eye for 9 months.

Neurological Examination. Vision 20/20 right and 20/400 left, with normal pupillary reaction and full extraocular movements. Atrophic appearance of left optic disc.

Skull Examination. Medial sphenoid wing hyperostosis.

Polytomography. Extensive granular hyperostosis and erosion involving the medial portion of the greater and lesser wings of the sphenoid and of the left side of the body of the sphenoid, with encroachment upon the sphenoid sinus from its lateral wall. Sclerosis extending to foramen ovale. Left anterior clinoid process erosion and posterolateral erosion of the left optic canal, with slight narrowing.

RN Scan. Tcp; normal dynamic and static scan. Tcd scan also normal.

CT Scan. Abnormal (Fig. 7.8, **B–E**).

Angio. Transfemoral selective internal and external left carotid studies showed no definite mass effect but suggested elevation of the left carotid bifurcation with slight narrowing of the precavernous segment of the internal carotid artery (suggesting encirclement by tumor), and considerably enlarged cavernous sinus branches of the internal carotid artery supplying an area of tumor blush in the antero-medio-inferior portion of the middle fossa adjacent to body of sphenoid and superior orbital fissure (Fig. **7.8A**). External carotid study was normal.

Operation. (Dr. Edward Tarlov.) Left frontotemporal craniotomy with decompression of optic nerve and extensive subtotal resection of tumor from the region of the superior orbital fissure and medial middle fossa. Tumor extended deeply around the internal carotid artery and into the cavernous sinus.

Histology. Meningioma, with bone involvement.

A. Left internal carotid angiogram, showing slight concentric narrowing of the precavernous segment of the internal carotid artery and hypertrophied cavernous sinus dural branches of the internal carotid artery (*arrowheads*).

B. L 30   W M.
Plain CT scan extending through the superior orbits and region of the sella. Bone density in the medial sphenoid wing region shows some thickening. An irregular area of high density (20–47), approximately 9–12 mm in width, extends from the region of the superior orbital fissure to the petrous bone in the left parasellar area.

C. L 16   W 30.
Scan following injection of 50 ml of Hypaque intravenously. The scan extends through the orbital roofs and sellar region. At this level, a dense mass (27–47) extends from the sphenoid sinus laterally for a distance of approximately 2 cm and extends from the superior orbital fissure to the petrous apex.

D. L 120   W M.
Scan through the orbits and inferior portion of the middle fossae. The high level setting reveals more clearly the thickening of the posterior wall of the left orbit and a dense calcific and/or osseous mass extending laterally from the left wall of the sphenoid sinus. There appears to be very little encroachment upon the orbit by hyperostosis.

E. L 0   W M.
This control setting reveals the posterior orbital fat (low absorption, extending down to approximately −50). The fat is bounded anteriorly by the globes and posteriorly by the posterior orbital wall, and confirms the lack of significant encroachment upon the orbit by hyperostosis and soft tissue tumor.

Although the meningioma was clearly identified on this CT study and the general extent of tumor and of hyperostosis were identifiable, polytomography and angiography were essential for confirmation of the diagnosis and for preoperative evaluation. Resolution of CT scans is suboptimal for complete evaluation of smaller basal lesions, even with use of the 160 x 160 system and 8-mm sections.

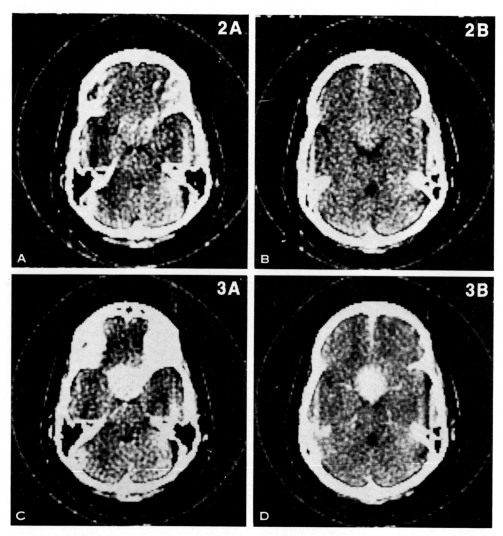

FIG. 7.9. MENINGIOMA, TUBERCULUM SELLAE, AND PLANUM SPHENOIDALE.

Clinical Features. A 59 y.o. woman who first noticed difficulty with vision in the left eye 1 year previously. There had recently been a more rapid deterioration of vision in the left eye and the onset of cloudy vision in the right eye. Examination revealed temporal hemianopsia in the left eye, with grossly reduced vision in the nasal field. There was suspicion of a small temporal field defect in the right eye.

Skull Examination. There was marked erosion of the upper third of the dorsum sellae, with loss of density and asymmetry of the contour of the lamina dura of the sella. In addition, hypocycloidal tomography revealed erosion, granular hyperostosis, and slight "blistering" of the planum sphenoidale, indicating the diagnosis of meningioma.

RN Scan. Tcp; dynamic and static studies, obtained 4 days before CT scan were normal.

CT Scan. Abnormal (Fig. 7.9).

Angio. A right retrograde brachial study with contralateral carotid compression, revealed elevation and stretching of both anterior cerebral arteries. A moderate homogeneous blush indicative of meningioma was demonstrated in the suprasellar region and above the planum sphenoidale.

Operation. (Dr. R. Ojemann.) Right frontal craniotomy, with microsurgical total excision of a tuberculum sellae meningioma.

Tumor extended below both optic nerves, which were displaced superiorly and laterally.

Histology. Meningioma of the meningoendotheliomatous type. **A** and **B.** Plain CT scans of 8-mm sections. 160 × 160 matrix system. A rounded mass of moderate absorption (15–30), 3 cm in diameter, is shown in the immediate suprasellar region, extending somewhat more to the left than to the right, and outlined bilaterally and posteriorly by CSF in the lateral extremities of the deformed carotid portions of the suprasellar cisterns and in the remaining portion of the interpedunuclar cistern.

C and **D.** Eight-mm scan sections similar to but not identical with those in **A** and **B**, obtained following intravenous infusion of 300 ml of Renografin 30%. There has been a striking increase in absorption by the meningioma (18–60). The diameter of the mass is now indicated to be 33 mm. The larger indicated diameter may be attributable to more favorable positioning of the section relative to the equator of the mass or to the overcoming of peripheral partial volume effects by the marked increase in absorption produced by the contrast medium. Without subsequent serial scans and concomitant blood iodine estimations, it is not possible to determine the relative parts played by tumor vascularity and by extravascular diffusion of contrast medium into the tumor.

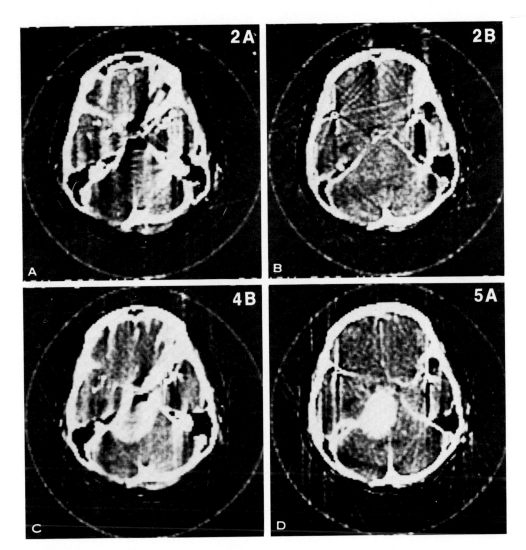

FIG. 7.10. MENINGIOMA OF THE CLIVUS; POST-OPERATIVE RECURRENCE.

Clinical Features. A 70 y.o. female, referred from another hospital for CT scan. She had a history of ataxia for several months, with falling to the right. She had had craniotomy and partial removal of a clival meningioma some 3 years previously. A ventriculoperitoneal shunt had been placed 9 months before CT scan, with temporary improvement.

Angio. Nine months before CT scan, studies had revealed hydrocephalus and a left posterior fossa mass.

A–D. Eight-mm sections. 160 x 160 matrix system.

A and B. Plain scan. Numerous artifacts are present in the posterior fossa on the section shown in **A.** In **B,** there is indication of narrowing of the CP angle and pontine cisterns. A large ovoid area of somewhat increased absorption (10–28) is evident in the region of the brain stem, extending to the left CP angle. Behind the region of increased absorption, in the midline

and extending broadly across the region of the left cerebellar hemisphere, is a triangular region of diminished absorption (5–14) consistent with edema. The fourth ventricle is not identified with certainty, suggesting that it is compressed.

C and D. Scan following injection of 300 ml of Renografin 30% by drip infusion. The scan planes are similar to but not identical with those in **A** and **B.** The large mass lying behind the clivus and extending posteriorly and into the region of the left CP angle has become very clear because of marked increase in absorption (34–65). The increase in absorption is presumed to represent a combination of circulating blood-pool iodine and extravascular contrast diffusion into the meningioma, but the relative contributions are not known. The small regions of very high absorption scattered in both temporal areas represent Pantopaque residues. More superior sections (not shown) showed the presence of the ventricular shunt, but moderate lateral and third ventricular dilation was present.

CHAPTER 8

Pituitary Adenomas and Craniopharyngiomas

Although a number of quite small lesions in the suprasellar region has been demonstrated by CT scanning, the method has distinct limitations in evaluation of this region. The complexity of anatomical structures within a relatively small anatomical space makes impossible the generally required detailed anatomical evaluation. Such evaluation requires pneumoencephalography with extremely high quality thin section laminography, which, when properly employed, can identify lesions producing distortion of local anatomy by as little as 2–3 mm. In the case of suspected vascular lesions of this region or when local surgery is contemplated, angiography is generally employed also. Additionally, in the evaluation of the lateral extension of pituitary adenomas, it is our regular practice to employ cavernous sinography from the anterior or posterior route. These contrast studies are employed only after meticulous evaluation of the osseous structures of the sella and perisellar regions, including polytomography. The relatively low resolution inherent in the present CT section thicknesses militates against requisite anatomical and pathological details of small lesions in this area. The use of 8-mm sections and low scan angles will improve diagnostic capabilities of the scanner in evaluating lesions of the perisellar region, and the improved horizontal anatomical resolution provided by the 160 x 160 matrix system is clearly advantageous.

The above notwithstanding, after detailed plain film radiographic studies, CT scanning offers a survey examination that may well be of value, and the method is certainly useful in evaluating larger lesions arising in this area. Certain features of the larger of such lesions, demonstrable by CT scanning, cannot be identified by any other currently available method short of surgery, and some of these features may be of considerable importance in surgical planning. The identification of calcifications insufficiently dense to be identified even on polytomography and the identification of the presence and extent of hemorrhage and/or cyst formation in lesions of the region may each be of considerable value in individual cases. The cases described in this chapter serve to illustrate certain of the advantages and disadvantages that have been noted.

PITUITARY ADENOMAS

Preliminary evidence indicates that high dosage intravenous contrast enhancement will improve CT capability in the diagnosis of suprasellar and lateral extensions of chromophobe adenomas (Figs. 8.3 and 8.4). Experience with magnification and subtraction angiography has indicated that the majority of such adenomas is sufficiently vascular to make such supplemental contrast-enhanced scans on a regular basis worthwhile. Additionally, evidence is accumulating that pituitary adenomas increase in density so strikingly following high-dose intravenous injection that a significant extravascular diffusion of contrast medium into these tumors is occurring. It is likely that differentiation of suprasellar extension of pituitary adenoma and suprasellar meningioma will be difficult on CT scans alone and will depend heavily upon detailed plain skull and laminographic examinations (Fig. 7.9). High quality angiographic studies will usually serve to distinguish these conditions. CT has the capability of revealing cystic changes within pituitary adenomas. The demonstration of major cyst formation in suprasellar extensions may influence a decision to operate via a transphenoidal approach rather than transfrontally. The former procedure carries about one-fifth of the mortality rate of the latter.

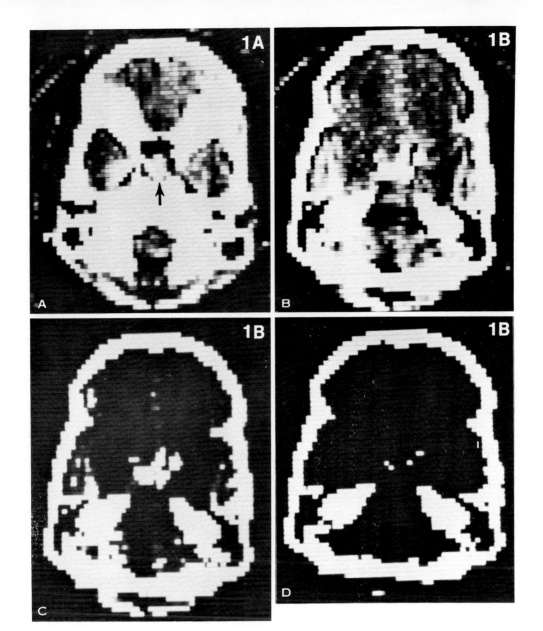

FIG. 8.1. CHROMOPHOBE ADENOMA, WITH SUPRA-SELLAR EXTENSION AND HEMORRHAGIC NECROSIS.

Clinical Features. A 19 y.o. male with progressive loss of vision in both temporal fields over a 2 month period. He also complained of headache.

Neurological Examination. Bitemporal hemianopsia. Decreased secondary sexual characteristics and growth were noted.

Skull Examination. The sella showed marked generalized expansion, indicative of a large intrasellar mass.

CT Scan. Abnormal (Fig. 8.1).

PEG. Revealed a suprasellar mass projecting 21 mm above the level of the anterior clinoids and indenting the anterior recesses of the third ventricle.

Operation. (Dr. William H. Sweet.) After aspiration of 5 ml of liquid blood from the tumor, an intrasellar and suprasellar chromophobe adenoma was extirpated.

Histology. Chromophobe adenoma with extensive hemorrhagic necrosis.

A. L 17   W 20.
Scan section through the inferior portions of the frontal lobes, sphenoid sinus, and sella. An irregularly rounded area of high absorption projects into the sphenoid sinus (*arrow*). The white area of high absorption to the left side of the sphenoid sinus has the characteristics of a local prominence in the floor of the middle fossa adjacent to the sinus.

B. L 17   W 20.

Thirteen-mm scan section immediately superior to that in **A**. An irregular distribution of high absorption is shown in the suprasellar region and extending bilaterally and posteriorly into the interpeduncular cistern. Absorption values through this region ranged from 20–41, consistent with hemorrhage.

C. L 24   W M.
These viewer settings clarify the regions of high absorption indicative of hemorrhage, lying in the area just anterior to the petrous apices. The width of this zone measured 32 mm. (Reprinted by permission from Radiology, 110: 109–123, 1974.)

D. L 46   W M.
This is also the same scan section as is shown in **B** and **C**. The higher window level settings reveal a few small densitites in the posterior portion of the lesion that may represent denser portions of the hemorrhage or partial volume representation of a little calcification in the posterior margin, probably the latter.

The CT diagnosis, based on the clinical presentation and the plain film findings, was that of chromophobe adenoma with hemorrhagic necrosis. The clinical manifestations had not raised suspicion of hemorrhage into the tumor. The high absorption values of what proved at surgery to be liquid blood were of considerable interest, since this was incompatible with previous statements regarding absorption values of blood (see Chapter 15).

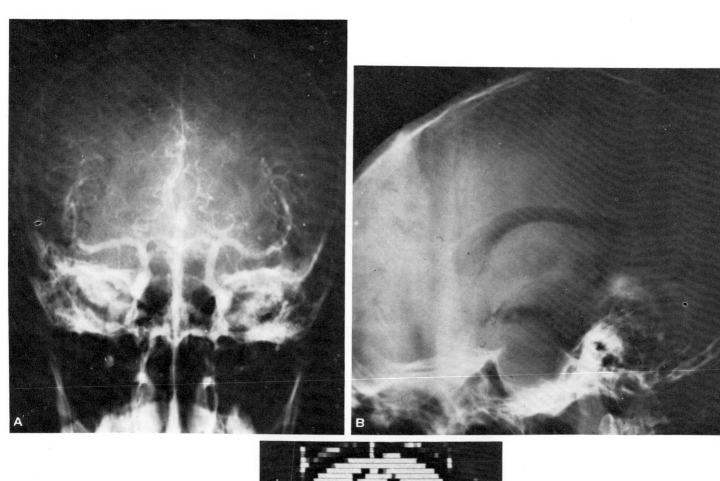

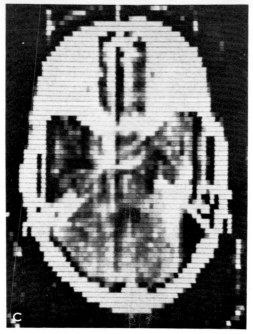

FIG. 8.2. CHROMOPHOBE ADENOMA WITH MARKED BILATERAL AND MODERATE SUPRASELLAR EXTENSIONS.

Clinical Features. A 19 y.o. male who had had a grand mal seizure and gave a history of headaches.

Skull Examination. Marked enlargement of the sella, with erosion and displacement of the anterior clinoids and dorsum sellae, indicative of a large intrasellar mass growing superiorly.

RN Scan. A recent scan performed elsewhere was interpreted as normal.

CT Scan. Abnormal (Fig. 8.2C).

Angio. Bilateral carotid angiograms indicated the presence of a large intrasellar mass, with at least anterior suprasellar extension (Fig. 8.2A).

PEG. This revealed a quite large suprasellar extension (Fig. 8.2B). No calcification was visible on laminography. A markedly expanded left temporal horn was demonstrated and was thought to be the result of atrophy following old cranial trauma.

Operation. (Dr. William H. Sweet.) Extirpation of a large chromophobe adenoma.

Histology. Chromophobe adenoma.

A. AP projection of early arterial phase of carotid angiography. The intracavernous siphons are bowed and each is displaced several millimeters laterally, the left being somewhat more displaced than the right. In addition, the anterior cerebral arteries are somewhat elevated.

B. PEG. Erect film, incompletely demonstrating the suprasellar extension. The marked enlargement of the sella is evident.

C. L 16   W 20.

CT scan through the orbital roofs, upper portion of the sella, and upper portions of the petrous pyramids. The ovoid density of the pituitary adenoma is visible, extending considerably in a lateral direction, further on the left than on the right. The transverse diameter of the mass was 36–39 mm, equivalent to the distance between the intracavernous carotid siphons at angiography. A higher scan section revealed the marked dilation of the left temporal horn. The marked bilateral extent of the tumor was of considerable interest. Although cavernous sinography has been used regularly to identify the lateral extent of pituitary adenomas, it has been found that marked lateral extension so compresses the cavernous sinuses that identification of the lateral contours of the adenoma may be difficult or impossible. Under these circumstances, CT scanning may be a valid alternative, especially with the use of thin sections and contrast enhancement.

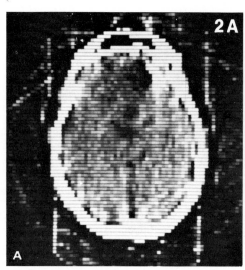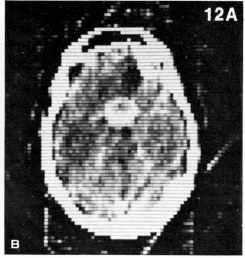

FIG. 8.3. CHROMOPHOBE ADENOMA.

Clinical Features. A 32 y.o. man with a 2 week history of diminished visual acuity in both eyes. Neurological examination was normal except for visual acuity of 20/200 bilaterally, without well-defined bitemporal homonymous hemianopsia.

Skull Examination. Markedly enlarged sella, with ballooned appearance and symmetrically concave floor.

Angio. Large suprasellar mass displacing A1 segments of anterior cerebral arteries superiorly, stretching and laterally displacing supraclinoid internal carotid arteries, and outlined in part by faint capillary blush, extending some 2 cm above the sella.

CT Scan. Abnormal (Fig. 8.3).

Operation. Total resection (Dr. J. Hanberry) of chromophobe adenoma extending 2–2.5 cm above the sella, with cystic necrosis centrally and a relatively vascular capsule.

L   18   W   30.

Corresponding sections before (**A**), and after (**B**), 300 ml of

Hypaque 30% was injected intravenously, passing through suprasellar cisterns at 10° to Reid's base line. A rounded mass occupies the suprasellar cisterns and encroaches upon the anterior aspect of the interpeduncular cistern. Before injection of contrast medium, the center of the mass has an absorption of 4–14, while the periphery of the mass has a range of 12–22 (which does not allow differentiation of anterior and lateral aspects of the mass from normal adjacent brain). After intravenous contrast, the mass is well defined, with a range of 23–34, except for the anterior central portion of the mass, which remains relatively low in absorption. The oval low absorption zone (3–12) in the right medial orbitofrontal region is immediately above the medial orbital roof; such a finding in this region is usually of no diagnostic significance, even when it appears quite asymmetrical, as in this case. Few of our cases of suspected chromophobe adenoma have been studied with intravenous contrast medium in the past, but contrast enhancement is now used routinely in such cases.

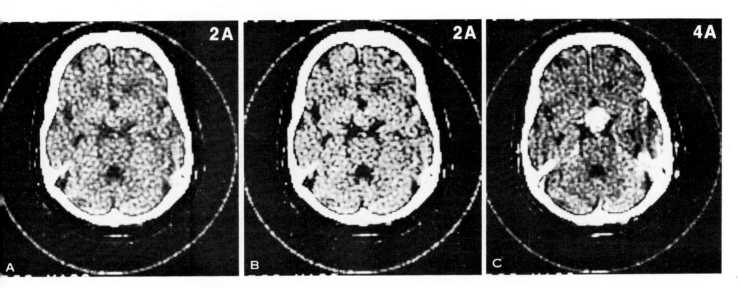

FIG. 8.4. A case similar to that described in Figure 8.3, further illustrating the markedly increased visibility of a large chromophobe adenoma with suprasellar extension, following intravenous contrast enhancement.

A. L 13 W 30 160 x 160 matrix system.
A soft tissue encroachment upon the interpeduncular cistern is visible. This has a convex posterior margin. Absorption values are virtually indistinguishable from those of surrounding brain, and the anterior and lateral boundaries cannot be distinguished from brain.

B. L 10 W 30.
Same section as in **A**. The lower L setting improves the contrast between the posterior surface of the suprasellar mass and CSF in the cistern.

C. Section very similar in level to that shown in **A** and **B** following intravenous injection of 75 ml of Hypaque 60 M. There has been marked generalized increase in absorption (peak 34 units) of the suprasellar mass. Similar increase in absorption was noted within the markedly expanded sella on a subjacent section (not shown). The distal portion of the carotid siphon and proximal portion of the middle cerebral artery are now visible on the left side, adjacent to the mass. The basilar artery is now more clearly visible as a small dense spot immediately adjacent to the posterior surface of the mass.

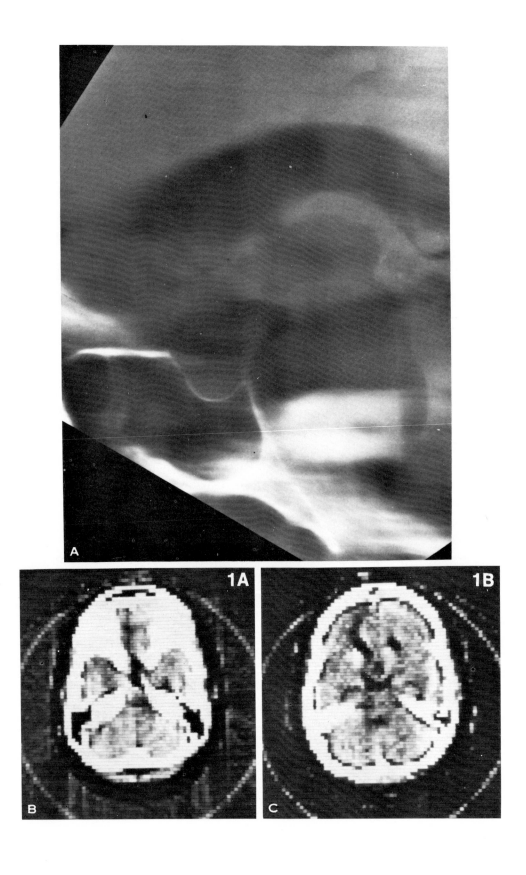

FIG. 8.5. CYSTIC CHROMOPHOBE ADENOMA.

Clinical Features. A 31 y.o. female with a 12 year history of galactorrhea and irregular menses. Four months before the present admission, she had noted visual disturbance in the right eye, followed by the left eye.

Neurological Examination. Revealed bitemporal visual field defects and bilateral central scotomas. She was noted to be slightly obese. A small amount of milk was expressible from both nipples.

Skull Examination. Gradually increasing changes had been noted in the sella over previous years. Recent examination showed slight but definite thinning and irregularity of the sellar floor and erosion of the dorsum consistent with an intrasellar mass.

CT Scan. Abnormal in the suprasellar region (Fig. 8.5).

Angio. Bilateral carotid studies revealed an avascular midline suprasellar mass.

PEG. A suprasellar mass was demonstrated, extending 2.5 cm above the sella (Fig. 8.5A).

Operation. (Dr. Raymond N. Kjellberg.) Transfrontal craniotomy, with intracapsular removal of a cystic chromophobe adenoma. The volume of the adenoma was estimated to be 3 ml, and approximately $2/3$ of the tumor was occupied by a cyst that contained brown fluid that coagulated rapidly following aspiration.

Histology. Cystic chromophobe adenoma.

A. Midline laminographic section at pneumoencephalography, brow-up position. The slight sellar expansion and the large suprasellar mass indenting and displacing the anterior recesses of the third ventricle are shown. The mass was noted to extend slightly more to the right than to the left above the sella.

B. L 16   W 30.
The scan extends in the plane of the anterior clinoids. No abnormalities are visible in this section other than possibly an abnormally low absorption in the region of the sella.

C. L 16   W 20.
A rounded mass, approximately 21 mm in diameter is shown immediately above the sella (just behind and medial to the white areas, which represent partial volume inclusions of the anterior clinoid processes). Posteriorly, the edge of the mass is shown encroaching upon the interpeduncular cistern (broad crescentic black region just anterior and medial to the petrous pyramids). Note that the central portion of the mass is of relatively low density ((absorption of the solid part of tumor, 8–15; of the central area, 6–11; of the interpeduncular cistern, 0–10; and of the temporal horns, 7–12 (partial volume)). Although at the time of interpretation this was thought to represent partial volume inclusion of a transversely "spread" anterior portion of the third ventricle, review indicates that this represents the large cyst within the adenoma. On each side of the interpeduncular cistern can be noted sections through the temporal horns, more clearly seen on the left side. Further posteriorly, the angled section extends through the fourth ventricle. A cystic change such as that exhibited by this tumor is generally not recognizable by other radiological methods, although very high quality magnification angiography subjected to subtraction may occasionally provide such evidence. Had the extensive cystic component of this adenoma been recognized before surgery, it might well have been opted to approach the tumor by the transphenoidal route.

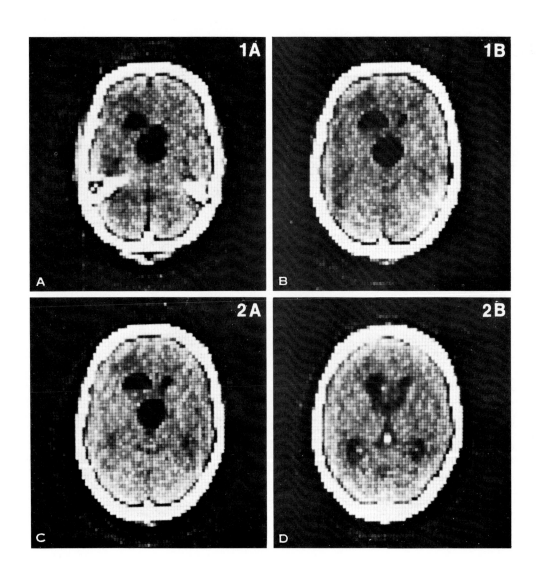

FIG. 8.6. CYSTIC CRANIOPHARYNGIOMA, WITH HIGH CHOLESTEROL CONTENT. (Case contributed by James Ambrose, M. D.)

Clinical Features. A middle-aged patient with a history of lifelong poor vision, lately becoming blind in the left eye.

A–D. Four contiguous scans, parallel to the orbitomeatal line at 4.5 and 6.0 cm. The scans reveal a large suprasellar cystic lesion, with a loculus extending into the left frontal lobe. The top of the cyst protrudes into the floor of the anterior aspect of the lateral ventricles and the third ventricle. Small specks of calcification (single white squares) are visible in the cyst wall (**C** and **D**). A computer printout of the scan at level 1A showed negative values (down to −52) within the cyst, indicating a considerable lipid (cholesterol) content. (Reprinted by permission from British Journal of Radiology, 46: 1023–1047, and from Journal of Neurosurgery, 40: June 1974.)

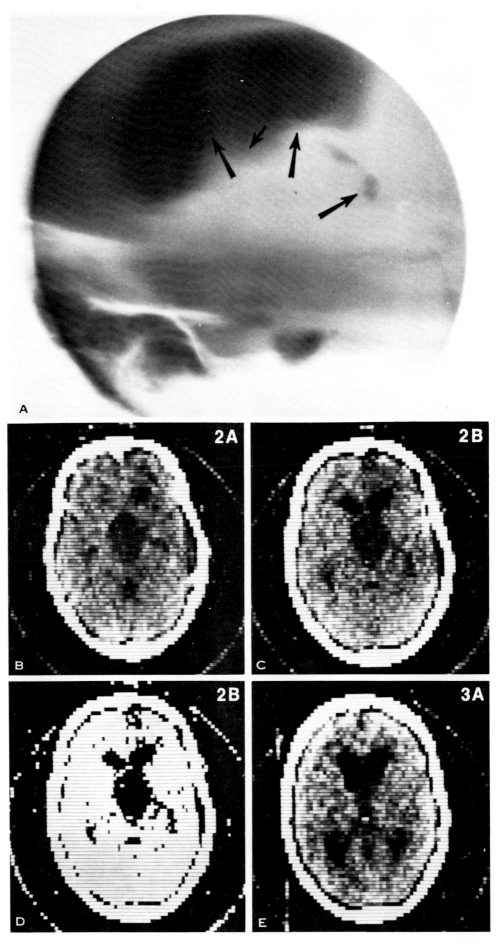

FIG. 8.7. CYSTIC CRANIOPHARYNGIOMA.

Clinical Features. A 35 y.o. male who had had operations with partial excision of craniopharyngioma 17, 10, and 3 years earlier. Current presentation with panhypopituitarism and recent onset of severe constant headache.

Skull Examination. Modest asymmetrical enlargement of the sella with increase in size over 10 years, erosion of the sellar floor, and marked truncation of the dorsum sellae. No calcification visible on laminography.

CT Scan. Abnormal (Fig. 8.7, **B–E**).

PEG. A large suprasellar mass was demonstrated. This projected 4 cm above the sella, causing gross indentation and compression of the third ventricle and encroachment upon the inferior aspects of the frontal horns. There was moderately severe enlargement of the lateral ventricles. The mass had enlarged since the PEG obtained 10 years earlier.

Histology. Craniopharyngioma with large cyst formation.

A. Brow-up projection obtained at recent PEG, showing a very large suprasellar mass grossly compressing the third ventricle and indenting the inferior portions of the frontal horns (*large arrows*). The region of the foramina of Munro is indicated by the *small arrow*. Obstruction in this region had produced moderately severe dilatation of the lateral ventricles, which had a frontal horn total span of 55 mm. The mass was shown to fill the interpeduncular cistern and extended into the upper pontine cistern. There was marked posterior displacement of the

aqueduct. The asymmetrically enlarged sella with destruction of the dorsum is also visible.

B–E. The large cystic craniopharyngioma is represented by an ovoid region of decreased absorption (2–14) measuring approximately 4.5 cm in maximum diameter and extending from the sella 25–30 mm superiorly (**B**, **C**, and **D**).

A. L 15 W 30.

The cyst is shown centrally, with modestly enlarged temporal horns on each side.

C. L 15 W 20.

The cyst is larger in cross section in this scan and lies immediately behind dilated frontal horns.

D. L 12 W M.

These control settings accentuate the cyst and portions of the lateral ventricles. There is evidence of some cerebral shrinkage in the right frontopolar region, probably resulting from previous surgery. The cyst contents were relatively homogeneous in absorption.

E. L 15 W 20.

This section, also 13 mm in thickness, is immediately above that shown in **C** and reveals the lateral ventricular dilatation. The third ventricle, although compressed in its vertical diameter, shows a "spreading" in transverse direction.

The cyst contents in this case evidently included insufficient cholesterol to reduce the absorption level below that of water. No tumor calcification was evident.

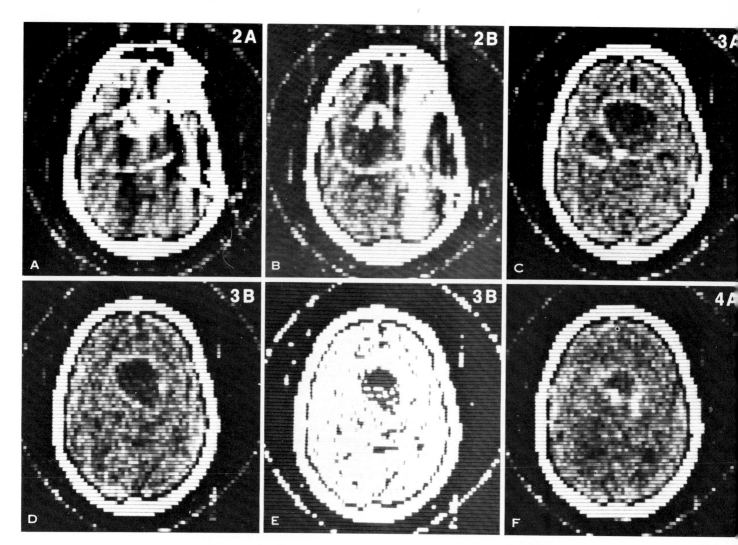

FIG. 8.8. LARGE CRANIOPHARYNGIOMA, WITH SOLID CALCIFIC AND CYSTIC COMPONENTS (NOT HISTOLOGICALLY VERIFIED).

Clinical Features. A 36 y.o. male who was noted to have decreased vision in the right eye 10 years earlier. He returned to medical care 2 years later with complaints of decreased vision in both eyes, impotence of 3 years duration, and frontal headache. He was found to be almost totally blind. Seven years earlier he was advised to undergo surgery but again refused.

Neurological Examination. Revealed evidence of pan-hypopituitarism. Severe bilateral optic atrophy was noted.

EEG. Diffuse bilateral slowing.

Skull Examination. Complete destruction of the region of the sella, with extensive calcifications in the region of the sphenoid sinus.

CT Scan. Abnormal (Fig. 8.8).

Angio. Right carotid study revealed an avascular mass in the region of the sella and in the suprasellar area, 5 cm in diameter. The patient again refused an operation.

Consecutive 8-mm CT scan sections. The two lowest scan sections (not shown) demonstrated extensive nodular calcifications in the sphenoid sinus and extending bilaterally.

A. A heterogeneous mass of calcification is shown in the immediate suprasellar area, with values extending up to 180. An arc of calcification extends transversely above the petrous apices. Between the two areas of calcification were heterogeneous values ranging between 0 and 16.

B. Arcs of calcification are shown anteriorly and posteriorly, more extensive to the left of the midline, where the lesion extends into the lateral portion of the temporal area. Between the calcifications lies a large area of generally low absorption value (8–22).

C. A bilocular cystic configuration is shown. The cyst content measured 8–28 and the dense capsule was mostly in the range 25–30, but with small areas of calcification being indicated by higher values posteriorly.

D. Only a single loculus in the midline area is shown at this level. Cyst contents measured 8–22 and most of the wall measured 25–30.

E. L 12   W M.

These control settings indicate separation of the cyst contents into a less dense superior material (5–12) and an inferior layering of more dense elements (8–15). This gravitational phenomenon has been observed in other cystic lesions and apparently represents settling of cellular debris during recumbency.

F. The most superior portion of the craniopharyngioma is shown here. Calcifications are present in the capsule posteriorly. Plain film skull examination failed to reveal any calcifications above the level of the destroyed sella.

190

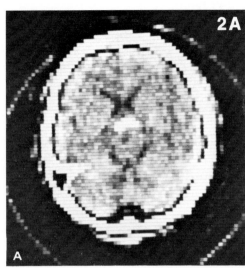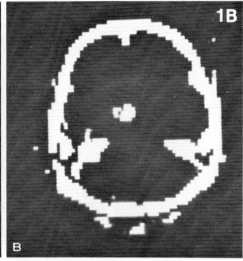

FIG. 8.9. CRANIOPHARYNGIOMA, LARGELY SOLID.

Clinical Features. A 33 y.o. male with decreasing vision in the left temporal field for 5 years, worse recently and associated with right temporal headache. Two weeks of episodic numbness in the left forearm.

Neurological Examination. Left homonymous hemianopsia, with bilateral optic atrophy and no other neurological findings.

Skull Examination. Amorphous suprasellar calcification and sellar erosion indicative of a chronic suprasellar mass.

RN Scan. Arsenic[74], abnormal.

CT Scan. Abnormal (Fig. 8.9).

Angio. Bilateral transfemoral carotid studies revealed a moderately large suprasellar mass.

PEG. Moderately large suprasellar mass containing calcification. Normal ventricular size.

Operation. (Dr. Robert G. Ojemann.) Right frontotemporal craniotomy, with total removal of craniopharyngioma containing dense calcification and a 2-ml cyst containing xanthochromic fluid.

Histology. Craniopharyngioma.

A. L 14　　W 20.

Section through the level of the inferior portions of the frontal horns and suprasellar region. The mass is clearly evident anteriorly, where there is a large amount of dense calcification. No calcification is visible in the remainder of the mass, which is outlined posteriorly by CSF in a considerably narrowed interpeduncular cistern. *Note that this plane of section is too low for this compressed and distorted interpeduncular cistern to be an ambient cistern, which it superficially resembles.* A small region of lesser density, approximately 2 squares in diameter, is seen in the central portion of the mass, and this probably represents the small cyst found at operation. The total mass extends a little more to the right than to the left of the midline. The anterior limit of the lesion was better shown than at PEG. The question of the extent of a cystic component could also not be answered by other radiological studies. However, the precise relationship of the mass to the third ventricle and circle of Willis could not be identified from the CT scan.

B. L 32　　W M.

Partial volume averaging of the calcifications in the section below that shown in **A**.

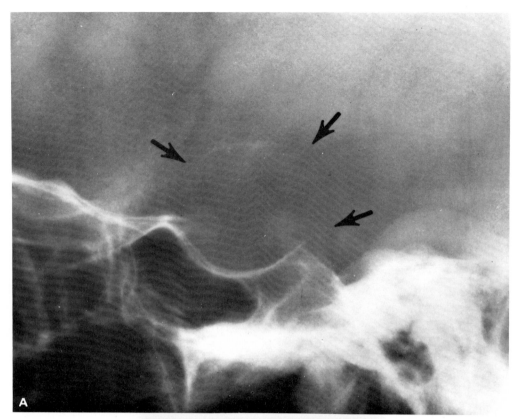

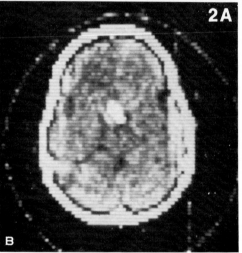

FIG. 8.10. CRANIOPHARYNGIOMA (NOT HISTOLOGI-CALLY VERIFIED).

Clinical Features. This 48 y.o. male had been evaluated elsewhere and clinical details are unknown.

Skull Examination. Including polytomography; suprasellar mass, with peripheral calcification (Fig. 8.10**A**).

CT Scan. Abnormal (Fig. 8.10**B**).

A. Lateral skull film of the region of the sella shows gross truncation of the dorsum sellae (*lower arrow*), a flat somewhat eroded sellar floor, and loss of density of the anterior clinoid processes. A fine curvilinear calcification was present superiorly (*upper arrows*) and bilaterally in the suprasellar region. There had been no change in these findings over a period of 3 years.

B. L 15   W 30.
A 21 x 12 mm ovoid calcific mass was demonstrated in the suprasellar area. No definite soft tissue tumor elements or cystic spaces were identified. The upper portion of the third ventricle and the lateral ventricles appeared normal. It was considered that the much greater sensitivity of the CT, in combination with its relatively low resolution, creates an appearance of a more or less homogeneous mass of calcification, whereas the high resolution but much less sensitive radiographic study shows fine bone texture, which adds an important parameter to evaluation in this and other cases.

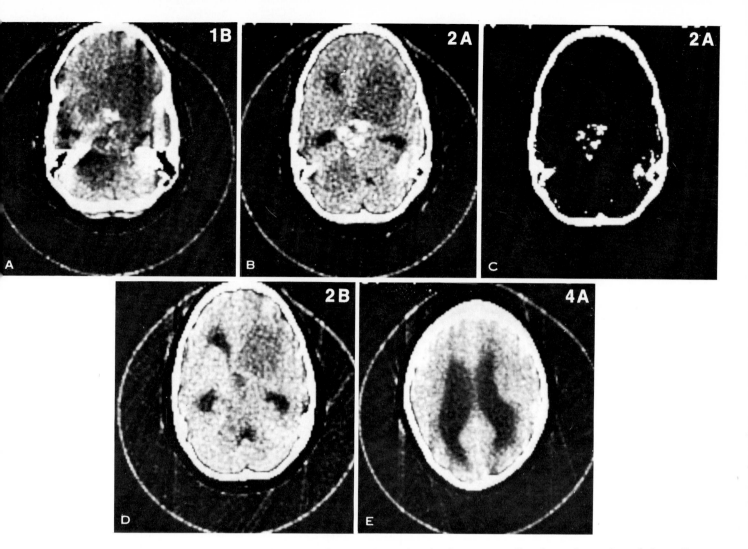

FIG. 8.11. CRANIOPHARYNGIOMA, MASSIVE, WITH CYSTIC SUPRA- AND INFRATENTORIAL COMPONENTS.

Clinical Features. A 12 y.o. girl with recent onset of acute headaches, nausea, and vomiting.

Neurological Examination. Papilledema, bitemporal visual field defects, and left fifth, seventh, and eighth nerve involvement.

Skull Examination. Moderate suture diastasis and "flat" sella, with diminished density of lamina dura and complete destruction of the dorsum. Small nodular and curvilinear calcifications were visible in the immediate suprasellar area and interpeduncular and upper pontine cisterns.

CT Scan. Abnormal (Fig. 8.11).

Operation. (Dr. Paul Chapman.) Right transfrontal approach with major excision of a very large cyst extending upwards and to the right from the suprasellar region. Fluid in the cyst was markedly xanthochromic but was not viscous and did not clot on standing. There was a large solid area of tumor in the suprasellar region and further cyst formation was visible extending into the interpeduncular region.

A–E. Plain CT scan.

A. Eight-mm section. Small spotty areas of calcification are present in the region of the interpeduncular cistern and upper pontine cistern. A streak of calcification is extending transversely in the region just medial to the left petrous apex. Behind this is a large region of abnormally low absorption (2–20) extending posteriorly in the left cerebellar region and to the midline. A very large circumscribed rounded area of diminished

absorption is shown extending from the region of the sella anteriorly and to the right into the inferior frontal and medial right temporal regions (absorption, −2 to +20).

B. Next 8-mm section above that in **A.** Larger nodules of calcification are shown in the region of the suprasellar and interpeduncular cisterns, also extending to the left, to abut the dilated temporal horn. The rounded area of diminished absorption in the posterior fossa is seen faintly (partial volume averaging). The lower portion of the fourth ventricle is markedly displaced to the right. The rounded low absorption region extending from the sella anteriorly and to the left is again visible (8–18). The inferior portion of the enlarged left frontal horn is shown to the left.

C. L 30 W M.

The central calcifications are visible. Due to partial volume averaging, peak absorption of these was in the region of 90 units.

D. The deformed and moderately displaced fourth ventricle is visible, as well as the dilated left frontal horn and dilated temporal horns. The right frontal cystic extension is again visible (10–19).

E. A 13-mm section at the level of the ventricular bodies and occipital horns. The lateral aspect of the right lateral ventricle is indented by the brain, which is markedly deformed due to the presence of the huge subjacent cyst.

The relatively high absorption of the fluid in the large supratentorial cyst is thought to be the result of an old hemorrhage into the cavity.

CHAPTER 9

Acoustic Neuromas

INTRODUCTION

CT scanning has proven to be of significant value in investigation of patients with suspected acoustic neuroma and other cerebellopontine lesions, such as meningiomas and epidermoid tumors. In the investigation of basal skull and intracranial lesions, it is of special importance to avoid all motion during scanning, since motion has a particularly deleterious effect upon such scans in regions where dense and irregular bone contours result in a less favorable signal to noise ratio than in more superior sections. The use of high angles (circa 30°) allows scanning of the posterior fossa with inclusion of less bone and air (nasopharyngeal and paranasal sinuses) than do shallower scan angles and therefore is indicated. Also, the use of 8-mm sections provides an opportunity for more detailed evaluation without apparent significant decrease in accuracy of absorption measurements. The use of preliminary high quality plain film skull examination and high quality laminography remains essential in the evaluation of basal lesions, which tend to produce highly characteristic bone changes. The employment of contrast enhancement is of great value in the study of basal neuromas (and meningiomas), although it is not always required. Some acoustic neuromas are sufficiently dense on plain CT scanning to be clearly identifiable. In other cases, the acoustic neuroma is insufficiently dense to be discriminated from surrounding anatomical structures until studied with contrast enhancement.

Using the above CT scan techniques, most acoustic neuromas are identifiable, even with the use of the 80 x 80 matrix system, down to approximately 1.5 to 2 cm in diameter (Table 9.1). Smaller tumors than this may be identified if they are highly vascularized and if contrast enhancement is employed, particularly with the 160 matrix system.

Acoustic neuromas of moderate or large size may have central lower absorption regions associated with necrotic changes. This broad, ring-shaped configuration may be seen on plain scan and can be accentuated with contrast enhancement (Fig. 9.3). This feature may permit differentiation from small rounded meningiomas, in which central necrotic change is unlikely, at least to the same extent as in neuromas, size for size. In cases of acoustic neuroma with typical bone erosion and a clear-cut demonstration on CT scan, the importance of further examination by angiography and/or pneumoencephalography will be debatable. Patients with clinical findings suggestive of acoustic neuroma, with or without bone changes, in whom the CT scan is not revealing will require additional study by posterior fossa cisternography, which is presently the most sensitive method for identification of very small acoustic neuromas. CT scanning should prove to be extremely valuable in differentiating true angle tumors from arachnoid pseudocysts resulting from local arachnoidal adhesions. Positive contrast cisternography should be employed only after CT scanning for the additional reason that even small residual Pantopaque droplets in the CP angle may cause artifacts sufficient to obscure anatomical details.

TABLE 9.1
Acoustic Neuromas: 7 Cases

	CT* scans (7)	RN scans (2)
Positive	5	1
? Positive	2	0
Negative	0	1

CT Cases:

2.0 cm, p̄ op;† moderate opacification; RN negative.

1.6 x 2.2 cm, p̄ op; clearly visible on plain CT scan.

1.5 x 2.0 cm, p̄ op; marked opacification.

? size, p̄ op; ? visible (plain scan only).

1.8 x 2.7 cm; marked opacification.   3.0 cm; decreased

3.0 cm; decreased absorption of cerebellum with no visualization of tumor itself and no opacification; RN positive.

2.0 x 3.0 cm; not visible until opacification.

* CT, computed tomographic; RN, radionuclide.

† p̄ op, CT scan following previous partial resection; opacification, increase in density following intravenous injection of 40–50 ml of Hypaque 60 M.

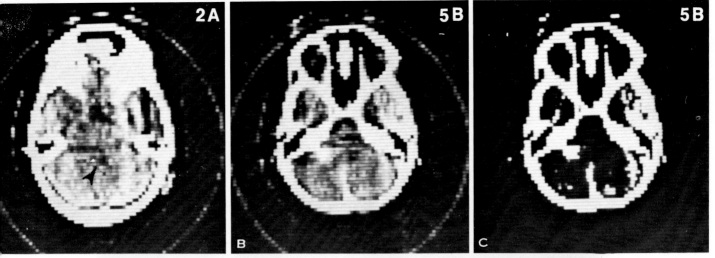

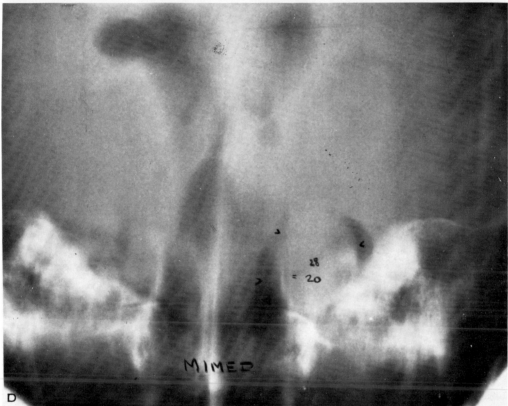

FIG. 9.1. ACOUSTIC NEUROMA.

Clinical Features. A 46 y.o. female with decreasing hearing associated with tinnitus in the left ear for 4 months. She also complained of a vague sense of uncertain balance. Over 4 months, numbness below the left eye spread to the left cheek and left side of the nose.

Neurological Examination. Markedly decreased hearing on the left side. Left-beating nystagmus with the eyes closed. Hypesthesia in the distribution of the trigeminal nerve. Normal facial nerve function. No caloric response on the left side.

Skull Examination. Studies included polytomography and revealed erosion of the left internal auditory canal.

CT Scan. Abnormal (Fig. 9.1, A–C).

PEG. A 2-cm diameter rounded mass in the left CP angle (Fig. 9.1 D).

Operation. Excision of tumor, approximately 2 cm in diameter.

Histology. Acoustic neurinoma.

Plain CT scan (**A**) revealed no evidence of abnormal absorption values in the region of the left CP angle (except for the typical horizontal low absorption artifact extending between the anterior portions of the petrous bones), even after intense scrutiny. However, moderate displacement of the fourth ventricle to the right was apparent (*arrowhead*). The study was repeated following intravenous injection of 50 ml Hypaque 60 (**B**; W 30). This 13-mm section, slightly below that shown in **A**, clearly reveals a rounded high absorption mass (22–40) in the left CP angle. The fourth ventricle is again shown to be displaced approximately 9 mm to the right.

C. L 27   W M.

The tumor is very obvious at these control settings.

D. PEG. Erect sagittal projection, linear laminographic section. The rounded mass in the left CP angle is very clearly outlined, and its corrected transverse diameter is 20 mm. Deformity of the configuration of the fourth ventricle, due to indentation of its left side and rotation, together with contralateral displacement of the fourth ventricle and aqueduct are clearly demonstrated.

(Fig. 9.1, **B** and **C** reprinted by permission from Radiology, 114: 75–87, 1975.)

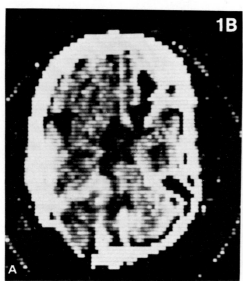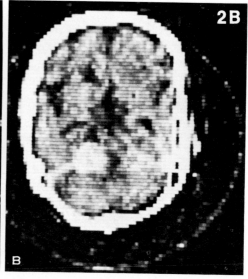

FIG. 9.2. ACOUSTIC NEUROMA, FOLLOWING PARTIAL RESECTION.

Clinical Features A 68 y.o. male who was referred for CT scan 4 months after subtotal resection of a left acoustic neuroma. Recent symptoms had raised suspicion of obstructive hydrocephalus.

A. Plain CT scan 4 months after limited resection. The right side of the head was tilted higher than the left and only the upper portion of the left petrous bone is included in the section. The left occipital craniectomy defect is visible. There is a quite "dense" mass in the left CP angle (18–31). Posteriorly, there is a relatively low absorption region within the mass, presumably representing the site of partial surgical resection. Medial to the mass is a 6–9 mm zone of low absorption, due to CSF between the mass and the pons, which is considerably indented on its left side and is displaced to the right. The low absorption of the fourth ventricle is visible. It is displaced to the right and

appears to be gaping in the region of its left lateral recess, adjacent to the tumor. It is most unlikely that the relatively high density of the neuroma on this plain CT scan is the result of hemorrhage into the tumor induced by surgery 4 months earlier. The wide CSF space between the tumor and the pons can be explained by appreciable surgical decompression and indicates clearly the marked pressure deformity created by the originally larger mass.

B. Contrast-enhanced scan obtained 11 months later (after intravenous injection of 50 ml of Hypaque 60). The scan is at approximately the same level relative to the left petrous bone as the initial scan. There is now insignificant head tilting. The tumor has grown considerably in the interval. Absorption range of the mass is 14–30. Enlargement of suprasellar cisterns and subarachnoid spaces is indicative of considerable cerebral atrophy. There was also considerable widespread enlargement of cerebral sulci, and the ventricles were moderately enlarged.

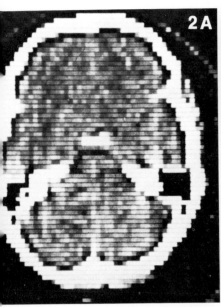
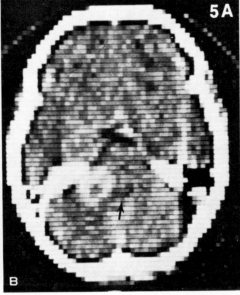
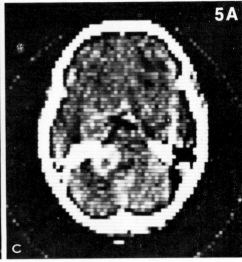

FIG. 9.3. ACOUSTIC NEUROMA.

Clinical Features. A 15 y.o. boy who had a 1½ year history of progressive decrease in hearing in the left ear, associated with tinnitus for the previous 6 months.

Neurological Examination. Marked reduction in hearing and caloric response in the left ear. Audiograms indicated severe sensorineural hearing loss. Tests of other cranial nerves were normal.

Skull Examination. Studies, including polytomography, revealed marked erosion of the left internal acoustic canal.

CT scan. Abnormal (Fig. 9.3).

Angio. Transfemoral selective left internal and external carotid angiograms and a selective left vertebral study revealed evidence of an *avascular* mass in the left *CP angle*.

Operation. Resection of a tumor in the left CP angle that was markedly indenting the brain stem. The tumor was firm and "slightly vascular." Its maximum diameter was approximately 4 cm.

Histology. Acoustic schwannoma, without cystic components.

A. Plain scan. **B.** Contrast-enhanced scan. W 20. Eight-mm sections.

A. The plain CT scan revealed only hints of slightly abnormal absorption values in and adjacent to the region of the left CP angle.

B. After intravenous injection of approximately 45 ml of Hypaque 60, the tumor was very clearly demonstrated as a quite large rounded mass (approximately 3 cm in transverse diameter). The fourth ventricle is slightly displaced to the right (low absorption area immediately to the right of the medial edge of the mass *arrow*). The bulk of the mass now shows quite high absorption (23–30). A small zone in its posterior central portion is appreciably less dense, measuring 14–22. The appearance of relatively ischemic central regions can be expected in CT scans of neurinomas following contrast enhancement, whereas they are infrequent in meningiomas, even of much larger size. This feature, together with the different plain film characteristics that are usually identifiable, aid in differentiating neurinomas from meningiomas. Extravascular diffusion of contrast medium is suggested as an important factor in enhancement in such cases.

C. L 10   W M.

Same section as in **B.** The narrower window display provides considerably higher contrast between the neurinoma and surrounding brain. (At our request, the viewer was fitted with an additional control, which permitted continuous adjustment of window width from 20 down to M. This replaced the window 100 setting. In practice, it appears that windows of 15, 10, and 5 would be sufficient.)

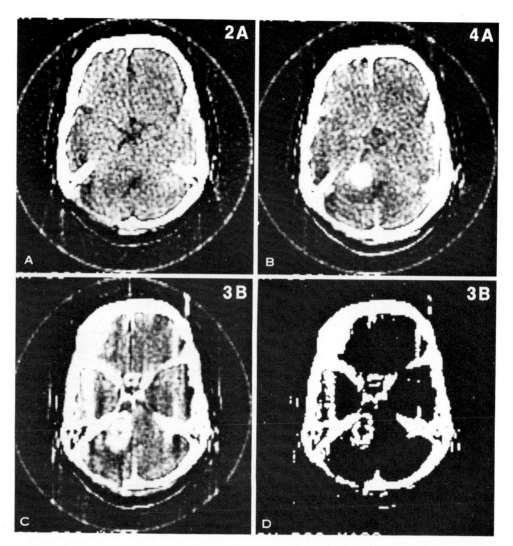

FIG. 9.4 ACOUSTIC NEUROMA; LARGE POSTOPER-ATIVE RECURRENCE.

A–C. Eight-mm CT sections. 160 x 160 matrix system.

A. L 15   W 30.

Plain scan section at the level of the fourth ventricle. The appearance of the fourth ventricle indicates indentation from the left anterolateral aspect, with some rotation and slight displacement towards the right. No definitely abnormal absorption values were evident in the posterior fossa on this or on adjacent sections, although there is a slight suggestion of a poorly defined region of diminished absorption in the cerebellum, to the left of the fourth ventricle.

B. L 18   W 30.

Scan section very similar to that in **A** after intravenous injection of 300 ml of Renografin 30%. The superior portion of the large recurrent left acoustic neuroma is very clearly visible, due to high absorption. At the periphery of the suprasellar cisterns, bands of increased absorption represent the circle of Willis. On the left side, the anterior cerebral, posterior communicating, and posterior cerebral arteries are quite clearly visible. Behind the tumor, slightly diminished absorption in the cerebellum is consistent with minor edema secondary to the mass. This stands out more clearly in contrast with the tumor and now higher absorption of normal portions of the cerebellum.

C. L 18   W 30.

Scan section immediately below that in **B**, through the region of the equator of the mass, which here shows a slightly irregular oval contour (peak absorption, 50). Areas of lesser absorption are present in the central portions of the mass, consistent with lesser vascularity and probably some necrosis. The osseous elements of the sella are clearly visible in the central area, and the upper portion of the basilar artery is visible just behind the dorsum sellae.

D. L 35   W M.

These settings more clearly reveal the less vascular and probably necrotic portions of the mass.

CHAPTER 10

Pineal Area Tumors

CT scanning readily identifies the hydrocephalus, which tends to be prominent at the time patients with pineal area tumors come to attention. At this time, the tumors are usually sufficiently large to be identified directly by this method. CT scanning also offers an opportunity to identify the gross character of the wide variety of solid and cystic tumors that occur in this region: cystic and solid teratomas; atypical teratomas, such as germinomas, gliomas of the pineal and adjacent structures, and the less commonly occurring true pineal tumors, pinealocytomas and pinealoblastomas. Calcification occurring in certain of these tumors, notably the teratomas and gliomas, is readily identified, but its characteristics are better evaluated by plain film examination, as is the displacement and rotation of pineal calcification that may be visible in some instances. If the tumor contains extensive calcifications, evaluation of the soft tissue components may be difficult on CT scans. Vascularity of the lesion is not readily evaluated by plain scans followed by contrast enhancement due to the component of enhancement that may be contributed by extravascular diffusion of contrast medium. Of particular value is the ease with which control of hydrocephalus by ventricular shunting and/or radiation therapy can be evaluated. The rapidity and degree of reduction in size or irradiated tumors can also be evaluated readily and can provide early indication of the probable type of pineal tumor present. Rapid and marked reduction in tumor size following irradiation is indicative of a very radiosensitive tumor, such as a germinoma, whereas poor response to radiotherapy is indicative of an insensitive tumor, such as a teratoma or glioma. Due to the close proximity of structures, it is likely to be difficult to distinguish some pineal tumors from tumors arising from the dorsal portions of the midbrain or from the posterior third ventricle. Angiography and pneumoencephalography are also likely to be required for satisfactory initial diagnosis.

TABLE 10.1
Pineal Area Neoplasms: 5 Cases + 1*
0 false negative
0 false positive

Age			
15	Glioma	2.0 cm + calc†	RN negative
12	Teratoma	Very large + calc†	RN positive
13	Endodermal tumor	Very large + calc†	RN positive
26	No histology	Small	
25	No histology	Small	
17	No histology	* Resolution p̄ radiation	

† calc., calcification; p̄, following.

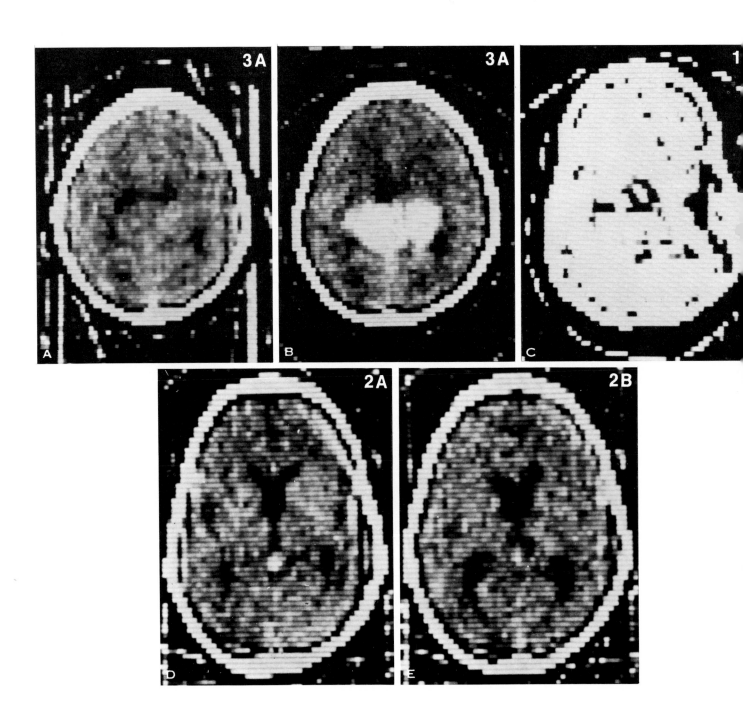

FIG. 10.1. ENDODERMAL SINUS TUMOR OF THE PINEAL (EXTRAGONADAL YOLK-SAC TUMOR).

Clinical Features. A 12 y.o. girl with a 10 day history of increasing lethargy and 3 days of nausea and vomiting. Growth had ceased at the age of 9 and no secondary sex characteristics had developed. Eighteen months earlier she was hospitalized with herpes simplex encephalitis, at which time diabetes insipidus was discovered and treated.

Neurological Examination. Normal. Moderate dehydration was noted. Repeated seizures developed, with lip smacking, roving eye movements, and movements of the right extremities. Papilledema, dilatation of the left pupil, right sixth nerve palsy, and right hemiparesis soon developed, with neck rigidity and bilateral Babinski signs. Mannitol and dexamethasone were given, with recovery.

Skull Examination. Questionable abnormal-appearing pineal calcification (not identified 18 months earlier).

RN Scan. Tcp; large well-defined area of increased activity in midline, posterior third ventricular region.

CT Scan. Abnormal (Fig. 10.1).

Angio. Transfemoral bilateral carotid and left vertebral studies showed a large well-vascularized tumor in the region of the pineal, with prominent irregular vessels and prolonged tumor blush.

Shortly after completion of radiotherapy (3000 rads to entire brain, with additional 1500 rads to the area of the third ventricle), she developed back and lower extremity pain, urinary retention, and motor and sensory signs of a dorsal spinal cord lesion. Myelography revealed extramedullary intradural masses in the spinal canal and complete obstruction at the sixth to ninth dorsal segments.

Operation. Decompressive laminectomy with tumor removal from subarachnoid space.

Histology. Endodermal sinus tumor of the pineal (extragonadal yolk-sac tumor).

A. Plain CT scan, showing a very large mass centered in the pineal region and causing gross compression of both trigones and the bodies of the lateral ventricles. The mass showed irregular areas of absorption slightly higher and slightly lower than normal white matter. On a lower section, calcification, presumably in a posteriorly displaced pineal gland, was evident.

B. Contrast-enhanced scan following intravenous injection of 30 ml of Conray 60 at a similar level to that in **A**. The absorption of the mass had increased from values of 10–15 and 14–20 on plain scans to a range of 20–31. The mass was now sharply defined and more homogeneous in absorption. Its maximum dimension was 8 cm. Surprisingly, the lateral ventricles were not significantly dilated by this huge mass lying above the aqueduct.

(Fig. 10.1, **A** and **B** reprinted by permission from Radiology, 110: 109–123, 1974.)

C. Plain CT scan through the suprasellar cisterns, showing an ovoid mass of approximately 9 x 12 mm in the suprasellar area, in the region of the hypothalamus and optic chiasm.

D and **E.** Contiguous 13-mm sections obtained 2 months after the initial study and approximately 6 weeks after completion of radiotherapy. The lateral and third ventricles are slightly enlarged. An area of calcification is noted in the region of the pineal, about 9 mm in diameter. There is no longer an appreciable mass effect and there is no convincing evidence of soft tissue tumor around the mass. The tumor was obviously highly radiosensitive.

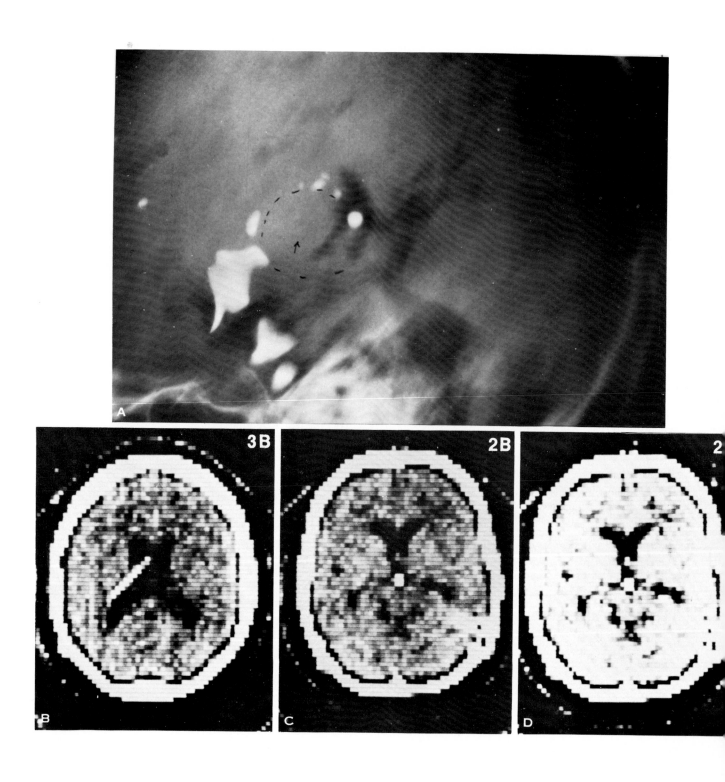

FIG. 10.2. ASTROCYTOMA, GRADE III–IV (GIGANTO-CELLULAR), OF POSTERIOR THIRD VENTRICLE-PINEAL.

Clinical Features. A 15 y.o. girl. Clinical onset 2 years and 10 months earlier, with headache and personality changes. Investigation with pneumography and Pantopaque ventriculography in another country led to a diagnosis of pineal area tumor of moderate size. She was treated by ventricular shunting and Cobalt 60 radiation, 4400 rads, at the MGH. Following this, reexamination with gas and Pantopaque in her home country revealed that the tumor had decreased only 25 to 30% in size. A further pneumoencephalogram several months before CT examination indicated that the tumor had returned to approximately the same size as at the original examination. Faint amorphous calcifications in a 1–1.5 cm area appeared in the pineal area following radiation. She was admitted for evaluation because of developing lethargy, with nausea and vomiting for 1 week. Parinaud's syndrome was not present. Extraocular movements were full.

Skull Examination and PEG, with residual ventricular Pantopaque, several months earlier; results as noted above. (Fig. 10.2**A**.)

CT Scan. Abnormal (Fig. 10.2, **B–D**).

Operation. (Dr. William H. Sweet.) The tumor was reached by an approach above the cerebellar hemispheres and below the tentorium. Apparently total excision of the mass was obtained, although it was adherent to the posterior portion of each thalamus and to the midbrain. Also, it encroached upon the third ventricle to become adherent to the massa intermedia.

Histology. Astrocytoma, Grade III–IV, with giant cells (gigantocellular).

A. Pneumoencephalogram. Erect lateral projection. Pantopaque remains in the lateral and third ventricles from previous examination. Faint amorphous calcification is noted in the region of the pineal (*small arrow*). No gas passed through the aqueduct. Gas is shown in slightly distorted retrothalamic cisterns and quadrigeminal cisterns. Synthesis of findings on the entire examination revealed a mass behind the third ventricle, as outlined by the *interrupted line*.

B. CT section through the lateral ventricles, which are slightly enlarged. The oblique, high density structure on the left side represents a portion of the ventricular shunt tube.

C. L 17   W 20.

At this level, the mildly dilated frontal and temporal horns are shown, and a moderately widened third ventricle lies just anterior to a calcific density, which lies anterior to the normal position of a pineal and at the anterior margin of a soft tissue mass projecting into a distorted quadrigeminal cistern. Absorption of calcification, 400 units; tumor absorption, 13–18 units.

D. L 14   W 10.

The higher contrast control settings more clearly reveal the contour of the mass projecting posteriorly into the quadrigeminal cistern. The third ventricle is encroached upon from the posterior aspect. There was a suggestion of slight bilateral indentation of the mesial aspects of the trigones. The mass measured approximately 2.5 cm in diameter, slightly greater than indicated by the pneumogram several months earlier. Repeat CT scan following intravenous injection of Hypaque showed no apparent increase in absorption of the mass.

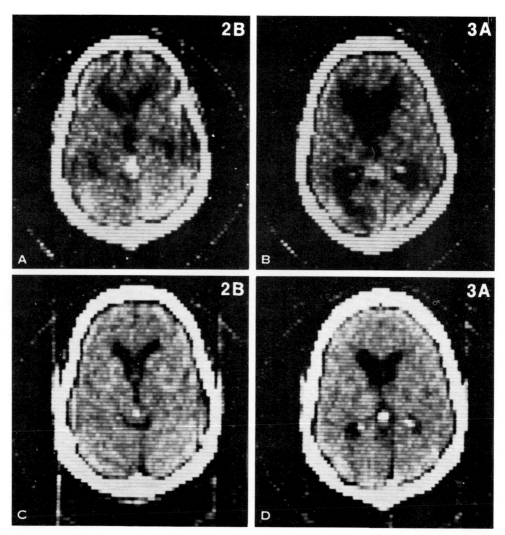

FIG. 10.3. TUMOR OF PINEAL AREA, CONTAINING CALCIFICATION AND SHOWN TO BE RADIOSENSITIVE (HISTOLOGY NOT OBTAINED).

Clinical Features. A 27 y.o. male with a 6 month history of headaches, increased by rapid movement of the head. Intermittent diplopia for 5 weeks, worse on upward and lateral gaze. Polyuria and polydipsia. Decreased libido.

Neurological Examination. Pupils equal in size, reacting to light. No papilledema. Conjugate upward gaze limited to 1 mm. Incomplete convergence, with nystagmus retractorius. Full downward gaze, with nystagmus.

EEG. Mildly abnormal, with bilateral slowing.

Skull Examination. Abnormally large area of calcification in the region of the pineal.

CT Scan. Abnormal (Fig. 10.3, **A** and **B**).

Angio. Avascular mass in the pineal area, with a cluster of small nodular calcifications in lower than usual position of the pineal. Marked lateral ventricular enlargement.

Dexamethasone relieved symptoms of increased intracranial pressure, and the patient was given radiotherapy.
A and **B.** A 12 × 15 mm region of high absorption (140) indicative of calcification was noted immediately behind the third ventricle. A surrounding zone 3–6 mm in width measured 21–30, indicating a soft tissue mass, which was difficult to separate from the calcification during analysis. Marked obstructive dilatation of the lateral and third ventricles was demonstrated. There appeared to be increased separation of the ambient cisterns on a lower section (not shown).
C and **D.** Scans obtained approximately 5 months after radiotherapy. Headaches were now rare and polydipsia had decreased. The lateral and third ventricles are now enlarged only slightly. The calcification in the pineal area is smaller and denser, and no definite soft tissue mass can be identified. No mass was identified in the region of the hypothalamus on either CT examination or in the angiogram.

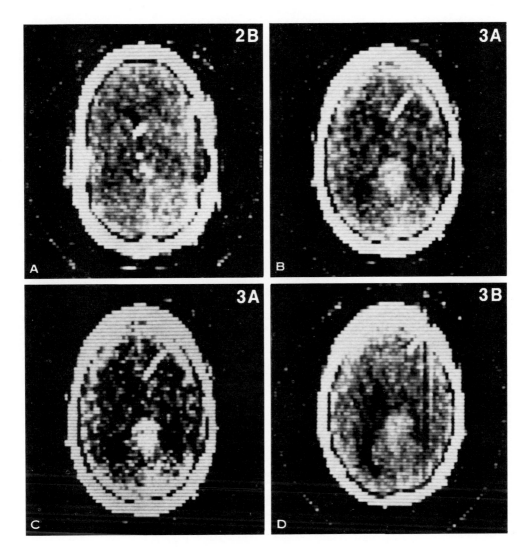

FIG. 10.4. PINEAL AREA TUMOR (HISTOLOGY NOT OBTAINED).

Clinical Features. A 25 y.o. male, in whom obstructive hydrocephalus had been satisfactorily controlled by ventriculoatrial shunting.

CT Scan. Abnormal (Fig. 10.4, **A–D**).

Angio. A large mass was shown in the pineal area, with slight tumor vessel formation, supplied partly by an enlarged left medial tentorial artery. A 3-mm calcification lay well anterior to the usual position of the pineal and several millimeters to the left of the midline.

A. L   18   W   20.

At this level, the tip of the shunt tube extends through the right frontal horn to the region of the left foramen of Munro. A minimally widened third ventricle appears indented posteriorly, where there is a 6-mm calcific absorption area that, with the third ventricle, lies several millimeters to the left of the midline. Additional calcific absorption zones are present a few millimeters posteriorly. These were not visible on skull films.

B. L   19   W   20.

A portion of the ventricular shunt tube is again visible anteriorly. A large area of increased absorption (18–20 and 20–30), approximately 3 cm in maximum diameter, is visible projecting superiorly from the pineal area to indent the posterior portions of the bodies of the normal-sized lateral ventricles.

C. L   10   W   10.

Same section as in **B**. The higher contrast control settings show the contours of the mass more clearly.

D. L   18   W   20.

The mass is still extensive in the section above that shown in **B** and **C**. At this level, there is marked local encroachment upon the posterior body and trigone of the right lateral ventricle. No calcific absorption values were noted in the scan sections above that shown in **A**.

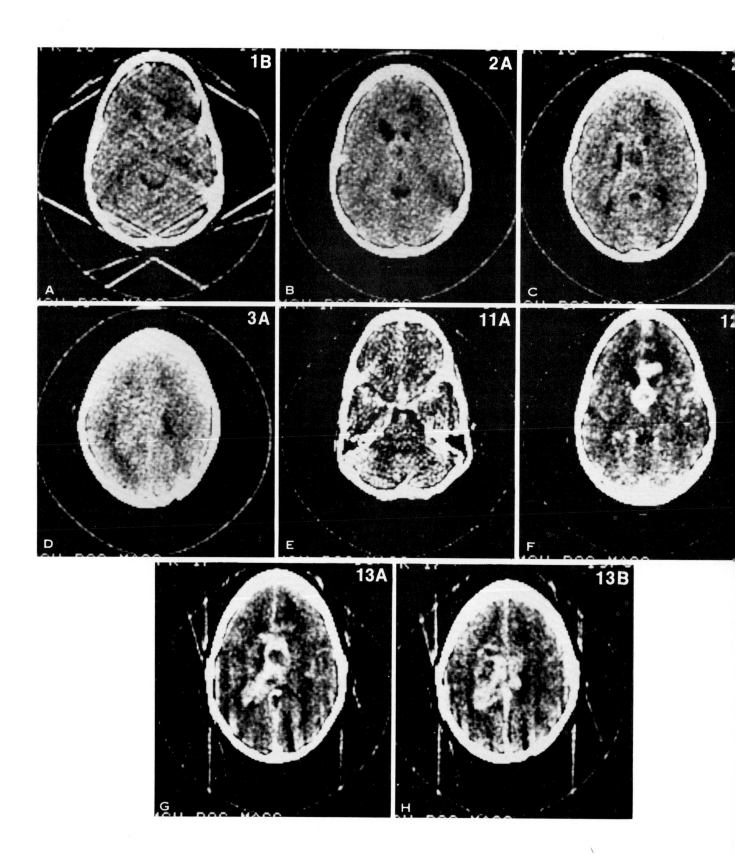

FIG. 10.5. GERMINOMA, ORIGINATING IN THE REGION OF THE ANTERIOR THIRD VENTRICLE.

Clinical Features. A 17 y.o. girl who was well until the age of 8, when it was noted that normal growth was not being maintained. Panhypopituitarism was identified at another hospital. Tcp scan and angiography were negative. Three years later she developed diabetes insipidus. PEG with laminography revealed minor changes in the region of the anterior third ventricle, leading to a diagnosis of chiasmal glioma. No radiation therapy was given. Increasing generalized headaches with occasional vomiting and right hemiparesis led to her first admission to the MGH. Her height was 4 feet 9 inches and there was absence of secondary sex characteristics.

Neurological Examination. Mental status was normal. Examination of the cranial nerves revealed no abnormality. There was a moderate right spastic hemiparesis. Sensory examination and cerebellar testing were normal. CSF total protein was 216 mgm % and contained many cells with the appearance of lymphocytes and a few large, questionably malignant cells.

CT Scan. Abnormal (Fig. 10.5).

Operation. (Dr. Robert Ojemann.) Right frontal craniotomy and biopsy of a grey-reddish tumor in the region of the right frontal horn.

Histology. Germinoma.

A–D. Plain CT scans. L 14 W 30. 160 x 160 matrix system.

A region of diminished absorption (5–12), with poorly defined margins, involves the grey and white matter of the anterior portion of the right frontal lobe. There is slight midline dislocation to the left and evidence of compression of the right frontal horn. The anterior and middle portions of the third ventricle are not visible. Irregular areas of slightly increased absorption (up to 20 units) are shown extending into the parathird ventricular regions and into the region of a thickened septum lucidum (**A** and **B**).

C. There is a generalized deformity and compression of both lateral ventricles from the frontal horns to the trigones, more on the right side. A broad irregular band of increased absorption (up to 24) surrounds the compressed left lateral ventricle and extends irregularly through the region of the superior frontal horn and body of the right lateral ventricle.

D. A very broad region of increased absorption extends through the region of the upper portion of the left lateral ventricle and across the midline through the region of the corpus callosum to terminate to the right of the markedly compressed body of the right lateral ventricle. The values through this region were heterogeneous, ranging from approximately 18 to 26.

E–H. Scan following intravenous injection of 300 ml of 30% meglumine diatrizoate.

E. An ovoid area of increased absorption lies in the region of the suprasellar cisterns.

F. The mass occupying the third ventricle and extending laterally into the medial portions of third ventricle and portions of the basal ganglia shows marked enhancement (22–39). Extension of the mass into the septum lucidum and much of the region of the right frontal horn is clearly apparent.

G and H. There is marked contrast enhancement (26–40) of the extensive mass surrounding the left lateral ventricle and, to a somewhat lesser extent, the right lateral ventricle. There appears to be extensive mass within these ventricles also.

The findings are indicative of very widespread para and intraventricular extension of the germinoma. Another case of paraventricular extension of germinoma is illustrated in Figure 10.6.

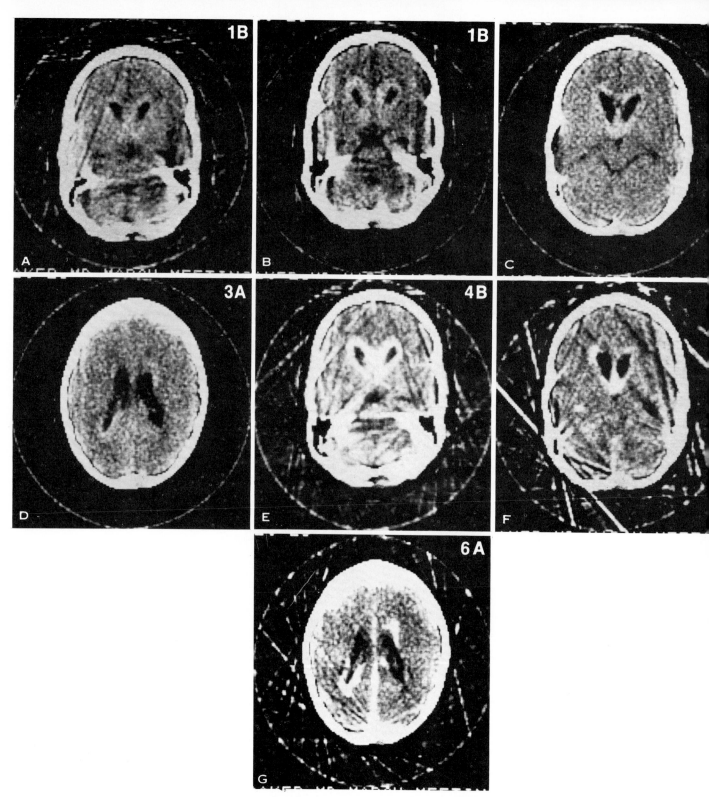

FIG. 10.6. PARAVENTRICULAR EXTENSION OF PINEAL TUMOR. (Case contributed by Hillier L. Baker, Jr., M.D.)

Clinical Features. A 14 y.o. boy who presented with signs and symptoms of increased intracranial tension.

Neurological Examination. Revealed diplopia on left lateral gaze and nystagmus retractorius on vertical gaze.

A CT scan and pneumoencephalogram revealed a mass in the pineal region. The pineal tumor was treated with radiation therapy. One year later, nausea and vomiting recurred. A plain CT scan was obtained, followed 1 month later by a contrast-enhanced scan (Fig. 10.6).

A–D. Plain CT scan. L 14 W 30 160 x 160 matrix system.

A broad, well-defined zone of moderately increased absorption (18–26) is shown encasing the lateral ventricles. This is most striking in the frontal horns but is also visible further posteriorly, particularly around the left occipital horn. A mass of similar absorption is shown involving the anterior portion of the third ventricle, anterior pillars of the fornix, and the widened septum lucidum.

E–G. Scan 1 month later, after intravenous injection of contrast medium. Marked enhancement of the absorption of the paraventricular tissue (up to 30–40 units) is revealed.

A third scan (not shown), obtained nearly 5 weeks later, demonstrated an increase in the thickness of the tumor encasing the ventricular system, particularly at the frontal horns. There was now evidence of seeding of tumor to the fourth ventricle. (Polaroid photographs obtained from magnetic tape records supplied by courtesy of Dr. Hillier L. Baker, Jr., Mayo Clinic, Rochester, Minnesota.)

CHAPTER 11

Miscellaneous Primary Neoplasms

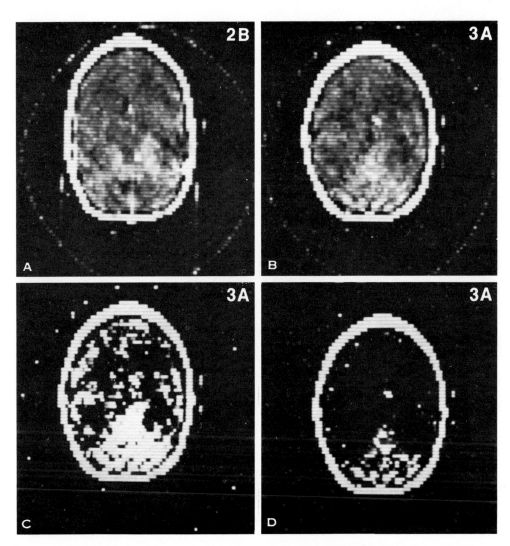

FIG. 11.1. MEDULLOBLASTOMA.

Clinical Features. A 2 ½ y.o. boy who presented at the age of 1 year with vomiting. Angiography and ventriculography were followed by posterior fossa exploration in another country. Medulloblastoma was found and a ventricular shunt was placed. He was referred to the MGH for radiation therapy, which was given to the posterior fossa only, because of his age, and therapy was completed at the age of 1 ½ years. Some months later he experienced difficulty walking, leg weakness, and gluteal pain. Myelography revealed extensive implants in the subarachnoid space of the dorsal and lumbar segments. He returned to the MGH and received radiotherapy to the spinal axis from D3 to S2. He returned for reevaluation after another 9 months because of recent headaches, head tilting to the right, irritability, and anorexia.

Neurological Examination. Holds head tilted to the right. Slight ataxia of left leg and slight hypotonia of the right upper extremity. No nuchal rigidity.

EEG. Normal.

Skull Examination. Posterior fossa craniectomy. No other significant features.

RN Scan. Tcp; no evidence of recurrent tumor. Some increase in activity in posterior fossa that was thought to be related to previous surgery or shunt tube.

CT Scan. Abnormal (Fig. 11.1).

A–D. Scans obtained only after contrast enhancement with 20 ml of Hypaque 60. The density of a right lateral ventricular shunt tube was noted. The lateral and third ventricles were very small. The fourth ventricle did not appear compressed but was posteriorly displaced (**A**). On the multiple 8-mm sections showing the posterior fossa, there was a very widespread and somewhat heterogeneous increase in absorption (19–25) that involved most of the cerebellum bilaterally and extended into the pons and midbrain (**A** and **B**). The areas of abnormal increase in absorption appeared to extend over the dorsal aspect of the midbrain in the quadrigeminal cistern to the regions of the retrothalamic cisterns, and there appeared to be extension into the area of the right thalamus (**B**) and third ventricle (**A** and **B**).

C. L 18   W M.   **D.** L 22   W M.

Same section as shown in **B**, further illustrating the wide extent of the abnormal absorption values in the posterior fossa and above the tentorial incisura.

Interpretation is hampered somewhat by previous radiotherapy and the lack of a plain CT scan. The findings are most compatible with widespread, somewhat vascularized, invasive tumor (medulloblastoma) throughout the cerebellum, brain stem, and third ventricular-right thalamic regions.

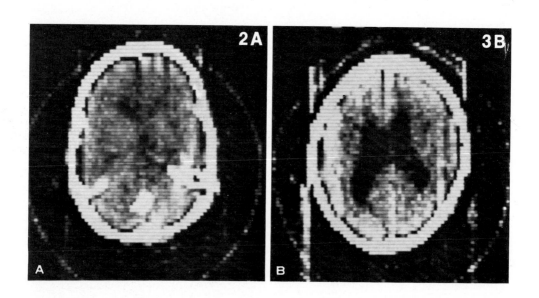

FIG. 11.2. MEDULLOBLASTOMA, CEREBELLAR VERMIS, WITH CALCIFICATION.

Clinical Features. An 18 y.o. female with a 3 month history of intermittent blurring of vision and occipital headaches.

Neurological Examination. Bilateral papilledema, otherwise normal. Clinical suspicion of obstructive hydrocephalus versus benign intracranial hypertension.

EEG. Mild generalized abnormality, with intermittent slowing.

Skull Examination. Initially interpreted as normal, but, in retrospect, faint granular calcification was evident in the area of the vermis (after CT scan).

RN Scan. Normal.

CT Scan. Abnormal (Fig. 11.2).

Angio. Transfemoral right carotid and vertebral studies demonstrated obstructive hydrocephalus and avascular mass in the inferior cerebellar vermis.

Operation. (Dr. Robert G. Ojemann.) Suboccipital craniectomy, laminectomy of C1; subtotal removal of medulloblastoma. The tumor was immediately apparent, having replaced the vermis. The tissue appeared relatively avascular and somewhat reddish. Large portions of the tumor were removed from the vermis and both cerebellar hemispheres. Tumor growth well beyond the excision was evident.

Histology. Medulloblastoma; soft mucoid grey-white tissue, with occasional hemorrhagic areas.

A. L 16   W 30.

A 13-mm scan section through the inferior frontal horns and the region of the fourth ventricle. A large, apparently solid area of calcification, approximately 24 mm in diameter, is present in the vermis, extending to the region of the fourth ventricle. The latter is not identified, apparently being markedly compressed. A few small (6–9 mm) areas of diminished absorption, 4–16, are present lateral and anterior to the calcification, suggesting islands of tumor. It is not clear whether the lesion originates in the fourth ventricle or in the vermis, with extension to the ventricle and adjacent areas. The CP angle and pontine cisterns appear compressed.

B. Third 13-mm scan section above that in **A,** showing marked dilatation of the lateral ventricles. The greater sensitivity of the CT scan was helpful in identifying calcification that was originally missed on skull examination. However, the lesser sensitivity and higher resolution of skull films revealed a granular texture to the calcification, which appeared as a single homogeneous mass on CT scan. *Radiographically* visible calcification is unusual in medulloblastoma, and the radiological findings in this case are more typical of ependymoma or subependymal astrocytoma of the region of the fourth ventricle. Thus far, medulloblastomas have generally shown higher absorption (20–30 range) than brain on plain CT scans. This may prove to be a helpful feature in differentiation from gliomas. Contrast enhancement of medulloblastomas occurs regularly.

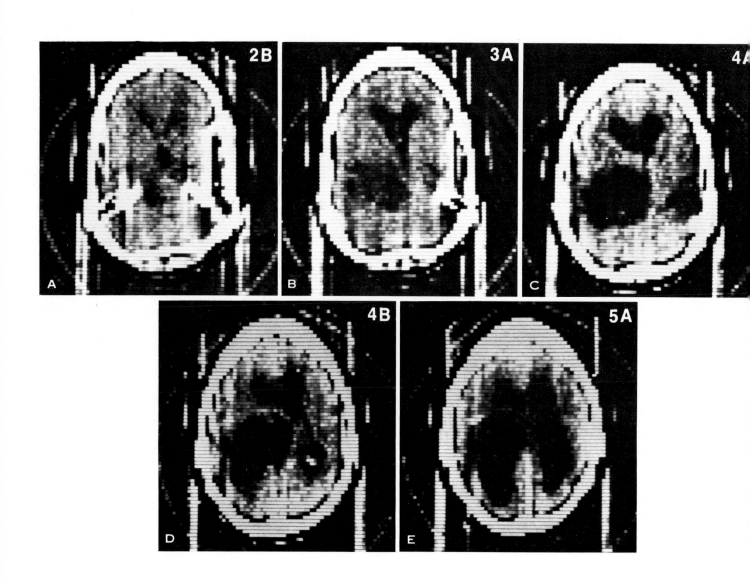

FIG. 11.3.   EPIDERMOID TUMOR.

Epidermoid tumors (pearly tumors, primary cholesteatomas). Experience with several such cases has indicated that the presence and extent of these tumors are readily determined on CT scanning. Due to very slow growth, they tend to be large at the time of clinical presentation. Of particular interest, however, is that the absorption values may be identical with or very similar to those of CSF-containing cavities. There is a real possibility, therefore, that these lesions may be confused with some varieties of leptomeningeal cyst

Clinical Features. A 32 y.o. female whose only complaint was that she had recently failed a visual test for a driver's license. She had not herself noted any difficulty with vision and denied having any other complaints.

Neurological Examination. Right inferior temporal homonymous quadrantanopsia. Slight right hyperreflexia, slight speech impairment, and confusion. General sensory and motor testing revealed no abnormalities.

EEG. Left temporal theta and delta slowing, with some sharp activity.

CT Scan. Abnormal (Fig. 11.3).

Angio. Transfemoral bilateral carotid and left vertebral studies revealed marked displacement of the internal cerebral vein to the right and marked lateral ventricular dilatation and suggested a large mass in the region of the left atrium (? dilatation of atrium). The anterior choroidal artery was displaced markedly superiorly and was stretched by a large mass in the region of the left atrium or adjacent deep structures. The vertebral angiogram suggested an extra-axial mass but did not exclude a mass within the atrium. The mass effect extended into the posterior fossa, with medial displacement of the superior cerebellar artery and lateral displacement of the posterior cerebral vessels. Although the mass was completely avascular, the study raised the suspicion of a tentorial meningioma.

Skull Examination, including polytomography of sella. Expansive and erosive changes at the sella, with obliteration of the dorsum, suggesting a long-standing increase in intracranial pressure with local pressure resulting from a suprasellar mass, such as a markedly dilated third ventricle.

Operation. (Dr. Raymond N. Kjellberg.) Left temporal craniectomy and total resection of a huge epidermoid tumor that elevated the temporal lobe and extended medially across the midline in the region of the quadrigeminal plate, to which it was somewhat adherent. After a 2-cm incision in the tentorium, the tumor was removed from the anteromedial portion of the posterior fossa.

Histology. Epidermoid with desquamated debris.

A–D. A huge, well-circumscribed, "cystic" appearing mass is shown in the inferior left supratentorial compartment, in the left temporal region, and bulging markedly into the region of the corpus striatum and to the considerably displaced and posteriorly compressed third ventricle (**B** and **C**). Low absorption values were present throughout this relatively homogeneous lesion and were not significantly different from normal absorption values of CSF (−2 to +10). The lesion extends approximately 15–20 mm to the right of the midline in the region of the posterior third ventricle and quadrigeminal cistern (**B** and **C**) and at the level of the internal cerebral vein (**D**). Inferiorly, the lesion extends to involve the anterior portion of the left CP angle cistern (**A**). Superiorly, the anterior and medial margins of the lesion are separated from the lateral ventricles by a narrow band of tissue (**D**). Posteriorly and superiorly, no demarcation from the greatly dilated lateral ventricle is visible, presumably due to the obliquity of the thin boundary, with resulting partial volume obscuration of differential absorption. The markedly displaced pineal is visible in **D**, adjacent to the wall of the mass and to the left of calcification in the glomus of the greatly dilated right trigone.

E. The huge, obstructed lateral ventricles are clearly shown. This feature, combined with the remarkable lack of symptoms, indicated an extremely chronic lesion, the absorption values of which suggested that this represented a leptomeningeal cyst, originating in the region of the left choroidal fissure.

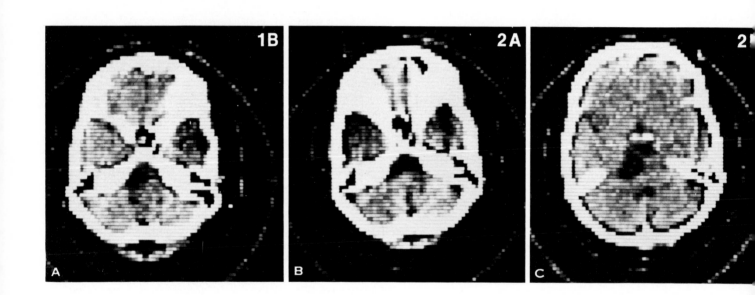

FIG. 11.4. EPIDERMOID (PEARLY) TUMOR, POSTERIOR FOSSA, WITH EXTENSION THROUGH THE TENTORIAL HIATUS.

Clinical Features. A 29 y.o. female with a history of paroxysmal facial pain and sensory loss of 2 years duration. She had also noted decreased vision in the peripheral fields and decreased sensation around the left side of her mouth. More recently there had been several abrupt short episodes of vertigo. There was a tendency to stagger to the right while walking.

Neurological Examination. Hypalgesia in the distribution of the third division of the left trigeminal nerve, extending to become hypalgesia and hypesthesia in the second and third division territories. Decreased peripheral vision, absent left corneal reflex, and wide-based gait with tendency to veer to the right on tandem walking. Finally, sensory loss in all three divisions of the left trigeminal nerve, hypesthesia in the right first division territory, and sensory loss over the C2 and 3 dermatomes bilaterally.

Skull Examination. Normal. Polytomography was also normal.

CT Scan. Abnormal (Fig. 11.4).

Angio. Transfemoral left carotid and vertebral studies revealed an avascular left CP angle mass extending to the retroclival region. The internal cerebral vein was displaced 2 mm to the right. Normal ventricular size was indicated, and no abnormal blood supply was noted on left external carotid study.

Operation. (Dr. Edward Tarlov.) Occipital craniectomy, with grossly total removal of epidermoid tumor from the left CP angle and pontine cistern, where it extended across the midline. Tumor was dissected away from the left fifth to twelfth cranial nerves and from in front of the basilar artery. It was noted that the brain stem had been rotated to the right. The tumor extended superiorly through the tentorial notch to the left infratemporal region. The left posterior cerebral and superior cerebellar arteries were encased. Adherent tumor was left in place superiorly.

Histology. Epidermoid (pearly) tumor.

Plain CT scan, with 8-mm sections of the posterior fossa.

A, B, and **C** show a low absorption (0–12) lesion of moderately large size in the left CP angle cistern and extending broadly across the prepontine space to the right side (**A** and **B**).

C. This section extends through the frontal lobes below the frontal horns and through the fourth ventricle posteriorly. The fourth ventricle is deformed by mild mass effect impinging upon its left anterolateral aspect. The low absorption mass is shown extending superiorly from the CP angle and pontine cistern to the superior portion of the dorsum sellae (irregular horizontal bone absorption region centrally). The entire lesion is quite sharply demarcated, and its extra-axial position is clearly demonstrated. The absorption values are very similar to those of CSF, although they extend slightly above the peak values for full-volume CSF. The anatomical arrangement of the lesion and experience gained from a previous case (illustrated in Fig. 11.3) led to the correct diagnosis from CT scans, although the possibility of a leptomeningeal cyst could not be excluded completely.

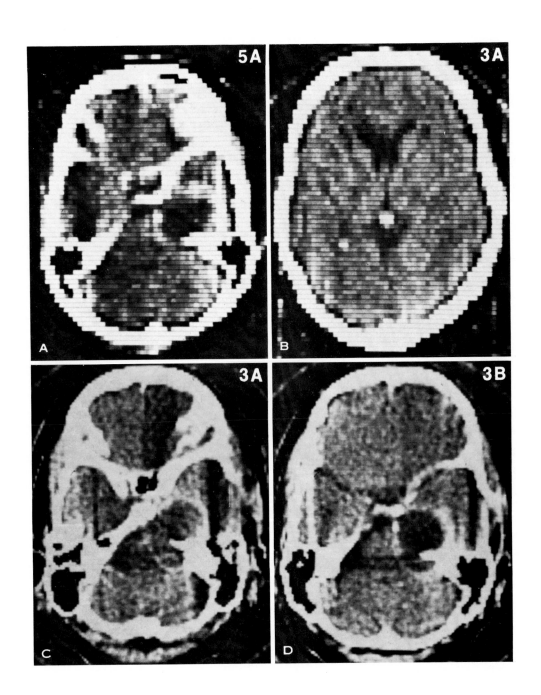

FIG. 11.5. EPIDERMOID CYST, BASAL EXTRADURAL.

Clinical Features. A 44 y.o. male with an 8 year history of numbness of the right side of the face and right-sided tinnitus with decreased hearing. Recently noted diplopia on right lateral gaze and, very recently, on forward gaze. Unsteady gait and progressive right facial palsy.

Skull Examination. Large area of bone destruction extending from the middle of the right petrous pyramid to involve the floor of the right middle fossa. Amputation of the medial extremity of the right internal acoustic canal and destruction of the anterior portion of the jugular foramen. Polytomography confirmed the above findings and revealed slight sclerosis of portions of the sharply defined margin of destruction, which extended to the posterolateral aspect of the right sphenoid sinus.

CT Scan. Abnormal (Fig. 11.5).

Angio. Transfemoral bilateral carotid and left vertebral studies revealed a generally avascular mass in the right CP angle, with extension into the middle fossa through the area of the eroded right petrous tip. Several small branches from the basilar artery appeared to extend to the mass, which was thought to be extradural and either a cholesteatoma or a trigeminal neurinoma.

Operation. (Dr. Robert G. Ojemann.) Right temporal craniectomy. A large cystic lesion was encountered in the extradural space in the region of the medial portion of the petrous pyramid and adjacent portion of the middle fossa. A thick brownish fluid was under increased pressure within the cyst. Yellow material, consistent with cholesterol crystals, was present. Small portions of the contents of the cyst were solid but freely removable from the very smooth thin fibrous capsule.

Histology. Epidermoid cyst.

CT scans were obtained before and after contrast enhancement with 50 ml of Hypaque 60; 13-mm sections.

A. No bone is visible in the region of the right petrous apex (although the right side of the head was tilted slightly higher than the left, as indicated by the relative amounts of the orbital roofs demonstrated anteriorly and by the appearance of the sella). Just behind the dorsum sellae is a small zone of osseous density (possibly displaced petroclinoid ossification or a portion of the clivus). A rounded area of diminished absorption, 36 mm in diameter, is shown extending from the destroyed petrous apex anteriorly to the middle of the lower portion of the middle fossa (absorption, 3–16). Bounding this anteriorly is a broad zone of greater absorption (19–30), which was less apparent in a very similarly positioned section before contrast enhancement (15–22). The nature of this "capsule" is not clear. It may represent vascularity of displaced dura around the lesion. In the light of the plain film skull changes, the CT findings were considered to be compatible with an epidermoid cystic tumor of the cranial base. The suggestion of a vascularized broad capsular zone also required consideration of the possibility of a large fifth nerve neurinoma, but the low absorption of the major central region (3–16) is lower than would be expected in a neuroma with central necrotic changes.

B. A higher CT section, showing the normal appearance of the lateral and third ventricles and a midline pineal.

C and **D.** Scan obtained with the 160 x 160 matrix system approximately 4 months after surgery. The patient had remained stable, except for pregression of the right sixth nerve paresis. These two sections were obtained following intravenous injection of 50 ml of Hypaque 60 M. Contents of the cyst have evidently reaccumulated. The absorption of the capsule measured 25–37 and the contents measured 3–16.

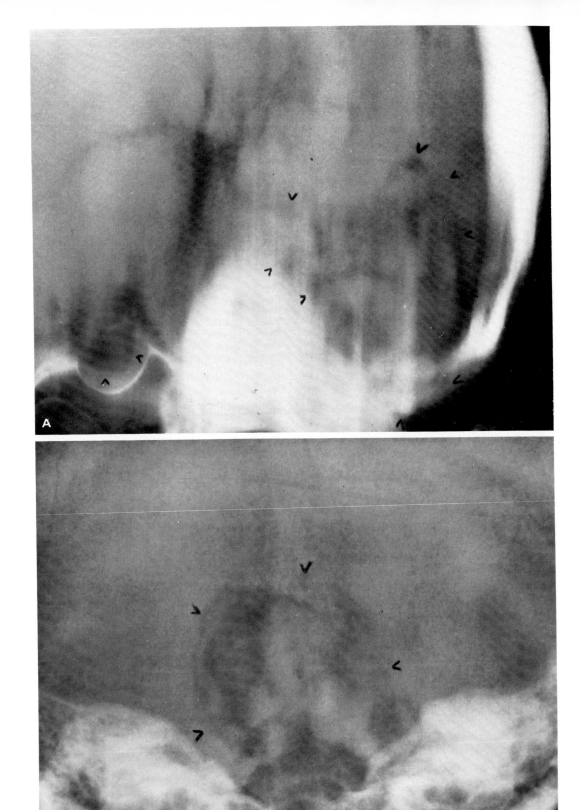

FIG. 11.6. EPIDERMOID TUMOR OF THE FOURTH VENTRICLE.

Clinical Features. A 35 y.o. female with a 6 year history of dizziness and occasional true vertigo. She had noted aching pains in the occipital region in the mornings and had occasional frontal headaches. She had had tinnitus and difficulty with balance.

Neurological Examination. Showed a normal mental status. The fundi were normal. There was fine rapid nystagmus on left lateral gaze and coarse nystagmus on right lateral gaze. There was bilateral coarse upward beating nystagmus on upward

gaze. There was mild left peripheral facial palsy and she consistently fell to the right on attempted tandem walking.

Skull Examination. The sella appeared slightly enlarged, with minor erosion and thinning of the dorsum.

CT Scan. Abnormal (Fig. 11.6, **E–G**).

PEG. A large, irregularly lobulated mass was shown to occupy a grossly enlarged fourth ventricle and lower cisterna magna (Fig. 11.6, **A** and **B**).

Angio. A transfemoral right vertebral study revealed evidence of an avascular moderately large mass posterior to the lower

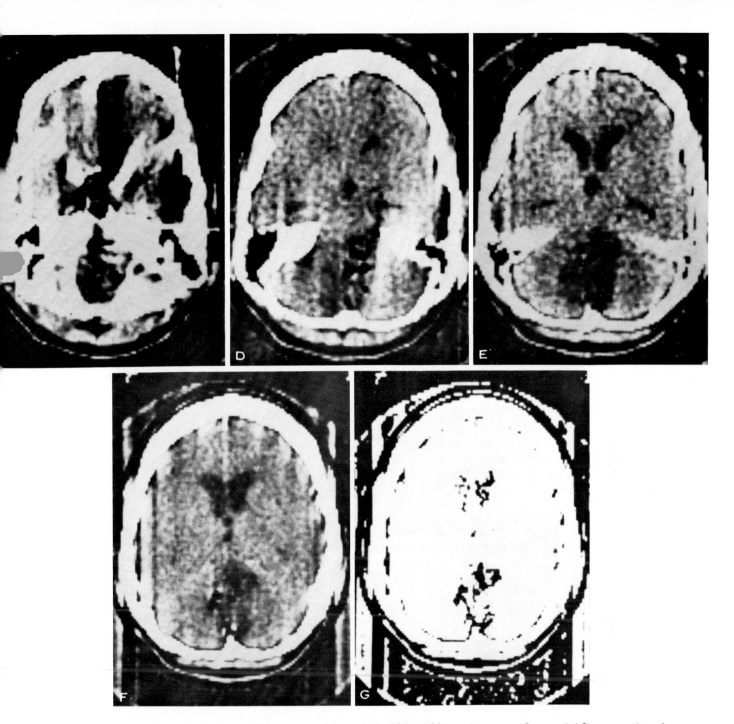

pons and medulla in the median area and extending more to the right than to the left.

Operation. (Dr. Robert G. Ojemann.) Suboccipital craniectomy and microsurgical total excision of a typical epidermoid (pearly) tumor of the fourth ventricle. The tumor extended up to the caudal portion of the aqueduct and, inferiorly, through the foramen of Magendie to the level of the first cervical vertebra. The cerebellar vermis was markedly compressed and displaced superiorly against the tentorium. The tumor had fibrous attachments to the wall of the fourth ventricle and extended more to the right than to the left of the midline.

A. Lateral median sagittal linear laminogram, and **B,** PA half axial projection, from the pneumoencephalogram. The large irregular mass, greatly distending the fourth ventricle and extending below the foramen magnum, is shown (*arrowheads*). Irregular congeries of gas outline the whorled tumor masses, characteristic of an intraventricular epidermoid tumor. The pontine cistern is narrowed and the sella is partly empty (intrasellar cisternal extension) (*arrowheads*).

C–F. 160 x 160 matrix system. Sequential 8-mm sections from below superiorly. No increase in absorption of the lesion was identified on a contrast-enhanced scan. The examination was obtained 2 days after the PEG, and gas bubbles (absorption down to less than −140) are shown scattered through the irregular mass in the region of the foramen magnum and more superiorly. The irregular contours of the tumor are shown (3–18) in the region of the fourth ventricle, which is markedly expanded in all directions. Owing to the admixture of CSF, tumor, and gas, partial volume averaging effects render absorption values of the elements unreliable. The third and lateral ventricles were modestly enlarged, due to obstructive hydrocephalus.

G. Same section as in **F**. W M. The serpiginous configuration of the masses of pearly tumor are suggested by this display, but the pneumoencephalogram reveals the characteristic features much more clearly.

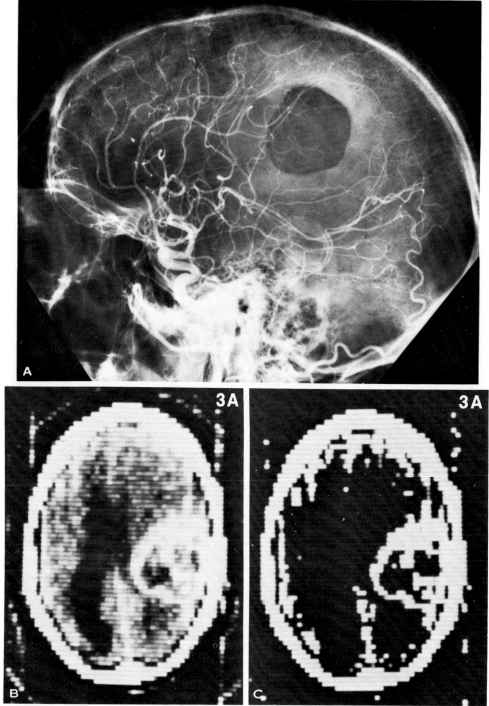

FIG. 11.7. CAVERNOUS ANGIOMA.

Clinical Features. A 39 y.o. male who presented with a firm soft tissue mass bulging in the right parietal region.

Neurological Examination. Normal.

Skull Examination. Large, sharply demarcated, rounded complete bone defect in the right parietal bone, showing poorly defined surrounding sclerosis without hyperostosis. Tangential frontal projection revealed well-defined beveled margins (broader inner than outer diameter). Marked erosion of the sella, with expansion, was indicative of prolonged increase in intracranial pressure.

CT Scan. Abnormal (Fig. 11.6, **B–F**).

Angio. Percutaneous right carotid study, with common and internal carotid series; very large, avascular, superficially situated mass, causing marked internal displacement of cortical branches, with stretching and bowing (Fig. 11.6A). Marked right temporal lobe herniation, apparently causing erosion of the dorsum sellae. Diagnostic considerations included epidermoid tumor with unusual appearance of the bone erosion and an atypical presentation of meningioma.

Operation. (Dr. Raymond N. Kjellberg.) Excision of a very large encapsulated mass, grossly indenting the parietal lobe.

Histology. Cavernous angioma; a brown rounded mass, 7 x 5 x 4 cm, with an external lobulated appearance. On section, numerous cyst-like spaces up to 2 cm in diameter were found. Some had contained brownish fluid and others contained dark clotted blood or whitish "colloid" material. No evidence of hair, bone, or other organized structures (Fig. 11.6G).

A. Early arterial phase from the lateral common carotid series, showing the large parietal bone defect and the striking displacement of many cortical branches by the very large avascular mass.

B and **D.** Contiguous 13-mm sections showing the huge, somewhat lobulated, intracranial mass in the parietal and posterior frontal regions. The lesion showed an encapsulated appearance, with multiple contained cystic spaces of varying size and absorption characteristics. The external capsular absorption ranged from 23–37, with minor variations in different portions and at different levels. The internal cystic spaces showed absorption ranges that varied from 9–20,

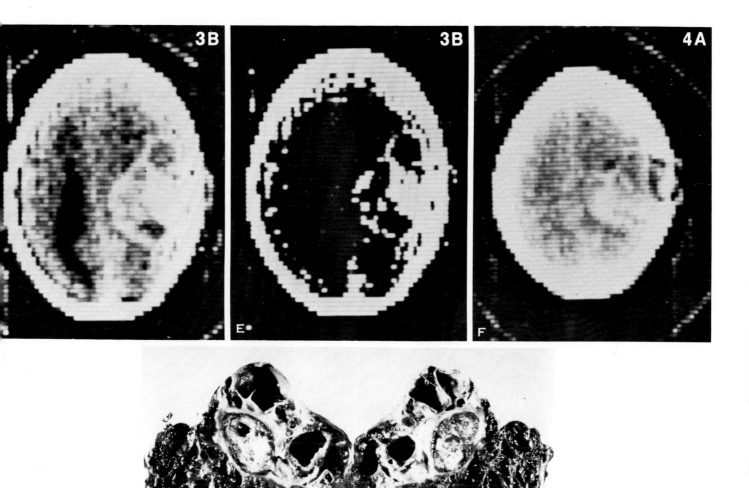

G

11–21, 13–24, 10–24, and 22–28. The spaces with the higher absorption values presumably represented those containing the whitish colloid-like material in the specimen. There is considerable right ventricular compression and midline dislocation, but these are quite moderate considering the very large size of the mass, indicating great chronicity and considerable cerebral pressure atrophy.

C and **E**. These are window M representations of **B** and **D**, respectively, accentuating the multicystic character of the lesion.

F. Section immediately above that in **E**, showing dense compartments in the superior portion of the mass at the level of the bone defect, which is visible on the right side and through which the tumor bulges.

G. Surgical specimen, sectioned and bivalved, showing the very numerous cystic spaces through the lesion, varying in size from tiny to 2 cm. The CT scan did not discriminate the very thin walls of many of the smaller cystic spaces, presumably due to their thin character, low absorption characteristics, and partial volume effects of oblique walls.

The CT scan was the only preoperative study that revealed the multicystic character of the lesion, which was then thought most probably to represent a form of teratoma with solid and cystic compartments but without bone, calcium, or frankly lipid components.

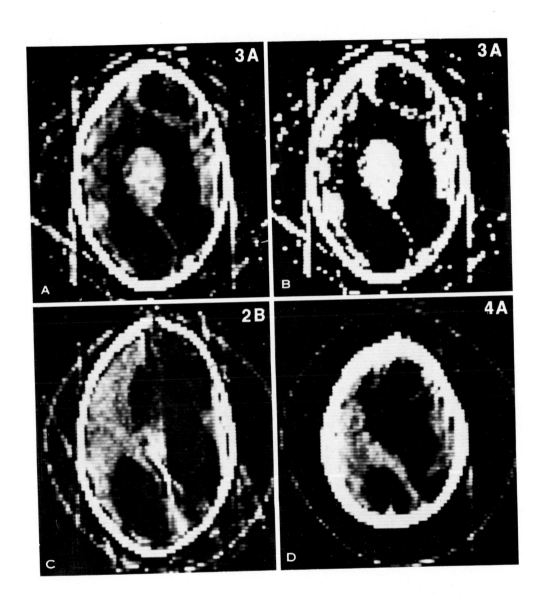

FIG. 11.8. CHOROID PLEXUS PAPILLOMA OF THE THIRD VENTRICLE; MASSIVE VENTRICULAR ENLARGEMENT AND PORENCEPHALIC CYST FORMATIONS.

Clinical Features. A 12 y.o. boy who was originally seen at the age of 6 months following a left-sided seizure. At that time, a third ventricular mass was biopsied through a right frontal craniotomy and was diagnosed as a form of hamartomatous malformation. He developed a left hemiparesis and a seizure disorder with poor control on medication. Recently, he started to complain of headaches.

Neurological Examination. Left hemiparesis and right homonymous hemianopsia. No papilledema, markedly decreased upward gaze, and poor conjugate gaze. Hemiparetic gait.

Skull Examination. Cranial vault enlargement, with slight coronal suture diastasis. Enlarged sella with posterior erosion of floor and marked thinning of the dorsum. Question of small amorphous calcification above the dorsum.

CT Scan. Abnormal (Fig. 11.8, A—D).

Angio. Transfemoral right carotid and vertebral studies revealed a huge, richly vascularized mass in the central supratentorial region. Further separate areas of increased vascularity were noted in the posterior frontal region and in the posterior parietal and occipital regions. A major avascular mass effect was noted through most of the right cerebral hemisphere.

Ventriculogram. Although 90 ml of oxygen were injected, the gas entered spaces so huge that only a limited amount of anatomical information was obtained. There was free communication between a very dilated right lateral ventricle, a mildly dilated left lateral ventricle, and right and left posteriorly situated porencephalic spaces. A filling defect was present in the third ventricle, through which gas did not pass. A huge midline mass was identified but poorly outlined, due to the size of the surrounding spaces.

Operation. (Dr. Howard Eisenberg.) Craniotomy with subtotal excision of a huge choroid plexus papilloma, with later ventriculoperitoneal shunting.

Histology. Choroid plexus papilloma.

A. L 18   W 20.

Fourth 13-mm section above the plane of the sella. A large ovoid mass with somewhat heterogeneous absorption values (general absorption, 8–18, but with areas extending up to 25) is shown in the central area, surrounded by huge low absorption spaces having CSF values. More of the mass is to the left than to the right of the midline. The spaces immediately around the mass appear to be greatly dilated lateral ventricles, but additional spaces having CSF absorption and demarcated from the ventricular cavities are noted in the frontal region (**A**) and parieto-occipital regions (**D**).

B. L 15   W M.

The demarcation of the central mass, the ventricles, and the frontal porencephalic space are more strikingly discriminated with these settings.

C. Section immediately below that in **A**. A lower portion of the mass is shown centrally. The right lateral ventricle is much more markedly enlarged than the left, except posteriorly, where it is not possible to distinguish between a grossly dilated left lateral ventricle and a porencephalic cyst on this section. There is very little cerebral mantle visible on the right side and in the parieto-occipital area and posterior temporal region on the left.

D. Second level above that in **A**. The upper portion of the right frontal porencephalic cyst and the posterior bilateral porencephalic cyst are visible. It is presumed that the anterior and posterior porencephalic formations arose from previous surgery and ventricular needling associated with chronic increase in intracranial pressure, although congenital cerebral maldevelopment and old infarction are also possibilities.

The study was obtained without contrast enhancement.

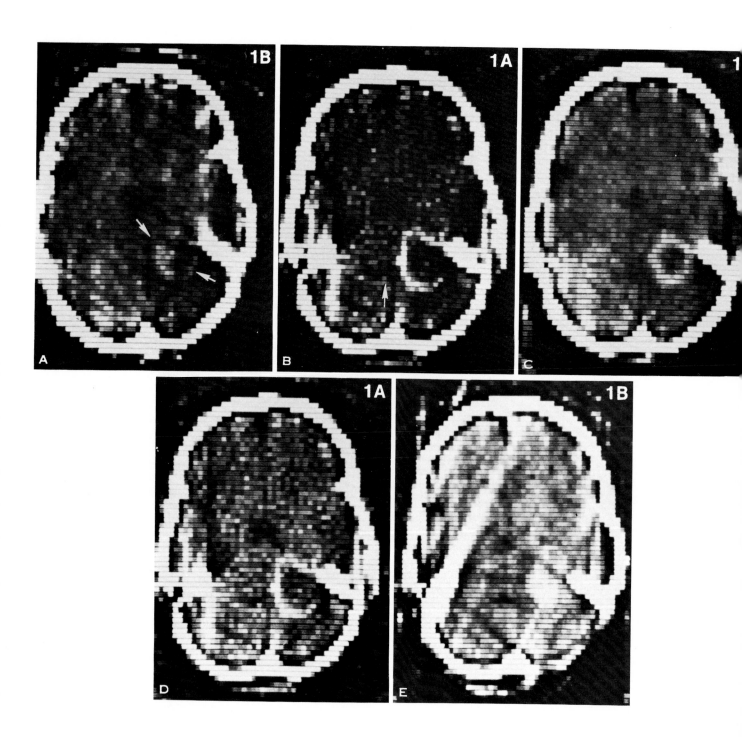

FIG. 11.9. CHOLESTEROL GRANULOMA, PRESENTING IN THE CEREBELLOPONTINE ANGLE. (Case contributed by Dr. Leon Menzer, Sabin and Mark, P. A., Boston.)

Clinical Features. A 60 y.o. male who had had bilateral mastoidectomies at the age of 13. He first noted decreased hearing and tinnitus in the right ear at the age of 55. Two years later, he began to suffer from intermittent right frontal and occipital headaches. Tingling paresthesias in the right side of his face and intermittent lancinating periorbital pain began at about this time. More recently, he had noted staggering gait, which had become worse over the past few months.

Neurological Examination. He was alert and oriented. There was tenderness to percussion over the right postauricular area. There was bilateral scarring of the tympanic membranes. Visual acuity was normal and there was no papilledema. The corneal reflex was absent on the right, and there was decreased pin and light touch sensation over the entire right half of the face. Moderate weakness of the upper and lower right face. No hearing in the right ear. Increased tone in the left lower extremity. Dysmetria of the right upper extremity. The patient fell to the right on tandem walking.

Skull Examination. This included laminography of the petrous bones and revealed a sharply defined destructive defect of the medial portion of the right petrous pyramid.

RN Scan. Tcp; slight abnormal uptake in the posterior fossa.

CT Scan. Abnormal (Fig. 11.9).

Angio. Right carotid study was normal. Vertebral angiography revealed evidence of an avascular mass in the right cerebellopontine angle. There was evidence of occlusion of normal venous channels, with collateral venous drainage posterior to the cerebellum to the posterior cervical venous system.

Operation. (Dr. Charles Poletti and Dr. Herbert Cares.) Right occipital craniectomy, with partial excision of a 3 cm diameter mass with a dense, fibrous capsule from the right CP angle. This contained yellowish material with the appearance of thick pus. No organisms grew in culture. The portion of the capsule adherent to the brain stem was left in situ.

Histology. Cholesterol granuloma. The thick dense fibrous capsule contained cholesterol clefts and multinucleated giant cells. The content was proteinaceous debris, not pus, and was sterile. (A. R. Wyler et al have described a similar case of this rare entity in a recent report, "Cholesterol Granuloma of the Petrous Apex." Journal of Neurosurgery, 41: 765–767, 1974.)

CT Scan. Postoperative scan at 1 month was abnormal (Fig. 11.9E).

A and B. Contiguous plain CT scan sections. The head is canted upwards on the right. A ring of increased absorption (13–26), measuring 36 mm in maximum diameter, is shown in the region of the right CP angle (*arrows*) and extending into the area of the pons and right cerebellar hemisphere. A small zone of absorption extending up to 60 units was noted in the medial portion of the lesion, indicating the presence of some calcification. The lesion extends into the region of bone destruction at the petrous apex. The central region of the lesion showed low absorption values (not recorded). The fourth ventricle is displaced considerably to the left (**B**, *arrow*).

C and D. Sections equivalent to those in **A** and **B** following intravenous injection of 50 ml of Hypaque 60 M. The overall absorption of the capsule of the lesion has increased, although the peak absorption increased only 2 units.

E. Scan obtained approximately 1 month after surgery. A homogeneous region of increased absorption (21–33), with a maximum diameter of some 24 mm, is visible in the region of the right CP angle. This represents the residual fibrotic capsule. There was no measurable change in absorption after contrast enhancement. The fourth ventricle is less displaced to the left than previously.

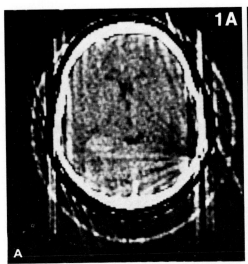 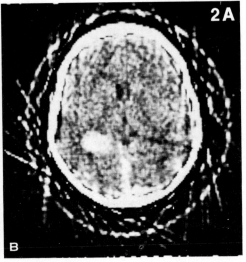

FIG. 11.10. CHOROID PLEXUS PAPILLOMA. (Case contributed by Dr. Jeffrey Gawler.)
Clinical Features. An 11 y.o. girl. Shortly after birth, her head had expanded rapidly and she had received a ventriculoatrial shunt for hydrocephalus, which was thought to be due to basal cisternal obstruction. She now presented with a 3 month history of headache. There were no abnormal physical signs.
CT Scan. Abnormal (Fig. 11.10).
Angio. A vascular blush was evident in the left trigone, supplied by choroidal vessels and typical of a choroid plexus papilloma.
PEG. A slightly lobulated mass was revealed in the left trigone.
A and **B.** L 13   W 30   160 x 160 matrix system.

A. Plain scan, undertaken to assess ventricular size. The lateral and third ventricles are of normal size. Radiating artifacts are due to partial inclusion of a shunt valve in the section. An oval region of moderately increased absorption (16–30) is evident in the area of the left trigone.
B. The scan, repeated after intravenous injection of 30 ml of Conray 60, shows marked enhancement of the area of abnormal absorption (23–35).
(Illustrations obtained from magnetic tape records, courtesy of Dr. Jeffrey Gawler, The National Hospital, Queen Square, London, England.)

CHAPTER 12

Benign Cysts

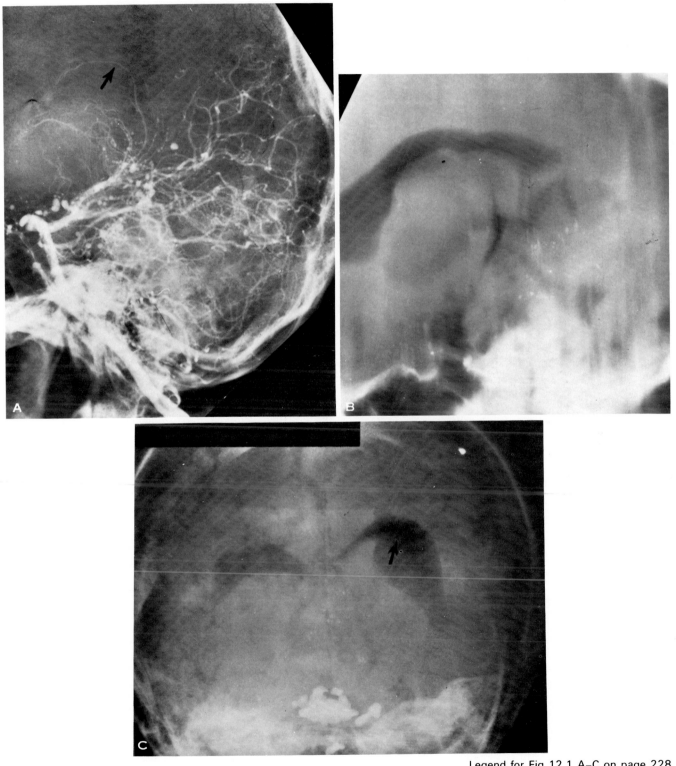

Legend for Fig 12.1 A–C on page 228

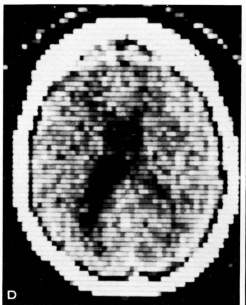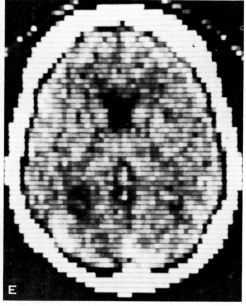

FIG. 12.1. EPENDYMAL CYST OF THE LATERAL VENTRICLE.

Clinical Features. A 32 y.o. male admitted for investigation of possible temporal lobe seizures. He had been observed to suffer from spells of automatic behavior, often associated with violent behavior and total amnesia for the episodes. The patient complained of acute paroxysmal headaches, some of which were said to be followed by these spells of automatism.

Neurological Examination. Alert, oriented, and coherent, without abnormal neurological findings.

EEG. Two examinations, including sleep studies, were normal.

Skull Examination. Normal, except for scattered Pantopaque residues.

RN Scan. Tcp; normal.

CT Scan. Abnormal (Fig. 12.1, **D** and **E**).

Angio. Transfemoral carotid and left vertebral studies, suggestion of a poorly defined avascular mass in the left temporal region and indication of a mass in the left thalamic and mesencephalic region on vertebral angiography (Fig. 12.1**A**).

PEG. A lobulated mass was shown projecting into the body and trigone of the left lateral ventricle from the floor, suggesting a tumor encroaching from the region of the thalamus. (Fig. 12.1**B**).

Operation. (Dr. James Wepsic.) Parieto-occipital craniotomy, with intraventricular exploration. A large, very thin-walled, blueish cyst was found almost filling the ventricle in the trigone and posterior body. Clear fluid was aspirated. No abnormal vessels or tumor tissue were identified and the cyst was fenestrated.

Histology. Thin-walled cyst, apparently of ependymal origin, from lateral ventricle or choroidal fissure. Birefringent material was found in the cyst wall, raising the question of the relationship between the cyst and residual Pantopaque from myelography performed several years earlier.

A. Lateral arterial phase of the left vertebral angiogram, showing elevation of the left lateral posterior choroidal artery (*arrow*). No neovasculature was identified.

B. Lateral erect film at PEG, showing a lobulated mass encroaching upon the inferior portion of the body and trigone of the left lateral ventricle. This was thought to represent a tumor extending upwards and posteriorly from the thalamus.

C. PA brow-down projection during PEG. A smooth convex mass encroaches upon the trigone from the inferior aspect (*arrow*). Note Pantopaque residues in the posterior fossa in **B** and **C**.

D. CT scan at the level of the bodies and trigones of the lateral ventricles. This was originally incorrectly interpreted as indicating a poorly-defined mass compressing the posterior portions of the *right* lateral ventricle. On review, the lesion is represented by a comma-shaped region of CSF absorption, slightly larger than normal ventricle, extending from the posterior body through the trigone and faintly demarcated by a narrow band of denser tissue from the body of the ventricle anteriorly and from the occipital horn posteriorly.

E. Section immediately below that in **D**, showing the posteroinferior portion of the cyst in the region of the occipital horn.

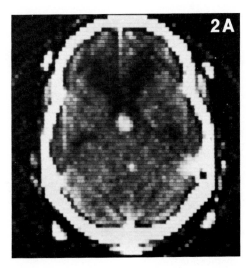

FIG. 12.2. COLLOID CYST. (Case contributed by Dr. Hillier L. Baker, Jr., Mayo Clinic, Rochester, Minnesota.)

Clinical Features. A 51 y.o. male who presented with a progressive decrease in mental functions, including alertness, work performance, ambition, drive, and energy. Severe intermittent frontal headaches for two years. Impairment of recent memory, shuffling gait, deterioration of handwriting, and incontinence.

Neurological Examination. Normal.
EEG. Normal.
Skull Examination. Normal.
RN Scan. Normal.
CT Scan. Abnormal (Fig. 12.2).

Operation. Transfrontal exploration of the right lateral ventricle. Greyish mass noted projecting into the lateral ventricle through the foramina of Munro. Following aspiration of a small amount of mucus-like material, the mass was peeled from the third ventricle and removed.

Histology. Colloid cyst of the third ventricle, measuring 1.5 x 1.3 x 1.0 cm.

CT scan through the frontal and temporal horns and the region of the foramina of Munro. A dense rounded mass (32–36 units), measuring approximately 12 x 15 mm, is shown in the midline in the region of the foramina. Dilatation of the frontal and temporal horns is shown.

(Illustration courtesy of Hillier L Baker, Jr., M.D.)

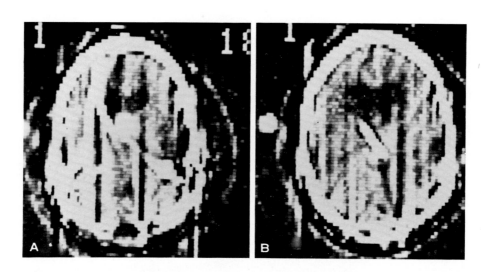

FIG. 12.3. MULTIPLE COLLOID CYSTS. (Case contributed by Dr. Hillier L. Baker, Jr., Mayo Clinic, Rochester, Minnesota.)
Clinical Features. A 50 y.o. male. Some 20 years earlier he developed headaches and blurred vision with vomiting following a blow on the head with a rifle. Six years later he was given a Torkildsen shunt following negative exploration for "posterior fossa tumor." After another 9 years, he had two attacks of numbness from the waist down, each lasting 24 hours. After a further 5 years, he noted the gradual onset of weakness in the right arm and had trouble walking. Four years later, he suffered from frequent falls, when stumbling and right foot drop developed. Two years later, an RN scan, left carotid angiogram, and myelogram were all said to be normal except for dilated ventricles. Three years later, he was told that he had myasthenia gravis. The right leg and arm became weaker and there was decreased libido.
Neurological Examination. Right leg weakness and bilateral Babinski signs.
CT Scan. Abnormal (Fig. 12.3).
Operation. Right frontal craniotomy. After entering a dilated ventricle, a large slate-grey cystic lesion was seen at the foramina of Munro. On puncture, the cyst was found to contain very thick gelatinous material, slightly yellow in color. The cyst was excised and a second, smaller cyst was removed from the choroid plexus of the left lateral ventricle.
Histology. Two colloid cysts, the larger 2 cm in diameter and the smaller 1.6 x 0.8 x 0.3 cm.

In spite of considerable motion artifact, the CT scans reveal modest enlargement of the frontal horns and a dense rounded mass (32–36 units) lying in the region of foramina of Munro **(A)**. This appears to be approximately 27 mm in diameter. The band-shaped density of a ventricular shunt tube is shown extending across the midline to the posterior portion of the left frontal horn **(B)**. While most colloid cysts so far described have absorption values in the 30's, an occasional purported example with lower values (similar to CSF) has been seen. These are apparently variant forms containing relatively "thin" fluid and are difficult to identify on CT scans. Dilatation of the lateral ventricles and a normal appearance of most of the third ventricle should localize the site of such a lesion, however.
(Illustrations courtesy of Hillier L. Baker, Jr., M.D.)
While the high absorption illustrated in Figures 12.2 and 12.3 seem to be the typical expression, there is some evidence to suggest that certain "colloid" (neuroepithelial) cysts, containing less dense material, will show lower absorption values. Such cysts may be difficult to distinguish from surrounding cerebrospinal fluid.

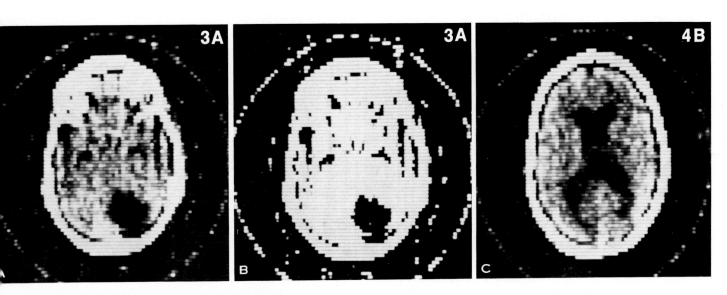

FIG. 12.4. GLIA-LINED CEREBELLAR CYST.

Clinical Features. A 27 y.o. female with a 9 month history of bursting headaches and slight unsteadiness of gait.

Neurological Examination. This was normal except for papilledema and very slight unsteadiness on tandem walking.

CT Scan. Abnormal (Fig. 12.4).

Angio. Retrograde brachial study revealed a large avascular mass in the posterior portion of the posterior fossa.

PEG. This revealed a mass in the region of the right cerebellar hemisphere, compressing the fourth ventricle and displacing it to the left.

Operation. Occipital craniectomy revealed a large right cerebellar hemisphere cyst with a smooth lining, which was finely corrugated anteriorly. The cyst fluid was thin and clear. No tumor tissue was identified.

Histology. Glia-lined cyst with no evidence of neoplasia.

A. L 15 W 20.

A slightly irregularly rounded cavity, approximately 40 mm in diameter, is shown in the right cerebellar hemisphere extending into the region of the vermis. Absorption values of the cyst contents ranged from -2 to $+10$.

B. L 11 W M.

Maximum contrast representation of the cyst, which clearly reveals the corrugated appearance of the anterior wall of the structure.

C. Higher scan section, showing the modest obstructive hydrocephalus produced.

The scan was taken to indicate a cystic glioma. In spite of the operative and histological findings, some suspicion remains, and long-term follow-up is planned.

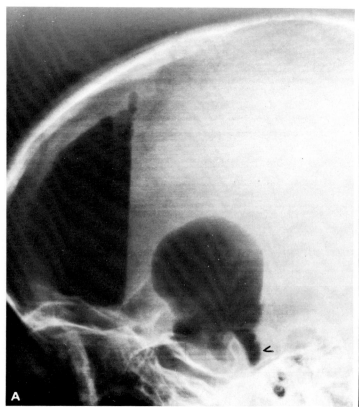

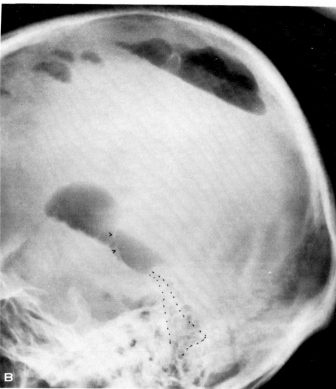

FIG. 12.5. SUPRASELLAR NEUROEPITHELIAL OR LEPTOMENINGEAL CYST.

Clinical Features. A 35 y.o. male investigated 7 years prior to CT scan for progressive mental deterioration and gait disturbance. He had developed a seizure disorder at the age of 6, after a purported attack of encephalitis. He had been retarded thereafter. There had been further mental deterioration since a severe head injury 18 months before this examination.

Neurological Examination. Eight years earlier he had an obviously enlarged head, bilateral optic atrophy, a broad-based gait, with a tendency to stagger to the right.

Skull Examination. Enlarged cranium (circumference 62.5 cm). The vault was relatively smooth internally and fairly thin. Enlargement involved particularly the supratentorial regions. The sella was enlarged, with a dense lamina dura, a depressed flattened tuberculum sellae, and a depressed corticated central portion of the superior surface of the dorsum. The appearance of the skull had been essentially unchanged for 17 years. The findings were consistent with a long-standing obstructive hydrocephalus at the level of the aqueduct or rostrad to this, with ballooning of the third ventricle onto the sella, or a very chronic noncalcified suprasellar mass.

Angio. A right carotid study 8 years earlier had demonstrated gross lateral ventricular enlargement, with considerable depression of the internal cerebral vein and no lateralized mass lesion.

PEG. Examination 8 years learlier revealed a thin-walled cystic suprasellar lesion (Fig. 12.5, **A** and **B**).

Operation. (Dr. William H. Sweet.) A ventriculoatrial shunt was placed. During the next few months immediately after the operation, he improved significantly, becoming more alert and talkative, with good recall of names and events. However, during the recent months before CT scan, his mental status had

declined significantly. He spoke little and was lethargic. Seizure activity had increased.

A and **B**. PEG obtained 8 years prior to CT scan.

A. Brow-up lateral projection showing massive enlargement of the frontal horns and a large rounded air-containing cystic mass in the suprasellar region. The cyst appeared to fill from the pontine cistern (*arrowhead*), although there appeared to be a thin velum between the lower portion of the cyst and the cistern.

B. Upright lateral projection, showing air filling of the posterosuperior portion of the cystic structure. The *small arrowheads* indicate a velum apparently separating the cyst from the posterior portion of the third ventricle. The anterior portion of the third ventricle could not be separately identified. The configuration of the aqueduct and fourth ventricle is indicated by *interrupted lines* traced from other films.

C–G. L 14   W 30.   160 x 160 matrix system. Contiguous 13-mm CT sections.

C. This section passes through the region of the suprasellar cisterns, and shows an abnormally large central space having the absorption characteristics of CSF that extends from the posterior subfrontal region to the upper pons. The latter appears somewhat flattened and displaced posteriorly, consistent with local mass effect of a fluid-containing suprasellar cyst. The junction of the carotid and left sylvian cisterns is suggested by a triangular extension laterally and there is a similar but less obvious configuration on the right at this point. Radiating artifacts from part of the shunt valve extend through the head from the right posterolateral scalp region.

D. This section shows the inferior portions of somewhat enlarged frontal horns, from which a broad ovoid region of decreased absorption extends posteriorly, again with CSF

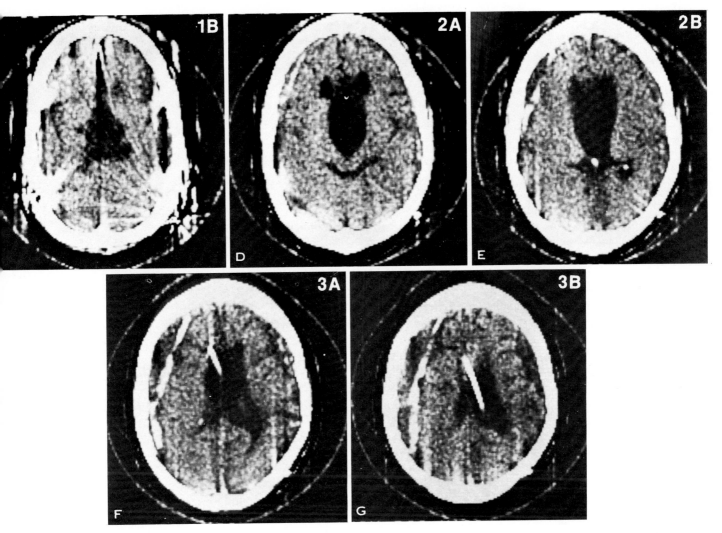

absorption values. This extends posteriorly to the region of the midbrain. Anteriorly, there is a suggestion of separation by a thin velum between this cystic cavity and the frontal horns. Posteriorly, the quadrigeminal plate and adjacent cisterns are clearly shown.

E. This section, through the level of the pineal, again shows the large central cystic cavity, merging indistinguishably with the frontal horns anteriorly. The cystic cavity extends posteriorly to the pineal. No demarcation between the cystic cavity and dilated posterior third ventricle can be identified. If the thin velum separating the cyst and third ventricle shown on the PEG 8 years earlier (A and B) still exists, it is not distinguishable on CT scan because of a curving configuration resulting in marked partial volume averaging with adjacent low absorption fluid on each side.

F and G. These sections reveal the configuration of the lateral ventricles. The right lateral ventricle is moderately enlarged and the left is within normal limits. Portions of the shunt tube are shown. This extends from the right parietal region anteriorly through the right lateral ventricle and septum lucidum to the left frontal horn. Portions of the shunt valve are shown posterolaterally on the right side in sections D, E, and F. The irregular thick plaques of high absorption (peak 90) extending over the left cerebral hemisphere (D–G) represent calcification in the internal portion of a very chronic subdural hematoma. Between this calcification and the inner table heterogeneous absorption values ranging from 0–25 units are apparent within the subdural collection. A smaller chronic subdural hematoma is evident on the right side.

A skull examination within a few days of the CT scan revealed paper-thin calcification surrounding the left subdural hematoma. A repeat PEG revealed that the cystic structure had enlarged considerably in the 8-year interval, with virtually complete obliteration of the posterior portion of the third ventricle. The cyst again appeared to fill directly from the basal cisterns.

CHAPTER 13

Metastatic Intracranial Neoplasms

INTRODUCTION

CT scanning has proven to be highly accurate in the diagnosis of intracranial metastatic tumors. In the first 600 consecutive CT examinations at the MGH, the accuracy of CT scan diagnosis surpassed that of radionuclide scanning, angiography, and pneumoencephalography (Table 13.1), and, although detailed comparative analysis has not yet been completed, the same appears to be true for the 2400 CT scan examinations to date. Paxton and Ambrose (51) have reported the identification of 34 of 35 histologically proven cerebral metastases on CT scans. The missed lesion was in the *high parietal convexity*.

Not only is CT scanning more accurate in identifying the presence of metastatic intracranial neoplasm than are the traditional radiological methods, but it provides a considerable amount of information concerning the *type* of metastasis present and, commonly, more information concerning tumor type than is provided even by cerebral angiography.

Metastatic adenocarcinomas have generally appeared on CT scans as small, medium, or large dense nodules, with absorption ranges from 12 or 15 up to 28 or 30, and the nodules are generally surrounded by very large volumes of diminished absorption (4-14) caused by edema. The smallest metastatic nodules identified have been in the order of 6 mm. In a number of cases, scanning before and after intravenous contrast injection has revealed a distinct increase in absorption of the nodules with contrast circulation. This renders the smaller vascular nodules easier to identify. Very small nodules occupying only a fraction of the full thickness of the slice and surrounded by low-density edema may, by density averaging, be rendered inconspicuous until the density is increased by contrast material (partial volume phenomenon).

The degree to which density is increased will be proportional to the blood level of iodine and to the vascularity of the nodule. Diffusion of contrast medium into the tumor is presumed to play a part in increasing density. Considerable increase in density of both small and large nodules of adenocarcinoma has been demonstrated following intravenous contrast injection, usually in the amount of 40-50 ml.

Occasionally, a small metastatic lesion will be invisible on a plain CT scan, but quite obvious following high-dose intravenous injection (see Chapter 27).

A number of cases of metastatic malignant melanoma has been studied, and these also tend to have high absorption values initially (sometimes ranging to the high 30's, a feature strongly suggestive of tumor hemorrhage). In other melanoma deposits, a considerable increase in density with intravenous contrast injection expresses their vascularity.

The larger nodules of metastatic adenocarcinomas and melanomas may contain irregular, less dense central areas representative of tissue necrosis.

In contrast with the above types of metastasis, metastatic squamous cell carcinoma generally presents a low density relative to brain (4-12 or 14) and rather smoothly rounded contours, with little or no evidence of surrounding edema. Marked cystic necrosis with sedimentation of heavier and higher absorption debris has been demonstrated in occasional cases (51).

Metastatic undifferentiated carcinoma has tended to resemble squamous cell metastasis, but exceptions have occurred.

A single case of metastatic rhabdomyosarcoma to the cerebellum showed low absorption values (8-14). Metastases treated by radiation therapy and chemotherapy generally show lowered absorption values, as compared with untreated lesions.

TABLE 13.1
Metastases: 24 Cases

	CT scans (24)	RN scans (12)	Angiograms* (12)	PEG (1)	PEG + Ventriculogram (1)
Positive	24†	11 (false diagnosis of single lesion in 3 cases)	≫8 (false diagnosis of single lesion in 1 case)	No diagnosis	"Cerebellar mass"
Negative	0	1	>4		

* ≫, CT very much superior to angiography; >, CT distinctly superior to angiography.

† Interpretation error in two cases; diagnosed as glioblastomas.

Of the 24 cases of metastasis in this series, there were no false positive diagnoses. Two cases, seen earlier in the series, were thought to represent glioblastomas, due to extensive confluence of multiple metastases. With greater experience, these errors would not be expected. It is therefore considered that, with some experience, the accuracy of CT scanning in the identification of metastases should approach 100% *in patients with related neurological signs or symptoms* and if contrast enhancement is employed when the plain scan is equivocal or negative. Radionuclide scans were obtained in 12 cases and were positive in 11 and negative in one. However, in three of the positive cases, only a single lesion was seen, whereas multiple lesions were demonstrated on the CT scans. Angiography was performed in 12 cases. CT scanning was considered to be very much superior in diagnosing the presence, size, and distribution of metastases in eight cases and distinctly better in four cases. In one case of multiple metastases revealed by CT scan, only a single mass was identified by angiography; multiplicity was always more clearly demonstrated by the CT scans. Pneumoencephalography was performed in only two cases. In one, no diagnosis was obtained. In the second case, supplemented by ventricular gas injection, a cerebellar mass causing hydrocephalus was correctly diagnosed.

Contrary to the opinion of Paxton and Ambrose (51), we have often found it possible to differentiate correctly between metastatic neoplasm and glioma. Multiplicity was the most helpful feature, but solitary metastases tend to have one or more of the following differential features: well circumscribed round or oval contours, rounded nodules with major volumes of surrounding edema, and a tendency to central necrosis of marked degree (which may be associated with layering of denser cellular debris). However, some gliomas may exhibit very similar or indistinguishable appearances and some metastases resemble gliomas, especially when contiguous deposits merge to appear as a single large lesion.

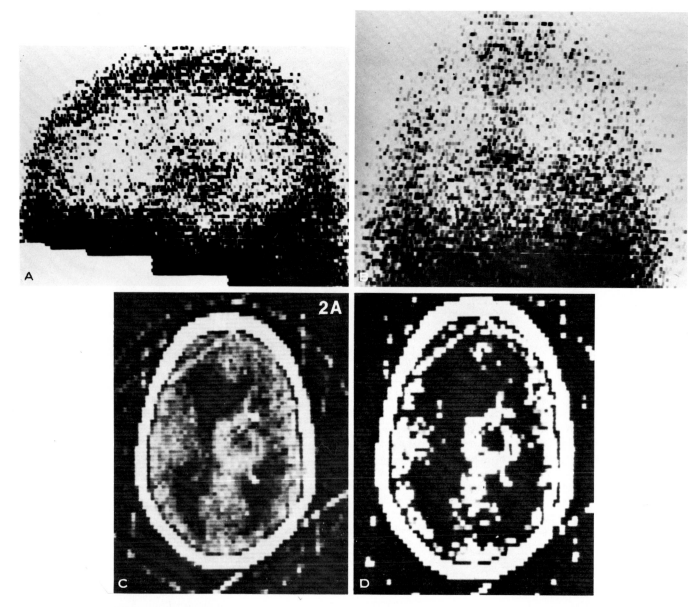

FIG. 13.1. SOLITARY METASTASIS: UNDIFFERENTIATED CARCINOMA.

Clinical Features. A 56 y.o. male without a known primary neoplasm had recently been explored (Dr. William H. Sweet) for biopsy of a vascularized mass demonstrated by RN scan and carotid angiography. The biopsy was reported to show only normal brain and the patient was referred for CT scan.

Skull Examination. Normal.

RN Scan. Tcp; obtained at another hospital; abnormal (Fig. 13.1, **A** and **B**).

Angio. A moderately vascularized mass of quite large size, containing irregular tumor vessels, was demonstrated in the region of the right internal capsule.

CT Scan. Obtained after negative biopsy; abnormal (Fig. 13.1, **C** and **D**).

Histology. Tissue culture resulted in the identification of multinucleate cells, characteristic of malignant neoplasm. Autopsy was obtained after a short interval and confirmed the CT scan findings. The histology was that of an undifferentiated carcinoma (from the lung) with central necrosis.

A. Right lateral scan view. **B.** Posterior rectilinear scan view. A large rounded area of considerably increased activity is noted in the region of the basal ganglia. Although obviously extending deeply in the right cerebral hemisphere, the contours of the area of increased uptake are not very well defined in the posterior view.

C. L 16   W 20.
A quite well circumscribed, rounded mass, 4.5 cm in diameter, is shown extending from a center in the anterior thalamic region to the posterior portion of the head of the caudate nucleus anteriorly, and into the third ventricle medially, where it crosses the midline. The major and peripheral portions of the mass showed a high absorption (20–28) and an eccentric central area had a relatively low absorption (12–20). The very high absorption of a metal clip was shown immediately adjacent to the anterolateral margin of the mass (the calcific absorption of the glomus of the choroid plexus is present just behind the mass). The third ventricle was markedly compressed and displaced to the left and was apparently invaded by the mass. The right lateral ventricle was extensively compressed in the region of its body and the contralateral ventricle was considerably dilated because of third ventricular obstruction. (Reprinted by permission from Radiology, 110: 109–123, 1974.)

D. W M. The mass is well discriminated from surrounding tissues and the lower absorption of central necrosis is accentuated. The regularly rounded configuration of this solitary lesion and the appearance of its central necrosis is much more typical of metastasis than glioma, though occasionally glioma will appear similar. The absorption characteristics are more typical of an adenocarcinoma than undifferentiated carcinoma.

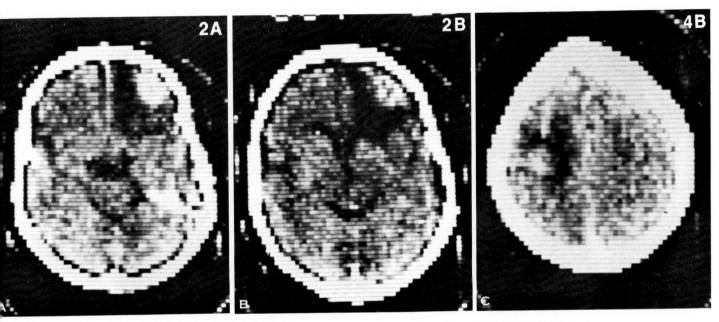

FIG. 13.2. METASTATIC ADENOCARCINOMA.

Clinical Features. A 58 y.o. female in whom a well differentiated carcinoma of the colon was diagnosed 1 year earlier and
treated by left colectomy. Metastases to bone and the epidural
space in the lumbosacral region had been identified. She then
had a grand mal seizure and developed pareses of the right side
of the face and the right arm.

CT Scan. Abnormal (Fig. 13.2).

A. A 2.4-cm circumscribed oval nodule of high absorption
(18–32) is shown in the right frontal lobe. The nodule extends
through the right frontal cortex to the surface and is surrounded
by a very large volume of low absorption (6–17), indicating
edema. (Reprinted by permission from Radiology, 114: 75–87,
1975.)

B. This scan section is immediately above that in **A** and shows
the superior portion of the peripheral nodule (appearing less
dense here because of partial volume averaging with adjacent

edema). The large volume of low absorption edema is clearly
shown. The right frontal horn is compressed by the mass effect.
The septum lucidum is displaced approximately 6 mm to the
left of the midline with the third ventricle, while the pineal
calcification lies in the midline.

C. The most superior section obtained, which reveals a dense
nodule in the left superior parietal region (15–25) with
considerable surrounding edema (6–15) extending mainly
medially and anteriorly from the nodule. The absorption
characteristics and general appearance of the nodules are
consistent with either metastatic adenocarcinoma or malignant
melanoma. However, such large volumes of associated edema
have not been observed in metastatic melanoma to date.
(Reprinted by permission from Radiology, 114: 75–87, 1975.)
The patient was referred directly for radiotherapy, without need
for angiography.

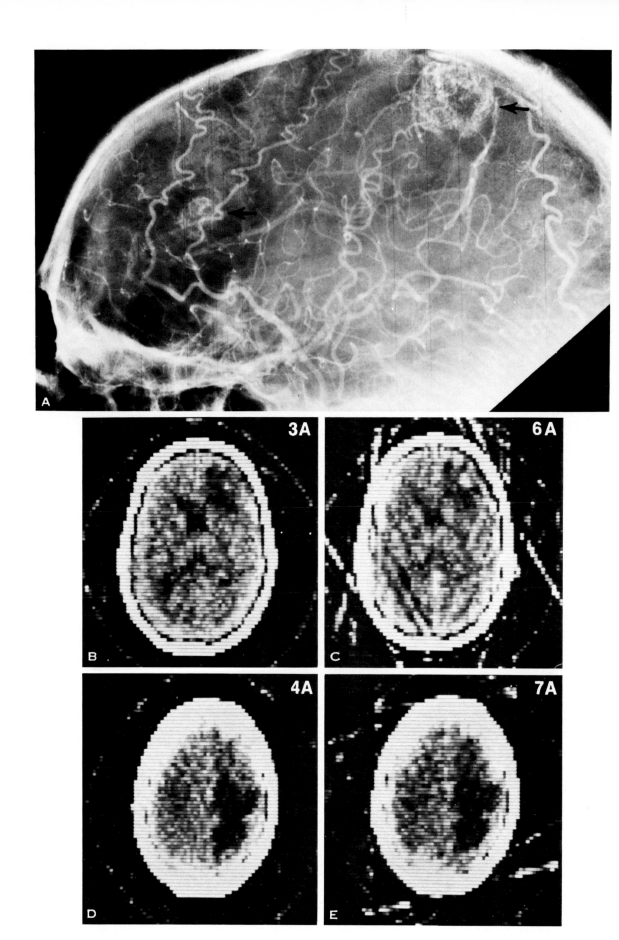

FIG. 13.3. METASTATIC HYPERNEPHROMA.

Clinical Features. A 59 y.o. man with a history of resected hypernephroma and evidence of rib metastasis. He had noted progressive numbness of the left side of the body for over 1 month and had had several focal motor seizures involving the left foot. There was a mild left hemiparesis.

Angio. Right carotid study revealed two vascularized nodules in the right cerebral hemisphere (Fig. 13.3A).

CT Scan. Abnormal (Fig. 13.3, B–E).

A. Right carotid angiogram; lateral view showing two rounded foci of malignant tumor vascularity (*arrows*). The smaller vascularized nodule measured 12 mm in diameter and lay at the level of the middle frontal gyrus. The larger nodule was approximately twice as large and lay in the anterior superior portion of the right parietal lobe. Around both nodules was evidence of additional mass effect, consistent with edema. There is questionable evidence of a third mass focus, avascular or poorly vascularized, more posteriorly in the right parietal lobe.

B. L 16   W 20.
Plain CT scan, revealing a large volume of decreased absorption (5–14) in the right frontal lobe, at the level of and compressing the right frontal horn. Within this edema is a small (apparently less than 6 mm) focus of considerably increased absorption (15–24).

C. L 16   W 20.
Scan repeated following intravenous injection of 50 ml of Hypaque 60 M. Scan quality was somewhat degraded by head motion, but there was no definite change in volume of

the region of reduced absorption. However, the small dense nodule (20–30) was now shown to be considerably larger, measuring approximately 12 x 15 mm in diameter. Increase in the general absorption of cerebral cortex and central grey matter is also evident. Apparently, a considerable proportion of the dense nodule of metastatic hypernephroma was obscured in the plain scan by the reduced absorption of the large volume of surrounding edema. After increase in density of blood following intravenous contrast injection, the density of the clearly quite vascular nodule was increased sufficiently to emerge more completely from the surrounding edema.

D. Plain scan. **E.** Contrast-enhanced scan. Both scans were through the superior portions of the parietal lobes. Two large rounded zones of diminished absorption are shown in the superior portions of the right parietal lobe. These have the appearance of originally separate zones of edema that have become confluent. No nodular, high absorption lesion is visible in the region of the posterior edematous zone. There appears to be only a minor partial volume inclusion of the vascular nodule shown at angiography, in the anterolateral portion of the more anterior zone of edema. The poor visibility of this nodule is explained by the scan sections extending insufficiently in a superior direction. Paxton and Ambrose have reported (51) that the only case missed in a series of 35 scan studies of metastatic malignancy was one in which the lesion lay high in the parietal lobe. Examination for suspected smaller lesions near the vertex should include scans that extend to the vertex.

(Fig. 13.3, **B** and **C**, reprinted by permission from Radiology, 114: 75–87, 1975.)

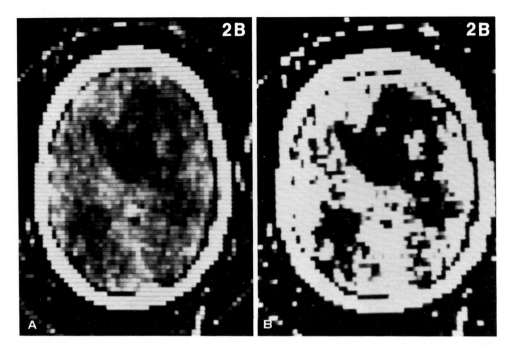

FIG. 13.4. METASTATIC ADENOCARCINOMA.

Clinical Features. A 54 y.o. man who presented with a short history of fatiguability and left-sided weakness.

EEG. Right-sided slowing.

Skull Examination. Normal.

RN Scan. [74]Arsenic; normal.

CT Scan. Abnormal (Fig. 13.4).

Angio. Right carotid study revealed a large avascular mass in the right frontal lobe, extending deeply and into the corpus callosum, suggesting the diagnosis of glioma.

Operation. (Dr. James Wepsic.) Modified right frontal lobectomy; necrotic edematous brain adjacent to firm tumor and several cystic areas containing proteinacious fluid. Necrotic nodules were excised as separate specimens.

Histology. Metastatic adenocarcinoma, with surrounding edema and gliosis. Multilocular cystic necrosis.

A. A large irregular area of decreased absorption (5–18) is shown in the right frontal lobe, extending to a distorted right frontal horn. Just lateral to the frontal horn is an irregular 2-cm nodular region of increased absorption within the region of edema. Smaller areas of similarly increased absorption are scattered around the more obvious focus and the region of decreased absorption extends posteriorly through the lateral basal ganglionic areas to reach the temporal lobe. The region of the septum lucidum is displaced moderately to the left, while the pineal appears midline in position. A quite large area of

decreased absorption, consistent with edema, is shown in the left posterior temporoparietal region, extending to involve the overlying cortex. There is also a patchy combination of decreased and increased absorption in the right posterior temporal and occipital regions. The scan was obtained approximately 1 hour after carotid angiography, at which time 20 ml of Conray 60 were injected. Thirty ml of Conray 60 were injected intravenously just before the scan. (Fig. 13.4, **A** and **B** reprinted by permission from Radiology, 110: 109–123, 1974.)

B. W M. The extensive bilateral abnormalities are more clearly visible. Contrast enhancement probably resulted in increased visibility of the multiple nodules of adenocarcinoma present in both cerebral hemispheres in this case. Experience indicates that vascularity insufficient to be identified at angiography may nevertheless be sufficient to result in increased absorption on contrast-enhanced scans, if sufficient contrast medium is injected. This study was performed at a time when experience was relatively limited. In retrospect, the presence of some cystic changes within the area of right frontal lobe edema might have been identified on the basis of regionally lower absorption and a suggestion of discreteness.

Right carotid angiography in this case revealed nonspecific features suggesting a single extensive avascular mass in the frontal region, probably a glioma. With the greater confidence now existing in the validity of CT scan findings, such a patient could have been spared additional contrast studies.

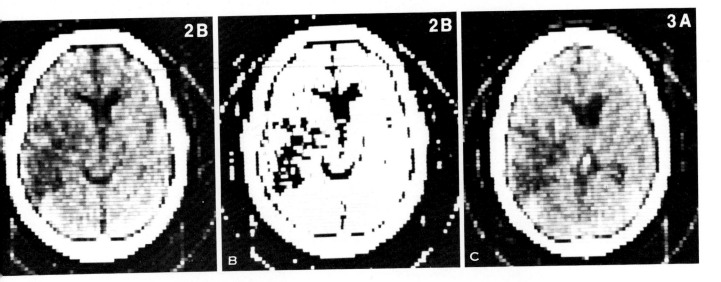

FIG. 13.5. METASTATIC ADENOCARCINOMA.

Clinical Features. A 66 y.o. male with a 1-month history of being "unable to find the right word," according to his wife. He had had a colectomy two years previously, for carcinoma of the colon. Amnestic aphasia, with emerging central aphasia, sparing praxic and speaking functions. No visual field defect. Clinical findings suggested a deep temporal mass, with glioma as the first consideration.

Skull Examination. No definite abnormality.

RN Scan. Tcp; dynamic and static studies. On the static study, a discrete area of increased activity was present in the peripheral portion of the left temporal region, suggesting a neoplasm. A Tcd cranial scan was obtained on the following day. This showed less activity in the temporal region than on the previous study, increasing the possibility of metastasis or glioma versus infarct or meningioma.

CT Scan. Obtained on the same day as the second RN scan; abnormal (Fig. 13.5).

Angio. Transfemoral left carotid and vertebral studies revealed marked elevation and anterior displacement of the sylvian triangle, with stretched retrosylvian branches. The middle cerebral artery was elevated and there was medial displacement of the sylvian branches. The study suggested a large avascular infrasylvian mass, probably a glioma.

Operation. (Dr. Robert G. Ojemann.) Craniotomy, with apparently complete excision of a discrete pseudoencapsulated, reddish avascular tumor, 2–3 cm in diameter, from the left temporal lobe.

Histology. Moderately well-differentiated metastatic adenocarcinoma.

Liver Scan. Tc sulphur colloid, 8 days after surgery; at least two large areas of decreased activity within the liver were consistent with metastatic disease.

A–C. Plain CT scan.

A. L 14   W 20.

A large region of decreased absorption, with a patchy variability in absorption levels, involves most of the left temporal lobe and extends into the region of the putamen and thalamus. Compression of the left frontal horn and 9-mm displacement of the septum lucidum and third ventricle to the right are visible. There is a rather poorly defined region of somewhat increased absorption in the temporal lobe, situated in the anterolateral portion of the zone of variably diminished absorption, suggesting a denser discrete nodule.

B. L 12   W M.

Same scan as in **A**. The heterogeneous region of diminished absorption (9–16) is more clearly visible. These settings suggest the presence of a rounded region of higher absorption approximately 3 cm in diameter, in the anterolateral temporal area.

C. Scan section immediately above that in **A**, revealing considerable displacement of septum lucidum and pineal to the right. The heterogeneous area of diminished absorption in the temporal and central regions is again visible. There is a suggestion of a nodular region of greater density laterally in the temporal area.

The poorly defined and irregular margins of the region of decreased absorption and the lack of a clearcut focal nodule of increased absorption suggested the diagnosis of an infiltrating neoplasm, probably malignant astrocytoma. A contrast-enhanced scan might very well have provided better discrimination of a focal nodular lesion, thereby increasing the possibility of a correct diagnosis.

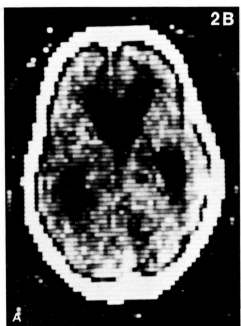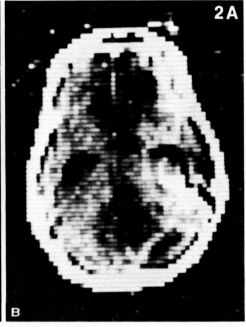

FIG. 13.6. METASTATIC ADENOCARCINOMA, PROBABLY FROM THE BREAST, WITH CYSTIC NECROSIS.

Clinical Features. A 56 y.o. female who presented with dementia, bifrontal signs, vertigo, diplopia, and abnormal gait. Six years previously, a breast carcinoma had been treated by radical mastectomy.

Skull Examination. Normal.

RN Scan. Tcp; increased uptake of isotope in the right posterior fossa. Repeat scan with [74]arsenic 5 days later was interpreted as showing probable abnormal slight uptake in the midline posterior fossa region.

CT Scan. One day after the second RN scan; abnormal (Fig. 13.6).

Angio. Transfemoral bilateral carotid and right vertebral studies revealed moderate hydrocephalus. There was a suggestion of anterior dislocation of the basilar artery, but no definite posterior fossa mass was identified.

PEG and Ventriculography. This combined study was performed 1 day after CT scan. No ventricular filling occurred with lumbar gas injection. By means of ventricular gas injection, a large right cerebellar hemisphere mass, extending towards the vermis and elevating the fourth ventricle, was identified. Moderately severe obstructive hydrocephalus was shown.

Operation. (Dr. Edward P. Baker.) Posterior fossa craniectomy. Tumor presented on the surface of the right cerebellar hemisphere, which was extensively discolored superiorly and laterally. Twenty ml of dark brown clear fluid was aspirated from the hemisphere, following which the hemisphere collapsed. Through a horizontal incision, an enormous cavity was revealed. This extended almost to the tentorial incisura medially and anteriorly. Radical excision of the cyst wall was performed.

Histology. Metastatic adenocarcinoma, with necrotic changes.

A and **B**. Contiguous scan sections, showing moderately severe hydrocephalus involving the lateral and third ventricles. A large, discrete but irregularly rounded zone of markedly decreased absorption (4–16) is shown in the posteromedial portion of the right cerebellar hemisphere, region of the cerebellar vermis and medial left cerebellar hemisphere. A high absorption band, apparently representing artifact, crosses the lesion obliquely. The very low absorption of the more central portions of the lesion extends anteriorly in the midline region to merge with what is probably an anteriorly displaced fourth ventricle (**B**). The superior portion of the lesion is included in the higher section (**A**), which also shows compression of the right side of the posterior third ventricle, which is displaced to the left of the midline. Also, the right temporal horn appears somewhat displaced and indented on its medial aspect. The latter features are consistent with superior cerebellar herniation.

The cystic necrosis of the large metastasis was correctly identified from the CT scan, but it was thought that the lesion represented a necrotic squamous cell metastatic tumor.

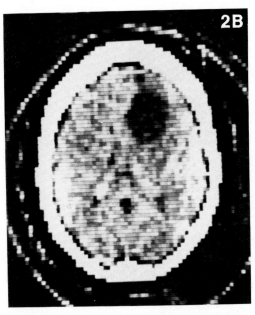

2B

FIG. 13.7. METASTATIC SQUAMOUS CELL CARCINOMA.

Clinical Features. A 68 y.o. female. Three months previously, a carcinoma of the larynx had been treated by laryngectomy and radiation therapy. Wedge resection of right lower lobe metastases had been performed. During the previous 2 weeks, clumsiness of the left hand, followed by unsteadiness of gait had been noted. For 1 week, she had had weakness of the left lower extremity, followed by retro-orbital headache on the left side. Hemiparesis had been increasing over the past 4 days.

Neurological Examination. Moderate left hemiparesis, involving face, arm and leg, without sensory or cerebellar signs or intellectual deficit.

EEG. Marked right-sided slowing.

Skull Examination. Pineal appeared slightly displaced to the left.

RN Scan. Normal.

CT Scan. Abnormal (Fig. 13.7).

A quite sharply-demarcated ovoid region of diminished absorption (4–14), approximately 4 cm in greatest horizontal diameter and about 5 cm in vertical diameter, is shown in the right frontal lobe. Within this region, numerous small spots of somewhat greater absorption are scattered. An obvious mass effect was present. On another section, a similar but smaller lesion was demonstrated in the left temporoparietal region on the left side (4–12) (not shown). The patient was referred for radiotherapy, without need for angiography or pneumography. The CT scan findings in this case are highly typical of squamous cell metastases in general. A relatively sharply circumscribed region of low absorption, within which are scattered small islands of slightly greater absorption, has been identified in most cases. In occasional cases, sufficient necrosis has been present to permit gravitation and posterior layering of cellular debris within the deposit. Surrounding edema has been absent or minimal.

(Reprinted by permission from Radiology, 114: 75–87, 1975.)

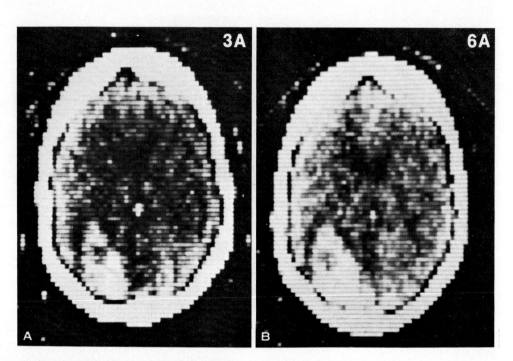

FIG. 13.8. METASTATIC MALIGNANT MELANOMA.
Clinical Features. A 53 y.o. female in whom a malignant melanoma was diagnosed 3 years earlier. Recent onset of right homonymous hemianopsia, which had increased noticeably in the previous few days.

CT Scan. Abnormal (Fig. 13.8).

A. A plain CT scan, at approximately 25° to the anatomical base line, passing through the frontal horns , third ventricle, and pineal, reveals a large ovoid area of increased absorption (22–34) in the occipital lobe and extending into the parietotemporal region. This measures 54 mm in maximum diameter and shows a narrow zone of peripheral diminished absorption, representing edema. A small zone of lesser absorption is shown within the large nodule and is consistent with a region of necrosis. There is minimal displacement of the calcified pineal to the right of the midline.

B. Scan after intravenous injection of 50 ml of Conray 60. A· modest increase in absorption of the mass (peak now 38) had occurred and the mass appeared somewhat larger, because of less obscuration of its periphery by partial volume averaging with edema. The lesser absorption of the presumed area of necrosis is somewhat overshadowed by the general increase in absorption of the mass, but is still visible. The narrow zone of surrounding edema is again visible. No other metastatic foci were evident and the patient was referred directly for radiation therapy.

(Reprinted by permission from Radiology, 114: 75–87, 1975.)

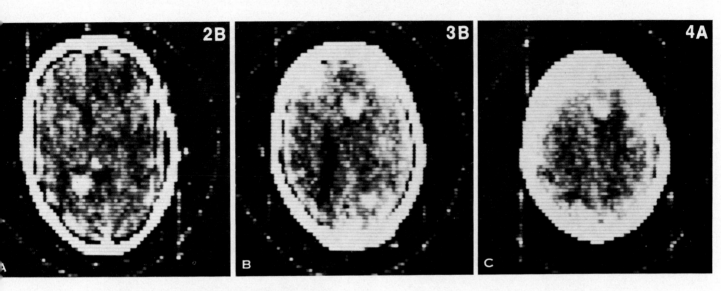

FIG. 13.9. METASTATIC MALIGNANT MELANOMA.

Clinical Features. A 51 y.o. man with known malignant melanoma. He had developed a right inferior homonymous quadrantanopsia with headache, and more recently had developed frontal lobe symptoms and signs, including abulia, apathy, and grasp and snout reflexes.

RN Scan. Tcp; 1 day before CT scan, showed a large area of *slightly* increased uptake in the left occipital region only.

CT Scan. Abnormal (Fig. 13.9).

A–C. Plain CT scan 1 day after an RN scan that showed only a single region of slightly increased activity.

A. L 18   W 20.

A 2-cm diameter, rounded area of markedly increased absorption (20–33) is visible in the left cerebral hemisphere just behind and to the left of the calcified pineal. The low absorption of CSF in a prominent quadrigeminal cistern lies immediately to the right of the lesion. Just lateral to the lesion is a partial volume inclusion of the left trigone. In addition, there is indication of a small amount of peripheral edema. Anteriorly, a compressed right frontal horn is visible and the frontal horns are displaced considerably to the left of the midline. Areas of diminished absorption are present in the right frontal lobe and in the area of the right insula. The calcified pineal is displaced markedly to the left, although less so than the frontal horns.

B. Second scan section above that in **A**. A high-absorption (23–38) lesion similar to that on the left is shown in the medial portion of the right frontal lobe and a smaller high absorption lesion is shown in the right occipital lobe. There is little evidence of edema around either lesion. Compression of the right lateral ventricle is apparent.

C. Section immediately above that in **B**. The frontal lobe lesion extends considerably into this section, which reveals diminished absorption attributable to a moderate amount of edema posterior to the nodule. A small high-absorption nodule is shown on the left side posteriorly, with a small peripheral zone of edema. There is also indication of a very small, high-absorption nodule in the anterior portion of the parietal lobe on the right side, also with a small adjacent zone of edema. At least four and probably five metastatic nodules are shown on the CT scan, whereas the RN scan indicated only one area of abnormal uptake. The high absorption of these nodules is indicative of hemorrhage into the tumor nodules, a not infrequent feature of metastatic melanoma. Other metastases of melanoma have shown nodules with absorption ranges indistinguishable from those of metastatic adenocarcinoma. However, the perifocal edema has generally been considerably less in melanoma than in adenocarcinoma.

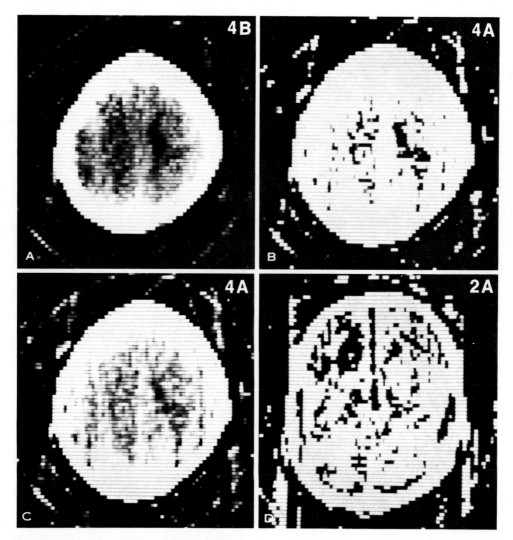

FIG. 13.10.   METASTATIC MALIGNANT MELANOMA.
Clinical Features. A 46 y.o. man. Several months previously, excision of axillary nodes had revealed malignant melanoma. In the previous 2 weeks, he had had seizures and had developed progressive weakness in the left upper extremity.
RN Scan. A Tcp scan obtained recently had shown a focus of increased activity in the right superior frontoparietal area. There was the suspicion of an additional area of abnormal activity on the left side also.
CT Scan. Abnormal (Fig. 13.10).
A–D. Plain CT scan.
A. L   23   W   30.
A rounded area of slightly increased absorption (16–25) was visible in the right parietal lobe. The lesion measured 3 cm in diameter. This was visible largely because of a zone of diminished absorption (6–16) surrounding it except on the lateral aspect where the nodule reached the cortical surface.

B. L   16   W   M.
The nodule, partly surrounded by edema, is accentuated.
C. L   15   W   20.
The appearance of the nodule (16–25) and surrounding edema (8–15) are visible on this section, which is immediately below that in **A**, increasing assurance concerning interpretation.
D. L   16   W   M.
An irregular region of diminished absorption (8–15) was noted in the left frontal lobe on this more inferior section. A very small nodule or pair of nodules (peak absorption, 17) is present within the region of apparent edema, consistent with additional metastasis. The majority of metastatic melanoma nodules have been denser than the lesions shown in this case. These nodules are not distinguishable from adenocarcinimas and from poorly differentiated carcinomas. Contrast enchancement no doubt would have considerably increased the absorption of the nodules, but was not performed.

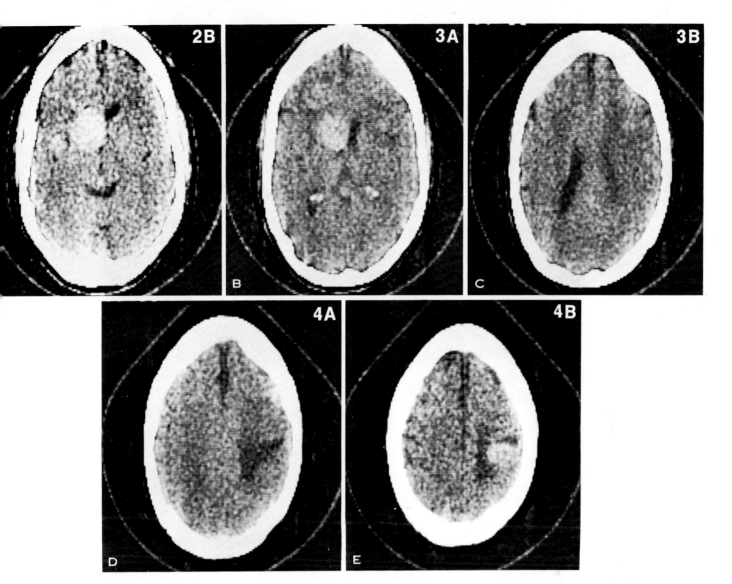

FIG. 13.11.   METASTATIC MALIGNANT MELANOMA.

Clinical Features. A 57 y.o. man who was well until 7 months prior to CT scan, when pleuritic chest pain led to an x-ray of the chest. This revealed a right upper lobe mass. Biopsies revealed metastatic malignant melanoma. He was treated with four courses of combined chemo- and immunotherapy. Four weeks before CT scan he started to complain of headaches and drowsiness, with occasional nausea and vomiting.

Neurological Examination. Rather slow mentation, fundic veins prominent, without pulsations. No definite abnormalities on neurological testing.

Skull Examination. Normal.

RN Scan. Tcd; abnormal, showing an area of increased activity in the right posterior parietal region and another in the right frontoparietal region, consistent with intracerebral metastases. No abnormal uptake was noted on the left side.

CT Scan. Abnormal (Fig. 13.11).

Histology. Bronchial and paratracheal node biopsies; malignant melanoma.

A–E. Plain CT scan.

A. W   40.   W   50.   160 x 160 matrix system.

A large discrete rounded mass is shown in the left frontal lobe, virtually obliterating the left frontal horn and indenting the medial aspect of the right frontal horn. There is almost no peripheral edema. The narrow third ventricle lies in the midline (**A**). The mass involves the region of the head of the caudate nucleus and the anterior limb of the internal capsule. Immediately lateral to the larger mass is a much smaller nodule of increased absorption in the region of the anterior portion of the insula (**A**). The pineal is largely noncalcified and is shown in the midline between the glomus calcifications (**B**).

C. Scan section immediately above that in **B**. The left lateral ventricle appears normal, but the right is compressed.

D. Section immediately above that in **C**. A roughly triangular region of diminished absorption is evident in the right parietal lobe. A slightly widened interfrontal fissure is evident, with the anterior falx.

E. Section immediately above that in **D**, showing a moderately large high absorption nodule in the right parietal lobe, with a moderate volume of surrounding edema. Several sulci are visible on the left side, but are not visible on the right, where they are evidently compressed by the metastatic tumor.

Note the more posterior appearance of the lesion relative to the vault in **E** compared with **D**, an effect produced by the obliquity of the scan section.

247

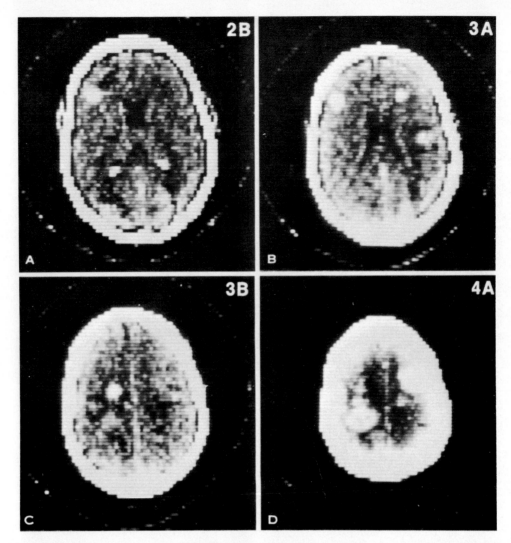

FIG. 13.12. MULTIPLE MALIGNANT ANGIOSARCOMA.

Clinical Features. A 57 y.o. male with a 2 week history of dysarthria and right hemiparesis, preceded by numbness and tingling in the right arm.

Neurological Examination. Oriented, but uncooperative in following instructions. Dysarthria, without dysphasia. Visual fields and extraocular movements were full and the fundi were normal. Right hemiparesis, with greater weakness of the arm than of the leg. Increased right lower extremity tone and equivocal right Babinski response. Sensation to pin prick was decreased in the left upper extremity. The gait was mildly ataxic, with failure to walk tandem. On the day after admission, he had a 20-minute episode of twitching of the right arm, with very brief twitching of the right side of the face and right lower extremity. He remained conscious but was incontinent. Right hemiparesis became marked and bilateral Babinski signs appeared.

RN Scan. Tcp; interpreted as showing foci of abnormal activity in the left occipital region and possibly in the right parasagittal region.

CT Scan. Obtained on the same day as RN scan; abnormal (Fig. 13, **A–D**).

Angio. Transfemoral bilateral carotid and left subclavian studies revealed bilateral avascular cerebral masses in the left anterior parietal parasagittal region and in the right frontal opercular area. Posterior displacement of the venous angles was noted, but the internal cerebral veins were not laterally displaced. The vertebrobasilar circulation was not shown optimally and no abnormality was detected in the posterior fossa. Metastatic malignancy was considered the most probable diagnosis.

Histology. The patient died 5 days after completion of the

angiographic study. Autopsy demonstrated multiple tumor nodules containing hemorrhage. A histological diagnosis of multiple angiosarcomas was made. A primary lesion was not identified.

A–D. Plain CT scan obtained on the same day as the RN scan and 1 day following carotid angiography.

At least eight focal lesions were identified in the cerebral hemispheres and one was noted in the cerebellum (not illustrated). The largest nodules measured 21 and 24 mm in diameter and lay in the left parietal and right frontoparietal regions superiorly (**D**). The remainder varied from a few mm up to approximately 15 mm in diameter. All of the lesions showed high absorption values, generally ranging from the low 20's to the high 30's and low 40's. There were only small perifocal zones of diminished absorption, consistent with edema. Metastatic melanoma and hypernephroma were considered the most likely possibilities on the basis of the CT scan. The small amount of associated edema is more consistent with melanoma.

A. CT section at the level of the frontal horns, showing a 15-mm dense nodule in the left frontal lobe, with minimal associated mass effect upon the frontal horn. Calcifications in the glomi of the choroid plexuses are symmetrically disposed posteriorly. Behind these, in each occipital lobe, are irregular areas of increased absorption, less clearly rounded, that merge with the density of cerebral cortex.

B. L 20   W 20.
Scan section immediately above that in **A**. The left frontal nodule is very clearly visible and slightly larger on this section. A smaller nodule is also clearly visible in the right frontal lobe in this section, surrounded by a small zone of diminished absorption representing edema. A slightly more irregular lesion

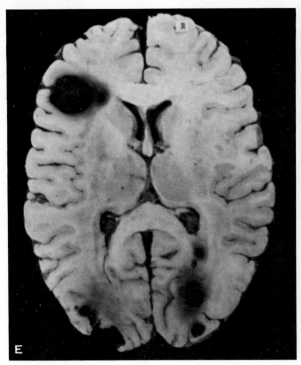

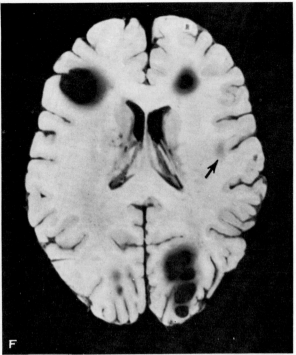

of similar size is evident in the right frontoparietal opercular region, surrounded by somewhat more edema. Only a single moderate-sized dense oval area is apparent in the right occipital lobe. Absorption values of these nodules were in the range of 22–45.

C. Scan section immediately above that in **B**. A 16-mm dense nodule with minor surrounding edema is visible just above the level of the anterior portion of the body of the left lateral ventricle.

D. L 30   W 20.
Section immediately above that in **C**. Large nodules are shown bilaterally and several smaller nodules, measuring only a few mm in size, are also visible.

In all, at least 9 and probably 14 nodules were demonstrated in the study.

E–G. Autopsy brain sections made at angles and levels corresponding approximately to those of the CT scan. However, *precise* correspondence is always very difficult to obtain and was not quite achieved in this case.

E. Brain section closely corresponding with the CT section shown in **A**. The hemorrhagic tumor nodule in the left frontal lesion is shown and there is a small satellite nodule mesially, which is not differentiated on the CT scan section (partial volume averaging effect?). The multiple lesions in each occipital region are more clearly discriminated than on the CT section.

F. Section corresponding closely with the scan section in **B**. The right and left frontal nodules are visible. The brain slice passes just below the right lateral lesion that is shown in the CT scan, and which is suggested here by a small area of staining (*arrow*). Four discrete contiguous nodules are shown in the right occipital lobe. These are incompletely discriminated on the CT sections shown in **A** and **B** (80 x 80 matrix system).

G. The 8-mm tumor nodule just lateral to the right dentate

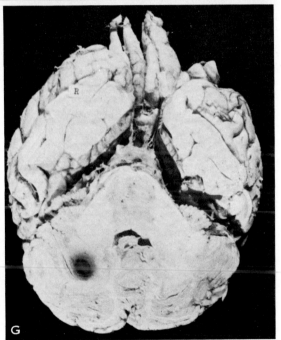

nucleus is shown. A 7-mm nodule in the posterior inferior cerebellar vermis was not identified on the CT scan.

Varying amounts of hemorrhage were noted in the multiple tumor nodules, some of which were almost completely destroyed by hemorrhage. This case offers additional evidence that markedly hemorrhagic lesions are better identified by CT scanning than by any other method short of autopsy.

(Fig. 13.12, **A, B, E,** and **F** reprinted by permission from Radiology, 114: 75–87, 1975.)

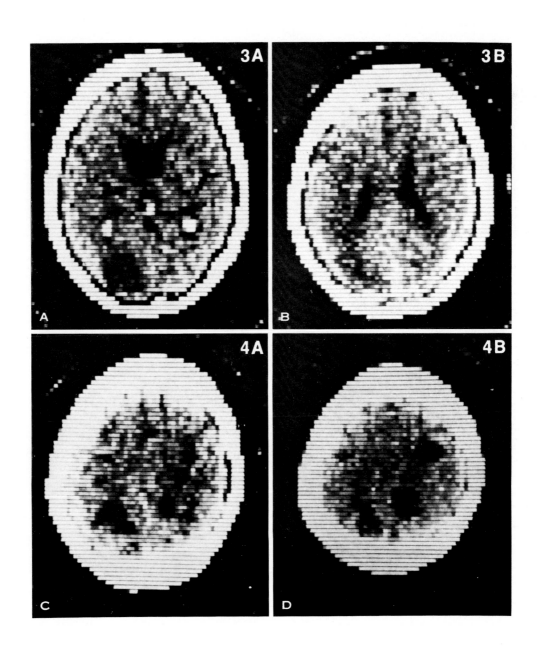

FIG. 13.13. METASTATIC LARGE CELL UNDIFFERENTIATED CARCINOMA.

Clinical Features. A 60 y.o. male, in whom a large cell undifferentiated carcinoma had been diagnosed by aspiration lung biopsies. Four months earlier, radiation therapy to the chest had been completed and he was started on a course of chemotherapy. He had recently developed focal seizures involving the left upper extremity and increasing weakness of the left arm.

RN Scan. Tcp; normal 4 months earlier. A second scan 4 days before CT examination demonstrated focal increase in activity high in the right parietal cortical region. The following day, Tcd scan revealed focal increase in activity in the same area, but activity was less than with Tcp, suggesting cerebral neoplasm rather than infarction. Both RN scans showed only a single focus.

Skull Examination. Normal, with normal pineal position, 2½ months before CT scan.

CT Scan. Abnormal (Fig. 13.13).

A–D. Consecutive CT sections from below superiorly. Four obvious focal low absorption lesions are shown, with absorption ranges between 7 and 20 units. The higher values were noted in the smaller lesions (greater partial volume effect). In addition, several very small low absorption lesions were also indicated.

A. A discrete rounded low absorption lesion, 3 cm in diameter, is present in the left occipital lobe. The calcifications of the pineal and choroid plexus glomi are not displaced, but there is indication of very slight compression of the right frontal horn and displacement of the frontal horns slightly to the left.

B. Slight displacement of the bodies of the lateral ventricles to the left is evident. There is partial inclusion of the superior portion of the left occipital lesion in this section. A low absorption region is evident in the lateral left frontal area (seen again in **C**).

C and D. A large low absorption lesion is visible in the posterior portion of the left parietal lobe. Two horizontal levels in the inferior portion are consistent with posterior gravitation of higher absorption debris within two confluent necrotic cavities (**C**). Two additional lower absorption lesions are present in the right parietal lobe (**D**). In both **C** and **D**, several smaller areas of reduced absorption are present in both posterior frontal regions and in the parietal lobes, consistent with multiple additional foci.

Due to the absence of a CT scan before commencement of chemotherapy, the possible contribution of the latter to the low absorption and probably necrotic change cannot be assessed in this case. The superiority of CT scan over RN scan in demonstrating the number and character of lesions present is clear.

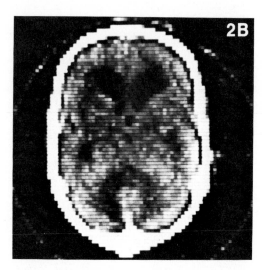

FIG. 13.14. METASTATIC POORLY DIFFERENTIATED ADENOCARCINOMA OF THE LUNG.

Clinical Features. A 62 y.o. man with a long history of chronic obstructive pulmonary disease. He was admitted for evaluation of a left hilar mass with peripheral infiltrate and recent difficulty walking. He had also noticed diminished memory.

Neurological Examination. Halting and wide-based gait, mild spasticity of the left lower extremity, diminished coordination of the left hand and past-pointing on finger to nose testing. Positive left Babinski sign. Normal position sense.

RN Scan. Tcp; normal. A bone scan was also normal.

CT Scan. Several days after RN scan; abnormal (Fig. 13.14).

Histology. Sputum cytology revealed poorly differentiated carcinoma. Scalene node biopsy showed several nodes replaced by tumor cells, with large vesicular nuclei and prominent nucleoli, consistent with metastatic carcinoma with giant cell features.

A very large rounded area of diminished absorption (figures not recorded) is clearly shown. This is centered in the upper vermis and extends into the region of both cerebellar hemispheres and arches forward into the brain stem area. The relative contributions of possible tumor nodule and residual vermis to the higher absorption more central region are not clear. An additional contrast-enhanced scan might have clarified this but was not obtained.

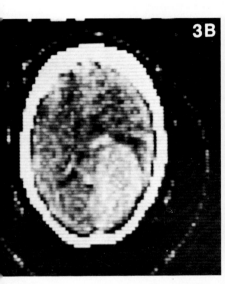
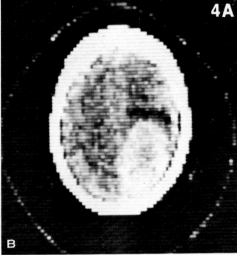
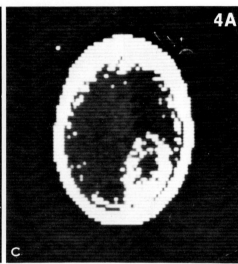

FIG. 13.15. METASTATIC UNDIFFERENTIATED LARGE CELL CARCINOMA FROM LUNG.

Clinical Features. A 58 y.o. female in whom a 2 x 3 cm nodule in the right upper lobe, associated with hilar and mediastinal node enlargement, had been noted on routine chest x-ray.

Neurological Examination. A dense and complete homonymous hemianopsia, with macular splitting, was noted shortly before CT scan. The optic discs were sharp, but the fundic veins did not pulsate. Pupillary responses were sluggish. There was a history of gait difficulty of uncertain duration.

A metastatic radiological series was negative.

RN Scan. Tcp; 2 days before CT scan, revealed a large area of increased activity in the right occipital region. The dynamic study revealed decreased perfusion in the posterior third of the right cerebral hemisphere, persisting throughout the series, suggesting a relatively avascular right parieto-occipital mass.

CT Scan. Abnormal (Fig. 13.15).

Angio. Transfemoral bilateral carotid and left vertebral studies, 4 days after CT scan, revealed an enormous almost avascular mass in the posterior frontal, parietal, occipital, and posterior temporal areas of the right cerebral hemisphere, thought to represent a glioma with considerable surrounding edema. A few irregular beaded vessels were noted in the right occipital pole.

Operation. (Dr. Robert G. Ojemann.) Parieto-occipital craniectomy, with apparently total excision of a 6 x 7 cm diameter firm

avascular somewhat necrotic-appearing mass.

Histology. Metastatic undifferentiated large cell carcinoma, similar to the histology of that found in a previous right paratracheal node biopsy.

A–C. CT scan obtained following intravenous injection of 50 ml of Hypaque 60 M.

A and B. W 20. Contiguous 13-mm sections.

A well-demarcated ovoid high absorption mass (20–31) is shown in the right parietal and occipital lobes. An irregular central to anterior zone showed a lower absorption (18–23), consistent with a large area of tumor necrosis. Anteriorly, a zone of reduced absorption (9–15) is indicative of partial volume representation of adjacent edema. In **A**, to the left of the tumor, are represented a grossly displaced choroid plexus of right lateral ventricle and a less displaced choroid of the left lateral ventricle. The mass measured over 8 cm in greatest diameter, and the zone of edema was 9–12 mm in width. Other sections revealed the gross compression of the right lateral ventricle and dislocation of the septum lucidum 6 mm to the left. The right ambient cistern was compressed. No other mass was identified. The findings were thought to be consistent with a huge metastasis or an unusual-appearing glioma.

C. L 24   W M.

Same section as in **B**, revealing more clearly the lower absorption necrotic region of the mass.

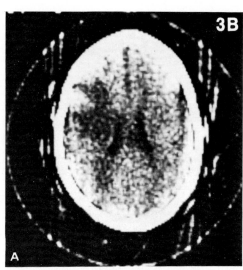 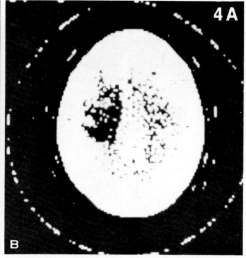

FIG. 13.16. METASTATIC POORLY DIFFERENTIATED LARGE CELL CARCINOMA FROM THE LUNG.

Clinical Features. A 55 y.o. male in whom a nonresectable squamous cell and a poorly differentiated large cell carcinoma of the lung had been diagnosed 2 years earlier and treated with palliative radiation therapy. He gave a 3 week history of weakness in the right extremities.

Neurological Examination. Right hemiparesis involving the upper extremity more than the lower. No sensory deficit was identified.

Skull Examination. A limited study was normal.

RN Scan. Tcp; showed increased activity in the left frontoparietal region.

CT Scan. Abnormal (Fig. 13.16).

Histology. Poorly differentiated large cell carcinoma of lung, previously diagnosed.

A and **B.** Plain CT scan.

A. L 17   W 20.

In the left cerebral hemisphere at the level of the midbody of the lateral ventricle, in the region of the postcentral gyrus, an irregular area of increased absorption (17–29) was evident. To what extent the higher absorption region at the cerebral surface represented tumor, cerebral cortex, and possibly some effect from partial volume inclusion of the adjacent vault is uncertain. Extending from this region of higher absorption is a large, quite well demarcated region of decreased absorption (6–14) consistent with edema, but possibly representing necrotic large cell tumor. There was no visible mass effect, suggesting that the low absorption region represented necrotic tumor rather than edema.

B. L 17   W M.

Section immediately above that in **A,** showing upward extension of the quite well demarcated low absorption region, occupying much of the parietal centrum semiovale. Two rather nodular-appearing islands of higher absorption are visible within the region, in addition to numerous smaller flecks, some of which may represent denser cellular portions of the tumor.

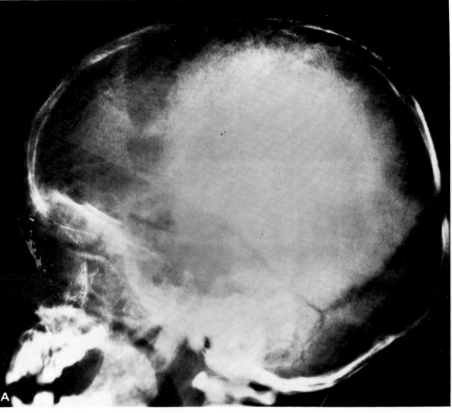
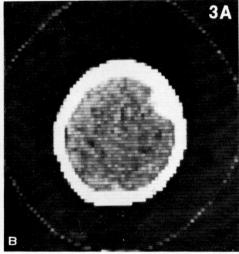

FIG. 13.17.   METASTATIC NEUROBLASTOMA.

Clinical Features. A 15-month-old girl with a 2 week history of left facial paresis and left otitis media. There was no history of trauma. Recent progressive bilateral proptosis and a nodular, hard enlarging liver had been noted. She had had a low grade fever and had been irritable for the previous few days.

Neurological Examination. Bilateral proptosis, left facial paralysis, and mild optic atrophy were noted. The left otitis media had been treated by myringotomy and antibiotics. There was clinical suspicion of brain abscess.

Skull Examination. Loss of aeration of the left mastoid air cells, diastasis of the major cranial sutures, and evidence of destructive changes involving the margins of wide coronal sutures (Fig. 13.17A).

RN Scan. Tcp; focal increase in uptake was present in the posterior frontal region superiorly and peripherally. There was also suspicion of a small area of increased activity in a similar region of the left side.

CT Scan. This was abnormal on the same day as the RN scan (Fig. 13.17B).

Angio. Bilateral internal carotid studies on the same day as the CT scan raised suspicion of an avascular mass in the region of the left frontal operculum and suspicion of a right frontal mass also. The study also raised suspicion of an extracerebral collection in the right midfrontal region. There was no midline dislocation.

Histology. Neuroblastoma with widespread metastasis was confirmed.

A. Marked widening of coronal sutures with evidence of extensive bone destruction at the suture margins is shown. There is also considerable simple diastasis of the lambdoid suture. The findings are characteristic metastatic neuroblastoma and increased intracranial pressure.

B. CT scan in the superior cerebral region. W   30.

A sharply demarcated region of homogeneous high absorption (18–40) and showing a convex inner margin is shown beneath the region of the right coronal suture. No definite abnormality is visible on the left side.

The CT findings are indistinguishable from traumatic epidural hematoma. However, there was no history of cranial trauma. Also the clinical features and the typical findings on skull films clearly indicated the diagnosis of metastatic neuroblastoma. The CT scan, in this context, indicates marked hemorrhage into metastatic tumor involving the epidural and possibly dural tissues. The CT scan did not reveal the less advanced metastatic involvement in the region of the left coronal suture, although this was shown on skull films and was suggested by the RN scan.

A short time later, CT examination of the orbit revealed bilateral metastatic involvement here also (Fig. 28.15).

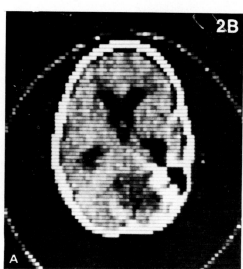 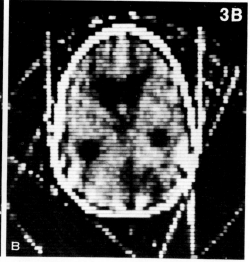

FIG. 13.18. UNDIFFERENTIATED MALIGNANT NEOPLASM, CONSISTENT WITH METASTATIC ALVEOLAR RHABDOMYOSARCOMA.

Clinical Features. A 3 y.o. boy who was seen at the age of 4½ months with left proptosis. A retrobulbar space tumor was found and diagnosed as rhabdomyosarcoma. The left eye was enucleated, and he was treated with radiotherapy and chemotherapy (vincristine and actinomycin D). He was well thereafter until 2 weeks before examination, when he developed occipital headaches.

Skull Examination. Suture diastasis.

CT Scan. Examination under general anesthesia; abnormal (Fig. 13.18).

Operation. (Dr. Paul Chapman.) A radical excision of the cerebellar mass was performed, but some tumor was known to remain. A 10-ml cyst containing greenish fluid was aspirated from the lateral portion of the right cerebellar hemisphere. The tumor was extensively necrotic.

Histology. Undifferentiated malignant neoplasm, consistent with metastatic alveolar rhabdomyosarcoma. The tumor was noted to resemble that removed from the orbit at the age of 4½ months.

A. L 15 W 20. **B.** L 18 W 20.
Plain CT scan, revealing a large, rather irregular area of diminished absorption (10–15) involving most of the area of the right cerebellar hemisphere and vermis at these levels. In **A,** a small region of lower absorption at the left anterior margin of the lesion suggests a deformed and displaced fourth ventricle. A crescent of higher absorption (20–25) arches from the posterior midline anteriorly and to the left around the region of lower absorption. This appears denser than normal vermis and suggests a denser cellular component of the tumor or a region of some hemorrhagic extravasation.

In **B,** the second 8-mm section above **A,** the low absorption regions of the lesion range from 8–12 units. These values suggest the presence of necrosis but could represent merely edema above the mass. The heterogeneous appearance is more suggestive of tumor necrosis. The posterior portion of the third ventricle is somewhat displaced to the left, and there appears to be some anterior displacement of the junction of the dilated right temporal horn and trigone, consistent with superior cerebellar herniation on the right side. However, the upward canting of the right side of the head may be contributory.

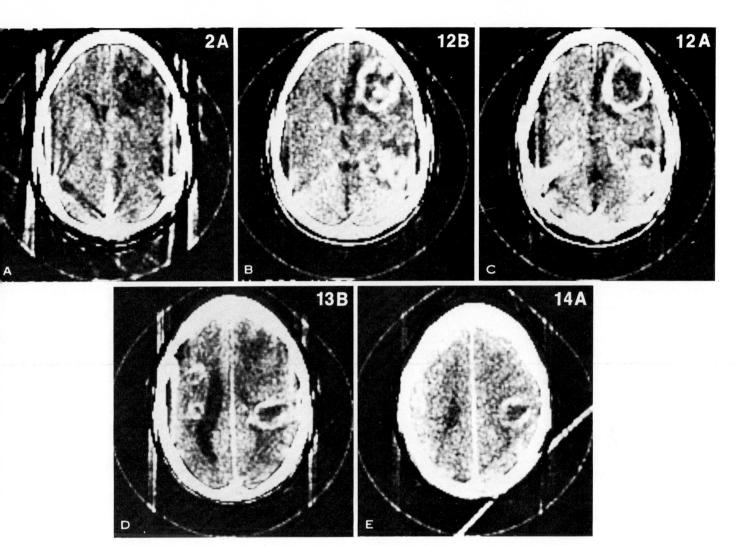

FIG. 13.19. METASTATIC LUNG CARCINOMA.

Clinical Features. A 51 y.o. man in whom a lung mass had been demonstrated by chest x-ray and who had recently developed bizarre behavior and slurred speech.

Neurological Examination. Bilateral papilledema, slight weakness of the right upper extremity, and bilateral equal hyper-reflexia. A left facial nerve palsy was present, but this had developed following an accident 7 years earlier. Sensory examination was within normal limits.

EEG. Right-sided slowing.

Skull Examination. The pineal was noted to be displaced 6 mm to the left of the midline, and there was very slight decrease in density of the lamina dura of the sella.

RN Scan. Tcp; multiple bilateral areas of increased activity were demonstrated on static imaging. Dynamic imaging revealed increased circulation in the right cerebral hemisphere, in the area of the large right frontal lesion noted on static imaging.

CT Scan. Multiple abnormalities (Fig. 13.19).

Sputum Cytology. Poorly differentiated carcinoma, possibly squamous cell.

A–E. L 15   W 30   160 x 160 matrix system.

A. Representative section from the plain scan series, which revealed multiple areas of generally diminished absorption of small and large size in both cerebral hemispheres. This section shows compression of the right lateral ventricle and displacement of the septum lucidum markedly to the left. A large, irregular area of diminished absorption is shown occupying much of the anterior portion of the right frontal lobe and extending into the region of the basal ganglia. A second, smaller area of diminished absorption is shown in the right temporal lobe, partly obscured by motion artifact.

B. Scan section similar to that in **A,** following intravenous infusion of 300 ml of 30% meglumine diatrizoate. Within the area of diminished absorption in the right frontal lobe, a large rounded area of strikingly increased absorption is now visible. An irregular area of lesser absorption is present within the mass, probably representing central necrosis within the tumor. A craggy nodular configuration of the denser elements is visible within the mass, which is now differentiated from the moderate surrounding cerebral edema. An irregular area of high absorption is also visible in the right temporal area, also surrounded by edema and containing a small area of presumed central necrosis.

C–E. More superior sections obtained following contrast enhancement. Additional masses of varying sizes are clearly visible as discrete nodules with presumed central necrosis in multiple areas that, on the plain scan, were represented only as poorly marginated irregular zones of diminished absorption, within which no clearly defined nodular masses were discriminated. Many of these foci could easily have been overlooked on plain scan alone.

CHAPTER 14

Lymphomas

INTRODUCTION

Cases of intracranial lymphoma studied by CT scanning at the Massachusetts General Hospital to date have generally been subjected to previous intracranial surgery and/or radiation therapy. Except in cases of extensive bilateral and approximately symmetrical cerebral involvement in reticulum cell sarcoma, no typical CT features have been identified to allow differentiation from the changes seen in many cases of low and intermediate grade astrocytoma (on plain CT scans), in which only irregularly marginated regions of decreased absorption are exhibited. Those cases having had radiation and chemotherapy have exhibited relatively large areas of markedly decreased absorption, generally poorly demarcated within the lesion, consistent with extensive tumor necrosis. For examples of lymphoma of the orbit, see Chapter 28, Figures 28.6 and 28.7.

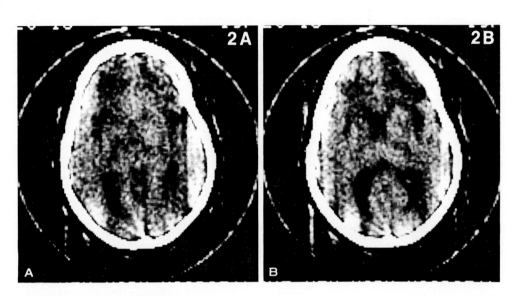

FIG. 14.1. RETICULUM CELL SARCOMA. (Case contributed by Michael D. F. Deck, M.D., The Memorial Sloan-Kettering Cancer Center, New York, New York.)

Clinical Features. A 30 y.o. female who had a reticulum cell sarcoma of the hard palate diagnosed by biopsy 1 year previously, and which had been treated with local radiation therapy. During the previous month, there had been a gradual onset of withdrawal and depression, with evidence on examination of bradykinesia, dementia, and Parkinson-like findings in the arms.

RN Scan. Increased activity bilaterally in the anterior basal ganglionic regions.

CT Scan. Abnormal (Fig. 14.1).

Angio. Diffuse bilateral basal ganglionic blushes, with early filling of the tributaries of the internal cerebral and basal veins. The lateral ventricles were small.

Treatment. By whole brain radiation therapy, with slight initial improvement.

A and **B**. Contiguous 13-mm plain scan sections. Very extensive irregularly marginated regions of diminished absorption are shown involving both frontal lobes, both in central areas and in cortical regions. The regions of diminished absorption extend posteriorly into the basal ganglia and insulae. At the level of the frontal horns (**B**) there is more striking involvement of the right frontal lobe than of the left and the septum lucidum is moderately displaced to the left, with more marked compression of the right frontal horn than of the left. There is modest enlargement of the trigones and occipital horns. The third ventricle is not discriminated, consistent with compression.

(Illustrations courtesy of Michael D. F. Deck, M.D.)

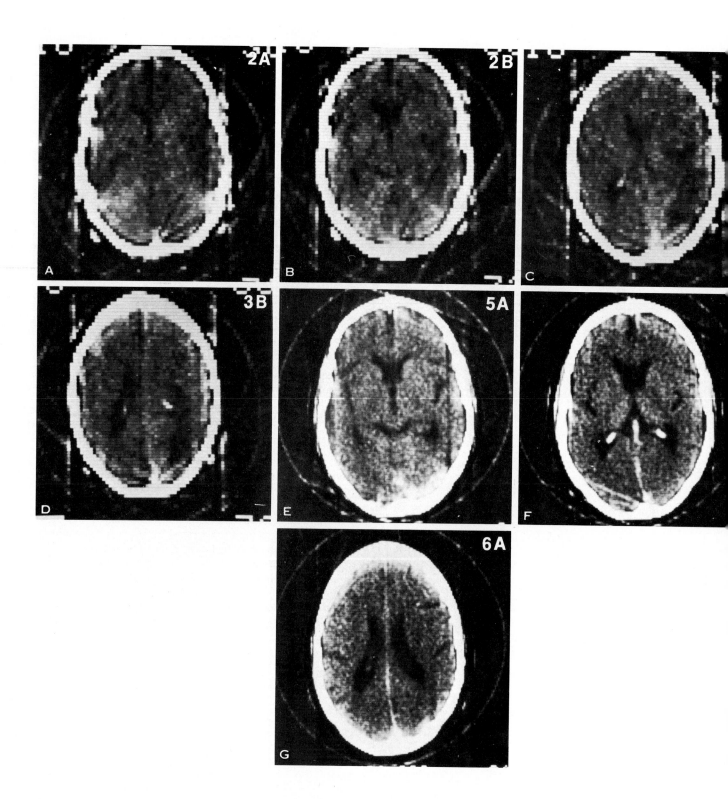

FIG. 14.2. MIXED CELL LYMPHOMA. (Case contributed by Hillier L. Baker, Jr., M.D., Mayo Clinic, Rochester, Minnesota.)

Clinical Features. A 69 y.o. male in whom an intra-abdominal mixed cell malignant lymphoma was diagnosed by biopsy 11½ months earlier. He was treated with radiation and chemotherapy. A few weeks before CT scan, he noted the onset of progressive dizziness, with staggering and falling. He then developed diplopia, blurring of vision, and headaches, followed by decreasing alertness.

Neurological Examination. The right pupil was larger than the left. There was bilateral nystagmus on horizontal gaze. Examination was otherwise not remarkable.

Skull Examination. Normal.

RN Scan. One week before CT scan, abnormal, with a discrete area of increased uptake in the right posterior fossa.

CT Scan. Abnormal (Fig. 14.2, **A–D**).

Angio. A right retrograde brachial study 1 day before the CT scan revealed an avascular mass in the posterior right medial temporal and thalamic regions.

Following a course of 6 meV radiation to the head through bilateral ports, to a total dose of 2400 rads, the patient improved and gained weight. His neurological symptoms abated markedly.

RN Scan. A repeat examination 6 months after the first showed no change from the original examination.

Neurological Examination. Thirteen months after the original CT scan; revealed a trace of unsteadiness and nystagmus.

CT Scan. Thirteen months after the original study; the scan had changed markedly (Fig. 14.2, **E–G**).

A–D. CT scan before cranial radiation therapy. A large area of nonhomogeneously diminished absorption, with moderately well defined margins, is shown involving the right temporal lobe and extending into the right basal ganglia and occipital lobe. There is moderate diffuse compression of the right lateral ventricle, and the third ventricle is displaced several millimeters to the left.

E–G. Scan 13 months later the following radiation therapy. 160 × 160 matrix system. No areas of diminished absorption within the cerebral parenchyma are visible now, and no mass effect is identified. There is modest enlargement of the lateral and third ventricles, enlargement of the sylvian and quadrigeminal cisterns, and enlargement of several cerebral convexity sulci on each side. Intravenous contrast enhancement also revealed no focal parenchymal abnormalities.

(Illustrations courtesy of Hillier L. Baker, Jr., M.D.)

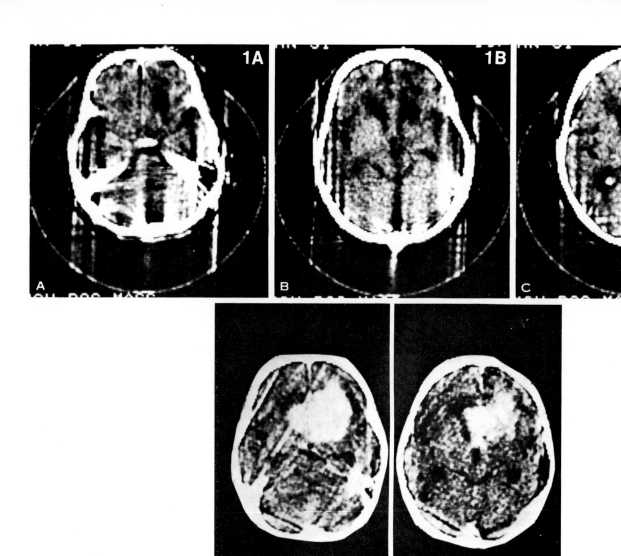

FIG. 14.3.   RETICULUM CELL SARCOMA.

Clinical Features. A 55 y.o. man admitted with a history of increasing lethargy over several days and involuntary shaking of the left arm. He gave a history of hospitalization for pneumonia 6 months previously, but had apparently recovered well. He had been at home with an upper respiratory infection for the past 2 weeks.

Neurological Examination. Stuporous, following only rare simple commands. The neck was not stiff. There was generalized increase in tone on the right side, which seemed stronger than the left side. Positive left Babinski sign. No gross sensory abnormality or ataxia where detected. LP revealed light yellow fluid in all tubes, 36 lymphocytes and 12 mononuclear cells. Opening pressure, 300 mm of CSF. Total protein, 135 mg, and sugar, 35 mg per deciliter. He was initially suspected to have a brain abscess or tuberculoma. On antibiotic and antituberculous chemotherapy plus steroids, he showed initial improvement and then progressively deteriorated.

Skull Examination. Normal, shortly after admission. Two and a half weeks later, polytomography revealed increased density of both frontal sinuses, consistent with sinusitis.

RN Scan. Several Tcp scans revealed a large area of increased activity in the right lobe area.

CT Scan. Two plain scans and a contrast-enhanced scan were abnormal (Fig. 14.3).

Angio. Transfemoral bilateral carotid studies revealed a large avascular right frontal lobe mass, extending deeply to the region of the lenticulostriate arteries. The internal cerebral vein was midline and no abnormality was noted on the left side.

Operation. (Dr. Charles Poletti.) Right frontal craniotomy, with biopsy of tumor.

Histology. Reticulum cell sarcoma.

A–C. L 14   W 30   160 x 160 matrix system.

The plain CT scan reveals a lesion in the right frontal lobe, consisting of patchy areas of diminished absorption (5–14) extending out to the frontopolar cortex and also involving the region of the head of the caudate nucleus. Minor involvement of the region immediately adjacent to the left frontal horn was also noted.

D and **E.** CT scan obtained after intravenous injection of 300 ml of meglumine diatrizoate 30%. A large and relatively homogeneous region of contrast enhancement (32–44) is shown extending through the right frontal lobe and basal ganglia, obliterating the right frontal horn. There is extension into the region of the left frontal horn. Regions of diminished absorption (6–15) are shown on the right and left sides of the lesion, presumably representing cerebral edema.

CHAPTER 15

Blood

ABSORPTION VALUES OF INTRAVASCULAR AND EXTRAVASATED BLOOD

At the inception of our work with computed tomography, no data were available to indicate the rapidity with which circulating blood (said to have a value of 6, based on the initial work of Ambrose and Hounsfield (1, 2, 4)) was altered to produce much higher absorption values upon extravasation into the brain. At that time it was believed that this increase in absorption was the result of the clotting process, with extrusion of serum and, consequently, more densely aggregated cellular elements and hemoglobin, possibly with some effect from an increased concentration of calcium ions. Our cases of intracerebral hematoma regularly showed a markedly elevated absorption (generally in the range of 20–45 and occasionally extending into the 50's). Several extracerebral hematomas were found to contain clotted blood and also showed similarly high absorption values. However, a chromophobe adenoma with suprasellar extension was noted to contain a large volume showing an absorption range of 24–41, which was interpreted as hemorrhage secondary to tumor necrosis (Chapter 8, Fig. 8.1). At surgery shortly thereafter, 5 ml of liquid blood were aspirated from the tumor. Another case, a chronic epidural hematoma that was seen to be liquid at surgery, also revealed a high absorption range preoperatively. Clotting, therefore, did not appear to be essential to a high absorption for extravasated blood. These findings stimulated further investigation.

CIRCULATING BLOOD

The absorption of circulating blood was investigated. Large arteriovenous malformations appeared to have areas of 6–8 units that were thought originally to represent the lumina of large draining veins. It seemed that these same areas increased to levels of approximately 40 units after intravenous injection of 40–50 ml of Hypaque 60. However, other large areas were noted to have values of about 20–30 before contrast material had been injected. Initially, the latter areas were thought to represent multiple areas of small extravasations of blood and/or gliotic reaction about the blood vessels of the vascular malformation. However, the complexity of the anatomical configuration of high and low absorption areas in these cases and the difficulty in obtaining precise correlation of the different areas in the scans before and after injection of intravenous contrast material prevented reliable conclusions. A large, incompletely thrombosed aneurysm of the basilar artery was examined. This had an absorption value of 36. A large intracranial aneurysm, however, is clearly an unreliable model for the study of the absorption value of circulating blood, since the presence of minute mural calcifications and/or thrombus, having a high absorption value, is likely to be averaged with the circulating blood to produce false values for the latter.

Therefore, the circulating blood of a dog was scanned by means of an arteriovenous bypass through a large diameter polyethylene tube, which was led into a glass bottle containing water. The bottle was placed within the head cap of the scanner, and the blood within the tubing, occupying the entire scan slice thickness of 8 mm, was found to have an absorption range of 13–28 units, with most of the volume of blood scanned being in the 15–25 range.

NONCIRCULATING BLOOD

The absorption values of noncirculating blood were studied using fresh unclotted blood, citrated blood, heparinized blood, a control normal saline-heparin sample, packed red cells, retracted clot, platelet-poor plasma, and serum. These samples were placed in polyethylene containers and scanned within a phantom (Table 15.1). These results were checked at intervals of several weeks on two subsequent occasions, with identical findings. The results indicated that the clotting process is not essential to the elevated absorption values of extravasated blood and that red cells are

TABLE 15.1
Absorption Values of Human Blood in EMI Units

Packed RBC'S (low calcium)	*13–43
Retracted clot	*13–42
Fresh unclotted blood	*13–31
Citrated blood (0–75 ml Na cit. to 15 ml)	*13–30
Heparinized blood (1 ml — 1000 U to 15 ml)	*13–30
Plasma (platelet poor, with low calcium)	2–13
Serum	1–12
Saline (normal)	1–8

* Partial volume effects gave rise to lower limit values. 120 kV
13- and 8-mm sections
5- and 14-ml volumes
Polyethylene containers } negative absorption values
Disposable syringes
In water, within thin plastic bottle or within central area of skull phantom.

These measurements were obtained with the 80 x 80 matrix system. With this system, the scanner used appeared to have an absorption measurement accuracy of approximately ±1 EMI unit, significantly better than the performance of the 160 x 160 matrix system, which appears to have a measurement accuracy approaching the guaranteed accuracy of ± ½% standard deviation. In the above experiments, the small diameter of the containers used resulted in peripheral partial volume averaging with the plastic container walls, which prevented satisfactory identification of the lower limits of the absorption ranges of the preparations.

responsible for the high absorption values of blood (Fig. 15.1).

An acute intracerebral hematoma was produced in a baboon. Two ml of blood were drawn from an arm vein of the anesthetized animal and injected immediately through a small burr hole in the parietal lobe. The mean time of the first scan obtained through the hematoma was 28 minutes. This showed an absorption range for the hematoma of 27–36. Serial studies were obtained at 68 minutes, 4 days, and 9 days. These revealed values of 25–38, 28–37, and 25–29, respectively. There was thus no significant change in absorption values of the hematoma from 28 minutes to 4 days, and there did not appear to be any important change in the size of the hematoma during this interval. However, at 9 days, most of the hematoma had been absorbed, and the very small remaining portion probably occupied only a partial volume of the slice thickness (13 mm). This factor could readily explain the modest decrease in absorption values on the final scan.

CONCLUSIONS FROM EXPERIMENTAL DATA

Based on the findings of these studies, it is concluded that clotting is not necessary to the production of high absorption values of extravasated blood. Circulating blood has a somewhat lower absorption than does

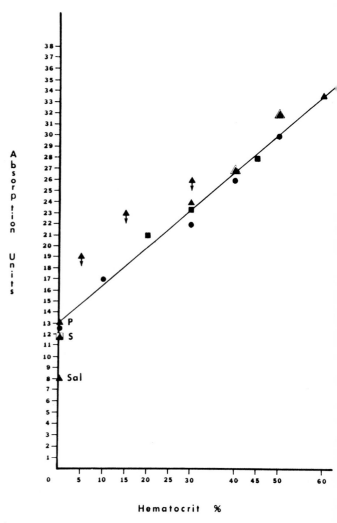

FIG. 15.1. Absorption values of various human blood preparations. The different *symbols* represent experimental results obtained with different sets of blood samples scanned on four separate occasions at intervals of many weeks. Absorption values (peak) in EMI units are plotted against hematocrit values. The regression line represents the peak values obtained for the different samples. *Sal*, normal saline, 8; *S*, serum, 12; *P*, plasma, 13. The remaining values plotted represent measurements on hematocrit preparations of 5, 10, 15, 20, 30, 40, 45, 50, and 60%. The measurements obtained show a remarkable consistency, with the exception of some measurements of the peak values of preparations of 5, 15, and 30% hematocrit. The scans of these preparations showed layering due to sedimentation, and this phenomenon was confirmed by examination of the tubes at the completion of the scan. It is interesting to note that the regression line of the peak absorption readings of the various hematocrits meets the ordinate at the peak value for plasma. From these results, it can be seen that the value of human blood of hematocrit 45% is 28 units. These figures are in satisfactory agreement with earlier in vitro blood studies (Fig. 15.2). (*The blood samples used were prepared by Dr. Angelina Cavalho, Head of the Special Clotting Laboratory at the Massachusetts General Hospital.*)

extravasated clotted or unclotted blood, and its relatively high values (13–28) are due to the red cells and, more specifically, to the iron content of hemoglobin. The experimental work suggests that there may be a modest further increase in absorption following extravasation, but the finding is not reliable in a single experiment, and the values for the circulating blood (dog), intracerebral hematoma (baboon), and in vitro blood samples (human) were obtained from different species. However, our experimental and clinical studies do indicate that there is probably an increase of 5–15 units in absorption values of blood in hours or a few days after extravasation of blood into the brain.

RELATIONSHIP OF ABSORPTION AND HEMATOCRIT VALUES

Samples of human serum and plasma and samples of heparinized human blood preparations at hematocrits varying between 5 and 60% were scanned in polyethylene containers surrounded by water. The results are shown in Table 15.2. In view of the importance of the absorption values of circulating blood in a wide variety of clinical scanning contexts, it is reassuring that these experimental results are in substantial agreement with the results obtained by Phelps (54, 54A), who has used monoenergetic beams of a variety of radioactive sources, to study the attenuation coefficients of a wide variety of substances including human blood of various hematocrit values.

CLINICAL CT SCANNING IMPLICATIONS

The findings described in the foregoing sections suggest that the appreciably higher absorption of cortical and central grey matter compared with white matter is likely to be due, in large part, to their much greater vascularity, although the higher myelin content of white

TABLE 15.2
Relationship Between CT Absorption Values of Blood and Hematocrit Values

Hematocrit (%)	Peak absorption (EMI units)
60	34
50	30
45	28
40	27
30	23
20	20
15	18
10	17
5	15
Plasma	13
Serum	12

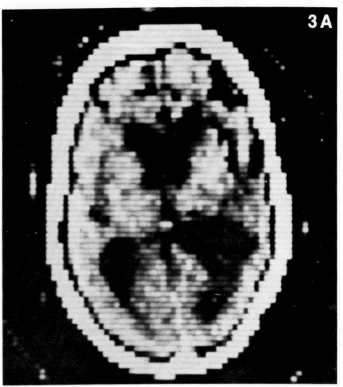

3A

FIG. 15.2. Cadaver scan. One of a series of scans obtained approximately 40 hours after death. Absorption values of the cerebral cortex and central grey matter were strikingly increased compared with the values obtained during life and those normally encountered. The increase in absorption was greater in cortical than in central grey matter. No change in the measurements of white matter was detected. Modest collections of gas were scattered in the subarachnoid spaces. The values for CSF were 5–14, several units higher than are normally found. Both the increase in absorption of grey matter and of CSF were possibly the result of loss of fluid from the smaller vessels on the one hand and from the CSF-containing spaces on the other, resulting in a greater concentration of hemoglobin and CSF protein, respectively.

matter is likely to be a significant contributing factor.

A cadaver was scanned approximately 40 hours after death (Fig. 15.2). It was found that grey matter had absorption values ranging up to 45–50 units, considerably above the upper limits obtained in that patient and in other individuals during life and presumably due to hemoconcentration. There was no obvious change in the absorption values of white matter. This finding is also consonant with the different vascularities of grey and white matter. These findings also reflect the rise in absorption values of cortical and central grey matter found after intravenous injection of contrast medium and the lack of any apparent change in absorption values of white matter under the same circumstances. It is of interest to speculate that the different absorption values in different areas of the cortex, and in the same area of

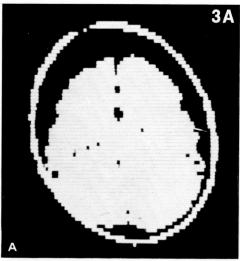

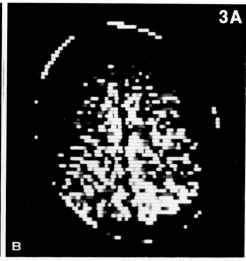

FIG. 15.3. Saline perfusion of brain. Representative section of a series of scans obtained following perfusion of the major cerebral vessels of a fresh brain with normal saline.

A. L 6   W M.

At this setting, the entire brain section is shown. As the window level was raised, portions of the cerebral cortex were progressively "lost" (changed to black).

B. L 15   W M.

At these control settings, almost all of the cerebral cortex has changed to black, indicating a significant reduction in the absorption values compared with the measurements normally found in life. Much of the cerebral white matter remains white at this level setting, and no definite change in absorption values in white matter was recognized compared with normal values in life. The findings further support the belief that the greater density of grey matter than white is partly an expression of the greater vascularity of the two regions, although the myelin content of white matter undoubtedly contributes to its lower absorption. *These scans were obtained without surrounding skull or skull-like high absorption phantom. Thus, the usual artifactual increase of 3–7 units in the external cortical zone caused by the thicker and denser areas of the skull was not present.*

cortex at different ages, may reflect, at least to some significant degree, changes in vascularity. At present, artifacts producing elevations of absorption values in a broad zone beneath the dense skull limit the precision of cortical measurements.

Fresh cadaver brains have been scanned following irrigation of the major vascular trunks with large volumes of normal saline. Scans of these preparations have demonstrated that the cerebral cortex, in which blood has been replaced by normal saline (of much lower absorption than blood), was now appreciably *less* dense than white matter instead of more dense, as is normally the case. Under these conditions, the peak density of the irrigated cortex appeared to be in the region of 15 units, rather than 30 units ± 6 (Fig. 15.3). However, for comparison of these measurements, up to 7 units (artifact) should be subtracted from the second figure, derived from scans of brain within skull. The *true* absorption of normal adult cerebral cortex appears to be 20 units ± 1 or 2.

Although postmortem changes may have affected the above results, these considerations suggest that carefully analyzed brain scans in life obtained before and after intravascualr injection of contrast medium, with careful serial measurement of the equilibrated blood pool level of iodine, may eventually provide a more accurate measurement of blood volume of different portions of the brain in life than is presently possible by other means. For such studies, it will be necessary to ensure highly precise matching of the scanned cerebral volumes before and after contrast medium injection. Careful account will have to be taken of regions where partial volume averaging may result in factitious measurements (see Chapter 27, pages 443, 445).

In considering various pathological conditions, the density of blood circulating in or about the lesion must be taken into account in evaluating the measured absorption in different portions of the lesion. Clearly, increased density in a lesion may be an expression of the physical density of the arrangement of cellular elements, an expression of a marked degree of vascularity of the lesion, the presence of hemorrhage into or about the lesion, or a combination of these factors. An additional consideration is the presence of such a distribution of psammomatous calcifications through the lesion that partial volume averaging may result in absorption values in the dense soft tissue range, considerably below the true absorption value of a full volume calcific aggregate.

Conversely, a diminished absorption measurement in an area of pathology may represent limited or absent blood flow through the region, an abnormally low cellular concentration relative to interstitial fluid, a considerable increase in the local fluid content (edema), or a combination of the above.

In consideration of the possibility of identifying pathological saccular or tubular spaces containing circulating blood, such as aneurysms and various forms of vascular malformations, it is apparent that, given an adequate dimension of the space, a sufficient absorption difference (contrast) between the vascular space and the surrounding tissues or fluids, and a high technical quality of the CT scan, such spaces should be recognizable, even in the absence of mural calcification and/or thrombus. A small aneurysm, which might be identified if surrounded by lower density white matter, could well be obscured if it projected into cortical regions, as is likely with the majority of aneurysms occurring intracranially. The basal location of the majority of these, where there is considerable irregular adjacent bone, also tends to create conditions disadvantageous to recognition. Recognition of aneurysms can be significantly enhanced by repeat scanning after intravenous contrast injection, with resultant considerable increase in the absorption values of the contained blood. Scanning of 8-mm (and eventually thinner) sections will further aid identification of such lesions, since this will reduce the possibility of partial volume averaging.

Scanning before and after the injection of contrast medium allows a reasonable estimate to be made of the vascularity of lesions themselves and/or the lack of integrity of the blood-brain barrier, as in neoplasms, and the vascularity of regions adjacent to lesions, such as the zones adjacent to cerebral infarcts. Knowledge of the absorption values of blood of different hematocrit values permits a reasonably accurate estimate of the amount of blood in certain extracerebral collections.

CHAPTER 16

Intracerebral and Intracerebellar Hemorrhage: Intraventricular Hemorrhage

INTRODUCTION

The reader is referred to Chapter 15 for a general discussion regarding the absorption values of blood in the circulation and following extravasation. The absorption values obtained by CT scanning of various blood fractions and changes in absorption values with variation in hematocrit values are also presented and discussed in that section.

Experience has amply demonstrated that CT scanning is overwhelmingly superior to any other technique in the diagnosis of the presence of hemorrhage within the brain and in the demonstration of its precise location and extent during life (41, 51, 59). CT scanning is the first technique to provide an accurate evaluation of the contributory role of cerebral edema in production of the mass effect associated with intracerebral hematoma. The method provides a relatively simple and absolutely hazard-free opportunity to study the natural course of such hemorrhages and accompanying edema. With this technique, the presence of an intraventricular clot can be determined with high accuracy. It has become apparent that extension of deeply situated cerebral hemorrhage into the ventricular system is by no means uncommon and that significant ventricular dilatation does not necessarily follow, even when an intraventricular blood clot is extensive.

Radionuclide studies in intracerebral hemorrhage have a relatively low yield. Indications of possible temporal relationships between the interval between hemorrhage and the appearance of occasional positive radionuclide scans suggest that the RN scan may become positive only with the development of a considerable amount of edema after a period of days (the case illustrated in Fig. 16.3 is of interest in this regard).

While high-quality angiography with magnification is relatively sensitive in the detection of medium-sized hemorrhages in the region of the putamen and the thalamus, the relative contributions of hematoma and associated edema cannot be distinguished. In more peripheral locations, particularly in the posterior portions of the cerebral hemispheres and in the posterior fossa, relatively large hemorrhages must be present for unequivocal angiographic identification of a mass. Angiography provides indirect evidence of intraventricular extension of hemorrhage only when there is considerable ventricular enlargement in association with appropriate clinical and other angiographic features.

The differentiation of intra-axial hemorrhage and pale and hemorrhagic embolic infarction (particularly in the cerebellum) can be a difficult clinical challenge. CT scanning offers a highly reliable means of differentiation. Although the present minimum CT section thickness is a limitation, experience has indicated that intra-axial hemorrhages only a few millimeters in diameter can be identified, provided that they are not limited to the cortical or immediately subcortical locations, where, at least in some cases, the absorption values may merge indistinguishably with those of the cerebral cortex.

A distinct limitation of CT scanning in the study of intra-axial hemorrhage is that the condition of the cerebral vessels is not revealed. Significant intrinsic vascular lesions, including developmental and mycotic aneurysms and small arteriovenous malformations, will generally not be identified. With the exception of certain typical clinical situations, such as those of intra-axial hemorrhages in classical locations in hypertensive individuals, cerebral angiography is required to complete the evaluation of patients who have been shown by CT scan to have an intra-axial hemorrhage.

TABLE 16.1
800 Consecutive CT Examinations

Infarcts	Ischemic	76	
	Hemorrhagic	11	87
Subdural hematomas			13
Extradural hematomas			4
Intracerebral hematomas	Hypertensive	27	
	AVM	4	
	Traumatic	2	
	Miscellaneous	12	45
Arteriovenous malformations	Without frank hematoma	6	
	With frank hematoma	4	10
Aneurysms			2
Total			162

TABLE 16.2
I.C. Hematoma

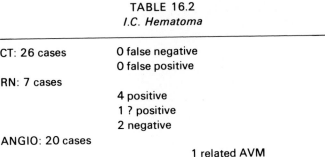

CT: 26 cases   0 false negative
              0 false positive

RN: 7 cases

        4 positive
        1 ? positive
        2 negative

ANGIO: 20 cases

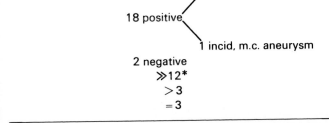

                1 related AVM
18 positive
                1 incid, m.c. aneurysm
2 negative
       ≫12*
       >3
       =3

*≫, CT very much superior to angiography; >, CT distinctly superior to angiography; =, CT equal to angiography.

The incidence of various cerebral and extracerebral vascular lesions in the initial 800 CT examinations is given in Table 16.1.

The relative value of CT scanning, radionuclide scanning, and angiography in the 26 cases of intra-axial hematoma examined in the first 600 CT examinations is presented in Table 16.2.

In the first 600 patients studied with CT were 23 patients with acute intracerebral and/or intraventricular hemorrhage. These cases included 14 with hypertensive hemorrhage, three with hemorrhage from arteriovenous malformations, one with hemorrhage complicating Coumadin therapy, and four with traumatic intracerebral hemorrhage, two of which were small hemorrhages associated with ventricular needling and one that was an extensive intraventricular hemorrhage in a premature neonate. Eight of the hypertensive cases were studied within the first 24 hours after onset, and the remainder were examined within 5 days. The hemorrhage appeared to have originated in the putamen in six cases and in the thalamus in six cases. The hematomas invariably extended beyond the limits of either the putamen or the thalamus. In many instances, both regions were involved. Two of the putaminal hemorrhages extended deeply into the temporal lobe, approaching the lateral temporal cortex, a feature that could not be deduced from cerebral angiography. Five of the six patients with thalamic hemorrhage had associated intraventricular clots, usually limited to the ipsilateral lateral ventricle. No patient with putaminal hemorrhage had evidence of ventricular hematoma. Mild to moderate lateral ventricular dilatation, apparently from partial obstruction of the foramen of Munro, was evident in one of six patients with putaminal hemorrhage and in three of six patients with thalamic hemorrhage. One hypertensive hemorrhage arose in the pons and extended eccentrically to the right. Four patients with clinically suspected hypertensive cerebellar hemorrhage were studied. One of the patients was found to have a small left posterolateral cerebellar hemisphere hematoma. In the other three patients, cerebellar infarction was diagnosed by CT and substantiated by subsequent clinical course. Each of the patients with hypertensive intracerebral hemorrhage presented a clinical picture strongly suggestive of the diagnosis, and four patients died. The location and extent of hematoma indicated by CT scans was confirmed in the only patient who had an autopsy. The two patients with major temporal lobe extension of hematoma had surgical evacuation of solid hematomas, with satisfactory postoperative improvement. The remaining patients had severe neurological deficits, with slow improvement occurring at the time of discharge.

The following CT features of hematomas were apparent, regardless of etiology. The absorption values of the hematomas generally ranged from the 20's to the 40's. A single large, acute hematoma had a small area that peaked at 60 units in its center. Almost all of the intracerebral hematomas had shapes of varying degrees of irregularity and slightly indistinct margins. The somewhat indistinct peripheral appearance is probably explained by the edge of the clot occupying less than the full thickness of the scan section. Repeat CT examinations in six patients demonstrated reduction in size of the high absorption hematoma after intervals of 10–30 days. One small thalamic hemorrhage lost its increased absorption completely over an interval of 32 days, leaving a very small area of decreased absorption.

Gradual reduction in the density of hematomas is evidently the result of progressive breakdown and removal of red cells and their contents. Eventually a cavity containing fluid with similar absorption to CSF may be identified in late CT scans. In other instances, a residual slit-like cavity may not be discriminated by scans. Scans of white clot (fibrin-platelet clot) in vitro have shown absorption in the 15–20 unit range (i.e., similar to normal brain values), depending on the extent to which serum has been extruded.

A low absorption zone of variable thickness was seen at the periphery of all of the intracerebral hematomas. This evidently reflects associated cerebral edema. The apparent edema was most prominent in those patients who had an onset of symptoms suggestive of hemorrhage more than 24 hours before CT study. Although heavy clinical demands upon the CT scanner have precluded a systematic study of the incidence, the rate of appearance, and the rate of regression of edema associated with intracerebral hemorrhage, there is evidence suggesting that such edema is minimal in the first 1–2 days and that a maximum edema volume may be reached in most cases after an interval of several days. At least in some instances, edema seems to persist for 3–4 weeks. The response of cerebral edema to osmotic agents and corticosteroid therapy merits detailed clinical and experimental studies with the aid of this new method.

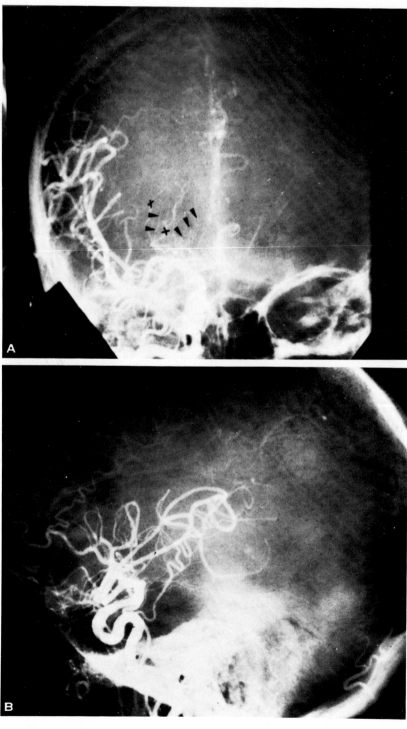

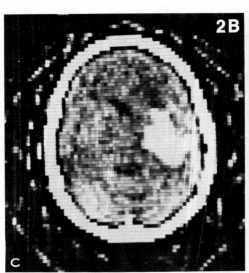

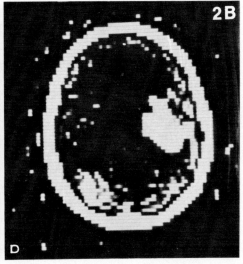

FIG. 16.1. HYPERTENSIVE PUTAMINAL HEMORRHAGE, EXTENDING SUPERFICIALLY.

Clinical Features. A 52 y.o. stuporous woman with left hemiparesis, left hemisensory defect, and left homonymous hemianopsia of 24 hours duration, whose CSF contained 44 red cells.

CT Scan. Abnormal (Fig. 16.1, **C** and **D**).

Angio. Right carotid study, which demonstrated a lateral centrosylvian avascular mass (Fig. 16.1, **A** and **B**).

Operation. (Dr. Robert G. Ojemann.) Clot was evacuated via a right temporal craniectomy. The patient had a good postoperative recovery.

Histology. Dark red gelatinous clot.

A and **B. A,** frontal, and **B,** lateral early arterial phases of the right carotid angiogram. Considerable medial displacement and disorganization of medial and lateral lenticulostriate arterial branches are shown (*arrowheads*). The insular branches of the middle cerebral artery are moderately displaced laterally, with crowding in a transverse direction and fan-shaped stretching

and arching with general elevation in the sagittal plane.

C and **D.** CT section in the plane of the maximum dimensions of the hemorrhage. The high absorption distribution of the hematoma is clearly visible. It is centered in the right putamen and extends laterally into the right temporal lobe to the subcortical region and deeply, to the internal capsule. The superficial extension, which was not identifiable on the basis of the angiogram, led to the decision to perform a surgical evacuation. There is a very small amount of edema (peripheral 3 to 6 mm zone of decreased absorption) associated with this recent hemorrhage. Compression of the right lateral ventricle and mild dislocation of the midline to the left were visible. However, there is a more diffuse slight decrease in absorption in the white matter of the frontal lobe anterior to the hemorrhage, also consistent with edema. **C** is W 20 and **D** is W M; display of the same section.

(Fig. 16.1C reprinted by permission from Radiology, 110: 109–123, 1974.)

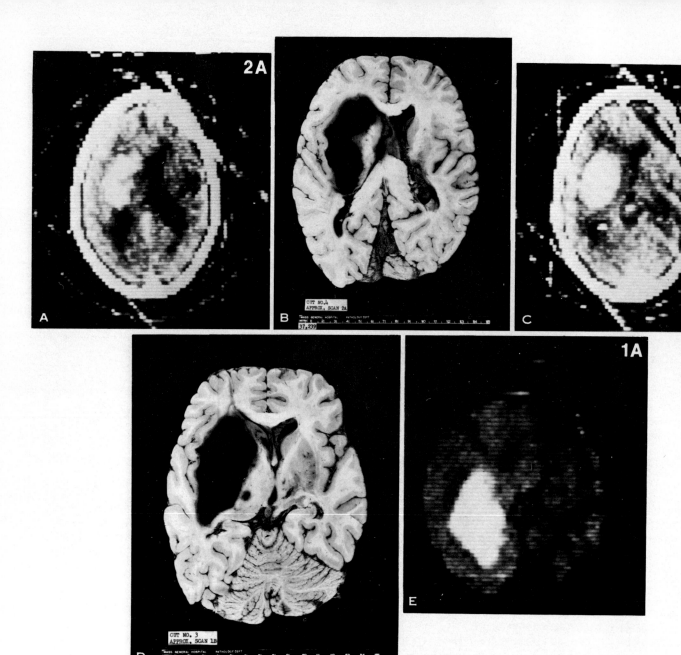

FIG. 16.2. HYPERTENSIVE INTRACEREBRAL HEMORRHAGE, MASSIVE, PUTAMINAL.

Clinical Features. A 68 y.o. male who, on the day before the CT examination, developed aphasia and right hemiplegia and then lapsed into coma. There was a past history of mild residual left hemiparesis from a poorly documented stroke 13 years earlier.

CT Scan. Abnormal (Fig. 16.2, **A** and **C**).

Angio. Transfemoral bilateral carotid studies revealed a large avascular mass in the region of the left putamen and a dilated right lateral ventricle.

Autopsy. Massive central left hemisphere hematoma (Fig. 16.2, **B** and **D**). The patient expired 24 hours after the CT examination.

A and **C**. Contiguous 13-mm scans revealed a large irregular ovoid region of hemorrhage, extending from the region of the left putamen anteriorly to involve the caudate nucleus and posteriorly to the anterior margin of the trigone. Considerable compression of the left lateral ventricle by the mass is visible, but there is only mild indentation of the third ventricle and mild displacement of midline structures to the right. Only a relatively

small amount of low absorption edema is visible adjacent to the recent hemorrhage, most prominent in the frontal lobe just anterior to the hematoma.

B and **D**. Sections of brain approximately corresponding in angle and level to the CT scan sections **A** and **C** demonstrated the extensive hematoma with the accompanying ventricular deformities. Although the hematoma had enlarged in the interval between CT scanning and death, there is a close correspondence in anatomical appearance between the CT scan and brain specimen sections. Enlargement of the right sylvian cistern is not as obvious in the brain specimen sections as in the CT scan (**A**), but an old infarction in the region of the right insula was confirmed pathologically.

(Fig. 16.2, A–C reprinted by permission from Radiology, 112: 73–80, 1974.)

E. CT scan of the fresh brain of the same patient. The high density and clear definition of the hematoma is apparent. Owing to difficulty in positioning the fresh brain in the scanner, the section does not correspond in level and angle with the scans in life and the sections of brain at autopsy.

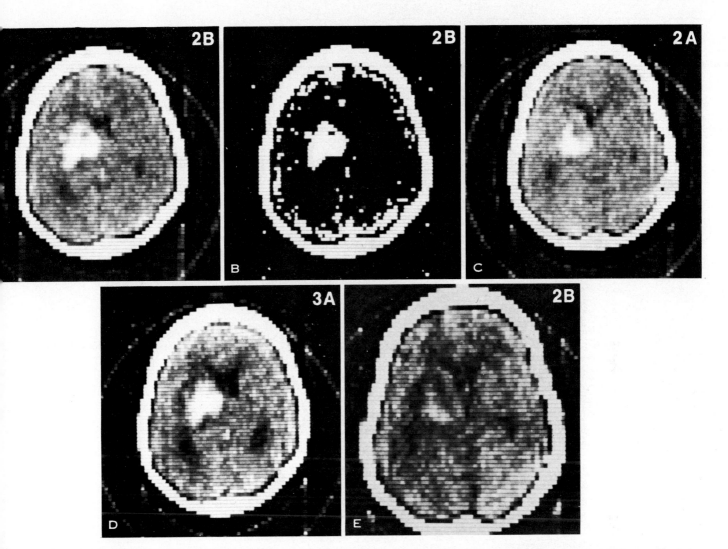

FIG. 16.3. HYPERTENSIVE PUTAMINAL OR THALAMIC HEMORRHAGE.

Clinical Features. A 27 y.o. female with known hypertension for 5 years and taking birth control pills. Sudden onset of complete aphasia, right hemiparesis, and right homonymous hemianopsia.

CT scan and angiography were both performed within a few hours of the onset.

CT Scan. Abnormal (Fig. 16.3, **A–C**).

RN Scan. Tcp; the day following the positive CT scan; normal.

Angio. Transfemoral bilateral carotid studies revealed lateral displacement of the left lenticulostriate arteries and the plexal portion of the anterior choroidal artery, indicating an avascular left thalamic mass effect. Confirmatory evidence was present in the form of increased convexity of the internal cerebral vein, which was displaced 3.5 mm to the right. There was delay in

arterial emptying in the distal anterior and middle cerebral branches. The angiogram and CT scan were both done on the day of the ictus.

By Day 2, the patient had improved and had begun to talk, although there was still severe dysphonia, dysarthria, and right homonymous hemianopsia.

CT Scan. This was repeated on Day 7 (Fig. 16.3, **D** and **E**).

RN Scan. Tcp; repeated on Day 13, abnormal (Fig. 16.3**F**).

CT Scan. Repeated on Day 17 (Fig. 16.3**G**).

A–C. CT scan, obtained on the day of the ictus. The high absorption (20–40) region of the left capsular hemorrhage is clearly visible. The hemorrhage extends from the anterior thalamic region through the putamen into the head of the caudate nucleus. There is mild midline dislocation to the right in the region of the frontal horns and the left frontal horn is moderately compressed. Note that absorption values surround-

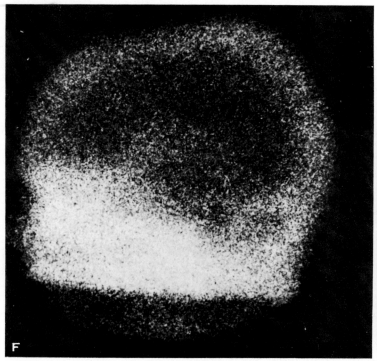

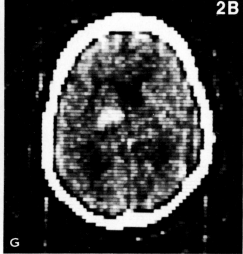

ing the hemorrhage are mostly in the normal range, indicating the presence of little or no surrounding edema.

B. L 20   W M.

Same scan section as in **A,** displaying the hemorrhage and portions of the cerebral cortex. The pineal is barely displaced from the midline.

C. Section immediately below that in **A.** The left capsular hemorrhage is less extensive at this level. There is no evidence of surrounding low absorption of edema.

D and **E.** CT scan obtained on Day 7. The hemorrhage has become slightly smaller. Displacement of the septum lucidum and of the pineal to the right has increased in the interval, with increase in the amount of edema.

F. RN scan obtained on Day 13; left lateral view showing a poorly defined area of modestly increased activity in the central region. The vertex view localized this to the region of the left basal ganglia.

G. CT scan on the seventeenth day. The hemorrhage has become reduced in size and the edema is clearing. There is now only a 3-mm displacement of the septum lucidum and pineal to the right.

This sequence of CT scans reveals the virtual absence of edema about the acute hypertensive capsular hemorrhage during the first hours following onset. Very well developed edema was present on the seventh day, and this clearly contributed to the total mass effect, although the patient had begun to improve several days earlier. Evidently, the abruptness of the development of the mass was a greater factor than was its total size in producing the neurological deficits. The RN scan was normal before edema developed. Whether the conversion to a positive RN scan was directly related to the development of edema or to other factors is not clear from this case. The final CT scan clearly revealed the progressing absorption of the hematoma and of the edema in this case.

274

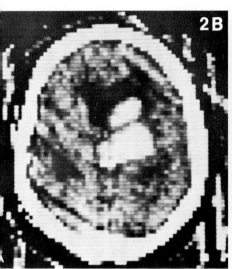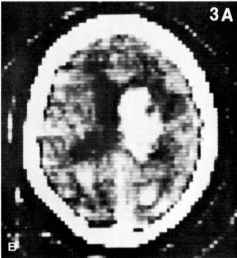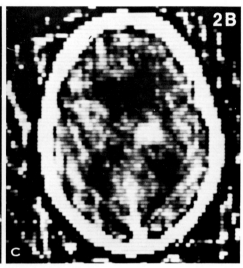

FIG 16.4. HYPERTENSIVE THALAMIC INTRACEREBRAL HEMORRHAGE.

Clinical Features. A 78 y.o. woman who was found comatose, with skew deviation of the eyes, a left hemisensory defect, and left hemiparesis. The CSF was bloody.

CT Scan. Abnormal (Fig. 16.4).

Angio. Right carotid study revealed marked ventricular dilatation and displacement of the internal cerebral vein to the left. A poorly localized, probably deeply situated mass was noted in the right cerebral hemisphere.

A and **B.** The high absorption region of hemorrhage is shown This appears to have originated in the thalamus, with extension into the internal capsule and caudate nucleus. The hemorrhage has extended into the frontal horn, the body of the right lateral ventricle, and the third ventricle. Some blood has accumulated in both occipital horns. Moderate enlargement of the lateral ventricles and minimal displacement of the midline to the left are also shown.

(Fig. 16.4A reprinted by permission from Radiology, 110: 109–123, 1974.)

This scan, obtained two days after onset, reveals a considerable volume of edema lateral to the hematoma.

C. CT scan obtained after an interval of seventeen days. The interval decrease in the size of the capsular hematoma and almost complete clearing of the intraventricular hematoma are revealed.

(Fig. 16.4, **B** and **C** reprinted by permission from Radiology, 112: 73–80, 1974.)

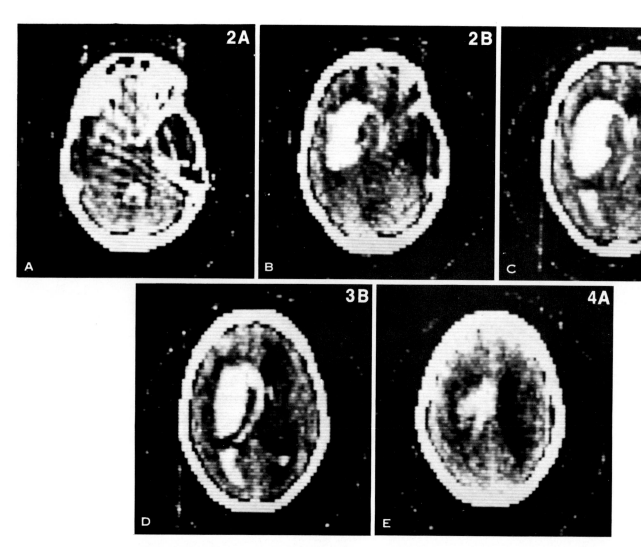

FIG. 16.5. MASSIVE HYPERTENSIVE HEMORRHAGE, CENTERED IN THE REGION OF THE PUTAMEN.

Clinical Features. A 56 y.o. female, known for several years to be mildly hypertensive but otherwise in good health, collapsed suddenly and became unresponsive.

Neurological Examination. Comatose, with minimally reactive pupils and slight deviation of the eyes to the left side. She soon developed bilateral decerebrate posturing and slightly disconjugate roving eye movements, with bilateral flaccidity and positive Babinski signs.

CT Scan. Abnormal (Fig. 16.5).

Angio. Transfemoral carotid and vertebral studies revealed major mass effect in the region of the left basal ganglia. The sylvian vessels were markedly compressed and displaced laterally.

A–E. Contiguous 13-mm scan sections from below superiorly.

A. This scan extends through the plane of the orbits and the fourth ventricle. The fourth ventricle is somewhat enlarged and is completely filled with a blood cast.

B–D. The massive hemorrhage is shown as a well-demarcated ovoid zone of increased absorption (23–44). There is a fairly broad zone of diminished absorption around the hematoma, best seen in **D**. Anteriorly, the hematoma has ruptured into the left frontal horn, which is largely filled with a blood clot that also extends through the body of the left lateral ventricle to fill the enlarged left occipital horn. Hematoma also extends in continuity through the left foramen of Munro to fill the third ventricle (**B**), and a small amount of blood has entered the right frontal and occipital horns. The lateral ventricles are markedly dilated due to obstruction of the third ventricle by a cast of blood. There is moderate midline dislocation to the right.

E. The superior extremity of the hematoma is shown, together with some of the blood in the body of the left lateral ventricle. The diminished absorption of edema is shown lateral to the hematoma.

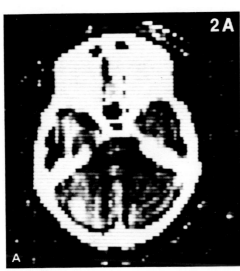

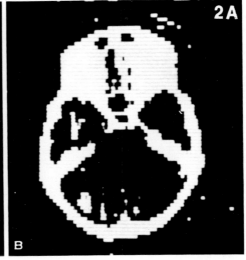

FIG. 16.6. HYPERTENSIVE CEREBELLAR HEMORRHAGE, SMALL.

Clinical Features. A 90 y.o. female with a long history of hypertension. Four months earlier, she had been admitted for treatment of atrial fibrillation. One day before the CT scan, she noted unsteadiness of gait, followed by vomiting and inability to walk.

Neurological Examination. Thick speech and clumsiness of the right hand. Blood pressure, 250/100.

CT Scan. Abnormal (Fig. 16.6).

A. L 22   W 20.   **B.** L 30   W M.

Two representations of the same scan, obtained from examination 1 day after the ictus. A 21 x 15 mm ovoid region of high absorption (28–37) is shown in the posterolateral portion of the left cerebellar hemisphere, extending internally from the surface. There is a narrow zone of surrounding decreased absorption consistent with minimal edema. No definite dislocation of the fourth ventricle is evident. A broad zone of low absorption extends between the anterior portions of the petrous bones, representing a machine artifact.

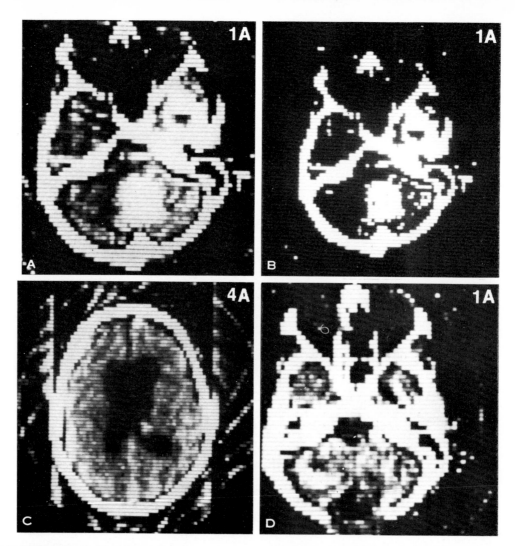

FIG. 16.7. HYPERTENSIVE CEREBELLAR HEMORRHAGE, MASSIVE.

Clinical Features. A 51 y.o. man with known hypertension for 10 years, untreated for the past 5 years. Sudden onset of vomiting 24 hours before admission.

Neurological Examination. Agitated and confused, with markedly dysarthric speech. Marked nystagmus on lateral gaze and vertical nystagmus on upward gaze. No paresis of extremities or any deficit on sensory examination. Wide-based lurching gait. Blood pressure, 240/130. A clinical diagnosis of hypertensive cerebellar hemorrhage was made, but there was also consideration of infarction and posterior fossa subdural hematoma.

CT Scan. Abnormal (Fig. 16.7, A–C).

Operation. (Dr. Edward Tarlov.) Posterior fossa craniotomy and laminectomy of C1, with removal of a large cerebellar hematoma under pressure. Parts of the hematoma were liquid fresh hemorrhage. Other portions were solid and partly organized. The hematoma had ruptured into the fourth ventricle. The hematoma lay in the medial portion of the right cerebellar hemisphere and in the vermis. After the operation, the patient's condition deteriorated considerably compared with the preoperative status. The pupils were small and reacted poorly to light. There were no extraocular muscle movements on passive head rotation, and movement of the extremities was minimal. Ventricular tap revealed a pressure of 510 mm.

CT Scan. Emergency postoperative study (Fig. 16.7 D).

Operation. Lateral ventricular drainage was instituted, with some initial improvement in neurological status. A ventriculoperitoneal shunt was performed several days later, but a few days after this he again became unresponsive and died.

A and **B.** Preoperative CT scan, obtained the day after the ictus.
A. L 16   W 20.   **B.** L 28   W M.
Two displays of the same scan section, which extends through the orbits, upper clivus, and torcula. A well-demarcated rounded area of high absorption (18–45) is shown in the central portion of the posterior fossa and extending into the right cerebellar hemisphere. The hematoma extends anteriorly beyond the normal position of the fourth ventricle, which is not identified. Surrounding the left half of the hematoma is a broad zone of diminished absorption (4–10), consistent with marked edema. There is also a generalized decrease in absorption throughout the remainder of the left half of the posterior fossa, suggesting more diffuse edema and/or ischemia. The hematoma measured approximately 4 cm in diameter and appears roughly centered in the region of the dentate nucleus. The posterior fossa sections were 8 mm in thickness.

C. A 13-mm scan section through the lateral ventricles, showing marked obstructive hydrocephalus.

D. First postoperative scan. This shows a cavity with CSF absorption values in the region of the vermis and the absence of residual or recurrent cerebellar hematoma. The grey matter of the left cerebellar hemisphere appears displaced anteriorly and shows higher than normal absorption values (possibly due to focal hemorrhagic changes). Supratentorial scans (not illustrated) revealed hematoma in the posterior third ventricle, obstructing the rostrad ventricular system, with marked dilatation. The third CT scan (also not illustrated) demonstrated reduced ventricular size following shunting, but the posterior third ventricular hematoma was still visible. This study also showed areas of infarction in both cerebral hemispheres.

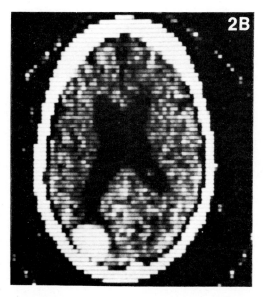

FIG. 16.8. OCCIPITAL LOBE HEMORRHAGE, DURING COUMADIN THERAPY.

Clinical Features. A 77 y.o. nonhypertensive male who was on Coumadin therapy for thrombophlebitis and pulmonary embolism. One day before admission, he casually noted loss of vision in the right visual fields. He had a grand mal seizure on the day of admission.

Neurological Examination. Right homonymous hemianopsia, dyslexia, and amnestic aphasia. Provisional clinical diagnosis: left posterior cerebral artery occlusion secondary to embolus; neoplasm to be ruled out.

Skull Examination. Normal, with midline pineal.

RN Scan. Abnormal, with increased activity on the left side in the posterior view and, questionably, also in the left lateral view (third hospital day).

CT Scan. Abnormal (Fig. 16.8).

Angio. Left carotid and vertebrobasilar studies on the second hospital day showed very slight medial displacement of the calcarine and parieto-occipital branches of the left posterior cerebral artery, with no pathological vessels. The left lateral ventricle was slightly enlarged, but no displacement of midline vessels was evident.

CT scan at the level of the lateral ventricles clearly reveals a smoothly rounded volume of increased absorption (25–42) within the left occipital lobe, immediately posterior to the occipital horn. The lateral ventricles are modestly increased in size. Minor widening of sulci is shown in both frontal lobes.

The pathology and its extent are very clearly revealed by the CT scan, whereas the angiographic studies were initially interpreted as normal.

(Reprinted by permission from Radiology, 112: 73–80, 1974.)

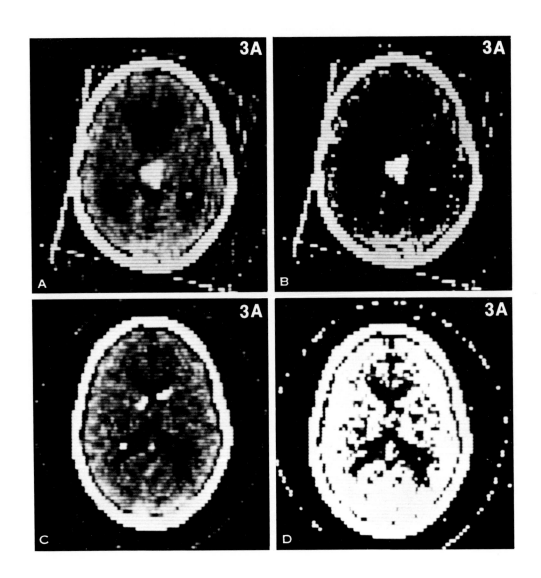

FIG. 16.9. HEMATOMA OF THIRD VENTRICLE, IDIOPATHIC.

Clinical Features. A 62 y.o. male admitted in stupor after an attack of vomiting and severe headache the previous evening. He had a history of frequent headaches for the previous 5 years, awakening him in the morning for the previous 2 years.

Neurological Examination. Stuporous; rousable by shout and pinch to follow simple commands. Very slow verbal and motor responses. Normal optic discs and pupils. Bilateral sixth nerve pareses and bilateral Babinski responses. Blood pressure, 230/120. He became progressively less responsive, and a lumbar puncture revealed an opening pressure of 190 mm and grossly bloody spinal fluid.

Angio. Due to difficulties with femoral catheterization, an emergency left brachial angiogram was performed. This was suboptimal in technical quality and no clear diagnosis was obtained. Following treatment with steroids and antihypertensive medications, he was still obtunded on the following day and a CT scan was then obtained.

CT Scan. Abnormal (Fig. 16.9, **A** and **B**).

Angio. The day after CT scan, transfemoral left carotid and vertebral studies provided a diagnosis of noncommunicating obstructive hydrocephalus and indicated a probable deep left avascular mass in the region of the basal ganglia, particularly the thalamus.

Operation. (Dr. Edward Tarlov.) Ventriculoatrial shunt, with bilateral ventricular tubes. Following this, there was rapid improvement in the level of consciousness and he became fully alert, ambulatory, with a normal mental status and essentially normal neurological findings.

CT Scan. This showed improvement (Fig. 16.9, **C** and **D**).

A. L 18   W 20.   **B.** L 24   W M.
Initial CT scan, showing marked dilatation of the lateral ventricles. The third ventricle appears markedly widened by a high absorption mass (24–42) consistent with blood clot. Immediately adjacent to the high density area on the left side is a narrow band of diminished absorption, approximately 6 mm in width, measuring 12–17. Immediately to the right of the posterior portion of the high density area is a small zone of diminished absorption measuring 16–24 on this section and 11–17 on the section immediately below.

These findings suggested the diagnosis of hemorrhage into a neoplasm within the third ventricle, probably an ependymoma.

C. L 18   W 20.
D. L 14   W M.

CT scans following shunting of both lateral ventricles (the ends of the dense shunt tubes are shown in **C**), obtained 15 days after the scan shown in **A** and **B**. The lateral ventricles are now virtually normal in size. The dense lesion in the third ventricular area has become much smaller and has considerably decreased in absorption (13–21). However, the lesion has not cleared completely and the ventricle still appears somewhat widened (**D**). The zones of decreased absorption on either side are no longer visible.

These findings indicated marked resorption of blood clot. It was uncertain whether the residual third ventricular density represented the residue of an absorbing clot or a neoplasm, and a further CT scan was planned to resolve the question. The third CT scan was obtained 4½ months later. This showed extremely small lateral ventricles (continuing effectiveness of shunt) and an entirely normal appearance of the third ventricle, in which there was no evidence of residual abnormal material. The shunt was therefore ligated.

Possible etiologies for this unusual form of hemorrhage include a subependymal origin of hypertensive hemorrhage and a subependymal cryptic vascular malformation (39).

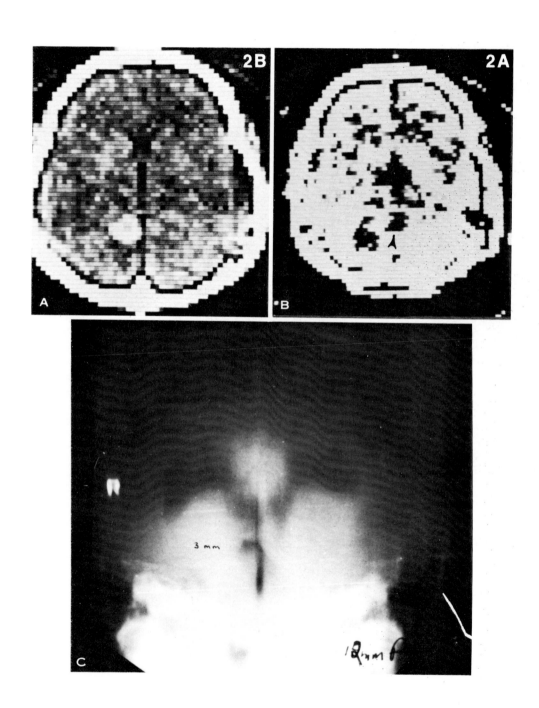

FIG. 16.10. HEMATOMA, SMALL CEREBELLAR, IDIOPATHIC.

Clinical Features. A 37 y.o. nonhypertensive physician who experienced the sudden onset of vomiting and staggering 2 days before the CT scan. He gave a history of slight slurring of speech for some time before the ictus.

Neurological Examination. Ataxia of the left extremities, with a tendency to fall to the left. A diagnosis of acute labyrinthitis was suggested.

Skull Examination. Normal.

CT Scan. Abnormal (Fig. 16.10, **A** and **B**).

Angio. Transfemoral left vertebral study revealed no evidence of a posterior fossa mass, although there was a suggestion of herniation of the left cerebellar tonsil. No pathological vessels were identified, even on review.

Operation. (Dr. William H. Sweet.) Occipital craniectomy with removal of old, dark red, largely clotted blood from a small cavity in the medial portion of the left cerebellar hemisphere and adjacent vermis. The volume of the clot was 5 ml; 1 ml liquid and the remainder semisolid. Careful examination of the walls of the cavity revealed no tumor or arteriovenous malformation.

Histology. Organizing blood clot. Material from the walls of the cavity revealed gliosis only. Tissue culture grew no tumor cells.

A. W 20. The section passes through the level of the frontal horns anteriorly and just above the central portion of the fourth ventricle posteriorly. A 2-cm diameter, quite rounded area of high absorption, indicative of hematoma, is shown extending from the midline to the left into the cerebellar hemisphere. A small zone of slightly less elevated absorption is shown centrally in the hematoma. The ventricular system was not dilated.

B. W M. Section immediately below that in **A**. This section extends through a small zone of edema just below the hematoma. This is shown as a low absorption black area slightly to the left of the midline. Just anterior and to the right of this is the black area representing CSF in the fourth ventricle. The appearance here indicates minor indentation of the left side of the fourth ventricle, which is displaced slightly anteriorly and to the right (*arrowhead*).

C. PEG. Sagittal projection in the erect position, hypocycloidal tomographic section. Although a firm CT scan diagnosis of intracerebellar hematoma had been given, there was considerable skepticism on the part of our colleagues, since this was the first scan of a hematoma obtained at the MGH. This additional examination was therefore obtained to confirm the presence of a mass. The fourth ventricle is shown slightly indented on the left side and displaced 3 mm to the right. Lateral projections showed slight anterior displacement of the ventricle.

(Fig. 16.10, **A** and **B** reprinted by permission from Radiology, 110: 109–123, 1974.)

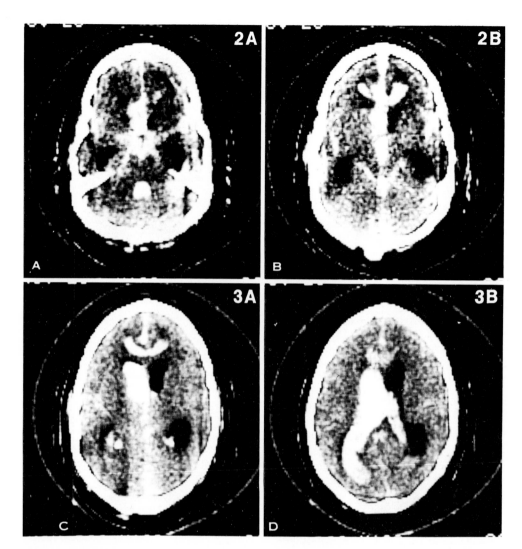

FIG. 16.11. MASSIVE SUBARACHNOID AND INTRAVENTRICULAR HEMORRHAGE.

Clinical Features. A 59 y.o. male who had undergone laryngectomy and right radical neck dissection for carcinoma of the larynx several years earlier. Three years before the present admission, the patient suffered a head injury, with later development of CSF rhinorrhea associated with probable cribriform plate fracture. The rhinorrhea ceased spontaneously, but recurred 6 weeks before the present admission. One day before CT scan, the patient underwent an operative closure of the CSF leak with a septal flap. Following this, the patient remained unresponsive in the recovery room, with bilateral Babinski and withdrawal responses and nonreactive pupils.

CT Scan. Abnormal (Fig. 16.11).

Rapid deterioration was followed by death on the day after CT scan.

Autopsy. A hemorrhage in the median inferior frontal region had dissected upwards through the frontal lobes to destroy the anterior portion of the corpus callosum, with the production of a large amount of blood in the ventricular system and subarachnoid spaces. Dura was intact over the nasal operative site. Dissection of the circle of Willis revealed no aneurysm, but the hemorrhage was thought to have originated from a small aneurysm of the anterior communicating artery.

A–D. Contiguous 13-mm sections from below superiorly. 160 x 160 matrix system.

A. Casts of blood fill the suprasellar and interpeduncular cisterns, and a blood clot is shown extending laterally into the sylvian cisterns and posteriorly into the crural and ambient cisterns. The fourth ventricle is somewhat enlarged and filled with a blood clot. In the midline subfrontal and inferior frontal region, a very dense collection of blood is shown extending anteriorly from the suprasellar region.

B. Blood is shown filling a considerably enlarged third ventricle and portions of the lower frontal horns. Blood is present bilaterally in the frontal lobes just anterior to the frontal horns. Between the frontal horns, blood is shown in the region of a widened interfrontal segment of the longitudinal fissure and in the region of the genu of the corpus callosum. Posteriorly, blood is shown in the posterior portions of the ambient cisterns and in the quadrigeminal cistern. More blood is shown in the sylvian cisterns. The markedly dilated temporal horns do not contain appreciable blood.

C and D. A blood cast of the considerably dilated left lateral ventricle is shown. There is less blood in the right lateral ventricle. A small amount of blood is visible in the left sylvian fissure. An arcuate zone of hemorrhage extends across the midline immediately anterior to the frontal horns, in the region of destruction of the corpus callosum noted at autopsy. The lower portion of this bifrontal collection of blood is shown in **B,** where it merges with blood in the frontal horns.

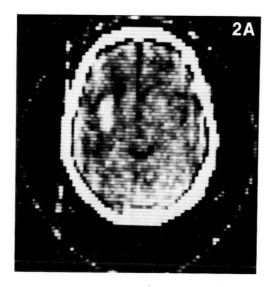

2A

FIG. 16.12. HYPERTENSIVE PUTAMINAL HEMORRHAGE.

Clinical Features. A 65 y.o. hypertensive man who had had the sudden onset of right hemiplegia, right hemisensory loss, and motor aphasia 11 days before CT scan. On clinical grounds, he was thought to have suffered a lacunar type of infarct.

CT scan, 11 days after onset. L 18   W 20.
An ovoid region of increased absorption (18–32) surrounded by an irregular zone of decreased absorption (4–14) provided the diagnosis of a 4 x 1.5 cm hemorrhage in the putamen, with surrounding edema. There was compression of the adjacent portions of the left lateral ventricle and slight displacement of the septum lucidum to the right of the midline.

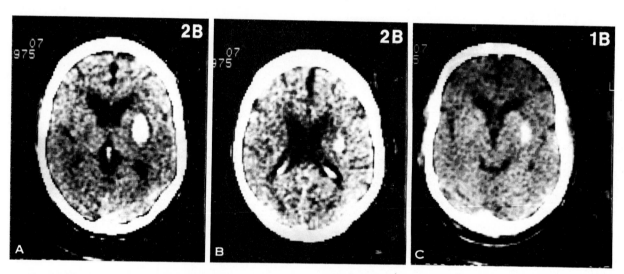

FIG. 16.13. HYPERTENSIVE PUTAMINAL HEMORRHAGE.

Clinical Features. A 66 y.o. hypertensive male who had a sudden onset of left hemiparesis.

CT scan. 160 x 160 matrix system.

A. An ovoid hematoma was demonstrated in the right putamen surrounded by a narrow zone of diminished absorption, indicating minor associated edema. The lateral ventricles and subarachnoid spaces were modestly enlarged. There was slight mass effect upon the right frontal horn and minimal midline dislocation to the left.

B. Scan section immediately above that in **A,** showing the upper pole of the very localized hematoma and a slight, localized pressure effect upon the lateral aspect of the right lateral ventricle.

C. Scan section immediately below that in **A,** showing the inferior pole of the hematoma and its relationship to the sylvian cistern laterally and the frontal horn and third ventricle medially.

CHAPTER 17

Extracerebral Hematomas

EXTRADURAL HEMATOMAS

Extradural hematomas are readily recognized by their uniformly high absorption, which generally lies in the range between the low 20's and the 40's. The configuration is characteristically lenticular, with a more or less prominently convex inner contour, sharply demarcated from underlying brain. The cases studied have ranged in duration from less than 24 hours to 2 weeks without apparent differences in appearance. Provided that scans of reasonable technical quality are obtained, diagnosis is sufficiently precise as to obviate the need for angiography before surgery. Such interesting features as extravasation from meningeal vessels and traumatic arteriovenous communications with superficial cerebral and/or diploic veins cannot, of course, be visualized without angiography. Also, as with many other posttraumatic conditions, difficulty in preventing patient movement short of extremely heavy sedation, general anesthesia, or brief paralysis with assisted respiration may make expeditious angiography more desirable. It is perhaps in the investigation of cerebral trauma, in which CT scanning has so much to offer and where patient motion is so likely to be a problem, that the greatest pressures will arise for the development of new equipment that will permit considerably reduced scan times.

If scan quality is satisfactory, very important information can be obtained by this method that is difficult or impossible to obtain by angiography. The differentiation of cerebral edema, cerebral contusion, and cerebral hemorrhage, alone or in combination with extracerebral collections, is readily made on the basis of CT scans. In addition, depression of bone fragments and the presence of denser foreign bodies can be identified and localized more accurately than by plain film cranial examination. It is even possible to identify some linear fractures by displaying the scan at high M levels, although this should not lead to the omission of plain film examination.

SUBDURAL HEMATOMAS AND HYGROMAS

In an early report, Ambrose (2) stated that, contrary to his expectation, the actual subdural hematoma was identified in only one of seven cases examined. This was because the hematoma fluid had an average density similar to that of the underlying brain. In each of the cases, the presence of a mass was revealed by displacement of the ventricular system or pineal. In the single case in which the subdural hematoma was identified directly, the hematoma was considerably denser than was the brain, and a typical superficial position and configuration were visible. In a later report by Paxton and Ambrose (51), thirty-five cases of subdural hematoma were diagnosed and confirmed at surgery. In each case, the EMI scan was positive. Twenty-one of the cases had high absorption values, 10 cases had absorption values lower than normal brain and were seen as low density peripheral bands, with midline displacement, and, in four cases, the scan did not reveal a clear-cut differential absorption compared with underlying brain, but experience permitted the correct CT diagnosis.

Our experience is consonant with the experience of these and other investigators. Acute subdural hematomas are found to have the high absorption associated with acute hematomas in general. Such an appearance is generally evident for 1–2 weeks or longer. The hematoma is readily differentiated from the underlying brain and shows a sharp demarcation from the brain, which generally maintains a convex or flattened contour. With further aging of the hematoma, breakdown and removal of hemoglobin and the entry of fluid by osmosis results in a gradual decrease in absorption values of the hematoma until the values closely resemble those of the underlying brain and differentiation becomes difficult. Such hematomas are generally of considerable size, and the obvious displacement of brain structures permits identification of a large mass lesion. Diligent analysis of the scans, provided that they are of satisfactory quality, generally permits the identification of inward deflection of the cerebral cortex in the marginal regions of the hematoma, and the presence of arching bands of slightly increased and slightly decreased absorption relative to brain can generally be identified (as in Fig. 17.4).

At the other end of the spectrum of subdural collections, subdural hygromas are very readily differentiated, since they have the very low absorption characteristics of CSF. Thin serosanguinous collections are also easily recognized (Figs. 17.5, 17.6 **F and G,** and 19.6). Some of these may show a quite striking band-like juxtaposition of regions with CSF absorption, or slightly higher, and zones of moderate density that stand out clearly (Fig. 17.5).

Interesting gravitational effects have been noted in occasional cases of chronic subdural hematoma (Figs. 17.6 and 17.10). In these cases, prolonged recumbency has allowed the denser constituents of the subdural collection to settle inferiorly, leaving a thinner supernatant fluid collection of much lesser absorption superiorly. This separation of the collection into high and low absorption fractions permits more ready identification of the extracerebral collection than if the elements are mixed. In the latter case, the admixture results in an absorption less readily differentiated from that of the underlying brain (Fig. 17.10). Intravenous injection of contrast medium may have a role in providing additional information by enhancement of thick subdural membranes in selected cases.

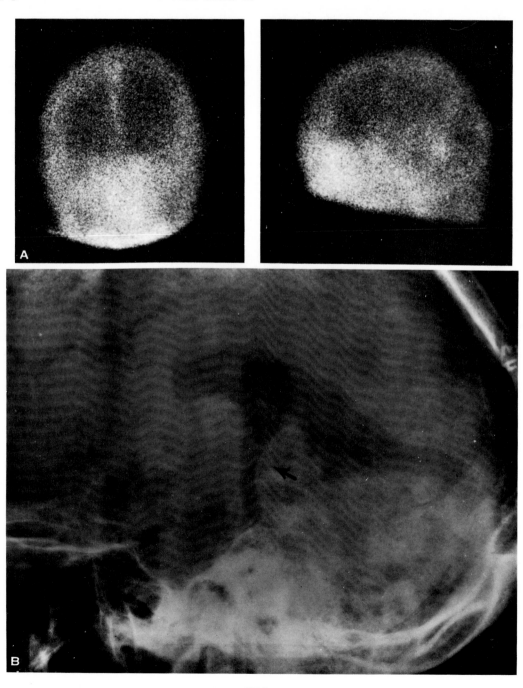

288

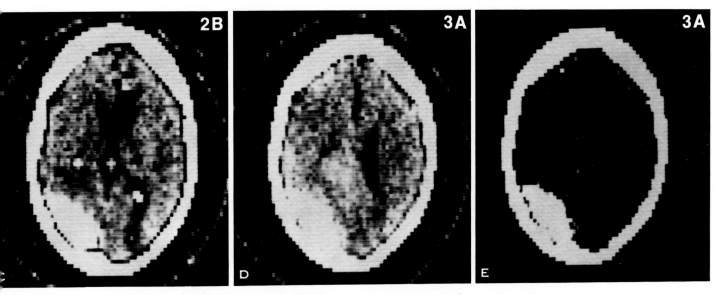

FIG. 17.1. EXTRADURAL HEMATOMA; VERY LARGE COLLECTION INVOLVING BOTH THE INFRATENTORIAL AND SUPRATENTORIAL COMPARTMENTS, AND ASSOCIATED WITH CONTUSION.

Clinical Features. A 43 y.o. chronic alcoholic male found unconscious on the street. Large hematoma of the left temporal scalp and positive Battle's sign at the left mastoid. Lethargic but arousable. No obvious visual, motor, or sensory findings. Over several days, alertness and orientation increased and there were still no focal signs. Six days after admission, there were left cerebellar signs and right homonymous hemianopsia. Lumbar puncture showed xanthochromic fluid at an opening pressure of 330 mm.

Skull Examination. Left basal skull fracture.

RN Scan. Fourth hospital day; positive (Fig. 17.1A).

Angio. Transfemoral bilateral carotid and vertebral studies on the sixth hospital day revealed a diffuse left parieto-occipital mass and was suggestive of a left cerebellar mass. Oblique projections were not obtained and an extracerebral collection was not identified.

PEG. A large left posterior fossa mass and a posterior left supratentorial mass were noted. Both appeared to be intraaxial, and metastatic malignancy was suggested (Fig. 17.1B).

CT Scan. This study was made for clarification, which was obtained (Fig. 17.1, C–E).

Operation. (Dr. Michael Scott.) The next day (14th hospital day), a left parieto-occipital craniectomy was followed by removal of a huge left parieto-occipital and left posterior fossa solid epidural clot, 4 cm in maximum thickness, extending inferiorly to the foramen magnum.

A. Tcp scan; frontal and left lateral views. A large area of rather patchy increase in uptake is present superficially in the posterior areas above and below the tentorium. This was interpreted as possibly due to scalp and bone trauma, "but it is not possible to exclude a small left sided subdural collection."

B. PEG; brow-down lateral projection. The posterior portion of the left lateral ventricle is dislocated anteriorly, and there is a local abrupt indentation of the region of junction of the left atrium and posterior portion of the temporal horn (arrow). A major mass effect was also demonstrated in the area of the left cerebellar hemisphere.

C–E. CT scan obtained after angiography and PEG. A large and well-demarcated area of high absorption (25–50) was demonstrated in the temporo-occipital and inferior parietal regions. This extended to occupy the left side of the posterior fossa down to the level of the foramen magnum. The region of high density had a lenticular shape throughout and its maximum thickness was in the posterior fossa. Note the apparent separation of the hematoma from the inner table of the skull by the "undershoot" artifact occurring at the interface between dense bone and soft tissue.

C. The frontal horns and third ventricle are moderately enlarged. The pineal is in the midline, but the calcified glomus of the left trigone is displaced markedly anteriorly and the posterior portions of the left lateral ventricle are grossly compressed. A lower section (not shown) revealed a disproportionately and markedly enlarged left temporal horn (confirmed on postoperative scan), probably the result of temporal lobe atrophy after previous injury. Although part of the generalized ventricular enlargement is probably due to the posterior fossa mass effect, it is likely that the patient had had preexisting ventricular and subarachnoid space enlargement from previous episodes of trauma. (Reprinted by permission from Radiology, 110: 109–123, 1974.)

D. Scan section immediately above that in **C**. The large extradural hematoma is evident as a lenticular zone of high absorption posteriorly. Compression of the left lateral ventricle is shown to be marked. Deep to the hematoma and adjacent to the lateral ventricles is a diffuse region of modestly increased absorption, consistent with cerebral contusion. There is some widening of the interfrontal portion of the longitudinal fissure.

E. W M. This control setting clearly reveals the high absorption and lenticular configuration of the hematoma.

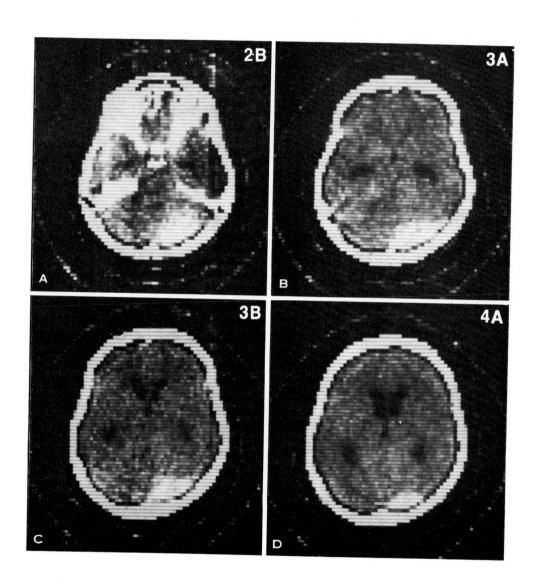

FIG. 17.2. EXTRADURAL HEMATOMA.

Clinical Features. An 18 y.o. girl who fell approximately 15 ft. On admission in the early hours of the morning, she was unresponsive to voice but moved all extremities appropriately and with excellent strength in response to pain. Pupils 2 mm in size and equal. Full range of ocular motion. Symmetrical deep tendon reflexes and negative Babinski signs. She was given steroids and observed closely. One and a half hours later, she was noted not to be moving spontaneously and shortly after was unresponsive to deep pain. Pupils had increased in size to 5 mm.

Skull Examination. Normal.

CT Scan. Emergency CT scan was abnormal (Fig. 17.2). She was taken directly to the operating room without further radiological studies.

Operation. (Dr. Robert Crowell.) Right posterior fossa craniectomy, with evacuation of a large epidural hematoma that extended to but not beyond the midline. During operation a fracture of the right occipital bone was noted. This had lacerated the lateral sinus and extended to the foramen magnum and jugular foramen.

A.–D. L 17   W 30.

Consecutive 8-mm sections, except **D**, which is a 13-mm section immediately above **C**.

The maximum thickness (20–25 mm) of the extradural hematoma is in the posterior fossa (**A**). The characteristic lenticular shape is visible at all levels. The fourth ventricle is inconspicuous but is probably visible as a low absorption area slightly displaced to the left and with a compressed appearance (**A**). The anterior margin of the extradural hematoma is not very clearly defined in **A**, suggesting the presence of frank contusion with small hemorrhages in the markedly compressed right cerebellar hemisphere. The hematoma extends from the midline almost to the right CP angle. Higher sections show gradually decreasing dimensions of the hematoma, with sharp demarcation from the underlying brain. The hematoma extends above the tentorium. There is slight but definite enlargement of the lateral and third ventricles, with no visualization of the cisterns of the posterior fossa or supratentorial region. No cerebral sulci were visible. These findings are indicative of early obstructive hydrocephalus associated with the very large hematoma. Hematoma absorption values ranged from 22–30 to 41–49 on the various sections. Note the undershoot artifact, which appears to separate the hematoma from the inner table of the skull.

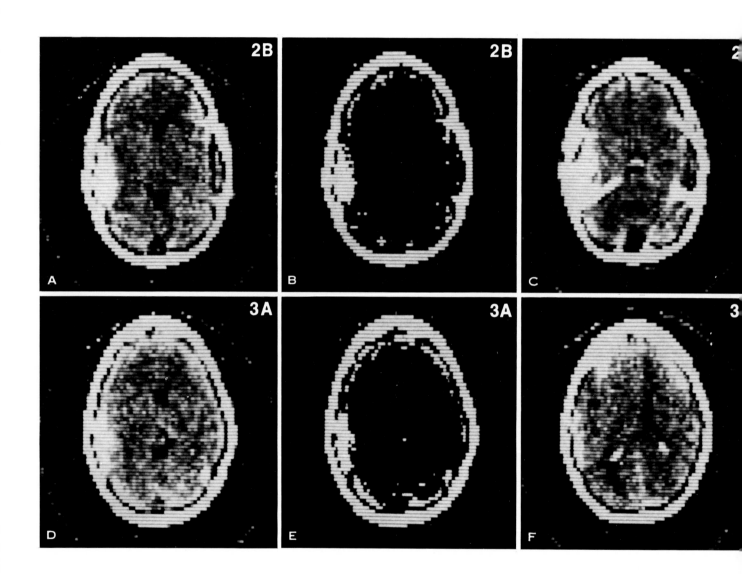

FIG. 17.3. EPIDURAL HEMATOMA.

Clinical Features. A 31 y.o. woman who was involved in an automobile accident 2 weeks earlier, hitting the left side of her head, without loss of consciousness. Malaise and generalized headache developed and she remained under observation in an outlying hospital for 1 week. Plain film skull examination, EEG, and radionuclide brain scan were said to be normal. She was admitted to the MGH for persistent, predominantly left-sided headache and difficulty in finding words and reading.

Neurological Examination. Alert and oriented, but with dysnomia and paraphasic errors on reading. Bilateral papilledema.

EEG. Repeat examination was normal.

RN Scan. Not repeated before operation.

CT Scan. Abnormal (Fig. 17.3).

Angio. Transfemoral bilateral carotid studies revealed an 8-mm thick extracerebral collection over the lateral aspect of the left temporal lobe "perhaps extending beneath the temporal lobe to some extent." A marked localized mass effect was noted in the posterior temporal region, with marked crowding and anterosuperior displacement of sylvian branches. This suggested an intracerebral hematoma or an epidural collection. The pericallosal artery and internal cerebral vein were displaced 8–9 mm to the right of the midline.

Operation. (Dr. Paul H. Chapman.) Left temporal craniotomy and evacuation of epidural hematoma. Large "current-jelly clot," extending from the superior aspect of the temporal lobe posteriorly to about 2 cm posterior to the external auditory meatus and anteriorly to the anterior wall of the middle fossa. The clot extended below the temporal lobe. Vascular granulating membrane was found on the external surface of the dura.

Histology. Dark red nonlaminated blood clot.

A. L 16   W 20.

This scan extends through the plane of the frontal horns and quadrigeminal cistern. The high absorption area (24–42) of the extradural hematoma is shown in the left temporal region. It is well demarcated from the indented subjacent brain. There is a 6–9 mm displacement of midline structures to the right. There is no associated intracerebral hematoma. A small zone of slightly diminished absorption is evident immediately deep to the collection, indicating the presence of edema, which is not very marked.

B. L 26   W M.

Same scan section as in **A.** At these settings, the extradural hematoma and some portions of the cerebral cortex remain white.

C. L 17   W 20.

The high absorption of the hematoma is shown extending into the inferior temporal region and the subjacent scan section revealed extension over the floor of the middle fossa.

D. L 16   W 20.

Scan section immediately above that in **A.** The hematoma is thinner at this level, which more clearly shows displacement of the frontal horns and pineal to the right.

E. L 26   W M.

Same scan section as in **D,** showing both the absorption region representing the hematoma and portions of the cerebral cortex. The pineal is also clearly discriminated.

F. L 16   W 20.

Scan section immediately above that in **E,** close to the superior extremity of the extradural hematoma. Compression of the left lateral ventricle and minor posteromedial displacement of the calcified left choroid plexus glomus are visible. This scan illustrates the ease with which a relatively thin extradural hematoma (9 mm in thickness) could be overlooked, particularly if the scan were suboptimal due to motion.

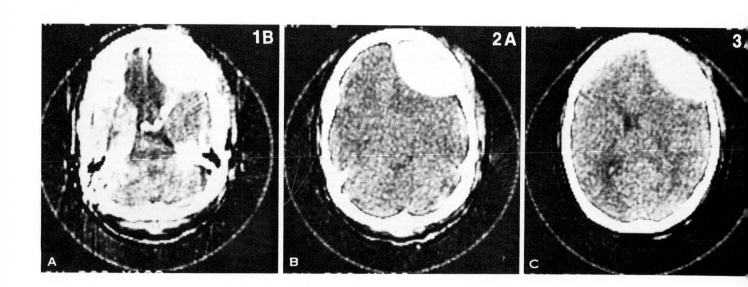

FIG. 17.3(1). EPIDURAL HEMATOMA.
Clinical Features. A 28 y.o. man, alledgedly hit several times about the head with a club without loss of consciousness. On admission to another hospital shortly after, he was found to have a 3-cm right frontal laceration. He was somewhat confused and had nausea and vomiting. The left pupil measured 4.5 mm and the right pupil measured 4 mm, both briskly reactive. Neurological examination was otherwise normal. The following day, a left arm drift was noted. This resolved on steroid therapy and his mental status became normal. He gave a history of a bleeding diathesis. A brother and a cousin were also reported to have bleeding dyscrasias (Factor XI deficiency).

Neurological Examination. Upon hospital transfer, he was complaining of some right-sided headache. Apart from the anisocoria noted above and a left-sided nystagmus to left lateral gaze, neurological examination was normal.

Skull Examination. Normal.

CT Scan. Abnormal (Fig. 17.3(1)), two days after injury.

Operation. (Dr. James Wepsic.) Right frontal craniotomy, with evacuation of a large right frontal epidural hematoma.

A–C. 160 x 160 matrix system.

The typical biconvex high-absorption appearance of a large epidural hematoma is shown in the right frontal region, extending from the orbital roof superiorly and from the anterior falx laterally. Marked displacement of the frontal horns to the left is shown (**C**). That the narrow, low-absorption zone just beneath the inner table is due to computer undershoot artifact and not subarachnoid space is illustrated by its persistence external to the hematoma in **B**.

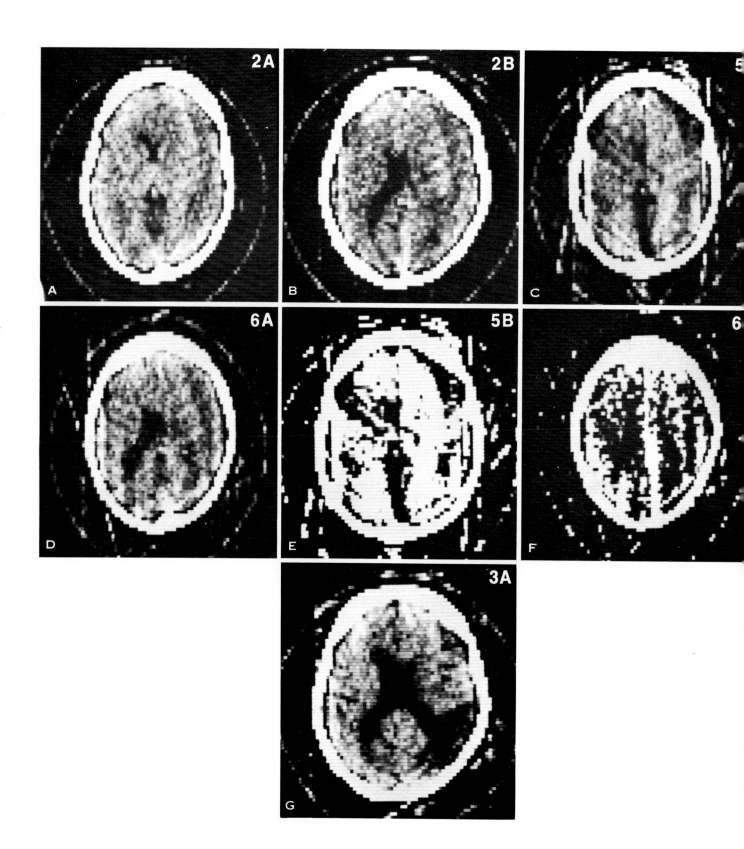

FIG. 17.4. BILATERAL SUBDURAL HEMATOMAS, VERY CHRONIC.

Clinical Features. An 87 y.o. physician with a 3 month history of a syndrome suggesting right parieto-occipital ischemia. The neurological deficits resolved. One week before the scan, he became intermittently lethargic, walked unsteadily, and experienced return of left homonymous hemianopsia. He had received Coumadin treatment.

Neurological Examination. Mildly lethargic, unconcerned; dense left homonymous hemianopsia, extinction of double simultaneous stimulation on the left side. No motor or reflex changes. The question of subdural hematoma was raised.

CT Scan. Abnormal (Fig. 17.4).

RN Scan. Because of difficulties with interpretation of the CT scan (31st clinical scan obtained at the MGH), an RN scan was suggested and this showed the typical findings of a large right and a small left subdural hematoma. There was quite high activity in a lenticular superficial configuration.

Operation. (Dr. Robert G. Ojemann) Evacuation of very large right and small left, typical, very chronic subdural hematomas with well-developed membranes.

A–F. Initial CT scans, plain (**A** and **B**) and after contrast enhancement with 40 ml of Hypaque 60 intravenously (**C–F**). A major mass effect extending from the right frontal to the right parietotemporal regions was immediately recognized. Poorly defined zones of somewhat increased absorption (18–27) and somewhat decreased absorption (10–16) were recognized in the right supratentorial regions, but the curved striated appearance of these abnormal regions was not appreciated at the time, and first consideration was given to a widespread malignant tumor of the right cerebral hemisphere. The scan was repeated after contrast enhancement, and this indicated that there had been a slight increase in absorption of a band lying just beneath the inner table (**D**), without evidence of increased absorption in more central regions. It was thought that the band of increased absorption represented the cerebral cortex. In fact, it probably represented an increase in absorption in the capsule of the chronic subdural hematoma. The appearance of inward displacement of both frontal lobes from the inner table, shown in **C**, was not appreciated at the original interpretation. Reanalysis with different control settings (**E**, L 13   W M; **F**, L 19   W M) more clearly revealed the bilateral inward deflection of the frontal lobe cortex near the inferior portion of each subdural hematoma (**E**) and the striated pattern of lower and higher absorption regions (**F**).

G. Repeat scan, several weeks after evacuation of the subdural hematomas. The large area of markedly reduced absorption (1–12) in the posterior portion of the right cerebrum, merging with the atrium, represents the porencephalic residue of a very old infarction in the territory of the middle cerebral artery. This cavity was so compressed by the subdural hematoma that it was not recognizable on the initial scan.

While inexperience with the method was primarily responsible for the incorrect diagnosis in this case, it is clear that some chronic subdural hematomas, particularly those that are smaller than in this case, may not be correctly diagnosed on CT scans unless they are of the highest technical quality and unless considerable care is taken in analysis.

(Fig. 17.4, **A**, **C**, and **E**) reprinted by permission from Radiology, 110: 109–123, 1974.)

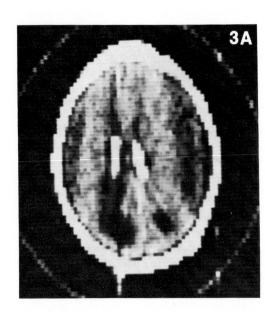

FIG. 17.5 SUBDURAL HEMATOMA, BILATERAL SERO-SANGUINOUS COLLECTIONS.

Clinical Features. A 15 y.o. boy in whom a small hypothalamic glioma had been diagnosed several years earlier and treated with ventriculoatrial shunting and radiation. His condition had been stable for a long time, but 1 month before CT scanning he deteriorated. Angiography at that time demonstrated severe dilatation of the lateral ventricles, and he underwent shunt revision. Following this there was slow resolution of obtundation and persistent headaches.

CT Scan. Initial CT scan was abnormal (Fig. 17.5). Following evacuation of the bilateral subdural hematomas (Dr. Robert G. Ojemann), a second CT scan revealed negligible residues of the hematomas, but revealed massive lateral ventricular enlargement. Following a further shunt revision, a third CT scan revealed a marked decrease in lateral ventricular size and minor hematoma recurrence on the right side.

Initial CT scan. The central high absorption bands represent the red rubber catheters in the lateral ventricles. The lateral ventricles are well decompressed, although there is considerable residual enlargement of the occipital horns. There is striking midline dislocation to the left and bilateral subdural collections of low absorption are shown, the right being much larger than the left. Within the low absorption collections are denser arching bands. Absorption of the collections ranged between 8 and 15 units. At operation, most of the hematoma contents represented markedly xanthochromic (8/10) fluid. The final CT scan, which was of better quality than the earlier scans, revealed evidence of a mass in the region of the anterior portion of the third ventricle, representing the 2–3 cm astrocytoma Grade III found at autopsy shortly afterwards.

This case illustrates well the value of sequential CT scans in identifying complications arising after treatment.

(Reprinted by permission from Radiology, 110: 109–123, 1974.)

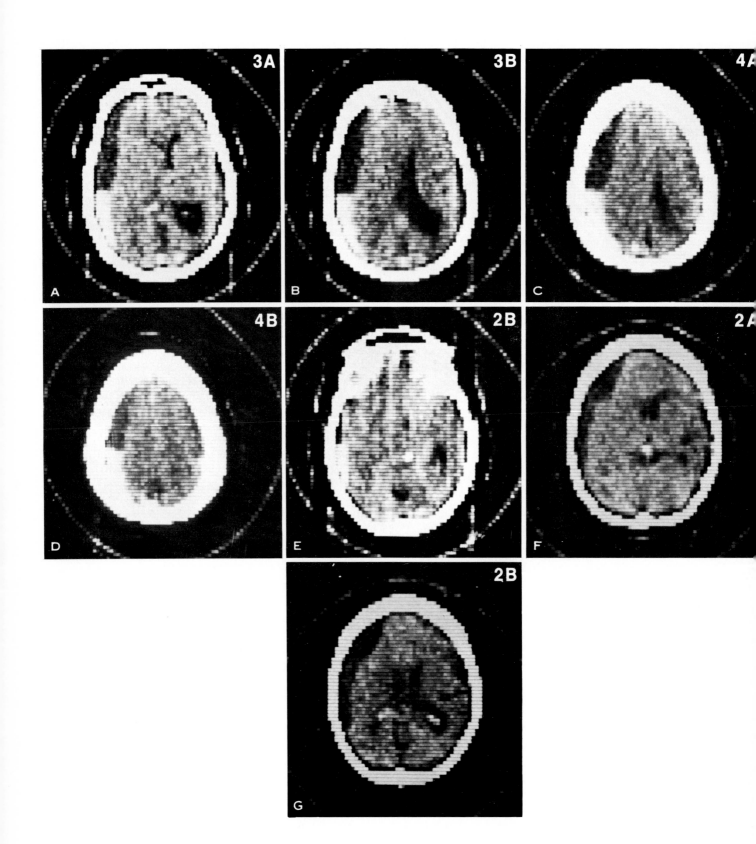

FIG. 17.6. BILATERAL SUBDURAL HEMATOMAS, EARLY CHRONIC.

Clinical Features. A 77 y.o. woman who was admitted following two sudden "drop attacks," decreased mentation, and difficulty with gait.

Neurological Examination. Bilateral cog-wheel rigidity and bilateral frontal lobe signs. Over a period of 24 hours, she became progressively more lethargic and then stuporous. Pupils remained equal and reactive, but she showed bilateral weakness and grasp reflexes.

CT Scan. Abnormal (Fig. 17.6, **A–E**).

Operation. (Dr. George Mendelsohn.) A burr hole was made in the left temporal area, through which a considerable amount of thin, straw-colored fluid under pressure was drained. A 1-inch trephine in the parietal area permitted removal of dark fluid with the consistency of crank case oil. A very thin outer subdural membrane was visible, but no inner membrane was seen. The cavity was fully irrigated with saline and the membrane coagulated. The brain expanded poorly. A smaller right subdural collection was evacuated through a parietal burr hole. The fluid was noted to be clearer than on the left side. The thin subdural membrane was coagulated, and bilateral subdural drains were left in place. Estimated size of the left collection was 75 ml and, of the right, 20 ml.

A–E. Preoperative CT scans; 13-mm sections. There is considerable midline dislocation to the right and compression of the left lateral ventricle. The posterior portions of the right ventricle are moderately dilated. The surface of the left cerebral hemisphere is obviously displaced inwards by a thick subdural collection that extends from the frontal to the occipital poles. The anterior portion of the collection is of low absorption (4–15 in **B**; 8–16 in **C**; and 10–18 in **D**) relative to the underlying brain. Note that the measurement is artifactually elevated in the high scan **D** due to inclusion of bone of the curving vault at this level.

The low density component of the collection changes abruptly at a fluid level just behind the middle of the sections. From this point posteriorly, the subdural collection has a high absorption (21–35 in **B**; 22–34 in **C**, and 25–35 in **D**). This interesting gravitational separation of elements of the subdural hematoma was evidently the result of prolonged recumbency in the supine position. From the graph illustrated in Fig. 15.1, it was determined that the supernatant portion of the hematoma had a hematocrit equivalent of approximately 15%, and the sedimented portion had a hematocrit equivalent of 65% prior to surgery.

E. Scan section immediately below that in **A**, showing the thin lower extremity of the subdural hematoma. This section illustrates that a hematoma measuring no more than 6–9 mm in width at any point could easily be overlooked, particularly if the scan was degraded by motion or if the hematoma had absorption values much closer to the underlying brain. The smaller right-sided hematoma, visible on **A–D** and showing a slight sedimentation effect (**D**), is not visible in this lower scan section.

F and G. Scan obtained several days after operation, showing considerable reaccumulation of low absorption subdural fluid on the left side and minor reaccumulation on the right side. There is significantly less midline dislocation to the right. Reevacuation revealed thin fluid with slightly brownish tinge, consistent with leakage of CSF into the subdural spaces.

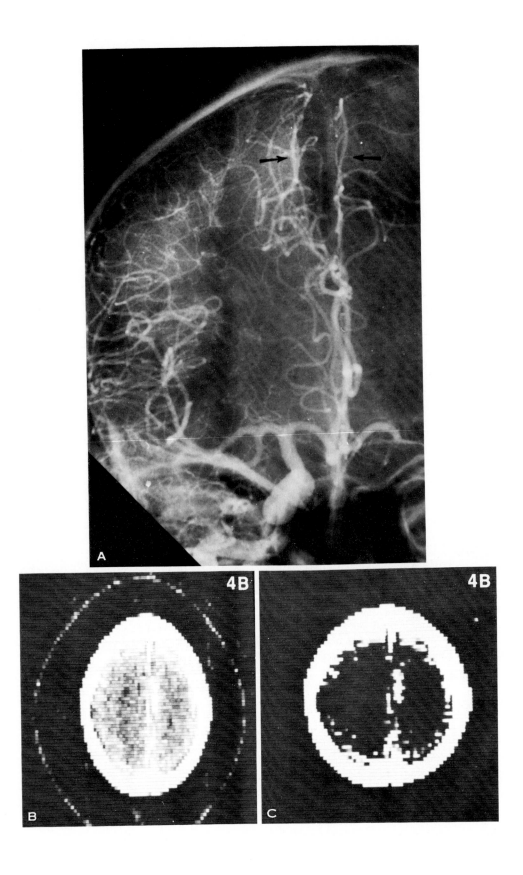

FIG. 17.7. SUBDURAL HEMATOMA, INTERHEMISPHERIC, EARLY CHRONIC.

Clinical Features. A 52 y.o. man who had hit his head on a steering wheel 16 days before the CT scan. He had not lost consciousness but developed severe headache. One day before CT scan, he developed weakness of his left leg that progressed so that he could not walk unassisted. He remained alert and oriented.

Neurological Examination. Marked spastic weakness of the left leg and left Babinski response.

Skull Examination. The pineal lay 2 mm to the left of the midline.

RN Scan. Tcp; showed a questionable increase in activity in the *left orbitofrontal region.*

CT Scan. Abnormal (Fig. 17.7, **B** and **C**).

Angio. Abnormal (Fig. 17.7**A**).

Operation. (Dr. Edward Tarlov.) Bilateral superior frontal bone flap. There was no subdural hematoma over the cerebral convexities, but, in the right superior interhemispheric region, thick shaggy subdural membranes were encountered and a 25-ml partially liquified subdural hematoma was removed.

A. Right carotid angiogram, sagittal projection. A small extracerebral collection is demonstrated superiorly in the posterior frontal portion of the longitudinal fissure, producing a concave lateral displacement of the regional cortical branches (*arrows*). The study was obtained 3 days after CT scan.

B. L 14   W 20.
Superior scan section as photographed at the time of the initial analysis. Lower scan sections had demonstrated considerable compression of the right lateral ventricle and slight midline dislocation to the left. This raised suspicion of a *laterally situated* extracerebral collection, but no definite focal abnormality was noted at the time. The band of increased absorption immediately to the right of the midline was noted but was thought to represent an area of dense cortex and was not analyzed further due to inexperience in this case seen shortly after acquisition of the scanner. After identification of the subdural hematoma by angiography, the disc record of the scan was studied further on the viewer.

C. L 26   W M.
One of several displays obtained on review of the scan that clearly revealed the small high-absorption subdural collection, the absorption of which peaked at 33. (The elongated configuration of the head in **B** is due to faulty adjustment of the viewer.) This case clearly illustrates the way in which small but significant lesions can be overlooked by inexperience or failure to use fully the available methods of analysis.

(Reprinted by permission from Radiology, 110: 109–123, 1974.)

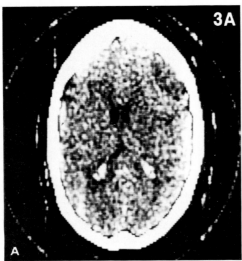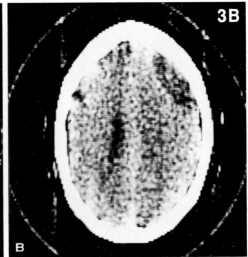

FIG. 17.8. CHRONIC SUBDURAL HEMATOMA.

Clinical Features. A 59 y.o. female with a history of atherosclerotic cardiovascular disease and myocardial infarction, who presented with left-sided transient ischemic attacks and possibly a completed small embolic right middle cerebral artery territory stroke. The patient had fallen some 6 weeks earlier and was hospitalized elsewhere for an occipital scalp laceration and cerebral concussion. Eleven days before CT scan, she noted the acute onset of numbness and weakness in her left hand and weakness in the left hip. The symptoms cleared completely in 4 minutes. Two similar attacks occurred during the ensuing 24 hours, associated with slurred speech and left facial drooping.

Neurological Examination. Left central facial weakness and slight left hemiparesis.

EEG. Right-sided slowing and sharp activity, more prominent over the right frontotemporal region.

Skull Examination. Interpreted as probably normal, but with question of slight pineal dislocation to the left.

RN Scan. Tcp; 1 day after the apparently completed stroke and 7 days before CT scan, the dynamic study was normal, but the static study revealed a large diffuse area of increased activity in the territory of the right middle cerebral artery, raising suspicion of infarction, hemorrhage, or tumor. Subdural hematoma was also suggested as a possibility. The RN scan was repeated on the same day as the CT scan and the findings were essentially unchanged.

Angio. Transfemoral right carotid study on the day of the apparently completed stroke revealed evidence of occlusion of

a Rolandic branch of the superior division of the right middle cerebral artery in the midopercular area.

There was no retrograde collateral flow or early venous filling. The anterior cerebral artery was displaced 5 mm to the left, with angular deformity indicative of subfalcial herniation. The internal cerebral vein was displaced a similar distance to the left. The possibility of an extracerebral collection on the right side was raised and it was suggested that the examination be repeated with appropriate oblique views.

CT Scan. Abnormal (Fig. 17.8).

At this time the neurological deficit had cleared completely on steroid therapy.

Angio. A repeat right carotid study the day following the CT scan confirmed the presence of a moderate-sized extracerebral collection in the right frontotemporal region.

As the patient was essentially asymptomatic at this point, it was decided not to operate and she was discharged to the care of a neurologist in her home state.

A. L 10   W 20.   **B.** L 8   W 30
160 x 160 matrix system.

These contiguous 13-mm sections clearly demonstrate the lenticular region of diminished absorption (3–11) in the right frontal region. The maximal thickness of the collection is slightly over 2 cm. The septum lucidum (**A**) is displaced 3–4 mm to the left of the midline, and there is evidence of some compression of the right lateral ventricle. An area of right cerebral infarction was not identified. Localized "atrophic" changes are noted in the left frontal lobe.

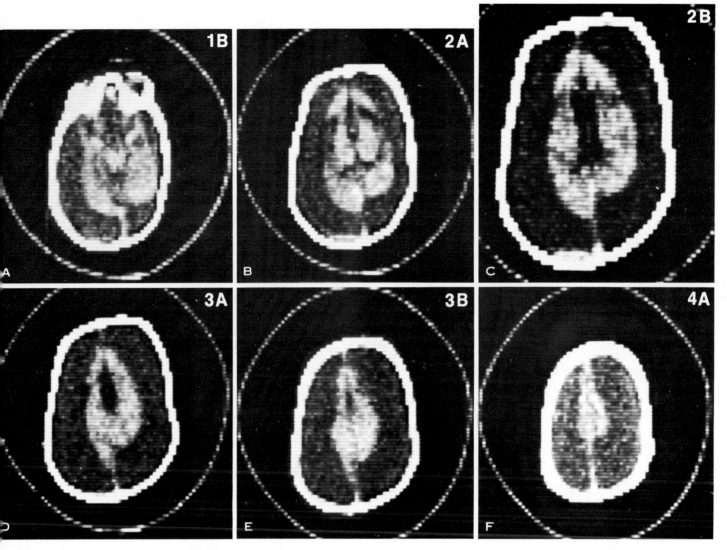

FIG. 17.9. SUBDURAL HYGROMA, MASSIVE BI-LATERAL.

Clinical Features. A 1 y.o. boy who began to have generalized seizures at the age of 6 weeks. His head had shown rapid increase in size from the age of 2½ months and marked transillumination appeared. At the age of 6 months, by which time a diagnosis of Menckes' kinky hair disease had been established, he had his first CT scan (see Fig. 24.8). This scan had demonstrated gross cerebral damage with considerable diffuse decrease in absorption values and marked nonobstructive ventricular enlargement. There was no clinical evidence of function above the brain stem, apart from seizures.

CT Scan. Second examination, 4½ months after the first (Fig. 17.9).

Treatment. In view of the child's overall condition, it was decided not to attempt drainage of the collections, and analysis of the fluid is therefore not available.

A–F. L 10–13   W 20.

Consecutive 13-mm scan sections from below superiorly. 10° to RBL.

The abnormal brain is now grossly collapsed and the lateral ventricles, although still enlarged, are much reduced in size compared with the initial scan. Huge bilateral extracerebral collections are demonstrated.

A. Scan section at the level of the orbital roofs anteriorly. In the central region, the configuration of the midbrain is evident, with slightly enlarged surrounding cisterns. The midbrain is displaced several millimeters to the right. At this level, the subdural collection is much larger on the left side than on the right, as it is in **B**.

C–F. On the higher levels of this series, the subdural collection is larger on the right side and the falx and collapsed malformed brain lie considerably to the left of the midline anteriorly. A mild scoliosis capitis is shown. Absorption of the subdural fluid was only slightly higher than that of ventricular CSF, indicating an essentially hygromatous consistency of the fluid. Absorption values of the cerebral hemispheres ranged between 10 and 20 units (see Fig. 24.8).

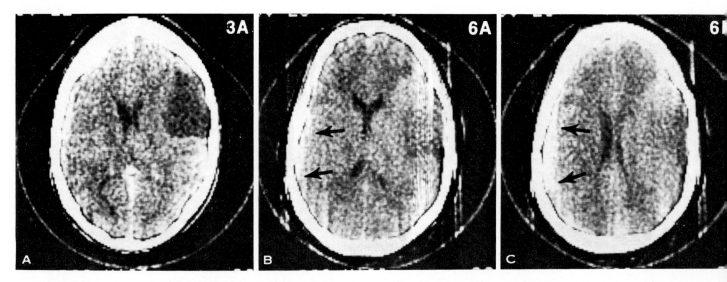

FIG. 17.10. BILATERAL CHRONIC SUBDURAL HEMATOMAS AND AGENESIS OF THE RIGHT TEMPORAL LOBE.

Clinical Features. A 22 y.o. man who was evaluated for headaches of several months duration.

Neurological Examination. No focal neurological findings were identified.

EEG. Abnormal, because of occasional left temporal slowing.

RN Scan. Tcp; abnormal, with increased activity in the right posterior inferior frontal region.

CT Scan. Abnormal (Fig. 17.10).

Angio. Transfemoral bilateral internal carotid studies, 3 days after CT scan, revealed an extensive extracerebral collection over the anterior half of the right cerebral convexity, with an average thickness of 2 cm and appearing to extend into the right temporal fossa. There was also evidence of a moderate-sized extracerebral collection over the left cerebral convexity, situated higher than the collection on the right, slightly more than 3 cm in maximum thickness, and not extending to the temporal fossa. The findings were believed consistent with subacute or chronic subdural hematomas.

Operation. (Dr. Paul Chapman.) Bilateral 2-inch trephine bone flaps revealed thin vascular outer subdural membranes and considerable amounts of dark red and brownish liquid old blood. On the left side, an additional blood clot was evacuated by irrigation, with good expansion of the brain. On the right side, absence of the anterior half of the right temporal lobe was evident.

CT scan. 160 x 160 matrix system.

A. Scan section following intravenous injection of 300 ml of meglumine diatrizoate 30%. A large, well-defined, cavitary-appearing lesion is visible in the right frontotemporal region, with an absorption range of 6–18 units. There is indication of a fluid level posteriorly, separating lower absorption material above and denser material (15–40) below. Considering the size of this lesion, there is a rather modest mass effect upon the ventricular system (suggesting an underlying loss of cerebral substance).

B. Plain CT scan obtained with the patient *prone*. The patient was placed prone shortly before the scan was obtained. There has been an admixture of the less dense and more dense elements; the latter are in the process of gravitating to the anterior, now more dependent, region, and the subdural hematoma is now less readily differentiated from underlying brain. In the left parietotemporal region, the inferior portion of denser extracerebral collection is just visible (*arrows*).

C. Section immediately above that in **B**, revealing the extensive, relatively high absorption (23–40) subdural hematoma on the left side.

This case and that illustrated in Figure 17.6 suggest that chronic subdural hematomas may be more readily identified if the patient is maintained in a supine position for some time (e.g., 1–2 hours) before CT scanning, so as to favor gravitational separation of the higher and lower absorption elements.

CHAPTER 18

Aneurysms

INTRODUCTION

The reader is referred to Chapters 15 and 27 for a general review of the potential role of CT scanning in the diagnosis of intracranial aneurysms. While angiography will remain supreme in the demonstration of intracranial aneurysms in the sites and sizes most commonly encountered and for demonstration of minute anatomy and circulatory variants required for treatment decisions, CT scanning offers an important means of assessing the effects on brain that may be associated. Recognition of cerebral ischemia and infarction, resulting from arterial spasm, of hematomas, both intra- and extra-axial, and of hydrocephalus, which may follow severe subarachnoid hemorrhage, generally is readily provided by CT scanning. Frequently, these complications are more readily identified by this means than by cerebral angiography. The relative simplicity of serial CT scanning is highly attractive for the identification and observation of progress of such complications.

CT scanning may also offer assistance in the determination of the source of hemorrhage in cases of multiple aneurysms, and in hypertensive patients with unruptured aneurysms associated with hypertensive intracerebral hemorrhage in the general vicinity. In the latter situation, CT examination provides a far more accurate localization of position and extent of intracerebral hemorrhage than is possible by angiography.

As improvements in equipment and technique are introduced, particularly the capability of obtaining high quality thin scan sections (2–4 mm thick; 27A and 27B) in conjunction with high-dose intravenous contrast medium injection, CT scanning will offer a preliminary "survey" method of diagnosing the presence of aneurysms only a few millimeters in diameter.

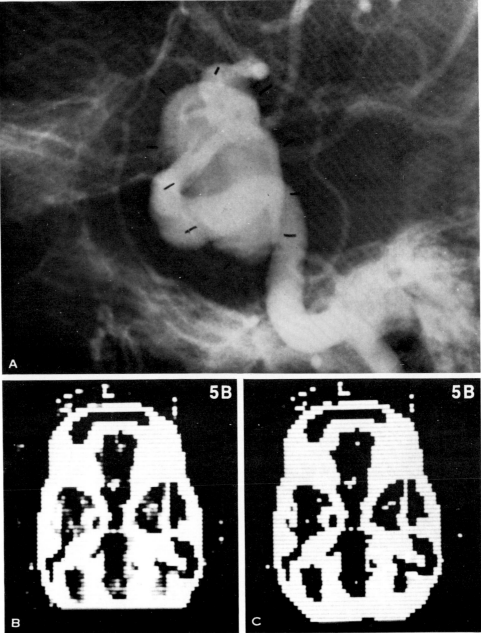

FIG. 18.1. LARGE ANEURYSM OF THE SUPRACAVERNOUS INTERNAL CAROTID SIPHON.

Clinical Features. A 77 y.o. female who had had a transient episode of right-sided weakness several weeks earlier. Nine days before CT scan she had developed severe aphasia and right facial weakness.

Skull Examination. Normal.

RN Scan. Tcp; 1 month earlier, normal; repeat exam 3 days before CT exam showed a definite focal lesion in left posterior inferior frontal region, extending from the periphery deeply into the insular region.

CT Scan. Abnormal (Fig. 18.1, **B** and **C**).

Angio. Eight days before CT, left carotid study revealed a supraclinoid internal carotid aneurysm projecting into the sella and left parasellar region, without mass effect. No vascular occlusions were noted. The aneurysm measured 23 mm vertically x 16 x 16 mm (Fig. 18.1**A**).

A. Left carotid angiogram. The aneurysm is shown superimposed upon the sella and carotid siphon, with projection into the suprasellar area (*short lines*). No vascular occlusions or further abnormalities were demonstrated in the remainder of the study.

B and **C.** Scan section at the level of the sella, after intravenous injection of 50 ml of Hypaque 60. No definite abnormality was detected in this section before contrast enhancement. The orbital roofs and sella structures are visible. Immediately to the left of the sella is an irregular ovoid abnormality with an absorption of 22–34. Its AP dimension is 15 mm, and there is a suggestion of extension into the left side of the pituitary fossa.

C. W M setting shows the aneurysm in high contrast. The white vertical band in the right middle fossa represents a common artifact. The density of the aneurysm was shown in the next superior section, which extended through the suprasellar cistern. In addition, there was an area of decreased absorption (7–14) in the left frontal lobe consistent with infarction (section not shown). A small area of diminished absorption in the right lower internal capsule region was noted and diagnosed as a probable lacunar infarct. In this case, angiography demonstrated the large aneurysm far better than did the CT scan but failed to reveal the relatively recent left frontal lobe infarct and the probable lacunar infarct. RN scan revealed the frontal lobe infarction but failed to reveal the aneurysm and probable lacunar infarct. It is important to recognize that partial volume inclusion of bone in the inferior parasellar area may mimic lesions. Also, without angiography it would be impossible on CT scanning to make the diagnosis of aneurysm with great confidence in such a case. Differentiation from a small parasellar meningioma would not be possible on CT scanning unless plain film cranial examination had revealed characteristic changes.

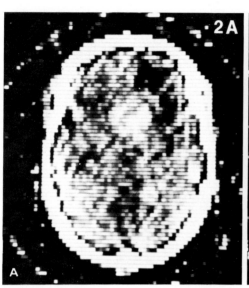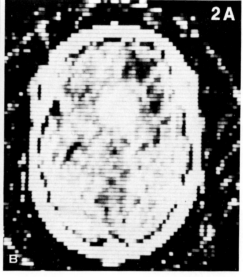

FIG. 18.2. ANEURYSM, LARGE AND THROMBOSED, ARISING FROM THE ANTERIOR CIRCLE OF WILLIS.
Clinical Features. A 52 y.o. male with a history of persistent moderate headaches, mostly in the right frontal area, for 2–3 months, and recent personality changes, consisting mainly of apathy and abulia. Difficulty with memory.
Neurological Examination. As above, with no other abnormality apart from a questionable left plantar response.
Skull Examination. Normal.
RN Scan. Tcp; abnormal uptake in the deep medial aspect of the right front lobe area.
CT Scan. Abnormal (Fig. 18.2).
Angio. Right carotid study only, which revealed an avascular mass in the right frontal lobe area.
Operation. (Dr. James Wepsic.) Based on the radiological studies, the preoperative diagnosis was inferior frontal meningioma. Right frontal craniectomy and partial right frontal lobectomy. Very firm hard grey mass was noted in the interhemispheric

fissure. Localized dissection of the mass revealed pulsations in the central portion. A 23-gauge needle resulted in the aspiration of bright red arterial blood. Excision appeared too hazardous, and oozing from the needle puncture was controlled with Oxycel and a small layer of aneurysm glue.
Pathology. Large aneurysm with considerable dense mural thrombus, in the region of the anterior communicating artery.
A. Scan section through the inferior frontal region shows a round lesion, about 3.3 cm in diameter, with an absorption range of 16–25. An irregular broad zone of markedly diminished absorption (8–13) in the right frontal lobe is consistent with edema or a relatively recent infarct. Plain scan only was obtained.
A. L 16 W 20. **B.** L 18 W 20.
The absorption values do not permit differentiation from other lesions, particularly meningioma, which was the CT scan diagnosis. However, the extremely rounded character of the mass should have indicated the possibility of an aneurysm.

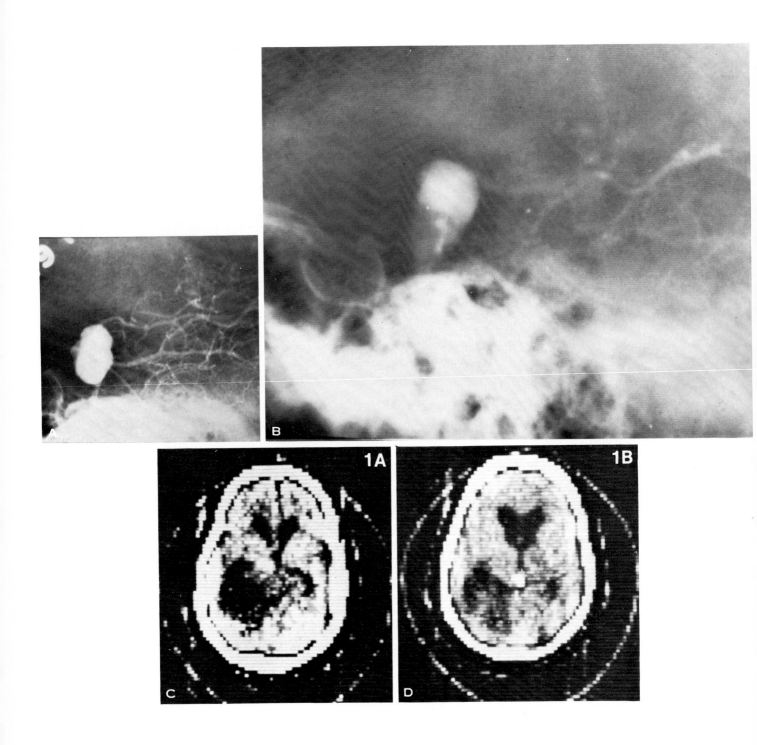

FIG. 18.3. ANEURYSM, DISTAL BASILAR ARTERY, BECOMING PARTLY THROMBOSED AND ASSOCIATED WITH EXTENSIVE INFARCTION.

Clinical Features. A 39 y.o. male with a history of headaches for several years, vertigo for several months, vertical diplopia, and mild, increasing dysarthria. One week before admission, there was increased diplopia and increased visual loss in the left eye. Shortly before admission, there was very severe headache, with sudden right hemiparesis and severe slurring of speech, with vomiting and sweating. Hemiparesis rapidly improved. Four days later there was an episode of respiratory arrest and decerebrate posturing and rigidity, which rapidly cleared with support of respiration, Mannitol, and Decadron. There was neck rigidity.

Angio. A retrograde right brachial angiography at another hospital 1 day before the respiratory arrest had demonstrated a 2 x 1.2 x 2 cm distal basilar aneurysm (Fig. 18.3A). Repeat brachial angiography 5 days later at the MGH revealed no filling of the aneurysm and local vessel deformities suggestive of a perianeurysmal clot. There was spasm of the basilar artery and of the right internal carotid artery and its branches. A further angiogram 6 days later showed partial filling of the aneurysm, with evidence of a mural thrombus. There was very slow emptying of the aneurysm, which was still partly filled at 9 seconds (Fig. 18.3B).

CT Scan. Obtained 1 and 4 days after the second angiogram showed extensive abnormalities (Fig. 18.3, C–D).

A. Initial angiogram, showing large distal basilar artery aneurysm with good filling of posterior cerebral circulation.

B. Third angiogram, showing incomplete filling of the aneurysm due to mural thrombus and poor filling of the basilar and posterior cerebral arteries due to spasm. Note the height to which the superior pole of the aneurysm projects above the dorsum sellae.

C. L 16   W 10.
A 2-cm ovoid area of increased absorption (peak, 36) is shown immediately to the left side of the midportion of the third ventricle, which is locally indented and displaced slightly towards the right on this section. A very large zone of diminished absorption (0–14) is shown extending laterally and posteriorly from the dense mass into the temporal and occipital lobes (higher sections showed extension into the parietal lobe also). A patchy appearance of diminished absorption is shown extending into the mesial posterior portion of the right cerebral hemisphere to the region of the lower portion of the right trigone.

D. L 15   W 20.
Scan section immediately above that in **C,** at the level of the most superior portion of the third ventricle and pineal. There is modest lateral ventricular enlargement. The extensive region of reduced absorption in the left posterior temporal and occipital lobes is again visible but is more heterogeneous and less sharply defined at this level. A small area of moderately diminished absorption is shown in the region of the right occipital pole also. The pineal is in the midline.

The small dense mass adjacent to the third ventricle indicates a thrombosed superior portion of the aneurysmal sac, extending above that portion of the aneurysm that was shown to fill on the first and third angiograms. However, a small hemorrhage from the upper portion of the aneurysm into the left thalamus could also produce this appearance. The large area of diminished absorption in the posterior portions of the left cerebral hemisphere is consistent with a relatively recent infarction, and there is evidence of smaller areas of infarction in the posterior portion of the right cerebral hemisphere. The first CT scan showed all of the above findings, in spite of the presence of considerable motion artifact. Because of these artifacts, the scan was repeated.

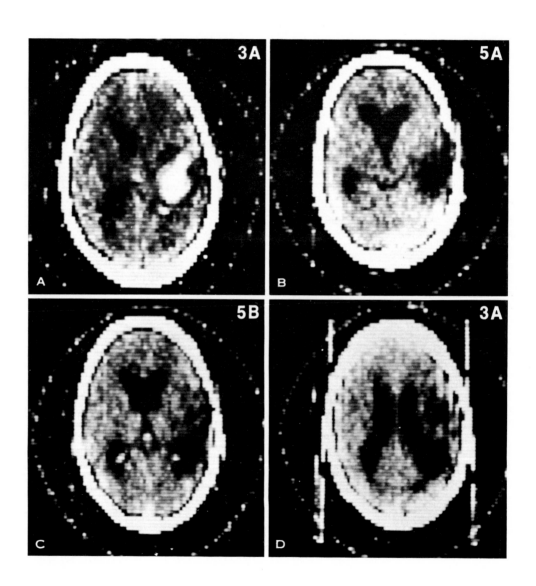

FIG. 18.4. HEMATOMA, LARGE SYLVIAN CISTERNAL, FROM PRESUMED MIDDLE CEREBRAL ANEURYSM.

Clinical Features. A 39 y.o. male with a history of mild, essentially untreated hypertension for 5 years. The day before admission he experienced severe headache and vomiting. Speech and behavior became progressively less appropriate. He was extremely agitated overnight at an outlying hospital and, next morning, was noted to have slurred speech and left hemiparesis.

Neurological Examination. At the MGH, approximately 28 hours after the ictus, he was disoriented but able to follow simple commands. Speech was very slurred. Left hemiparesis with bilateral Babinski signs and decreased left corneal reflex were noted. Lumbar puncture showed an opening pressure of 420 mm and bright red fluid.

Skull Examination. Normal.

CT Scan. Abnormal (Fig. 18.4A).

Angio. Transfemoral bilateral carotid and left vertebral studies revealed a deeply seated avascular mass in the right putaminal region, extending laterally into the frontal operculum and posteriorly into the temporoparietal area, and indicated a probable putaminal hemorrhage. Narrowing of middle cerebral branches over the frontal operculum was consistent with spasm. The lenticulostriate branches were displaced mesially, and the sylvian middle cerebral branches were displaced laterally. There was slowed circulation through the middle cerebral territory. No aneurysm was identified.

Three days later he abruptly became less responsive, with dilatation of the right pupil, and was immediately taken to the operating room.

Operation. (Dr. Robert G. Ojemann.) A large hematoma was evacuated from within the sylvian cistern. The hematoma surrounded the insular branches of the middle cerebral artery that were situated in the lateral portion of the mass. No aneurysm was identified, but fibrotic changes surrounding an insular branch suggested old extravasation from an aneurysm here.

Angio. A repeat transfemoral right carotid study approximately 1 month after the operation revealed occlusion of several opercular and retrosylvian branches of the middle cerebral artery, with retrograde collateral flow from the anterior and posterior cerebral vessels. A residual mass effect in the same area as originally, but less in degree. A 4-mm aneurysm was now visible at the origin of the posterior communicating artery.

CT Scan. Repeat CT scan was abnormal (Fig. 18.4, **B–D**).

A. The characteristic appearance of a hematoma is illustrated by the large, inverted comma-shaped high absorption lesion (25–38) in and adjacent to the region of the right sylvian cistern. Anteriorly, this merges imperceptibly with the cerebral cortex. Surrounding the hematoma is an irregular, generally quite broad zone of diminished absorption, indicative of perifocal edema. There is considerable compression of the right lateral ventricle and moderate midline dislocation to the left. The density of calcification in the pineal is visible medial to the hematoma, and that of the glomus lies just behind it (see Fig. 2.11**B** for the numerical printout of this scan section). Whether the bulk of the hematoma is in an expanded sylvian cistern or in the lateral putamen, with lateral extension and displacement of the cistern, cannot be determined from the CT scan.

B–D. CT sections from the postoperative scan obtained approximately 1 month after surgery. At this point, the patient had memory difficulties and severe residual hemiparesis. The scan shows no evidence of residual hematoma. The lateral and third ventricles are moderately dilated, and there is marked focal dilatation of the right trigone. There is slight midline dislocation to the left. A large, fairly sharply demarcated region of diminished absorption is demonstrated in the temporal and parietal lobes. Higher sections show some extension into the most posterior portion of the frontal lobe. Absorption values of the lesion ranged between 5–13, 8–15, and 9–15 on different sections. Right trigone measurements were 2–12. Some small low absorption areas extend into the right corpus striatum. The findings indicate extensive infarction, becoming demarcated by phagocytosis. This feature and the absorption values together suggest that the infarction occurred more than 3 weeks and less than 6–8 weeks earlier. The ventricular enlargement is presumably due to a degree of obstructive communicating hydrocephalus secondary to the very severe subarachnoid hemorrhage.

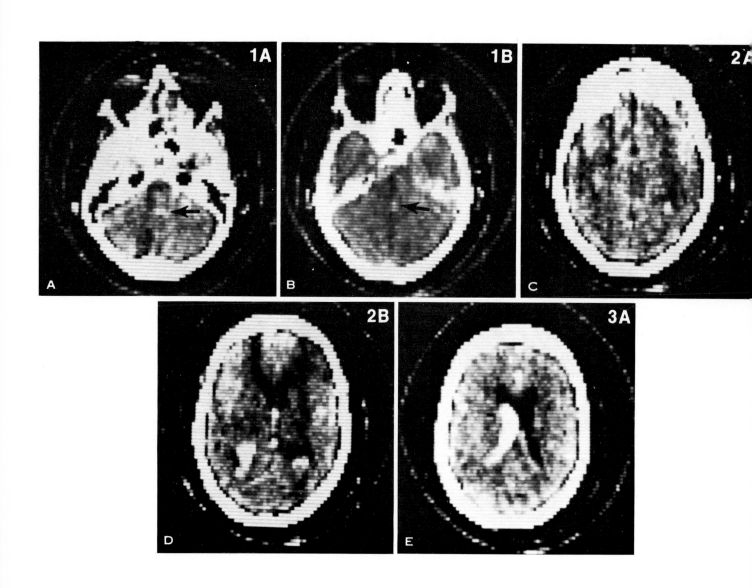

FIG. 18.5. EXTENSIVE SUBARACHNOID AND INTRA-VENTRICULAR HEMORRHAGE, FROM RUPTURED ANEURYSM.

Clinical Features. A 73 y.o. female with a history of hypertension who suffered a sudden collapse with flaccid paralysis and cardiorespiratory arrest. She was comatose on admission.

Neurological Examination. Unable to follow commands, eyes deviated to the left, prominent frontal lobe signs with grasp, suck, root, and snout responses bilaterally. Neck rigidity. Lumbar puncture showed an opening pressure of 370 mm, with bloody CSF.

CT Scan. Abnormal (Fig. 18.5).

Angio. Bilateral carotid studies revealed 5 aneurysms: a 6 x 9 mm aneurysm at the knee of the right middle cerebral artery, a 3 x 4 mm aneurysm of the left intracavernous carotid siphon, a 6-mm aneurysm at the origin of the left posterior communicating artery, a 2.5-mm aneurysm of the right pericallosal artery, and a 9-mm aneurysm originating at the knee of the left middle cerebral artery (diameters corrected for magnification). There was moderate narrowing of the right middle cerebral arteries and markedly delayed filling of the branches of the left middle cerebral artery due to partial occlusion near the site of the aneurysm. Slight collateral circulation from the anterior and posterior cerebral distributions entered the left middle cerebral branches, which appeared generally spastic. No ventricular enlargement was visible. The internal cerebral veins were displaced 9 mm to the right. The findings suggested that subarachnoid hemorrhage had originated from the left middle cerebral aneurysm.

A–E. Consecutive 13-mm CT scan sections from below superiorly.

A. A small zone of increased absorption (30–39) is evident in the fourth ventricle (*arrow*). The vertical zone of decreased absorption in the pons and cerebellum to the left of the midline has the appearance of an artifact.

B. A very small zone of increased absorption (16–27) is probably a partial volume representation of blood in the aqueduct (*arrow*).

C. Numerous patchy areas of increased absorption are evident in the region of both sylvian cisterns, suprasellar cistern, subfrontal region, around the midbrain in the ambient and quadrigeminal cisterns, and in the region of the superior cerebellar cistern. These areas of density had absorption ranges between 20 and 38 and are consistent with blood clots in the subarachnoid spaces. They are somewhat more prominent to the left of the midline. None of the aneurysms can be distinguished in this examination without contrast enhancement.

D. The ventricular system is normal in size for the patient's age. A high absorption (22–32) zone is present in the third ventricle, extending posteriorly to a calcified pineal (60 units). Blood clots are evident in the left trigone and occipital horn (28–40) and in the right occipital horn (28–40). High density areas are shown in both sylvian cisterns at this level. What appear to be low density artifacts are shown in both frontal lobes and in the right corpus striatum on this section.

E. An extensive blood cast of the left lateral ventricle (21–40) is shown, and there is indication of some blood extending along the mesial wall of the body and trigone of the right lateral ventricle. Small areas of increased absorption are noted in the upper portion of the left sylvian cistern anteriorly and in the posterior portion of the interfrontal longitudinal fissure.

The distribution of the subarachnoid and intraventricular blood suggests that the aneurysm responsible for subarachnoid hemorrhage was one of those on the left side. No intracerebral hematoma was apparent, and the route of blood to the ventricular system is not clear. In the absence of blood cast in the left temporal horn, entry through the anterior third ventricle appears most likely. CSF values in areas not involved in obvious accumulations of blood were 1–12, slightly higher than usual. In most cases of severe subarachnoid hemorrhage, no elevation of absorption values of CSF have been noted. Only three cases with evidence of accumulations of blood in the cisterns and subarachnoid spaces have been encountered, presumably due to the more usual dilution and diffusion of blood entering the subarachnoid space. Since it is not unusual to find generalized ventricular enlargement soon after a major subarachnoid hemorrhage, the relatively normal size of the ventricular system in this particular case is surprising.

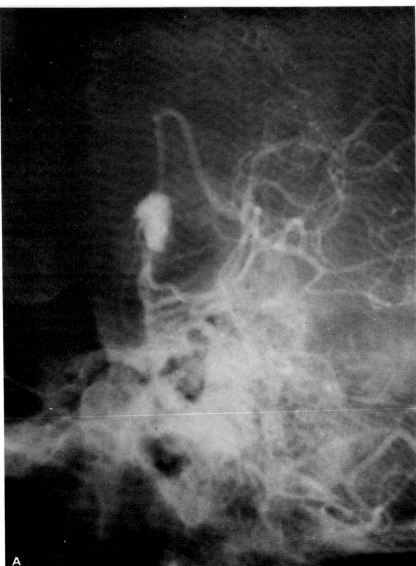

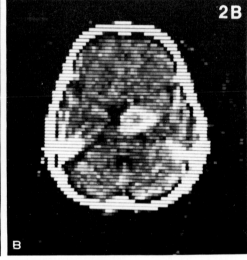

FIG. 18.6. BASILAR ARTERY GIANT ANEURYSM, PARTIALLY THROMBOSED.

Clinical Features. A 60 y.o. old male who had a history of subarachnoid hemorrhages 12 and 4 years previously. Mental decline was partly improved by a ventriculoatrial shunt (Dr. J. Hanberry) for communicating hydrocephalus 3 years previously. Persistent headaches had been unchanged recently.

Neurological Examination. There was a static deficit consisting of markedly decreased vision bilaterally, worse on the left, with absent upward gaze and a mild left hemiparesis.

Skull Examination. Normal, except for right ventricular shunt.

Angio. Studies 1 and 3 years previously had demonstrated a distal basilar artery aneurysm, with evidence of partial thrombosis (Fig. 18.6A).

CT Scan. Abnormal (Fig. 18.6B).

A. Left vertebral angiogram, lateral projection. An aneurysm with an irregular contour is shown arising from the top of the basilar artery, projecting superiorly and, on AP projection (not shown), to the right. A much larger thrombosed component of the aneurysm is indicated by the marked upward (and medial, on AP projection) displacement of the right posterior cerebral artery and inferior displacement of the superior cerebellar artery. The right anterior choroidal artery was displaced superiorly and laterally on the carotid angiogram (not shown).

B. L 18 W 20.

The CT section passes through the suprasellar cisterns and fourth ventricle. A 27 x 33 mm mass is shown occupying the right interpeduncular and posterior suprasellar cisterns, projecting into the superior portion of the right upper pons and the inferior medial portion of the right middle fossa. Absorption measured 20–35 in the peripheral portions of the mass (thrombus) and 15–25 in the central region (circulating blood in residual aneurysmal lumen).

CHAPTER 19

Arteriovenous Malformations: Vein of Galen Aneurysm

ARTERIOVENOUS MALFORMATIONS

For a general review of CT scanning in arteriovenous malformations, the reader is referred to Chapters 15 and 27.

Cerebral angiography remains the primary method for demonstration of the presence and detailed anatomical and circulatory characteristics of arteriovenous malformations. Plain film cranial examination is occasionally capable of indicating the presence of large arteriovenous malformations, particularly those with dural components, by revealing enlarged meningeal arterial channels, prominent internal carotid canals and parasellar sulci, and greatly enlarged and abnormally distributed diploic venous channels. CT scanning is capable of revealing the presence of complex abnormalities of both increased and decreased absorption relative to brain resulting from vascular malformations within cerebral substance.

Our experience with arteriovenous malformations uncomplicated by hemorrhage includes only the larger varieties (more than several centimeters in diameter), but the experience of others indicates that it may be possible by CT scanning alone to identify the presence, although not necessarily the nature, of arteriovenous malformations as small as 1.5–2.5 cm in diameter. The possibility of identifying such small malformations is considerably increased if studies include scans with contrast enhancement. CT scanning therefore offers a worthwhile preliminary examination in cases suspected to be harboring a vascular malformation. When the clinical features are highly localizing, examination with 8-mm sections and including high volume contrast enhancement will be advantageous.

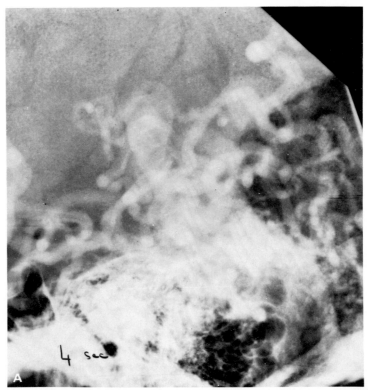

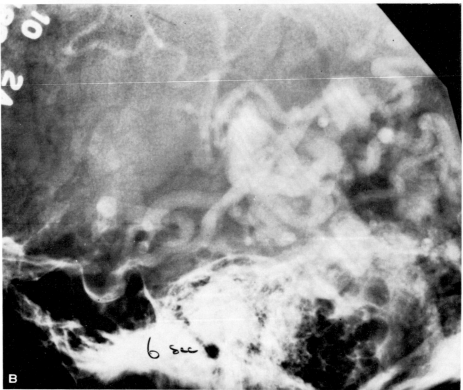

FIG. 19.1. ARTERIOVENOUS MALFORMATION, LARGE AND DIFFUSELY ARRANGED, INVOLVING BOTH PARIETAL AND OCCIPITAL LOBES AND CERE- BELLUM, WITH DURAL COMPONENTS IN ADDITION.
Clinical Features. A 23 y.o. male. Clinical onset was at 17 years of age, with headaches and seizures. He had had two decompressive craniectomies and ligation of external carotid arteries, occipital arteries, and multiple meningeal branches, with little change in the malformation.
Neurological Examination. Upper left homonymous hemia- nopsia, slightly decreased hearing in the left ear, and normal motor, sensory, and cerebellar tests.
CT Scan. Abnormal (Fig. 19.1, **C–G**).

Angio. Multiple studies, including transfemoral bilateral carotid and vertebrobasilar series (Fig. 19.1, **A** and **B**).
Treatment. Dr. Raymond N. Kjellberg. Stereotactic Bragg peak proton beam radiation to two areas of the malformation to totals of 4500 rads (4 portals) and 10,000 rads (8 portals).
A and **B.** Lateral angiograms showing the very numerous hypertrophied arteries and extremely large draining veins of the extremely extensive diffuse arteriovenous malformation. The lesion was principally cerebral in location, but numerous dural components were present also.
C–G. CT scans at similar levels before and after contrast enhancement with 45 ml of Hypaque 60 intravenously.
C and **D.** Plain CT scan. Numerous irregularly rounded areas of

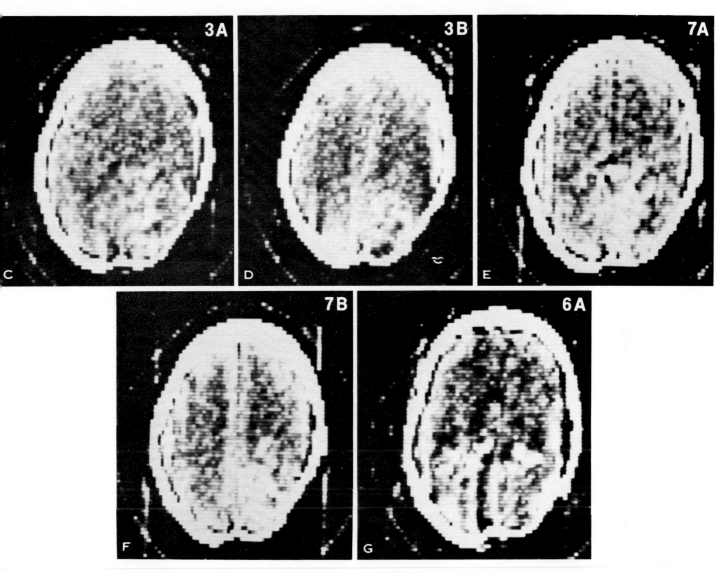

increased absorption (17–30) are distributed through the parietal and occipital lobes bilaterally. Adjacent to these regions are small irregular areas of diminished absorption, in the ranges 8–14 and 11–20. The large rounded or ovoid areas of increased absorption are consistent with blood circulating in the greatly dilated tortuous vessels of the malformation. The regions of decreased absorption presumably represent areas of cerebral atrophy secondary to the mechanical and circulatory effects of the malformation. A more diffuse background of slightly increased absorption in the region of the malformation may represent gliosis with hemosiderin deposition from previous extravasations.

E–G. Scans obtained following contrast enhancement, showing an obvious increase in absorption of rounded and ovoid regions, similar in appearance to the discrete regions of higher absorption in the plain scan. Due to the marked tortuosity of the malformation vessels, it is impossible to reproduce precisely the spatial orientation of these vascular spaces on repeat scan, but the findings are most compatible with the increase in absorption of blood circulating through the malformation that results from the injected iodine. Obstructive ventricular dilatation and frank hematoma formation were excluded by the scans.

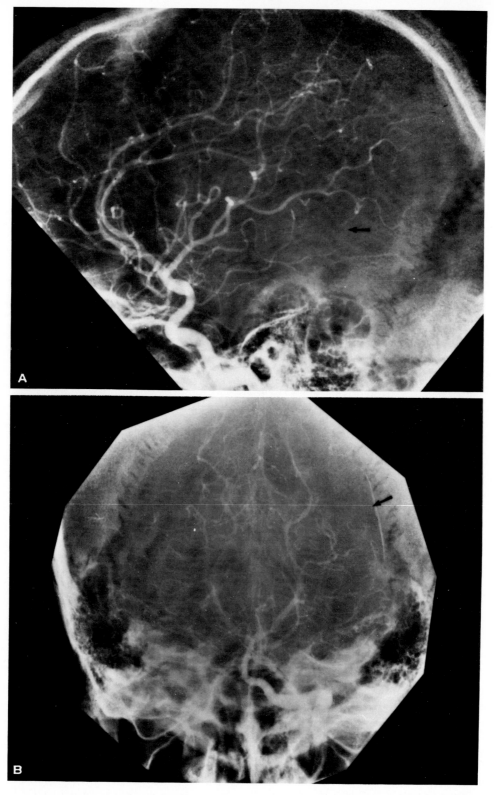

FIG. 19.2.   ARTERIOVENOUS MALFORMATION, WITH INTRACEREBRAL, INTRAVENTRICULAR, AND SUB-ARACHNOID HEMORRHAGE.

Clinical Features. A 22 y.o. male who had a sudden onset of severe midline frontal headache and diminished vision to the right side. He denied loss of consciousness, change in mentation, and strength, and other symptoms. There was no relevant past history. At another hospital, lumbar puncture revealed grossly bloody fluid and he was transferred to the MGH.

Neurological Examination. Suffering severe headache, but alert and cooperative. Blood pressure, 108/50. Normal speech, slow but accurate calculations. Amnesia for the events of the past 2 days. Right homonymous hemianopsia, with normal optic discs. The remainder of the neurological examination was

normal. He shortly became slightly disoriented. Lumbar puncture showed grossly bloody fluid with an opening pressure of 300 mm.

Skull Examination. Normal.

Angio. Transfemoral bilateral carotid and left vertebral studies 1 day after the ictus revealed a poorly marginated left parietal mass. Initially, no abnormal vessels were identified. After CT scan, review suggested the presence of a few small abnormal vessels in the parietal lobe area (Fig. 19.2, **A** and **B**).

CT Scans. One day after angiography, abnormal (Fig. 19.2, **C**–**F**).

Operation. (Dr. Michael Scott.) Parieto-occipital craniotomy with removal of a large parieto-occipital hematoma; evacuation of blood from the left lateral ventricle, which was in communi-

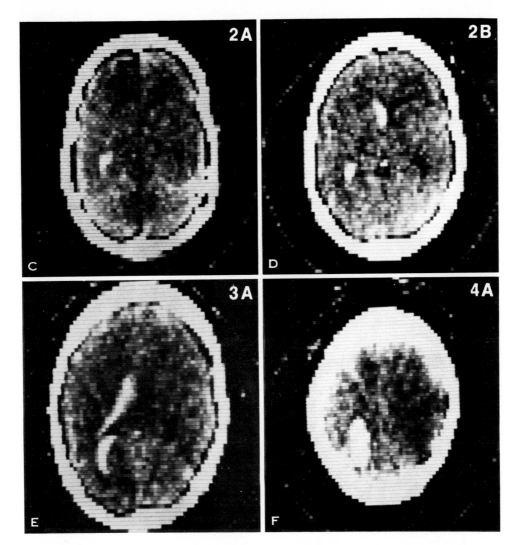

cation with the hematoma. A 2-cm diameter vascular malformation adjacent to the occipital horn was found and was noted to contain circulating blood following decompression. This was excised. The patient did well following operation, with gradual improvement in recent memory and slow resolution of the hemianopsia.

Histology. Small arteriovenous malformation (8 mm in diameter in collapsed state).

A postoperative CT scan revealed a modest sized porencephalic cavity at the site of the evacuated hematoma, some residual hematoma superiorly in the parietal lobe, and evacuation of most of the left ventricular blood cast.

A. Lateral early arterial film of the carotid angiogram, showing a diffuse mass effect in the parieto-occipital region, with a minor mass effect separating the retrosylvian branches and displacing the sylvian triangle anteriorly (*arrow*). No definite pathological vessels are evident, although there is suspicion of a few small abnormal vessels just above the arrow.
B. Frontal arterial phase projections of the vertebral angiogram. There is a very slight, poorly localized mass effect upon the branches of the left posterior cerebral artery, from the superolateral aspect (*arrow*).
C–F. L 17   W 20.
A cast of blood measuring 24–37 is shown filling most of a

nondilated left lateral ventricle (**C–E**, which represent contiguous 13-mm sections).

C. This section passes obliquely through the left temporal horn, which at this point is filled with blood.
D. The section passes through the frontal horns, the left being almost filled with a blood clot and the right, also not dilated, filled with CSF. Posteriorly on the left, the section passes through the region of the junction of the temporal horn and trigone, which is blood filled. The midline structures are not displaced.
E. This section shows the body, trigone, and occipital horn filled with blood. The trigone and occipital horn are displaced anterolaterally, and behind the occipital horn is the lower extremity of the parieto-occipital hematoma. (Reprinted by permission from Radiology, 110: 109–123, 1974.)
F. Second section above that in **E**. This and the subjacent section showed the greatest dimensions of the parieto-occipital hematoma, which measured 45 mm in greatest diameter. Absorption values of the hematoma ranged up to 55 units. A 20-ml hematoma was removed from this region and blood clots were sucked out of the ventricle, which was open to the hematoma cavity at the occipital horn. The most superior portion of the hematoma was not removed, as was shown on the postoperative CT scan.

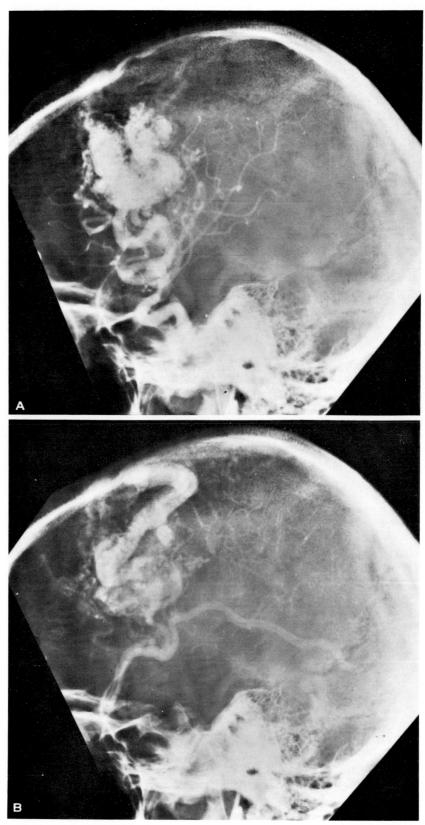

FIG. 19.3.   A and B (see legend on page 325).

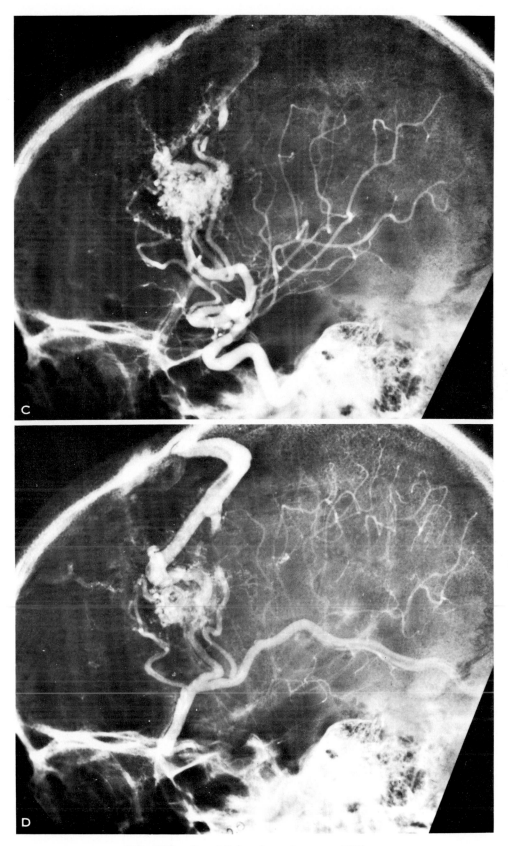

FIG. 19.3.   C and D (see legend on page 325).

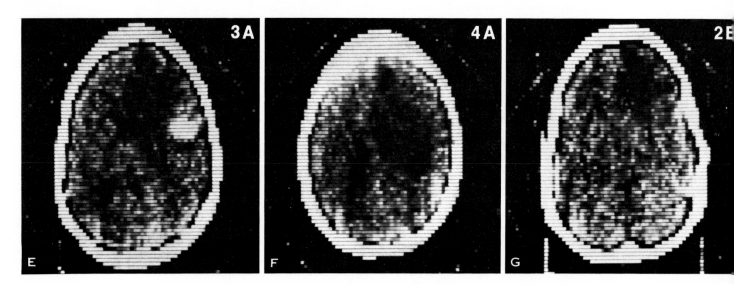

FIG. 19.3.   E–G

FIG. 19.3. ARTERIOVENOUS MALFORMATION, STATUS AFTER PROTON-BEAM RADIATION THERAPY.
Clinical Features. A 16 y.o. female with a known right posterior frontal arteriovenous malformation, reevaluated approximately 1 year after proton beam radiation therapy because of headaches and visual symptoms. There was clinical suspicion of recent intracerebral hemorrhage.
CT Scan. Abnormal (Fig. 19.3, E–G).
Angio. Angiography 13 months earlier, before treatment, had revealed a large posterior frontal arteriovenous malformation (Fig. 19.3, A and B). Recent angiography, approximately 1 year after radiotherapy, revealed a significant reduction in size of both the large and small vessel elements of the vascular malformation (Fig. 19.3, C and D). The malformation now measured 4 cm in width, 3.2 cm in height, and 3.5 cm in AP diameter (corrected for magnification). The volume of shunting had been reduced. There was now evidence of a striking right suprasylvian mass effect, with depression of the sylvian triangle and 9 mm displacement of the internal cerebral vein to the left. This was diagnosed as a sizable hematoma.
A and B. Initial right carotid angiogram; lateral films at 1 and 2 seconds. The malformation is fed by several greatly dilated frontal opercular branches of the middle cerebral artery.
C and D. Lateral views of the recent right carotid angiogram, at the same time intervals as in **A** and **B**. Reduction in size of the feeding branches, the smaller vessels of the nidus, and the superiorly draining cerebral vein is visible. There is now a striking suprasylvian mass effect.

E–G. L 15   W 20.
E. A very large volume of diminished absorption is shown in the right frontal lobe. This involves widely the overlying cortex and extends across the midline just anterior to the left frontal horn. There is considerable dislocation of the septum lucidum to the left. A rounded volume of high absorption (2 x 2.5 cm in diameter, peaking at about 40 units) is evident in the region of the posterior frontal operculum and extending deeply.
F. The region of markedly diminished absorption is again evident in the frontal region and extends posteriorly to involve the parietal lobe in this section, which is 2.5 cm above that in **E**. Midline dislocation to the left is again evident.
G. This scan section is immediately below that in **E** and again shows the widespread low absorption region in the frontal lobe, involving the cortex and white matter.
The low absorption area is quite sharply, although somewhat irregularly, demarcated. The absorption value of this lesion extended down to approximately 4 units, and it is therefore consistent with a large area of severe encephalomalacia, probably with some cavitary changes. The findings suggest an area of old infarction, possibly with a contribution from radiation necrosis in the region of the vascular malformation. A relatively recent and moderate-sized area of intracerebral hemmorrhage has clearly occurred. This and associated edema explain the contralateral midline dislocation that is present in spite of the malacic changes.

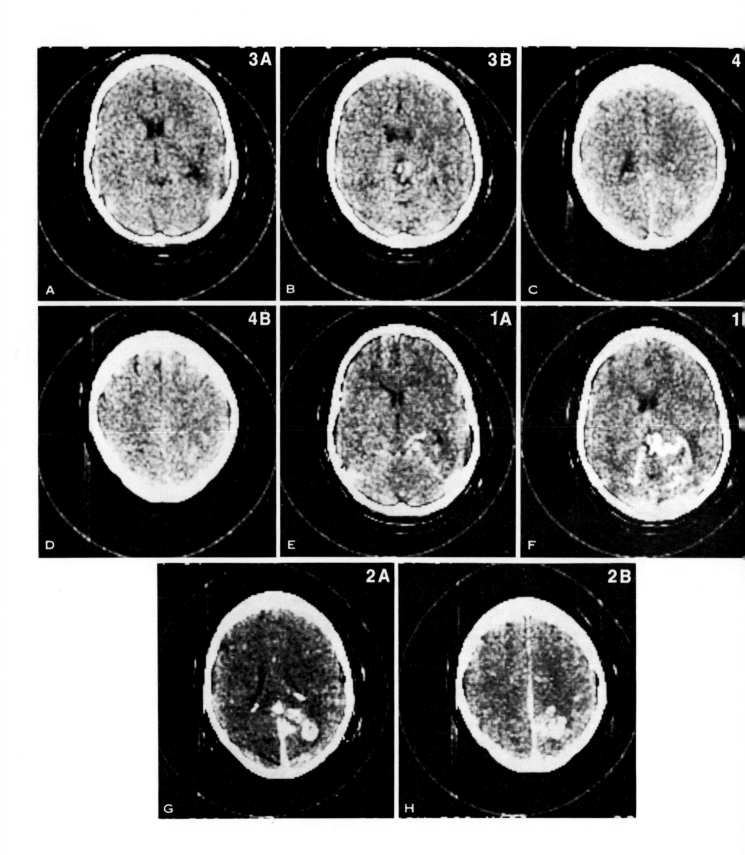

FIG. 19.4. ARTERIOVENOUS MALFORMATION.

Clinical Features. A 49 y.o. female who 3 months earlier had begun to experience episodic subjective vertigo, especially with change in her head position. The surroundings would appear to spin and she experienced loss of balance.

Neurological Examination. Alert and well oriented. Normal fundi. Nystagmus on lateral gaze, more marked on gaze to the left. Full visual fields. Examination was otherwise normal.

EEG. Borderline abnormal, symmetrical tracing, without focal abnormalities.

Skull Examination. Normal.

RN Scan. Tcp; positive on two recent occasions. Dynamic scan showed asymmetrical activity in the early phase and abnormal prolongation of increased activity in the posterior right cerebral area, near the midline. Static scan showed increased uptake in the occipital area, just to the right of the midline. These findings suggested a vascular neoplasm or arteriovenous malformation.

CT Scan. Abnormal plain and contrast-enhanced scans, typical of arteriovenous malformation (Fig. 19.4).

A–D. Consecutive 13-mm sections from below superiorly, without contrast enhancement. 160 x 160 matrix system.

A. Slight enlargement of the posterior portion of the right temporal horn is evidenced by a low absorption region lateral to the quadrigeminal cistern. Between the cistern and the temporal horn are small focal areas of slightly increased absorption.

B. The pineal is included in this section and is displaced approximately 4 mm to the left of the midline. Immediately to the right of the calcified pineal is a comma-shaped circumscribed region of increased absorption (peak, 30). Extending laterally in an arcuate fashion from the latter is a band of increased absorption extending to the region of confluence of the right temporal horn and trigone, the position of which is just suggested by the presence of tiny areas of low absorption.

C and D. In the posterior parietal and anterior occipital regions, irregularly rounded zones of increased absorption (peak, 30) are visible. The trigone and posterior portion of the body of the right lateral ventricle are inconspicuous and appear compressed. In **C,** calcification in each lateral ventricular glomus is evident and that on the right appears dislocated anteriorly.

On the plain scan, the peak absorption and form of the regions of increased absorption are indicative of a vascular malformation. Adjacent regions of diminished absorption, seen with some larger arteriovenous malformations and thought to be due to cerebral atrophy and areas of gliosis, are not identified in this case.

E–H. Consecutive 13-mm sections obtained after injection of 300 ml of meglumine diatrizoate 30% by drip infusion. Two hundred ml of the contrast medium were infused rapidly before scanning and the remaining 100 ml were infused slowly during the scan. The sections correspond approximately in level and angle with those in **A–D,** respectively. The vessels of the malformation are now very clearly identified, including smaller channels lying in the quadrigeminal and ambient cisterns, both immediately behind and to the right of the midbrain (**E** and **F**), a large vessel extending posteriorly from the quadrigeminal cistern through the region of junction of the left temporal lobe and upper cerebellum (**F**), and serpiginous and saccular large vascular channels involving the right posterior temporal, parietal, and occipital regions (**F–H**). In **G** are visible an enlarged great vein of Galen and straight sinus. The choroid plexuses of the lateral ventricles are also clearly visible extending anteriorly from the partly calcified glomi. Local mass effect, displacing the right trigone anteriorly, is more obvious in **G** than in **C.** The falx has become very dense with contrast enhancement, as expected (**H**). Absorption in the vascular malformation ranged up to 49 units, and there appeared to be a small focus of calcification within the malformation (peak, 70 in **H**).

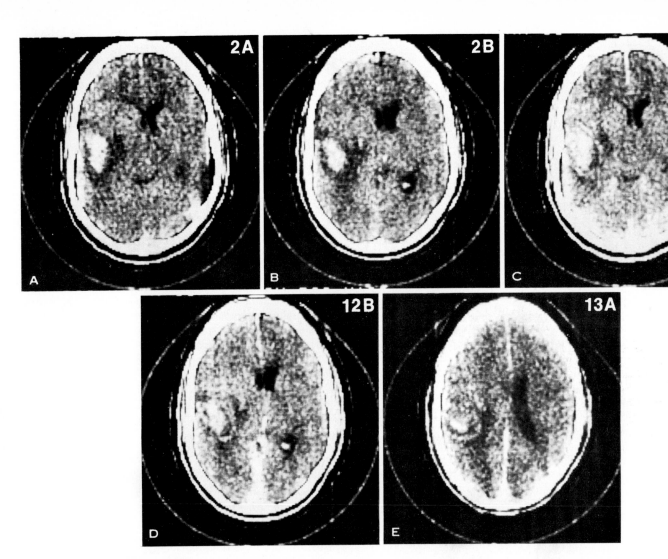

FIG. 19.5. ARTERIOVENOUS MALFORMATION WITH HEMORRHAGE.

Clinical Features. A 20 y.o. male who had an acute onset of severe pain in the left frontotemporal region and behind the left eye, at times sharp and steady and at other times throbbing in character. He had difficulty in finding words and in pronunciation of some words. A few hours later, he developed nausea and vomiting. There was no previous history of headache or seizure disorder. Early motor and intellectual development were entirely normal.

Neurological Examination. Oriented and alert. Literal and verbal aphasic errors. Poor capacity to read and write, although calculations were performed well. Right superior homonymous quadrantanopsia. No motor or sensory abnormalities.

EEG. Abnormal, with left-sided slowing.

Skull Examination. Normal.

RN Scan. Tcp; dynamic and static imaging revealed no abnormality.

CT Scan. Abnormal (Fig. 19.5, **A–E**).

Angio. Arteriovenous malformation and mass effect (Fig. 19.5 **F**).

A and **B.** L   14   W   30.   160 x 160 matrix system. Contiguous 13-mm sections.

This scan without contrast medium reveals a fairly discrete region of increased absorption (peak, 38 units) in the anterior and middle portions of the left temporal lobe. This is surrounded by a zone of diminished absorption (6–14). These features are indicative of a hematoma with surrounding cerebral edema. In both sections, there is a faint suggestion of curved narrow bands of slightly greater density within the zone of edema. A moderate mass effect is indicated by generalized compression of the left lateral ventricle and displacement of the septum lucidum some 6 mm to the right of the midline. The pineal (**B**) is not dislocated.

C and **D.** L   14   W   30.

Scan sections corresponding with those in **A** and **B**, respectively, following intravenous injection of 300 ml of Renografin 30% by infusion. No change in absorption of the hematoma and surrounding edema has occurred, but there is now clear demonstration of narrow arcuate bands of increased absorption (peak, 24, with partial volume phenomenon) in the area of surrounding edema. (A diffuse increase in density of the tentorium is indicated in **C**, which also shows opacification of vessels in the region of the posterolateral tentorial margins. Opacification of the upper portion of the sigmoid sinus is visible on the right in **C**. These are commonly visualized normal features following high-dose contrast enhancement). In **D**, an unusually broad straight sinus is shown.

E. Contrast-enhanced section immediately above that in **D**, showing the posterior portion of the temporal hematoma, behind which an arcuate band of increased absorption (peak, 30) is visible in the zone of edema. Anteriorly, small rounded areas of increased absorption (peak 24–28) are indicative of additional enlarged vessels. The compression of the body of the left lateral ventricle is well shown. The enhanced density of the falx is visible anteriorly and posteriorly, and it shows slight angulation towards the right.

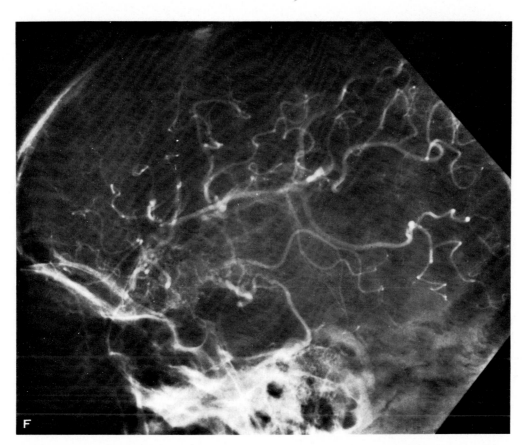

F

F. Left carotid angiogram, lateral midarterial phase. There is moderate general elevation of the sylvian branches of the middle cerebral artery. The small vessel type of arteriovenous malformation is projected in the anterior temporal area. The frontal series revealed that the malformation lay in the insula and was supplied by many small branches of the sylvian vessels in the anterior portion of the sylvian cistern. The vein draining posteriorly and inferiorly from the malformation arose antero-medially and evidently represents the most obvious arching vascular shadow shown on the CT scan (**C–E**). The lenticulostriate, anterior choroidal, and posterior cerebral branches were displaced medially by the temporal lobe hematoma. There was no blood supply to the malformation from the vertebral circulation, and no abnormal vessels were observed in the region of the tentorium.

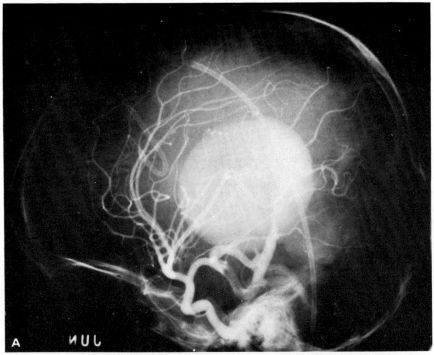

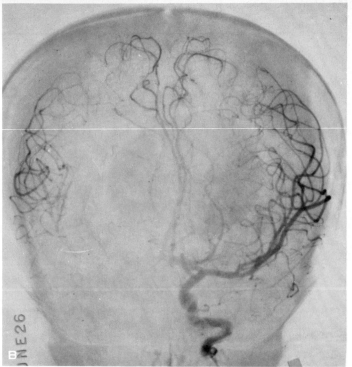

FIG. 19.6. ANEURYSM OF THE GREAT VEIN OF GALEN, ASSOCIATED WITH OBSTRUCTIVE HYDRO-CEPHALUS AND BILATERAL SUBDURAL HEMATO-MAS AFTER VENTRICULAR SHUNTING (Case contributed by Dr. Derek C. Harwood-Nash, The Hospital for Sick Children, Toronto, Ontario.)

Clinical Features. An 11-month-old boy who presented an enlarged head and increased general somatic growth (body size equivalent to a chronological age of 2½ years).

Neurological Examination. Normal, except for the enlarged head. No Parinaud's sign and no papilledema. Endocrinological tests were normal.

Skull Examination. Enlarged head and slight diastasis of cranial sutures.

CT Scan. Obtained after ventricular shunting, abnormal (Fig. 19.6, **C–H**).

Angio. Transfemoral bilateral carotid and vertebral studies showed a huge ovoid cavity in the region of the great vein of Galen, supplied by two very large arterial branches of the posterior cerebral artery (Fig. 19.6, **A** and **B**).

Operations. A ventricular shunt was placed prior to CT scan and angiography. Following these studies, bilateral subdural hematomas were evacuated. These contained serosanguinous fluid, and there was a suggestion of a very thin early membrane on the pial surfaces. The two arteries supplying the varix were ligated at their site of entry. Postoperative angiograms revealed complete occlusion of the feeding arteries.

A. Lateral early arterial phase film of the carotid angiogram, showing filling of the left posterior cerebral artery from the internal carotid. Two huge posterior cerebral branches have filled the massive ovoid Galenic aneurysmal varix (note jet effect posteroinferiorly). Although the lateral ventricles are decompressed by the ventricular shunt, the pericallosal arteries are considerably elevated and stretched by the mass. There was a striking steal effect from the normal carotid and vertebral branches.

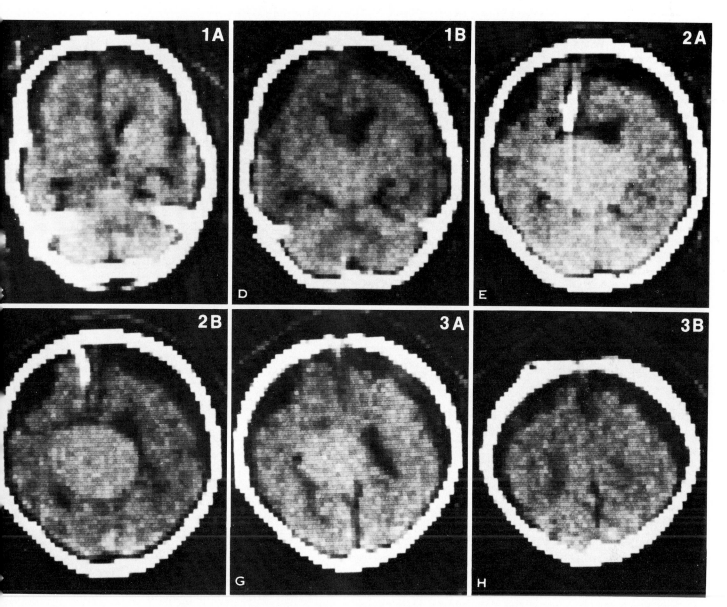

B. Arterial phase frontal subtraction of the left carotid angiogram. The pericallosal arteries are moderately bowed to the left. The marked and extensive separation of cortical branches of both cerebral hemispheres from the inner table is apparent. The density of the faintly filled Galenic varix is visible centrally and projecting more to the left side than to the right.

C–H. Contiguous CT scan sections from below superiorly. The interfrontal longitudinal fissure is displaced a few millimeters to the left and the septum lucidum is displaced a few millimeters to the right. The high absorption of a shunt tube extending to the left frontal horn is noted. The lateral and third ventricles are now dilated relatively mildly. Widespread separation of the cerebral cortex from the inner table is evident, and the configuration of the bilateral subdural collections is indicated very clearly. Absorption values of the subdural collections ranged from 0–9, with most values being in the 4–7 range. The smooth ovoid configuration of the Galenic varix is clearly demonstrated. Absorption values in this structure ranged between 13 and 21. This compares with cortical readings of 18–21 laterally and 20–23 posteriorly. The structure is clearly denser than white matter. The compression and distortion of the lateral ventricles by the mass are obvious.

Absorption of the serosanguinous subdural collections is slightly higher than CSF. Reference to Fig. 15.1 indicates that the hematocrit equivalent of the Galenic varix contents is between 25 and 35%. Actual hematocrit measurements on this boy at the time of CT scan are not available.

CHAPTER 20

Infarcts

INTRODUCTION

Our data regarding the overall accuracy of CT scanning in the diagnosis of infarction have thus far been analyzed less completely than in the major neoplastic categories. One reason for this is the lack of completely satisfying proof of the pathology in a significant number of cases.

Clinical criteria, RN scans, and angiography have been used in various combinations to provide a basis of diagnosis against which to measure the apparent efficacy of CT scans in the diagnosis of infarction. In a few instances, autopsy confirmation and correlation of large infarcts has been obtained, and good correlation of the character and distribution of the lesion with CT scan diagnosis has been found.

While precise figures are still lacking in our series, it is reasonably clear that CT scanning provides an important new method of assessing cerebral ischemia sufficient to produce appreciable edema and for the recognition of cerebral infarction in both the earlier and later stages. Overall accuracy in detection of all but the small lesions is likely to be greater than 80% and quite possibly higher than this if serial scanning is employed. Small infarcts appear to be more readily identifiable in the acute stage (first 7–10 days) than subsequently, when edema is resolving or has resolved. O'Brien et al (50) have measured the water content of brain samples obtained from cats 4 hours to 20 days after occlusion of one middle cerebral artery. Maximum water content was found in infarcted tissue at 2 days. These findings are consistent with our experience that smaller infarcts may not be visible as areas of reduced absorption when scanned on the first day or two after insult but may become visible if rescanned between 2 and 7–10 days. If such small infarctions remain as cavities of 1 cm or greater in size and are not collapsed but remain filled with fluid of the same absorption as CSF, late CT scanning has been shown capable of demonstrating the residual tissue defect. Slit cavities are likely to go undetected. Lack of detection of an infarct scanned in the first few days and/or lack of visibility after 1 to 2 weeks suggests that the infarct has been relatively small.

In our series of CT examinations, a review of cases diagnosed as cerebral infarcts on the basis of clinical features and frequently with supporting evidence from other studies indicated an overall incidence of positive CT scans in 62% (63). Most of the negative studies were in cases with presumed small infarcts and those scanned in the initial 2 days. Serial scans were obtained in only a few of these cases.

Paxton and Ambrose (51) found that CT scans were positive in 27 of 55 patients with occlusive cerebrovascular disease. CT scans were positive in each of the 15 cases studied in the first 7 days after the ictus, in 8 of 17 cases examined at 7–21 days, and in only 4 of 23 cases scanned after 21 days. Lateral ventricular enlargement was found in 11 of the 40 cases examined after 7 days. In no case of occlusive cerebrovascular disease studied by Paxton and Ambrose was an increase in absorption found at the boundaries of infarcted tissue on scans after intravenous injection of Conray (see Fig. 20.10). Our experience with as yet relatively few cases scanned after high-dose intravenous contrast medium injection suggests that irregular peripheral and central areas of increased density can be expected in a modest percentage of cases of infarct. Peripheral neovascularization is presumed to be the cause of enhancement in those scanned after 7–10 days. Extravascular diffusion of contrast medium may be responsible for central enhancement in the first days after onset of the lesion.

ISCHEMIA AND PALE INFARCTS

During the acute phase (first few days), the severely ischemic cerebral territory appears as a region of reduced absorption involving white matter and cortex or central grey matter. At this stage, it is the volume of cerebral edema that is being detected, and the area of infarction itself cannot be distinguished separately, and indeed, in certain instances, the ischemic condition may not progress to actual tissue necrosis. In the early phase, the typical lesion has an irregular, poorly defined margin and within this is a nonhomogeneous, patchy appearance of varying degrees of lowered absorption. The typical absorption range is 6–14 units. The clinical features, the somewhat lower absorption range, nonhomogeneous character, generally relatively minor or absent mass effects, and frequently, a typical vascular distribution, taken together, generally permit differentiation from most primary and secondary neoplasms. If the clinical presentation and course are atypical, a further examination of the region after 7–14 days should permit differentiation. The infarct will generally then show some diminution in the territory of diminished absorption, some increase in homogeneity, and some increase in definition of marginal contours. The latter feature, consistent with phagocytic activity in removal of necrotic tissue, is more often clearly identified after 2–3 weeks. The earliest CT scan obtained in cerebral infarction in our series was at slightly more than 24 hours after the ictus and was positive. Paxton and Ambrose (51) have recorded identification of reduced absorption in a large infarct examined 8 hours after onset. Additional scanning of the patient at 3 and 6 days revealed increasing marginal definition and some increase in homogeneity of the reduced absorption in the territory.

With the typical absorption range, the mean absorption of an acute infarct of considerable size is in the order of 10 units, some 5 units lower than the mean absorption of white matter. With smaller infarcts, significant partial volume averaging effects with surrounding normal or near normal brain will increase the apparent absorption of the infarct, raising the values and rendering the lesion more difficult to discriminate from normal structures.

In the case of larger lesions, increasing demarcation of the lesion is most frequently identified after 2–3 weeks, although it may be identified earlier. Homogeneity of the lowered absorption, combined with a further lowering of absorption values, is commonly progressive from the first week to a stable state, usually at 4 weeks or more. At this stage, a relatively well demarcated parenchymal cavity may be observed, typically with ab-

sorption characteristics identical with those of CSF. When such cavities extend deeply to become adjacent to a ventricle, it is likely that a distinction cannot be made between communication with the ventricle and separation by a thin velum. In other cases, the cavitary area is more or less completely collapsed and the adjacent portion of the ventricular system is expanded towards the lesion. The overlying surface of the brain may be observed to collapse inward, with visible enlargement of the overlying subarachnoid space. A variety of combinations of the above possibilities may be seen.

In a very few cases, CT scans of hypertensive patients with a typical past history of lacunar stroke have shown irregular cavities in the basal ganglia, with fluid content having the same absorption as CSF. Acute lacunar infarcts have been scanned but not identified by this method. It is clear that only the atypically large old lacunar infarcts will be visible, since partial volume considerations indicate that the lesion must approach 1 cm in diameter. The use of 8-mm sections should improve detectability of these small old lesions.

HEMORRHAGIC INFARCTS

While the foci of increased absorption are clearly of higher value than central grey matter and can commonly be distinguished in cortical regions, the peak absorption range tends to be appreciably less than in a typical acute parenchymal hematoma, probably due to partial volume averaging of the extravasated blood with the adjacent edema. In some instances, larger solitary foci of extravasated blood are found, more closely resembling a typical cerebral hemorrhage. In the early case, the lesion may be distinguished from the usual cerebral hemorrhage on the basis of the larger volume of surrounding edematous brain, the distribution in grey matter, and the less regular and homogeneous appearance of the extravasated blood.

Tables 20.1–20.3 indicate the results of retrospective studies of the efficacy of CT, RN and angiographic studies in the diagnosis of infarction.

TABLE 20.1
Recent Ischemic and Old Infarcts. CT Visibility in Relation to Interval between Ictus and Scan

Days	Negative	Equivocal	Positive
0–2	1 (20%)	2 (40%)	2 (40%)
3–7	2 (18%)	3 (27%)	6 (55%)
0–7	3 (19%)	5 (31%)	8 (50%)
8–14	2 (12%)	2 (12%)	13 (76%)
15–21	1 (8%)	4 (33%)	7 (59%)
22–28	0	1 (17%)	5 (83%)
More than 28	1 (2%)	7 (13%)	47 (85%)

These figures are derived from a total of 107 CT scans of 93 patients diagnosed as having had a recent (within 28 days) or old infarct on the basis of clinical and/or angiographic findings. In a few cases, autopsy confirmation was available. Thirty-seven cases of recent ischemic infarct had single scans and 7 cases had serial scans. Forty-seven cases of old infarction had single scans and 2 cases had serial scans. Individual numbers of cases scanned in the periods 0–2 days and 3–7 days were too small for reliable comparisons, but there was a suggestion that fewer cases show positive results when scanned in the first 2 days as compared with the 3–7 day period. Two cases with positive scans in the first few days showed equivocal or negative findings when re-evaluated a few days later.

TABLE 20.2
CT and RN (Static) Scans in 20 Cases of Infarct

Days from Onset	CT Scans			RN Scans		
	Negative	Equivocal	Positive	Negative	Equivocal	Positive
0–7	0	50%	50%	47%	20%	33%
8–21	16%	24%	60%	58%	8%	34%
15–21				100%	0	0
>22	0	10%	90%	55%	28%	17%

Twenty cases of acute infarction, all having one CT and one RN scan each, except for one patient who had two RN scans. Nineteen cases of old infarcts, with three patients having two RN scans each. The positive RN scans after 28 days from onset were obtained at 1 month, 37 days and 8 months, respectively.

TABLE 20.3
Correlation of CT Scan Visibility and Angiography* in Recent Ischemic† and Old‡ Infarcts. Only CT Cases with Angiogram Included. RN Results also Included

Days from onset	Angiography			CT Scan			RN Scan		
	Negative	Equivocal	Positive	Negative	Equivocal	Positive	Negative	Equivocal	Positive
0–2	4 (2)	1 (5%)	14 (74%)	2 (50%)	1 (25%)	1 (25%)	1 (50%)	0 (0%)	1 (50%)
3–7	2 (22%)	2 (22%)	5 (56%)	1 (14%)	2 (29%)	4 (57%)	3 (37.5%)	3 (37.5%)	2 (25%)
8–14	2 (33%)	0 (0%)	4 (67%)	2 (12%)	3 (18%)	12 (70%)	2 (25%)	2 (25%)	4 (50%)
15–21	0 (0%)	0 (0%)	1 (100%)	1 (17%)	3 (50%)	2 (33%)	0 (0%)	0 (0%)	0 (0%)
22–28	0 (0%)	0 (0%)	0 (0%)	0 (0%)	0 (0%)	2 (100%)	0 (0%)	0 (0%)	0 (0%)
More than 28	6 (42%)	2 (16%)	6 (42%)	1 (5%)	1 (5%)	20 (90%)	4 (50%)	3 (38%)	1 (12%)

* Angiographic findings related to occlusive disease, mass effect associated with infarction, and spasm in cases of infarction with subarachnoid hemorrhage.

† Twenty-nine cases of recent ischemic infarction with angiography. Thirty-seven CT scans (one patient with four serial CT scans, one patient with three serial CT scans, and three patients with two serial CT scans). Includes 15 RN scans, no serial scans, and 14 patients without RN scans. Includes 30 angiograms, one per patient, except for two angiograms in one case.

‡ Eighteen old infarct cases. Angiogram in each case, two angiograms on one patient (total of 19 angiograms). Total of 22 CT scans, each patient having at least one CT scan and two patients receiving three serial scans. Nine patients receiving RN scans, and a repeat scan in two of the patients.

334

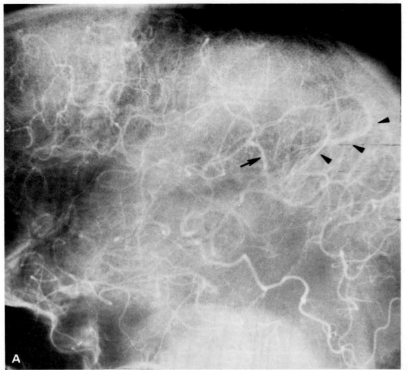

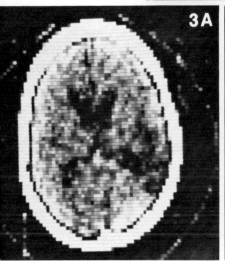
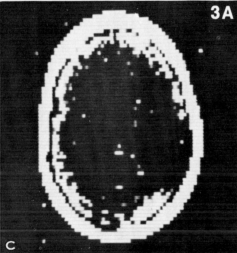
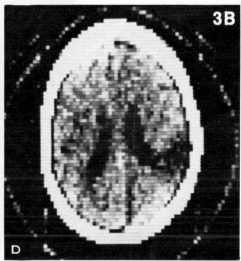

FIG. 20.1. RECENT INFARCTION, RIGHT MIDDLE CEREBRAL ARTERIAL TERRITORY, PROBABLY EMBOLIC AND 2 DAYS OLD.

Clinical Features. A 72 y.o. man who noted numbness and weakness of the left hand 2 days before CT scan. This rapidly improved.

Neurological Examination. Slight residual numbness in the left hand. No motor findings or other abnormal findings.

EEG. Mild right temporal slowing.

Skull Examination. Normal.

RN Scan. One day after CT scan, Tcp dynamic study was normal, but the static imaging showed a moderately well defined area of increased activity, with a rather wedge-shaped configuration, in the right superior parietal convexity area.

CT Scan. Abnormal (Fig. 20.1, B–D).

Angio. Direct puncture right carotid study revealed some atheroma at the common carotid bifurcation, without evidence of ulceration or important stenosis. There was circulatory abnormality in the right parietal region (Fig. 20.1A).

A. Lateral projection from the right carotid angiogram obtained 1 day after the ictus. Stagnation of circulation was revealed in cortical arterial branches in the parietal region (*arrow* and *lower arrowhead*). There was premature filling of the regional superficial ascending parietal vein (*upper 2 arrowheads*). No mass effect was identified. The findings were considered indicative of embolic infarction in the anterior parietal lobe.

B–D. CT scan obtained 2 days postictus.

B. L 18   W 20.

A wedge-shaped region of rather patchy diminution in absorption (8–14) is shown extending from an apex in the region of the trigone, anterolaterally to the lateral putaminal region and sylvian fissure, and also laterally and posterolaterally to involve the region of the superior and middle temporal gyri. The pineal is displaced about 3 mm to the left.

C. L 22   W M.

This display of the same section as in **B** shows the region of reduced absorption in the cortex of the temporal lobe. This appearance of considerably diminished cortical absorption was present in the adjacent sections, where the extent was smaller.

D. L 18   W 20.

Section immediately above that in **B**. The wedge-shaped region of diminished absorption (7–14) is shown extending laterally from the right trigone to the superior and middle temporal gyri. The two 13-mm sections above this (not shown) revealed a slighter patchy diminution of absorption in the parietal lobe.

The findings are typical of a recent infarct in the middle cerebral arterial distribution. The volume of tissue involved was considerably greater than was suggested by the clinical features.

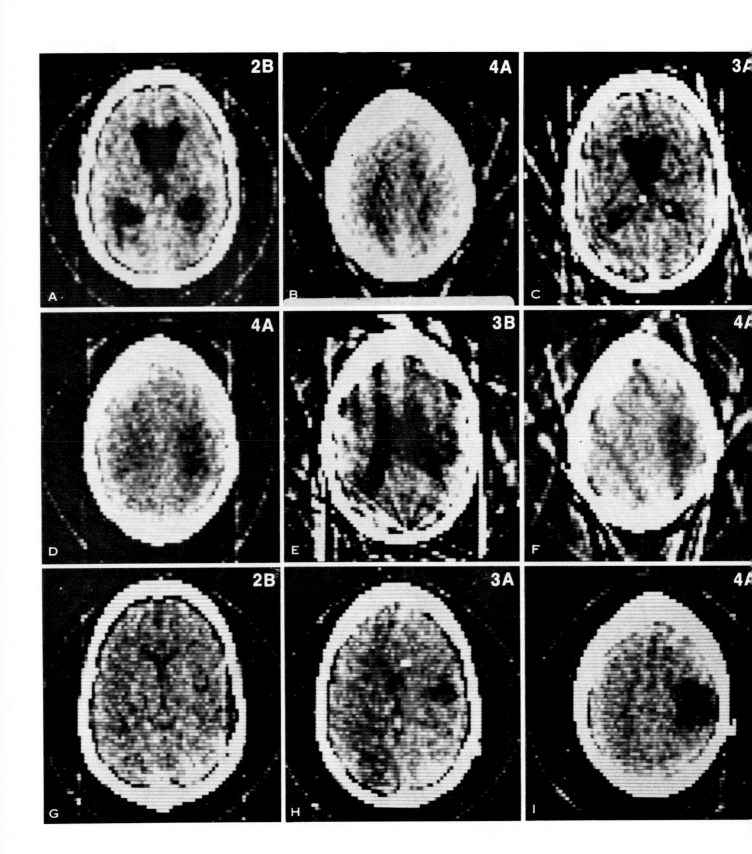

FIG. 20.2. COMMUNICATING OBSTRUCTIVE HYDROCEPHALUS AND PARIETAL INFARCTION AFTER SEVERE SUBARACHNOID HEMORRHAGE.

Clinical Features. A 46 y.o. man who developed severe bifrontal headache and collapsed the afternoon before CT scan. He was known to be hypertensive.

Neurological Examination. Initially very restless and then drowsy, complaining of severe frontal headache. Neck rigidity. No focal neurological deficit. Blood pressure was 220/150. Lumbar puncture revealed a pressure of 265 mm, with grossly bloody spinal fluid.

Skull Examination. Normal.

During the first hours after admission, he gradually became stuporous and no longer spoke or followed commands. Plantar responses became extensor.

Angio. Transfemoral bilateral carotid studies revealed moderate lateral ventricular enlargement. No definite aneurysm or mass lesion was identified.

CT Scan. Abnormal (Fig. 20.2, **A** and **B.**), 45 minutes after angiography. He continued to have episodes of agitation, but remained obtunded. Two days after the first CT scan, he had a focal seizure involving the left upper extremity. No further change in condition occurred before the second CT scan.

CT Scan. The second scan (not shown) showed slight decrease in lateral ventricular size and a questionable slight reduction in absorption in the right frontal region, raising suspicion of early infarction.

Eight days after the ictus, paresis of the left upper extremity was noted and this progressed to a left hemiplegia. Lumbar punctures showed pressures of 340 and 270 mm, with xanthochromic fluid. Speech gradually improved, but left hemiplegia persisted.

CT Scan. The third scan, 19 days after the ictus, showed further abnormality (Fig. 20.2, **C** and **D**).

Angio. Transfemoral carotid and vertebral studies 1 week after the third CT scan revealed an aneurysm in the region of the anterior communicating artery and an aneurysm at the distal extremity of the basilar artery, which showed moderate spasm. A zone of hyperemia associated with regional early venous filling was noted in the right frontoparietal region, where there was suspicion of slight diffuse swelling.

CT Scan. A fourth scan was obtained 11 days after the second angiogram (Fig. 20.2, **E** and **F**).

During this period, there was minimal improvement in the left hemiplegia. He spoke little and inappropriately. He followed few commands and evidently had a severe memory deficit.

Operation. (Dr. Robert G. Ojemann.) Twelve days after the fourth CT scan, a ventriculovenous shunt was placed, using a medium pressure Hakim valve. There was immediate improvement and his speech became much clearer, of better volume, and much more appropriate. Memory improved also. During the next month, there was increasing movement in the left leg and slight movement of the proximal portion of the left upper extremity. There was still difficulty with recent memory and more complex calculations at the time of the final CT scan.

CT Scan. Fifth scan, some 3 months after the ictus (Fig. 20.2, **G–I**).

A. L 19 W 20.
B. L 22 W 20.

First CT scan. Moderate symmetrical enlargement of the lateral ventricles and considerable widening of the third ventricle are shown. No mass effect is visible. A small region of somewhat increased absorption is evident in the region of the right sylvian cistern, raising question of a small amount of blood in this cistern. Similar areas just behind the pineal could also represent a small amount of blood in the quadrigeminal cistern. No intraparenchymal areas of abnormal absorption are visible.

C and **D.** Third CT scan. The lateral ventricles are slightly smaller than at the initial scan (**C**). There is slight dislocation of the right lateral ventricle and pineal towards the left. A large area of moderately decreased absorption, with fairly well defined boundaries and a few patchy areas of greater absorption within, is shown in the right parietal lobe (**D**). Absorption in this region was 6–16. There was only slight diminution in absorption in the overlying parietal cortex.

E and **F.** Fourth CT scan, revealing modest enlargement of the left lateral ventricle and further enlargement of the right lateral ventricle, which now bulges into the region of diminished absorption in the right parietal lobe. The third and fourth ventricles had remained unchanged in size (fourth ventricle slightly enlarged). The region of diminished absorption in the right parietal lobe is again shown. Absorption values were unreliable because of considerable head movement.

G–I. L 16 W 20.

Fifth CT scan, obtained after ventriculovenous shunting. The lateral and third ventricles are now within normal limits and the pineal is in the midline. The tip of the shunt tube is shown in the right frontal horn (**H**). The region of diminished absorption (**H** and **I**) is now much more sharply defined than on the earlier scans and shows further lowering of absorption (3–13). The findings are now indicative of a cavitated infarct.

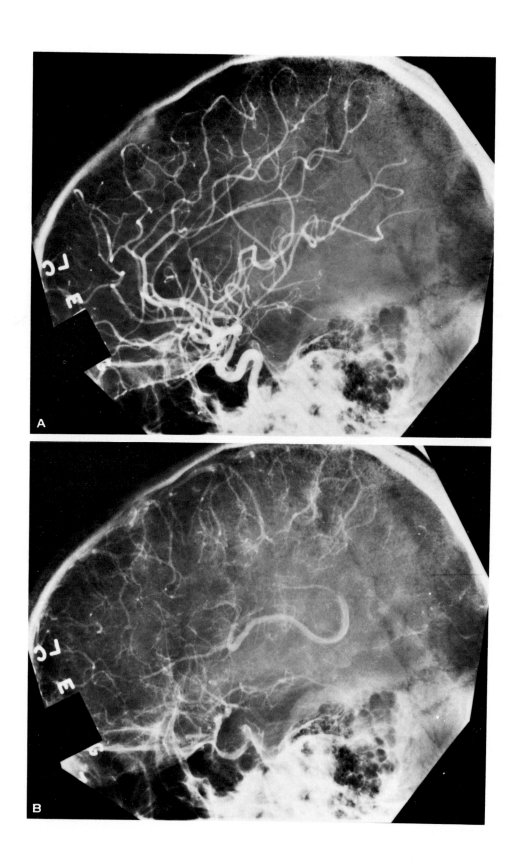

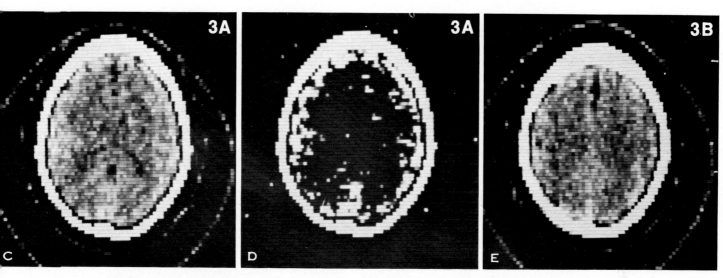

FIG. 20.3. RECENT PARIETO-OCCIPITAL INFARCTION, PRESUMED TO BE THE RESULT OF POSTPARTUM CORTICAL VEIN THROMBOSIS.

Clinical Features. A 31 y.o. female, 14 days postpartum. She had been having headaches for 12 days. Four days earlier, she became confused, dysphasic, and lethargic.

Neurological Examination. Full visual fields. No focal motor or sensory findings.

Angio. Transfemoral left carotid and left vertebral studies showed striking abnormality (Fig. 20.3, **A** and **B**).

CT Scan. Subtle abnormality, 2 days after initial angiogram (Fig. 20.3, **C–E**).

CT Scan. Repeated 10 and 17 days after the first, indicating regression of abnormality and return to normal appearances, respectively.

A. Lateral early arterial phase. **B.** Lateral midvenous phase of the initial angiogram. There was delayed filling of the posterior parietal, angular, and posterior temporal branches of the left middle cerebral artery. Subsequently, very poor perfusion of most of the left parietal lobe was noted and there was extremely poor filling of superficial parietal veins in the later phases. No mass effect was identified. The findings were thought to be consistent with cerebral infarction, probably on the basis of venous thrombosis.

C. L 16   W 20.
The scan, obtained in the third week of our experience with the method, was originally interpreted as normal. Subsequent review indicated the presence of slight lowering of absorption in the left posterior temporal and adjacent parietal lobe regions. On the original scan section illustrated here, a wedge-shaped zone of very slightly diminished absorption extends peripherally from the region of the inconspicuous left trigone.

D. L 18   W M.
Same scan as in **C**. This display reveals evidence of diminished absorption, with a patchy appearance, in the posterior portion of the left temporal lobe. There is suspicion of abnormally reduced absorption in a small portion of the region of the *right* lateral occipital gyrus.

E. Section immediately above that in **C**. There is again indication of slight diminution in absorption involving the cortex of the angular gyrus and immediately subjacent white matter. On the repeat CT scan 10 days later, abnormalities were barely detectable in the regions described, and on the final scan no abnormality whatsoever could be identified. The patient made a very good clinical recovery.

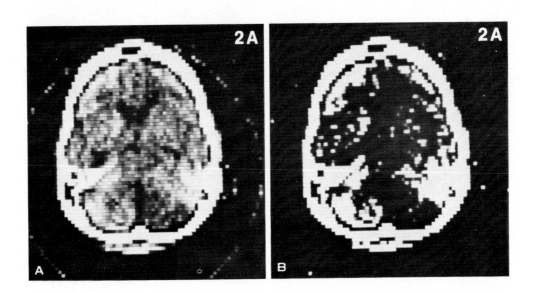

FIG. 20.4. RECENT CEREBELLAR INFARCTION, IN THE TERRITORY OF THE RIGHT POSTERIOR INFERIOR CEREBELLAR ARTERY.

Clinical Features. A 60 y.o. man who experienced acute vertigo, nausea and vomiting, and inability to stand or walk 8 days before CT scan.

Neurological Examination. Nystagmus on right lateral gaze and mild right facial weakness. Severe ataxia of stance and gait, falling to the right. Increasing severity of cerebellar signs on observation.

Skull Examination. Normal.

CT Scan. Abnormal (Fig. 20.4, **A** and **B**).

Angio. Transfemoral left carotid and vertebral studies, followed by right retrograde brachial study, revealed occlusion of the right posterior inferior cerebellar artery, without collateral flow into its territory.

CT scan obtained 8 days after the ictus.

A. L 18   W 20.

The scan shows a wedge-shaped region of appreciably decreased absorption (11–17) in the right cerebellar hemisphere, extending to the midline and to include the superficial regions. There is no visible differential absorption of the right side of the vermis or of the cerebellar grey and white matter in the involved region. The area involved corresponds with the territory of the right posterior inferior cerebellar artery. Normal absorption and differential features are visible in the left cerebellar hemisphere. The anterolateral portion of the right cerebellar hemisphere shows a normal appearance (territory of the anterior inferior cerebellar artery). (Reprinted by permission from Radiology, 110: 109–123, 1974.)

B. L 18   W M.

Same section as in **A**. The wedge-shaped area of decreased absorption on the right side is more strikingly displayed at these settings.

A repeat CT scan 16 days after the stroke (not shown) revealed a considerable decrease in the territory showing reduced absorption, and there appeared to be better-defined areas of actual tissue necrosis in the posterior portion of the cerebellar hemisphere.

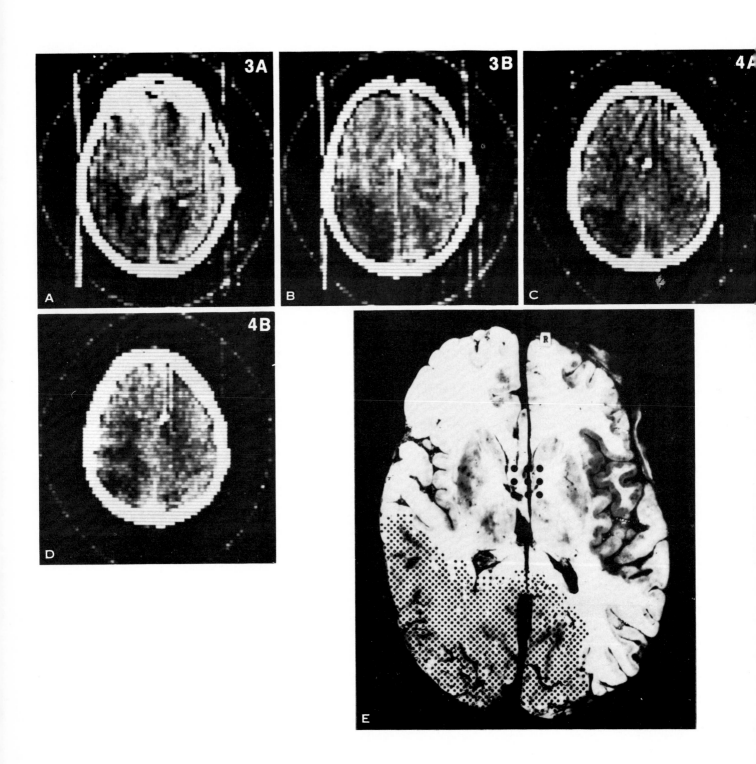

FIG. 20.5. EXTENSIVE RECENT POSTOPERATIVE BILATERAL CEREBRAL INFARCTION.

Clinical Features. A 54 y.o.female with complaints of increasingly severe headaches and memory loss of 2 years duration. Twenty-four years earlier, she had been admitted with headaches, poor memory, and double vision. At that time, she had horizontal gaze diplopia, unsteady gait, vertigo, polyuria, and polydipsia. Bilateral papilledema and superior visual field defects were noted. A ventricular shunt was performed, which ceased functioning because of adhesions and was later removed. She received radiation therapy (3000 rads). For the next 23 years, she was followed annually in clinic. There was little change in visual acuity, no diplopia, and only rare headaches. There was no further memory loss. Optic atrophy was present. One year previous to the present admission, increasingly severe bifrontal headaches and deterioration of memory were noted, associated with increasing fatigue, polyuria, and polydipsia. Polytomography of the region of the sella revealed a calcific suprasellar mass, and a ventriculoatrial shunt was introduced. Final admission was due to persistent bifrontal headaches and further deterioration of memory and gait.

Neurological Examination. Disoriented to time and place, with very poor memory and markedly reduced visual acuity bilaterally.

RN Scan. Tcp; 1 day after CT scan; normal.

CT Scan. Abnormal, with suprasellar calcifications, consistent with craniopharyngioma. No ventricular dilatation.

Operation. Partial removal of the tumor was attempted. After the operation, the patient remained obtunded. Right hemiplegia was noted 11 days after surgery.

Angio. Right carotid study 6 days after surgery revealed spasm of the middle cerebral branches and a suggestion of frontal lobe edema. There was questionable evidence of a mass in the region of the third ventricle.

CT Scan. Repeat examination 13 days after surgery showed additional abnormalities (Fig. 20.5, **A–D**).

During the next 2 weeks, she became increasingly obtunded, lapsed into coma, developed evidence of pneumonia, and died 40 days after surgery.

Histology. Autopsy revealed residual craniopharyngioma and extensive pale infarctions of the cerebral hemispheres (Fig. 20.5E).

A–D. Second CT scan, obtained 13 days after operation and 27 days before death. Sequential 13-mm sections from below superiorly.

A. Section obtained through the inferior portions of the frontal lobes, pineal, and trigones (calcified glomi). Extensive areas of reduced absorption (6–14), with a patchy nonhomogeneous appearance, are shown extending throughout the left temporal lobe and occipital lobe. The calcified right glomus is displaced somewhat anteriorly and mesially, but the pineal is midline. A similar region of diminished absorption is shown extending from the region of the right trigone posteriorly and mesially through the posterior portion of the right temporal lobe to involve the region of the posterior cingulate gyrus and posteromedial portion of the right occipital lobe. The vertically oriented band of decreased absorption in the medial anterior right frontal region has the appearance of partial volume inclusion of the subarachoid space beneath the frontal lobe.

B. The densities of shunt tubes are shown in the midline region anteriorly. The region of diminished absorption is shown again on each side.

C. The right and left shunt tubes are visible (peak, 80). The zone of diminished absorption is still visible, involving the posterior temporal and the occipital lobes. A smaller but similar region of low absorption is visible in the mesial portion of the right occipital lobe at this level. The high absorption values of shunt tubes are present in the anterior portions of the lateral ventricles.

D. At this level, very irregularly distributed regions of considerably decreased absorption are shown extending widely through the left parietal lobe to the occipital lobe. Less obvious regions of similarly decreased absorption (10–15, partial volume effect) are visible in the right parietal and occipital lobes.

E. Brain sections corresponding with a level between CT sections shown in **A** and **B**. Calcified craniopharyngioma is shown in the area of the anterior columns of the fornix, head of the right caudate nucleus, and genu of the right internal capsule (*large dots*). The extensive areas of bland (pale) infarction in the cerebral hemispheres are indicated by the *small dots*. The infarction on the right had evidently extended to involve more of the right occipital pole since the CT scan 27 days before death.

(Fig. 20.5, **A** and **E** reprinted by permission from Neurology, 25(3): 201–209, 1975.)

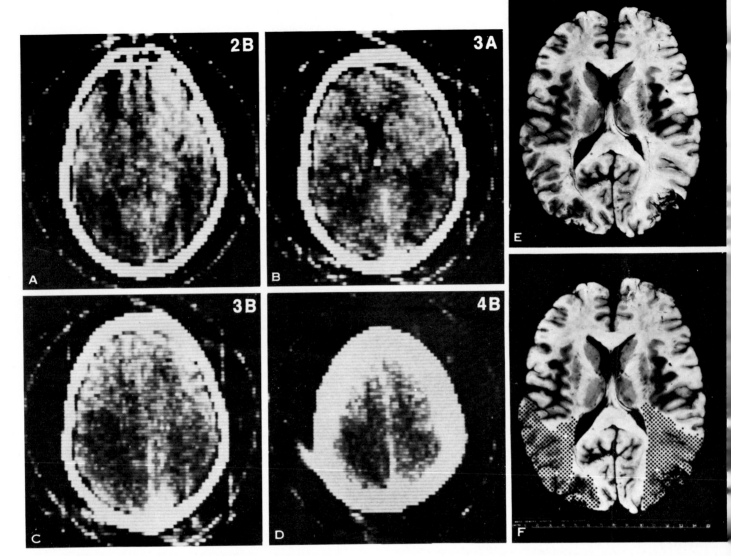

FIG. 20.6. EXTENSIVE BILATERAL CEREBRAL IN-FARCTION, FOLLOWING SUBARACHNOID HEMOR-RHAGE.

Clinical Features. A 59 y.o. male who suddenly lost consciousness 11 days before death. Postictus vomiting, headache, and neck rigidity were noted. Lumbar puncture revealed a grossly bloody spinal fluid, under a pressure of 170 mm. Seven days after the ictus, the patient had a 10-minute period of unconsciousness. Abulia, snout reflex, and mild right long tract signs were noted.

Angio. Transfemoral bilateral carotid studies 8 days after the ictus revealed an aneurysm at the termination of the left internal carotid artery and aneurysms at the primary division point of each middle cerebral artery. There was moderate spasm of the terminal portion of the left internal carotid artery, spasm of the left middle cerebral trunk and of the right anterior cerebral artery. There was also evidence of a mass effect in the region of the left basal ganglia.

CT Scan. Abnormal, 3 days after angiography (Fig. 20.6, A–D). The patient died on the day of CT scan.

Autopsy. Extensive bilateral pale infarction in the territory of each middle cerebral artery (Fig. 20.6, E and F).

A–D. Thirteen-mm CT sections from below superiorly, obtained 11 days after the ictus. There was some patient motion during the scan. The dense area in the inferior right frontal region in **A** represents partial inclusion of the orbital roof. The low density area in the inferior portion of the left frontal region on this section probably represents a combination of artifact and subarachnoid space below the frontal lobe. Extensive areas of diminished absorption are shown bilaterally, involving the cortex and white matter of the temporal lobes. The diminished absorption shows a nonhomogeneous pattern and ranged from 4 to 15 units in different areas and on different sections. The more superior sections demonstrate extension of the low absorption zones into the right and left parietal and occipital lobes. There is more striking and extensive change in the left parietal lobe (**C**). The pineal was displaced 6 mm to the left and patchy areas of decreased absorption are shown extending into the basal ganglia (**B**). The pineal also appears displaced anteriorly.

E. Brain section corresponding approximately with the level of the CT scan shown in **B** as far as the frontal region is concerned and passing at a slightly higher level than that scan posteriorly. There is extensive bilateral pale infarction in the parieto-occipital regions. Histological changes in these regions were consistent with infarction of one week duration.

F. The areas of infarction are shown schematically by small dots. Comparison with the extent of diminished absorption shown in **B** suggests that the CT scan demonstrated edema extending anteriorly on both sides, beyond the region of actual infarction. The CT scan does not differentiate between the region involved in infarction and the region of adjacent edema. (Fig. 20.6, **B**, **E**, and **F** reprinted by permission from Neurology, 25(3): 201–209, 1975).

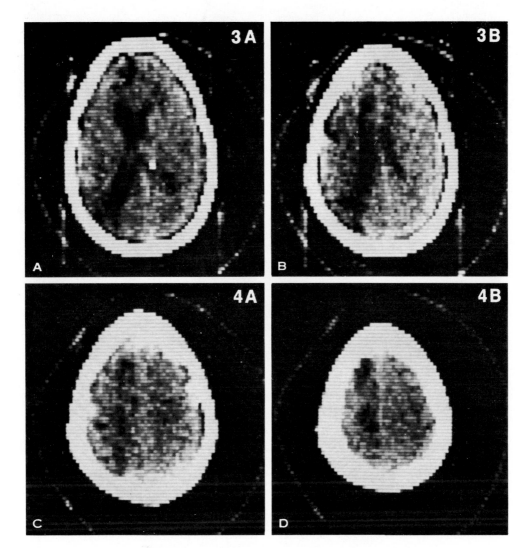

| 3A | 3B |
| 4A | 4B |

A

B

C

D

FIG. 20.7. DISTAL FIELD (WATERSHED) INFARC-TION.

Clinical Features. A 52 y.o. female who had presented in the previous year with left cerebral transient ischemic attacks. At that time, angiography had demonstrated left carotid occlusion. Subsequent to this, there had been several further episodes, with residual aphasia and right hemiparesis. Seven days before the CT scan, she had developed transient ischemic attacks or seizures, with increased weakness of the right limbs.

Neurological Examination. Mild aphasia. Dysgraphia and dyslexia, with right hemiparesis.

RN Scan. Tcp; 6 days before CT scan; dynamic study showed decreased perfusion of the left cerebral hemisphere. Static scan was suggestive of increased uptake in the left parietal area.

CT Scan. Abnormal (Fig. 20.7, A–D).

A–D. Contiguous 13-mm sections from below superiorly, 7 days after increase in right hemiparesis.

A and B. L 18   W 20.

The right lateral ventricle is normal in appearance. The left lateral ventricle shows modest generalized enlargement. The left frontal horn and left occipital horn are each enlarged towards an area of diminished absorption (frontal, 5–12; temporo-occipital, 7–12). A small region of diminished absorption is shown in the frontal white matter adjacent to the frontal horn.

C and D. Patches of obviously diminished absorption (4–16) are distributed in a broad band in the left parasagittal region, corresponding with the watershed zone. The findings are consistent with infarction in the watershed areas of the junctions of the left middle and anterior and left middle and posterior cerebral arterial territories. In addition, there is indication of small areas of infarction in the anterior territories of both right and left anterior cerebral arteries.

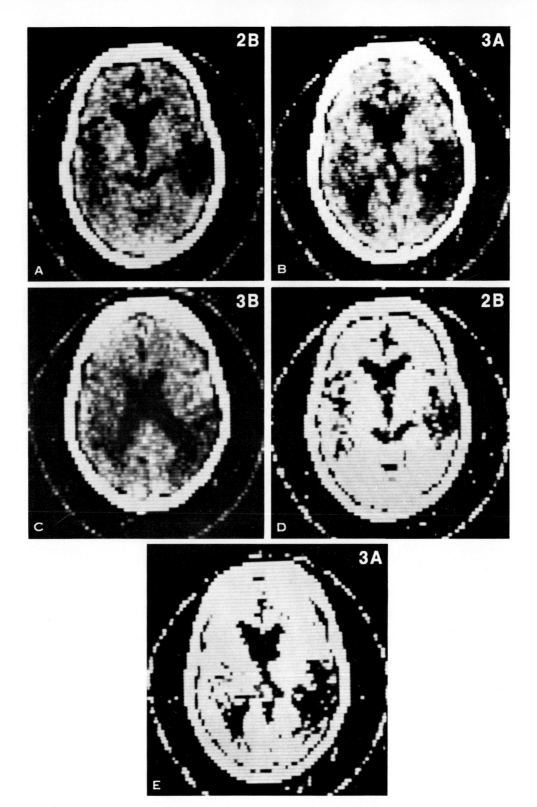

FIG. 20.8. REMOTE AND RECENT MIDDLE CERE-BRAL ARTERY TERRITORY INFARCTS.

Clinical Features. An 87 y.o. cardiologist who suffered an embolic infarct in the territory of the inferior division of the right middle cerebral artery, 5 months before death. Fifteen days before death, he developed the acute onset of aphasia and right hemiparesis.

CT Scan. Initial scan 2½ months after onset had revealed a right-sided mass, found to be a chronic subdural hematoma (Fig. 17.4).

Angio. A left carotid study, 10 days before the final CT scan, revealed occlusion of the inferior division of the left middle cerebral artery, with some collateral flow into its distal territory.

CT Scan. Abnormal (Fig. 20.8, A–E).

The patient died 5 days after the final CT scan.

Autopsy. Brain sections in the approximate planes of the CT scan showed a cavitated bland (pale) infarct, consistent with several months duration, in the right cerebral hemisphere, and softening in the left cerebral hemisphere, consistent with infarction occurring 15 days before death (Fig. 20.8, **F** and **G**).

A–E. CT scan obtained 5 days before death. There is mild enlargement of the lateral and third ventricles and enlargement of the interfrontal portion of the longitudinal fissure and of the quadrigeminal cistern, indicative of cerebral atrophy.

A and **B.** A large and quite well-defined zone of markedly diminished absorption (1–12) is shown in the area of the right temporal lobe and insula. The area merges with the right trigone, which is drawn towards the area of cavitated infarction. Although no separation between the trigone and the cavitated infarct is visible on CT scan, a thin velum was present at

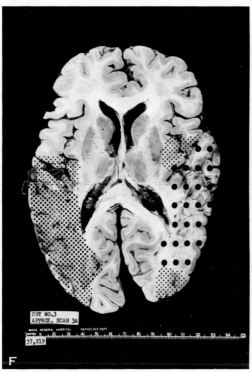

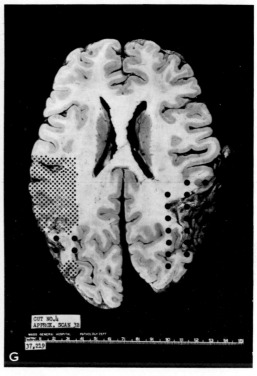

autopsy. A patchy and less sharply-demarcated region of diminished absorption (9–15) extends widely through the left temporal lobe and into the adjacent portion of the left frontal lobe. The appearance is consistent with a relatively recent infarction (10 days old by history). The cortex of the superior and middle temporal gyri does not show a marked general diminution in absorption. This may be an expression of the slightly hemorrhagic appearance of the cortex noted at autopsy. High absorption features of hemorrhage were not noted in these regions on the CT scan.

C. At this level, the patchy diminution in absorption on both sides extends into the parieto-occipital regions. Absorption values are higher because of partial volume averaging. The right occipital horn appears continuous with the deep portion of the cavitated infarct on the right side, although it was not so at autopsy.

D and **E. L 12   W M.**
Additional displays of the sections shown in **A** and **B**, respectively. The irregular encroachment by fronds of gliotic tissue upon the cavity of the old right sided infarct is indicated more clearly.

F and **G**. Brain sections corresponding approximately with the CT sections shown in **B** and **C**, respectively. The area of the remote right cerebral infarction is indicated by *large dots*. The cavity has collapsed. The surrounding associated neuronal loss and gliosis is indicated by *small dots*. The region of softening in the left cerebral hemisphere is indicated by the *medium-sized dots*. There is close correspondence with the CT scan findings on both sides.

(Fig. 20.8, **B** and **F** reprinted by permission from Neurology, 25(3): 201–209, 1975.)

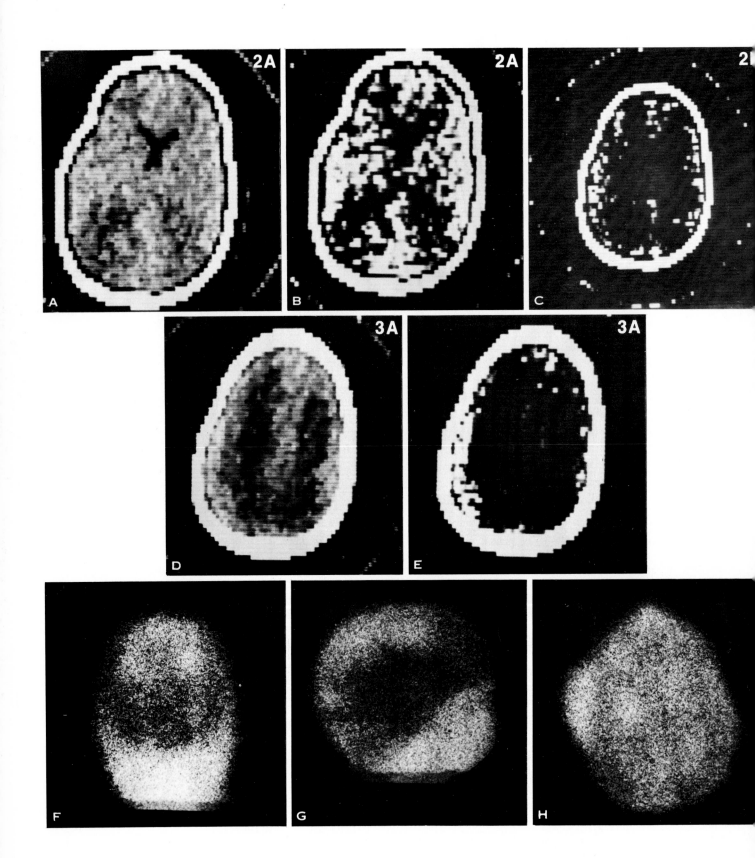

FIG. 20.9. BILATERAL DISTAL FIELD (WATERSHED) INFARCTION AND HYPOXIC ENCEPHALOPATHY.

Clinical Features. A 5½ y.o. girl who had had a left nephrectomy for Wilms tumor 8 months previously. A recent chest radiograph had demonstrated metastasis in the right middle lobe. Eight days before CT scan, the patient aspirated and was anoxic and probably hypotensive for a considerable time. Tracheostomy was performed, but she showed decorticate posturing subsequently and had remained comatose.

CT Scan. Abnormal (Fig. 20.9, A–E).

RN Scan. Tcp; 3 days after CT scan; abnormal (Fig. 20.9, F and G).

The child made a considerable recovery. Eight months later, she was generally alert and cooperative, but rather bland of affect and showing spells of inattention. She responded readily to simple questions, speaking slowly, distinctly, and articulately. The extremities were dystonic and weak, but she could ambulate with a walker.

A–E. CT scan 8 days after anoxia and probable hypotension.

A. L 15 W 20.

Extensive, rather wedge-shaped and poorly-marginated zones of decreased absorption are shown extending anteriorly from the frontal horns to the paramedian frontal lobe cortex and from the regions below the trigones to the posterior temporal, parietal, and occipital cortex. The scan was performed at a shallow angle to the baseline.

B. L 17 W M.

Same section as in **A**. At these settings, the areas of diminished absorption in white matter are exaggerated, but the patchy diminution in absorption in the cortex of the anterior portion of the left frontal lobe and on both sides posteriorly is clearly visible.

C. L 20 W M.

Section immediately above that shown in **A** and **B**. This was the best representation of cortex obtainable at this level. There is indication of widespread patchy diminution of cortical absorption, especially in the frontal lobes and in the parieto-occipital regions. Similar features were present in cortical representation at other levels.

D. L 15 W 20.

In this superior section, broad longitudinal bands of diminished absorption are shown in the superior paramedian regions of each cerebral hemisphere, indicative of bilateral watershed infarction.

E. L 20 W M.

Same section as in **D**. Cortical representation is quite well preserved in the left parietal lobe, but there is marked decrease in cortical absorption in remaining areas, particularly in the superior frontal and parieto-occipital parasagittal zones.

F–H. Static RN images obtained 3 days after the CT scan.

F. Anterior view. **G.** Right lateral view. **H.** Vertex view. Increased activity is demonstrated in broad longitudinal zones in the paramedian regions of the frontal, parietal, and occipital lobes on each side, corresponding with the watershed zones. The increased activity is a little greater on the left side.

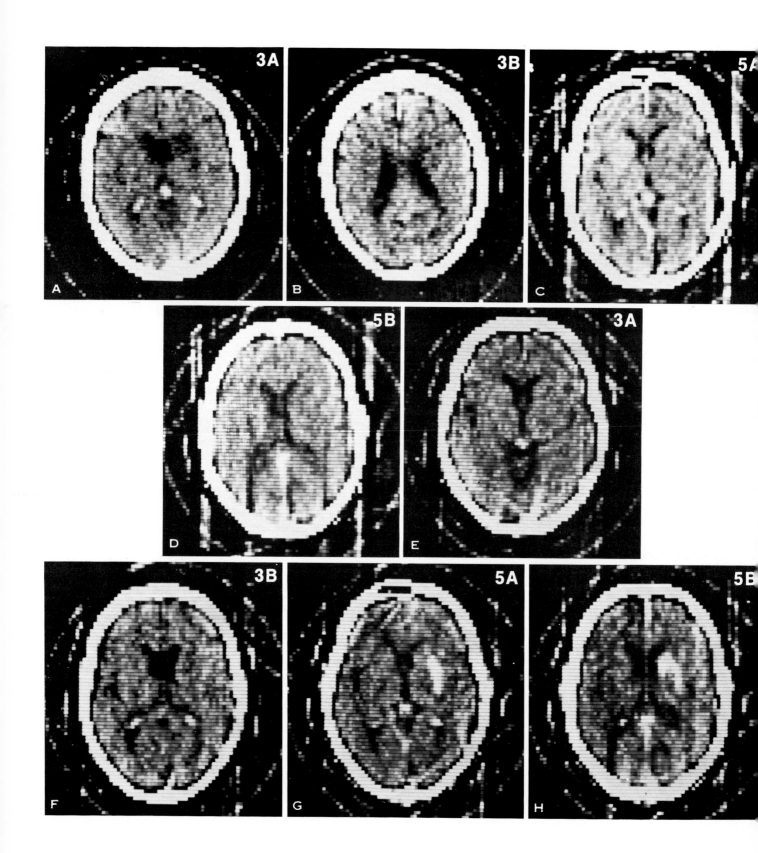

FIG. 20.10. RECENT PALE INFARCT INVOLVING BASAL GANGLIA, SHOWING INCREASED ABSORPTION FOLLOWING CONTRAST INJECTION.

Clinical Features. A 74 y.o. hypertensive male who was found comatose with left hemiparesis.

Angio. Right retrograde brachial study on the day of presumed onset revealed a recent-appearing occlusion of the right internal carotid artery from the carotid sinus to the origin of the ophthalmic artery. Flow from the basilar artery through the right posterior communicating artery entered the partially clotted right supraclinoid internal carotid segment, to proceed slowly into the right ophthalmic artery and right middle cerebral arterial stem. There was almost complete occlusion, embolic in appearance, of the right middle cerebral artery main stem, with anterograde escape of several superior and inferior division branches. The right posterior cerebral artery supplied the inferior division of the right middle cerebral artery in a retrograde direction. A left carotid study was not obtained.

CT Scan. Abnormal, 5 days after angiography (Fig. 20.10, **A–D**).

The clinical course was one of moderate improvement, with residual deficit.

CT Scan. Twelve days after angiography (Fig. 20.10, **E–H**).

A–D. CT scan obtained 5 days after presumed onset of infarction.

A and B. Scan at approximately 25° to RBL. There is a fairly well-demarcated zone of diminished absorption (8–13) lateral to a somewhat compressed right frontal horn and extending through the region of the head of the caudate nucleus into the putamen (**A**). The septum lucidum is slightly displaced to the left. In **B**, the region of decreased absorption (11–16) is hardly visible, because of partial volume averaging.

C and D. Two contiguous scan sections obtained at 0° to RBL after injection of 100 ml of Hypaque 60 M. Although the angle is different, the sections include the region of diminished

absorption adjacent to the right frontal horn shown in **A**. There was an increase in absorption of cortex and the left central grey matter. The region of decreased absorption previously demonstrated on the right side has been obliterated by a diffuse local increase in absorption, which is less than the increase in absorption shown in the equivalent and presumed normal regions on the left side. A minimal mass effect is expressed by compression and slight displacement of the right frontal horn and lateral aspect of the body of the right lateral ventricle. The change following intravenous contrast medium injection suggests that there has been an extravascular diffusion of contrast medium into the area of infarction, because of increased capillary permeability at the margins of the infarct.

E and F. Plain CT scan obtained 12 days after the presumed ictus. There are clearly appreciable small regions of slightly diminished absorption in the region of the head of the caudate nucleus and in the putamen on the right side. No mass effect is evident and there is now indication of slight enlargement of the right frontal horn in **F**.

G and H. Scan sections similar in level and angle to those in **E** and **F**, following intravenous injection of 100 ml of Hypaque 60 M. There is now a zone of striking increase in absorption (21–42) in the region of the head of the right caudate nucleus and arching into the putamen. The region showing this striking change is quite similar in position and extent to that represented by low absorption in **A**. There has apparently been a more striking diffusion of circulating contrast material from the microvasculature into the infarcted area. A small region of slightly diminished absorption is present just medial to the high absorption region in **G** (globus pallidus) and another small area of diminished absorption just lateral to the high absorption region in **H**. The appearance therefore does not suggest that the increase in absorption is attributable to marked hyperemia or neovascularization at the periphery of an area of infarction.

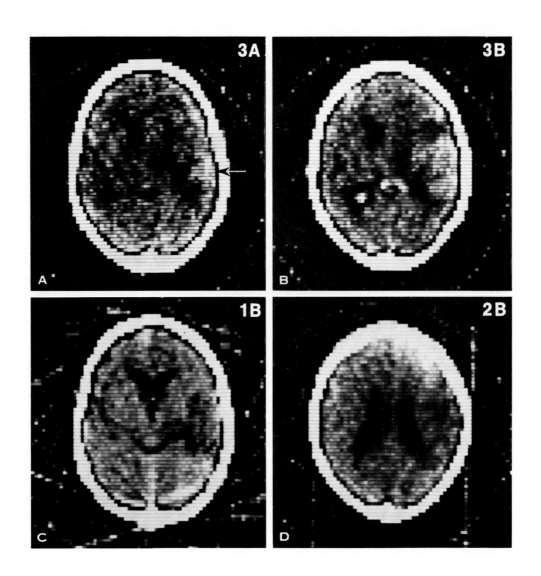

FIG. 20.11. HEMORRHAGIC INFARCTION, 8 DAYS OLD.

Clinical Features. A 75 y.o. male with a previous history of an old myocardial infarct, atrial fibrillation and diabetes, who presented with sudden onset of left hemiparesis and left hemisensory deficit, left hemianopia, and left facial weakness, 8 days before CT scan.

Neurological Examination. Alert, with neurological deficits as noted above. No carotid bruits.

Angio. A right retrograde brachial study on the day of the ictus showed a right middle cerebral artery stem embolic occlusion, with anterograde escape of frontopolar and pre-Rolandic middle cerebral superior division branches. The inferior division of the middle cerebral artery was supplied by retrograde leptomeningeal collaterals from the right posterior cerebral artery. Lumbar puncture was negative at this time.

Treatment with Heparin was started. Over the next few days, the level of consciousness decreased and hemiparesis became more severe. Lumbar puncture now showed xanthochromic fluid, which become bloody on subsequent taps.

CT Scan. Abnormal, 8 days after onset (Fig. 20.11, **A** and **B**).

Angio. Transfemoral right carotid study, after the first CT scan, revealed clearance of the embolic obstruction, a diffuse right cerebral mass effect and spasm of the middle cerebral artery and several of its branches, presumably resulting from subarachnoid hemorrhage.

CT Scan. Second examination, 18 days after the ictus (Fig. 20.11, **C** and **D**).

The patient subsequently showed a low and minimal neurological improvement.

A and **B**. Contiguous 13-mm sections from the scan obtained 8 days after the ictus.

A. There is marked displacement of the frontal horns to the left, with compression of the right frontal horn. Patchy areas of decreased absorption (8–17) are distributed through the central portion of the right frontal lobe, right putamen, right thalamus, and deeper portions of the right temporal lobe, around the posterior portion of the temporal horn. In addition, there is evidence of increased absorption in the region of the right post central gyrus (*arrow*) with an appearance of broadening of the cortical absorption in this region, fading off as it extends to the deeper region of diminished absorption. There is also a suggestion of local increase in absorption in the cortex in the area of the right middle frontal gyrus and precentral gyrus, without apparent broadening of the cortical zone.

B. Marked displacement of the frontal horns to the left is again shown, with compression of the right frontal horn. The pineal is less displaced to the left. The right glomus is displaced considerably in a medial direction. Patchy areas of diminished absorption are distributed through the central portion of the right frontal lobe and extend deeply from the region of the central fissure. Additional areas of decreased absorption are present in the basal ganglia and about the right trigone. A broad zone of increased absorption (24–33) involves the cortex in the regions of the superior and middle temporal gyri and extends deeply from these regions. This increase in absorption is diffuse, but with additional patchy areas of greater absorption scattered within.

These appearances are considered to be relatively typical of hemorrhagic changes in a large embolic infarct in the middle cerebral arterial territory.

C and **D**. Scan obtained 11 days after that shown in **A** and **B**. The lateral ventricles are now enlarged, the left more than the right. The right cerebral hemisphere mass effect is now slight. Patchy areas of diminished absorption are present in the region of the insula, temporal lobe and widely through the cortex and white matter of the parietal lobe (7–14). Small areas of diminished absorption are also visible extending deeply to the right thalamus and the third ventricle is moderately widened. No areas of abnormally high absorption are visible now.

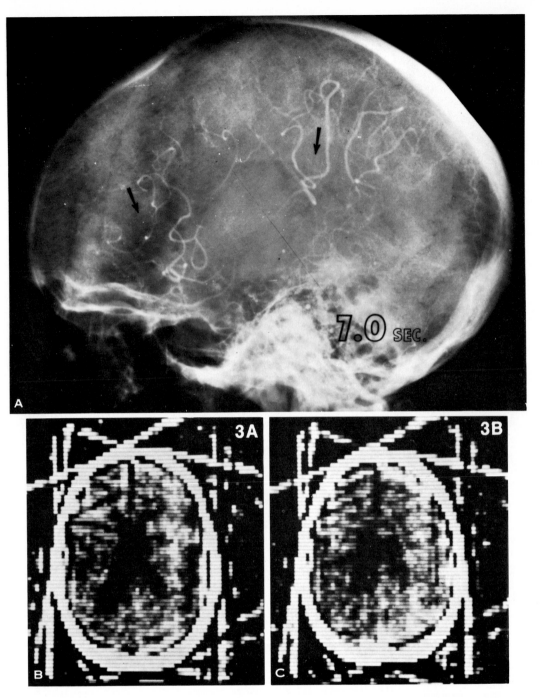

FIG. 20.12. HEMORRHAGIC INFARCT, MIDDLE CERE-BRAL ARTERIAL TERRITORY.

Clinical Features. A 49 y.o. female who had had mitral valve surgery 4 years previously. She had a history of atrial fibrillation and an old embolic infarction in the left middle cerebral territory, with mild residual right hemiparesis. Fifteen days before CT scan, she had the sudden onset of left hemiparesis, consistent with an embolus to the right middle cerebral artery. While on heparin therapy, there was progression over 36 hours to complete hemiplegia and hemisensory defect, with left homonymous hemianopsia.

Angio. Right retrograde brachial study 1 day after the ictus, showed complete occlusion of the stem of the right middle cerebral artery, with retrograde collateral flow into the middle cerebral territory from the anterior cerebral artery. There was no midline dislocation (Fig. 20.12A).

RN Scan. Tcp; normal, 3 days after the ictus.

CT Scan. Abnormal (Fig. 20.12, **B** and **C**).

A. Angiogram, lateral projection at 7 seconds, showing delayed and incomplete retrograde collateral circulation into the middle cerebral branches from the anterior cerebral circulation (*arrows*).

B and **C.** Contiguous CT sections, obtained 15 days after the ictus. There was still a dense left hemiplegia, left homonymous hemianopsia, and expressive aphasia. The patient was being treated with Coumadin. There is some degradation of scan quality because of head motion. There is slight enlargement of the body and atrium of the left lateral ventricle and the body of the right lateral ventricle appears slightly compressed. Patchy areas of increased absorption (3**A**, 20–33; 3**B**, 22–32) are shown in the area lateral to the body of the right lateral ventricle. Patches of increased absorption extend out to the opercular cortex. Focal areas of decreased absorption (2–15) are distributed medially and especially laterally to the higher absorption regions in **B**. The findings are consistent with extensive infarction in the territory of the superior division of the right middle cerebral artery, associated with hemorrhagic features.

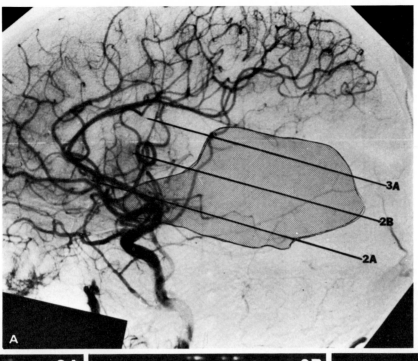

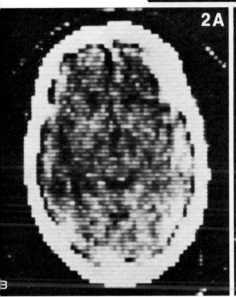
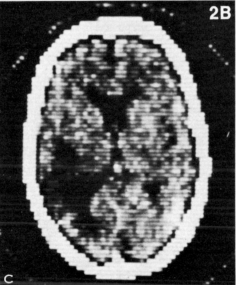
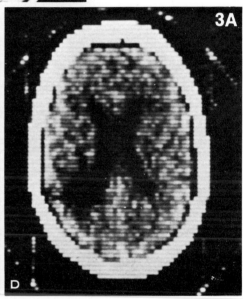

FIG. 20.13. A 7-WEEK-OLD EMBOLIC INFARCT IN THE MIDDLE CEREBRAL ARTERIAL TERRITORY.
Clinical Features. A 55 y.o. male who, 7 weeks prior to CT examination, suddenly developed confusion of speech and fell to the right, with questionable weakness of the right leg.
Neurological Examination. Sensory aphasia, hemianopsia, and contralateral hemisensory deficit.
CT Scan. Abnormal (Fig. 20.13, **B–D**).
Angio. Left common carotid study, on the day of onset; abnormal (Fig. 20.13**A**).
There was persistence of aphasia and hemianopsia 7 weeks later, at the time of the CT scan.

A. Lateral arterial phase projection, showing nonfilling of the inferior division branches of the middle cerebral artery (posterior parietal, angular, and posterior temporal branches). There was no indication of mass effect or of regional hypervascularity and early venous filling. The *shaded area* represents a reconstruction of the region of abnormal absorption demonstrated on the CT scan obtained 7 weeks later (L. R. Altemus, unpublished work).

B–D. Consecutive 13-mm sections from below superiorly, from the CT scan obtained 7 weeks after the ictus.
B. Patchy areas of diminished absorption are shown in the left temporal lobe, representing the inferior extremity of the region of infarction.
C. Section through the central portion of the region of infarction, represented by a relatively well defined zone of markedly diminished absorption. Most of this region had values ranging from 0–8 units. Medially and posteriorly, the area of infarction extended to the left trigone and occipital horn, which were enlarged. No boundary zone between the ventricle and the cavitated infarct was apparent. The third ventricle appeared displaced some 3 mm to the left, but no displacement of the pineal was identified.
D. Section through the upper portion of the infarct, which is represented by an irregular zone of diminished absorption extending anteriorly and posteriorly for a short distance beyond a moderately enlarged trigone. There is mild enlargement of the body of the left lateral ventricle also.

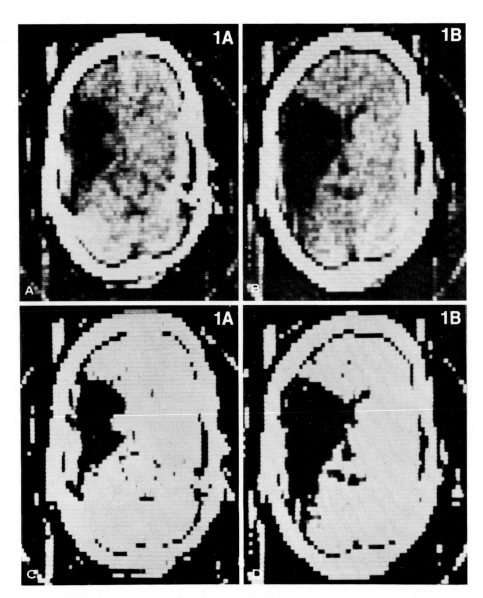

FIG. 20.14. MAJOR CAVITARY RESIDUE OF IN-FARCTION FROM MIDDLE CEREBRAL ARTERIAL OC-CLUSION 9 YEARS EARLIER.

Clinical Features. A 23 y.o. male who 9 years previously had suffered a left middle cerebral occlusion of unknown etiology.

Neurological Examination. Static residual severe aphasia and paralysis of the right arm and right side of face, with relative sparing of the right leg.

CT Scan. Abnormal (Fig. 20.14).

Angio. Left carotid study 9 years earlier had demonstrated occlusion of the left middle cerebral artery.

CT scan 9 years after middle cerebral arterial occlusion.

A and **B.** Adjacent 13-mm sections, revealing a large, sharply marginated region of markedly diminished absorption (absorption identical with that of CSF) involving the lateral portion of the left frontal lobe, temporal lobe, and centrosylvian region in continuity. In **A,** a shrunken representation of the basal ganglia projects into the large porencephalic cavity from its medial aspect. **B** shows the cavity extending without visible demarcation to include the left frontal horn. There is considerable displacement of the septum lucidum and third ventricle to the left.

C and **D.** L   12   W   M.

These control settings provide maximum discrimination of the porencephalic cavity, lateral and third ventricles, and perimesencephalic cisterns.

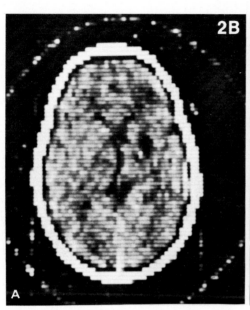 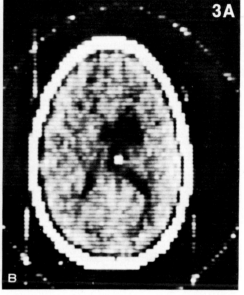

FIG. 20.15. EMBOLIC INFARCTION INVOLVING THE BASAL GANGLIA 1 YEAR BEFORE CT SCAN.

Clinical Features. A 6½ y.o. boy who developed left hemiplegia after open heart surgery 1 year previously.

Neurological Examination. Mild residual left hemiparesis, with considerable dystonia, involving the upper extremity more than the lower.

CT Scan. Abnormal (Fig. 20.15).

CT scan 1 year after the ictus.
A. L 17 W 20. **B.** L 19 W 20.

These contiguous 13-mm sections reveal a well-defined region of markedly lowered absorption involving a portion of the head of the right caudate nucleus, the anterior limb of the internal capsule, and adjacent anterior portion of the putamen. Absorption values were identical with those of the ventricles (4–12, partial volume representation of CSF and fluid in the cavitated infarct). The septum lucidum, third ventricle, and pineal were shown to be displaced several millimeters to the right. A small spot of high absorption is shown in the region of the posterior medial margin of the cavity in **A** and is consistent with partial volume representation of a very small calcification.

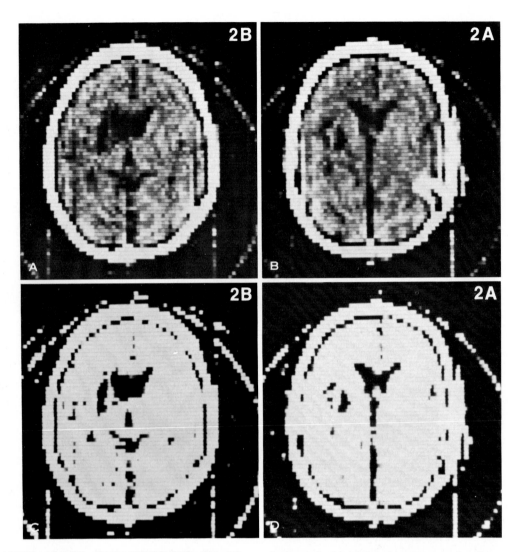

FIG. 20.16. VERY LARGE OLD INFARCTS OF LA-CUNAR TYPE, INVOLVING THE BASAL GANGLIA.
Clinical Features. A 67 y.o. hypertensive male who had suffered the sudden onset of right hemiparesis and motor aphasia 13 months prior to CT scan.
Neurological Examination. Minimal improvement since onset. Dystonic and severe right hemiparesis. There had been no new symptoms recently.
RN Scan. Tcp; normal, 3 months prior to CT scan.
CT Scan. Abnormal (Fig. 20.16).

CT scan 13 months after the ictus.
A and **B.** W 20. Contiguous 13-mm sections.
A. A sharply defined irregular oval area of markedly diminished absorption (0–10) extends through the region of the head of the left caudate nucleus across the anterior limb of the internal capsule to involve the putamen. A narrow zone of demarcation is present between the anterior portion of this cavity and the lateral wall of the frontal horn. The latter is expanded in the direction of the cavity. A poorly defined irregular region of decreased absorption is apparent in the region of the left sylvian cistern, which suggests that there may be additional malacic areas in this region.
B. Section immediately below that in **A**, showing a discrete oval region of diminished absorption (0–10) in the left putamen. Immediately lateral to this are several quite sharply defined regions of similarly diminished absorption, which may represent widening of the sylvian cistern. At this level, the head of the caudate nucleus appears intact.
C. L 8 W M. **D.** L 9 W M.
These are the same sections shown in **A** and **B**, respectively, displaying the ventricular system, cavitated central infarcts, and subarachnoid spaces more prominently.
The use of 8-mm sections would provide better discrimination of extremely small old infarcts and might permit demonstration of the larger forms of *acute* lacunar infarcts (in the order of 4–6 mm diameter). Acute lacunar infarcts have not been identified on 13-mm sections thus far.
(Fig. 20.16, **A–C** reprinted by permission from Radiology, 110: 109–123, 1974.)

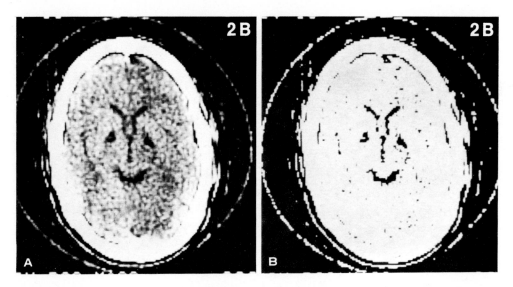

FIG. 20.17. BILATERAL SYMMETRICAL GLOBUS PALLIDUS INFARCTS, OLD.

Clinical Features. A 24 y.o. man with a history of multiple drug use for at least several years. Four months before CT scan, after an overdose of pills thought to be barbiturates, he lost consciousness and suffered an indeterminate period of apnea. After this he had been confused, with loss of memory, generalized loss of coordination, and anisocoria. Three weeks after the above event, bilateral carotid angiography revealed no abnormality. Disturbed mental status, poor memory, and marked difficulty with writing and calculations persisted.

Neurological Examination. Frequent involuntary movements of choreiform character, principally in the head and neck, but also involving the fingers and toes. Generalized hyperreflexia and right-left confusion.

CT Scan. Abnormal (Fig. 20.17).

A. L 15   W 30.   13-mm section. 160 x 160 matrix system.

The only CT scan abnormality identified is shown on this section. Triangular and quite symmetrical well-demarcated regions of low absorption (equivalent to CSF) are visible in the region of each globus pallidus. These have the character of cavitary lesions, consistent with small old infarcts. The lateral and third ventricles were not definitely abnormal in appearance, although possibly minimally enlarged for the patient's age.

B. L 12   W M.

Same section as in **A,** with control settings for maximum discrimination of the bilateral lesions and CSF-containing spaces.

The scan was repeated with 8-mm sections, which again clearly revealed the bilateral cavitary lesions. Injection of 300 ml of 30% meglumine diatrizoate produced no significant change in the appearance of the lesions, except that the partial volume averaging effect with surrounding brain was increased, due to the expected increase in absorption of the central grey matter resulting from the circulating contrast medium.

MIGRAINE

With one probable exception (Fig. 20.18), the patients with a typical history of migraine scanned by us have shown nothing remarkable on CT scans. However, the majority of these patients was not scanned during or shortly after a severe migrainous attack. According to Baker (6), several cases of migraine scanned at the Mayo Clinic at the time of a severe attack demonstrated relatively large volumes of diminished cerebral absorption, consistent with edema.

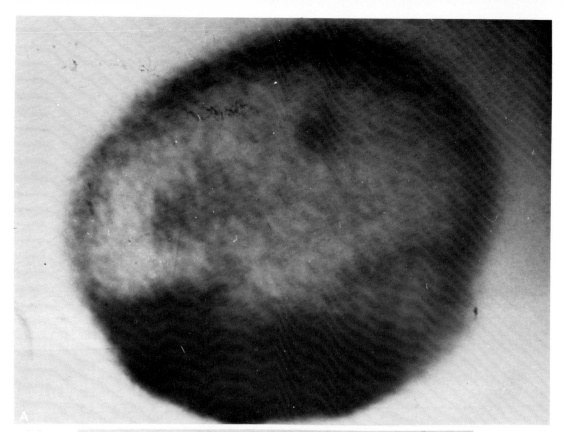

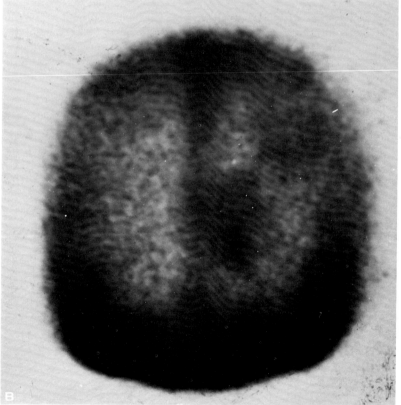

FIG. 20.18. PROBABLE MIGRAINE.

Clinical Features. A 5⁵/₁₂ y.o. girl with a 5 months history of severe occipital headaches, admitted to the Children's Hospital Medical Center under the care of Dr. Michael J. Bresnan. There was nothing unusual in the child's earlier medical history, but the mother gave a history of classical migraine. One month before admission, during a 2–3 day febrile illness, the child had become unresponsive, with drooling from the left side of the mouth and vomiting. She appeared normal in 2–3 hours. Headaches had recurred in the occipital and right or left frontal regions. These had a pounding character, tending to appear in the morning, with clearing in about 1 hour. She was apyrexial during hospitalization.

Neurological Examination. Alert, with normal memory. Bilateral papilledema, with full visual fields. Left facial weakness was present. Examination was otherwise normal.

EEG. Two examinations were abnormal, with continual, paroxysmal right frontal theta and delta slowing.

Skull Examination. Normal on two recent occasions.

Lumbar Puncture. Normal findings.

RN Scan. Tcp: markedly abnormal (Fig. 20.18, **A** and **B**). RN

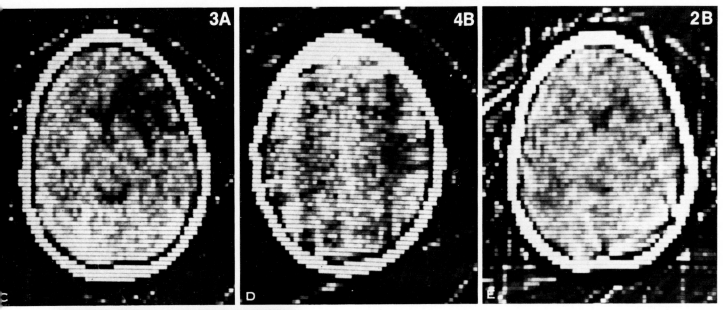

3A   4B   2B

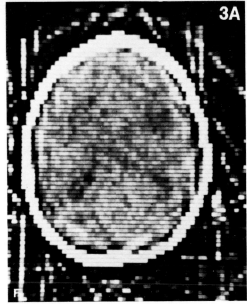

3A

scan was repeated 5 days later, following treatment with Decadron (3 mg every 6 hours) and was then normal.

CT Scan. Performed 2 days after the second RN scan; markedly abnormal (Fig. 20.18, **C** and **D**).

Angio. Transfemoral bilateral carotid and left vertebral studies following the initial RN scan revealed evidence of a very poorly localized minor right frontal mass effect. No definite intrinsic vascular abnormality was detected (Dr. Roy Strand).

PEG. Obtained 8 days after CT scan. Slight dislocation of the septum lucidum to the left, indicating a nonspecific diffuse mass effect in the right frontal lobe and, in addition, evidence of a slight mass effect in the region of the right corpus striatum.

Repeat CT scan 6 weeks later, during which time the child had done well. This showed a very slight residue of the changes observed earlier (Fig. 20.18, **E** and **F**). A few weeks later, there was recurrence of severe headaches, associated with transient attacks of *right* hemiparesis, which cleared after each episode after a nap. These attacks were followed by the onset of severe right hemiparesis and she was readmitted.

RN Scan. Dynamic and static scans, at the second admission. Dynamic scan showed slowing of circulation in the left cerebral hemisphere, with normal circulation on the right side. The static

study showed areas of increased uptake of isotope in the region of the left basal ganglia and in the frontal and parietal regions. The hemiparesis cleared rapidly in a few days on treatment with Decadron.

A. Right lateral view. **B.** Anterior views from the first RN scan. A quite discrete rounded area of increased uptake, 2–3 cm in diameter, is shown in the right anterior parietal convexity region, appearing subcortical. A large and less discrete region of considerably increased activity is visible in the area of the right frontal horn.

C and **D.** Initial CT scan. A large, irregularly marginated region of diminished absorption (6–14) is shown extending through the right frontal lobe and into the putaminal and opercular regions. The region of low absorption extends to merge with the right frontal horn, which is slightly compressed. Laterally, the lesion extends through the cortex in three different areas, producing striking diminution in cortical absorption locally. The frontal horns and third ventricle were displaced moderately on the left. The more superior section shows that the region of diminished absorption extends superiorly and posteriorly to merge with a more rounded and discrete region of diminished absorption in the anterior portion of the parietal lobe. This area measured approximately 2.5 cm in diameter, with narrow extensions laterally to involve the parietal cortex. There is considerable similarity in the configuration of the two somewhat different appearing regions shown here with the appearances on RN scan, although both lesions are shown to extend further than is indicated by the latter examination.

The initial diagnostic considerations on the basis of the CT scan were infiltrating glioma and edema associated with a cerebritis. Insufficient weight was given to the absorption range of 6–14, which is rather characteristic of extensive edema and less than is expected in most cases of infiltrating glioma.

E and **F.** CT scan 6½ weeks after the first. There has been marked improvement in the abnormalities previously demonstrated. Small, poorly defined regions of diminished absorption (8–13) are visible adjacent to the right frontal horn and extending superiorly into the two superjacent sections. No mass effect is visible now and no further abnormalities were detected in the scan. It was felt to be unnecessary to repeat the CT scan at the time of the later attack associated with severe right hemiparesis.

CHAPTER 21

Inflammatory Disease

INTRODUCTION

Cerebral Abscess

Our experience of CT findings in cerebral abscess has been derived from the study of some eight cases. In general, cerebral abscesses present in plain CT scans as regions of relatively low absorption, similar to the absorption of cerebral edema and representing a combination of the lower than cerebral absorption of contained pus and perifocal cerebral edema. In general, even a relatively well developed abscess capsule has not been differentiated within the region of diminished absorption on plain scan, presumably due to the averaging of the absorption of a capsule with the well-developed surrounding edema. During the initial stages of development of an abscess capsule, the use of intravenous contrast enhancement, particularly with higher doses (vide Chapter 27), may reveal the developing zone of higher absorption. As the capsule becomes better developed, contrast enhancement reveals a rounded zone of considerably increased absorption between the pus and the poorly marginated perifocal edema. In the more acute abscesses, this contrast enhancement is likely to be due predominantly to extravascular diffusion of contrast medium, whereas in more richly vascularized abscess capsules, intravascular (circulating) contrast medium will contribute more significantly to the enhancement.

Paxton and Ambrose (51) have reported CT scans in six patients suffering from cerebral abscess. The lesion was seen in every case. Three cases exhibited an extensive, poorly defined low density region, with marked displacement of midline structures. The other three cases showed, in addition, a ring of high absorption surrounding a central area of lower absorption. Enhancement of the ring density (capsule) occurred with injection of contrast medium.

It is likely that, in very chronic abscesses, with densely cellular capsules, the capsule itself may be discriminated on a plain CT scan. Identification of an abscess capsule obviously facilitates surgical excision of the lesion with minimum damage to uninvolved cerebral tissue and, in this respect, a CT scan is markedly superior to angiography in the many cases in which an abscess capsule is not sufficiently opacified to be visible at angiography. In such cases, relatively diffuse mass effects due to the often extensive perifocal edema may make precise localization of the abscess itself extremely difficult.

Multiloculation of abscesses seems to be rather readily identifiable by contrast-enhanced CT scanning, a point of obviously great importance in planning the surgical approach.

The plain and contrast-enhanced CT patterns found in cerebral abscesses can mimic extremely closely those visible in certain extensively necrotic metastatic neoplasms and even in some necrotic and cystic primary tumors. However, the clinical contexts will usually serve to differentiate the cases of abscess. In Figure 21.1, the abscess contained gas, which could readily be identified by its very low absorption characteristics. Such a finding is obviously a most important differential feature and may prove to be more commonly recognizable by CT than was possible heretofore.

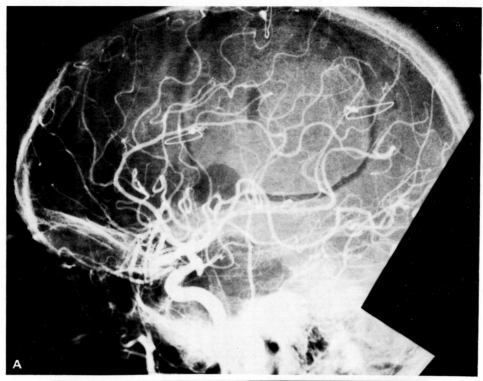

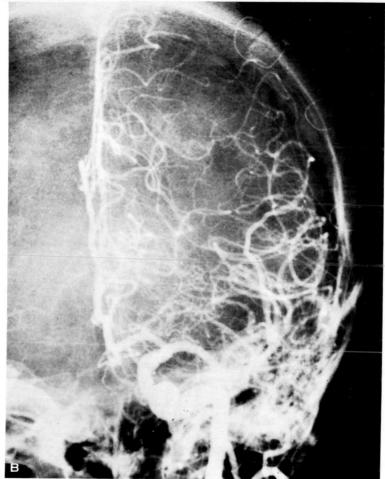

LEGEND FOR FIG. 21.1 A.B ON PAGE 364

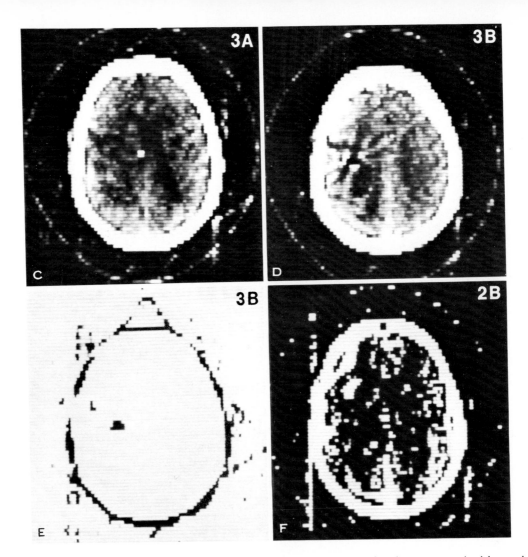

FIG. 21.1. LARGE GAS-CONTAINING CEREBRAL ABSCESS AND RECURRENT CHRONIC SUBDURAL HEMATOMA.

Clinical Features. A 69 y.o. female with aphasia and right hemiparesis. Two months earlier, a left subdural hematoma was diagnosed by angiography and evacuated. Three weeks later, recurrence of the hematoma was demonstrated by angiography and the hematoma was re-evacuated. The patient improved, but 6 days before the present admission aphasia and hemiparesis had increased.

CT Scan. Abnormal (Fig. 21.1, **C–F**).

Angio. The third angiographic study, obtained on the same day as the CT scan, revealed a left frontoparietal subdural hematoma, 13 mm in maximal thickness, and indicated in addition an intracerebral mass in the suprasylvian region (Fig. 21.1, **A** and **B**). This gave rise to suspicion of an intracerebral hematoma.

Operation. (Dr. William H. Sweet.) A large frontoparietal abscess was excised. Cultures grew anaerobic micrococci.

A. and **B.** Lateral and frontal projections, respectively, from the left carotid angiogram obtained on the same day as the CT scan. Separation of cortical branches from the inner table is visible in the frontoparietal region (**B**). The sylvian vessels are disproportionately depressed and the posterior opercular branches are focally stretched and dislocated, with separation of branches above the posterior half of the sylvian triangle (**A**). The bone flap from previous surgery for earlier evacuation of subdural hematoma is visible. The presence of a collection of gas within the cerebral hemisphere was recognized on the angiogram only after its presence had been demonstrated on the CT scan.

C and **D.** These scan sections show an extensive area of reduced absorption (6–12) in the posterior portion of the frontal lobe and extending into the parietal lobe. The lesion shows heterogeneous absorption, with multiple irregular regions of very low absorption, with intervening regions showing a lesser decrease in absorption.

C. There is marked compression of the right lateral ventricle and displacement of the midline several millimeters to the right. At the wall of the posterior body of the left lateral ventricle is a small region of high absorption (58), indicating calcification. The nature of this lesion is uncertain, but the patient had a history of old tuberculosis and this may represent a small calcified tuberculoma.

D. A small collection of gas is evident within the parietal lobe (absorption, −340). Overswing computer artifacts have resulted in local areas of high absorption readings immediately adjacent to the gas and there is some radiation of artifacts from the collection.

E. L −10 W M.

Air is shown around the head, and the pocket of gas in the parietal lobe stands out as a black zone, showing a fluid level posteriorly. There may be another, much smaller gas collection in the subcortical region further anteriorly.

F. Section immediately below that shown in **C.** The high absorption (18–30) of recurrent subdural hematoma is shown bulging internally from the inner table in the left frontal region (*arrow*).

364

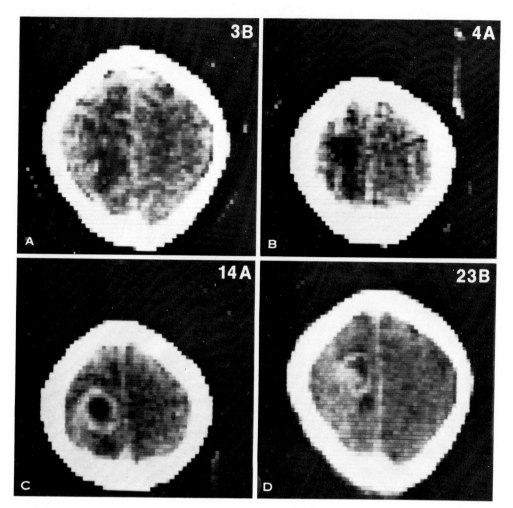

FIG. 21.2. CEREBRAL ABSCESS. (Case contributed by Dr. Leon Menzer, Sabin and Mark, P.A.)

Clinical Features. A 28 y.o. male with known Kartagener's syndrome (total situs inversus, bronchiectasis, and chronic paranasal sinusitis). He had had a right-sided motor seizure and a generalized seizure on the 2 days before admission.

Neurological Examination. Right-left confusion, finger agnosia, and inability to read or write (Gerstman's syndrome). The right plantar response was extensor.

RN Scan. Tcp; a rounded discrete region of high uptake was noted in the superior parietal convexity region on the left side.

Angio. There were signs of a not very discretely localized avascular mass lesion in the superior portion of the left cerebral hemisphere.

CT Scan. Abnormal (Fig. 21.2, A–C).

Operation. (Dr. Herbert Cares.) Craniotomy and excision of a chronic cerebral abscess from the left parietal lobe. The capsule was very thick and appeared generally avascular at surgery. One small vein was noted extending from the capsule in a superficial direction. The abscess contained approximately 8 ml of not very viscous pus, which was not foul smelling. No organisms grew in cultures (the patient had been on long term antibiotic treatment for his bronchiectasis and dosage had been increased because of suspected cerebral abscess). He did well after surgery, with no residual neurological deficit.

A and **B.** Plain CT scan sections through the superior portions of the cerebral hemispheres. In **A,** there is an irregular, heterogeneous low-absorption region involving the posterior portion of the left frontal lobe and a more discretely rounded and more homogeneous, low-absorption region in the parietal lobe. Absorption range was 9–16 units. In the next superior 13-mm section (**B**), the rounded low-absorption (6–15) lesion in the left parietal lobe is more clearly visible. No peripheral high-absorption region is visible.

C. Scan section following intravenous injection of 100 ml of Hypaque 60 M. The section is slightly below that shown in **B.** There is now a very clearly defined ring of increased absorption (11–22) at the periphery of the low absorption region, representing the abscess capsule. Increase in absorption of the capsule may be partly attributable to very slight vascularity, but is probably also the result of extravascular diffusion of contrast medium.

D. CT scan obtained approximately 1 month after surgery, also following intravenous injection of 100 ml of Hypaque 60 M. No plain scan was obtained on this occasion. A less dense and somewhat thinner ring of increased absorption and a patch of similar increase in absorption are visible at the resection site. As no plain scan was obtained, it is not clear to what extent these increases in absorption represent residual gliosis alone and to what extent minor residual hyperemia was contributory.

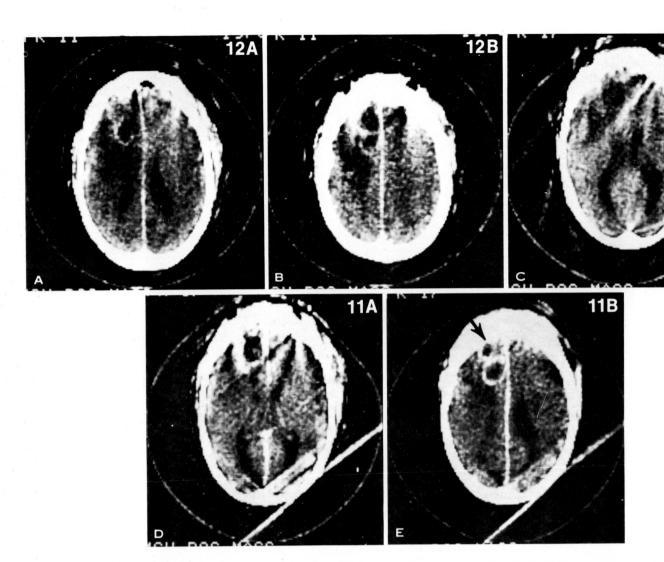

FIG. 21.3. BILOCULAR FRONTAL LOBE ABSCESS.

Clinical Features. A 65 y.o. man who had been investigated at another hospital during the previous month for evaluation of persistent headaches, abulia, and gait apraxia. There had been recent onset of right-sided weakness.

Neurological Examination. He was drowsy, without spontaneous speech. There was marked right hemiparesis.

Angio. Transfemoral bilateral carotid studies revealed bilateral superior frontal extracerebral collections.

At operation, a left epidural abscess and a right subdural abscess were evacuated.

CT Scan. The first CT study was obtained 7 days after the initial surgery (Fig. 21.3, **A** and **B**) and the examination was repeated 6 days later (Fig. 21.3, **C–E**).

Skull Examination. After the first operation, the examination showed thickening and sclerosis of bone adjacent to the frontal sinuses and opacification of these sinuses.

Second Operation. (Dr. Robert M. Crowell.) Two days after the second CT examination, a left frontal corticectomy was performed, with microsurgical excision of a bilocular left frontal lobe abscess, which extended to the pial surface anteromedially. The abscess wall was tough and thick and contained pus in which alpha streptococci and anerobic, Gram-negative

organisms were identified (similar to those obtained from the extracerebral purulent collections).

CT scans obtained 8 days (**A** and **B**) and 2 days (**C–E**) before excision of the frontal lobe abscess. 160 x 160 matrix system.

A and **B.** Scan obtained after injection of 300 ml of meglumine diatrizoate 30%. Thin arcuate rings of increased absorption are shown in the left frontal lobe. There is a very extensive surrounding region of decreased absorption (5–14) representing edema, which is also present in the anteromedial portion of the right frontal lobe (**B**). Moderate compression deformity of the anterior portion of the left lateral ventricle was visible. Before contrast enhancement, only decreased absorption was visible in the left frontal lobe and the abscess capsules were not visible.

C. Plain scan revealing only an irregular area of decreased absorption (4–17), involving much of the left frontal lobe.

D and **E.** Adjacent sections after contrast enhancement. The walls of the bilocular left frontal abscess have become very dense (16–48 in **D** and 21–35 in **E**). Absorption of the abscess contents ranged from 8–17 units, mostly in the lower portion of this range. The thick dense frontal bone is visible on these three scans. Burr holes are visible in **C** and **D** and surgical wire has produced radiating artifacts in **C** and **D**.

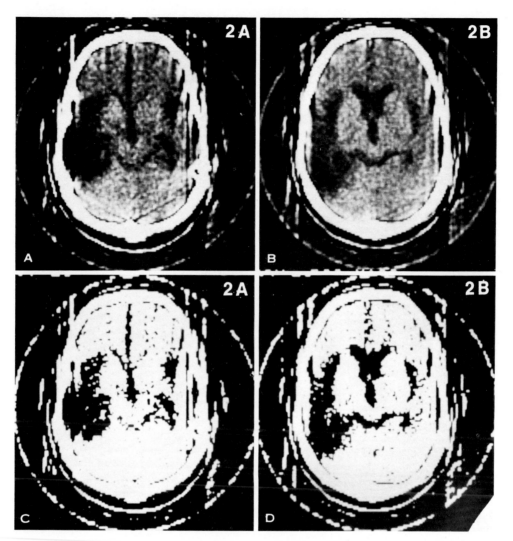

FIG. 21.4. POSTENCEPHALITIC ENCEPHALOMALA- CIA, WITH PORENCEPHALY.

Clinical Features. A 28 y.o. male diagnosed as having viral encephalitis (probably Herpes simplex encephalitis) 1 year previously at another hospital. He was in coma for 60 days and was left with residual severe language disorder and impotence.

CT Scan. Abnormal (Fig. 21.4).

A. L 16 W 20. **B.** L 12 W 30.
Contiguous 13-mm scan sections, demonstrating a large region of markedly diminished absorption replacing most of the left temporal lobe and extending into the lateral portion of the frontal lobe. Mesially, the lesion extended to the ambient cistern and choroidal fissure. The insular cortical region has been destroyed and the lesion extended to the lateral border of the putamen. On more superior sections, the lesion extended into the region of the frontal and parietal opercula. The lateral and third ventricles were slightly to moderately enlarged and the fourth ventricle appeared normal. Absorption range through the lesion was 1–12 or 13, indicating a cavitary lesion with very irregular walls.

C. L 13 W M. **D.** L 12 W M.
Same scan sections as in **A** and **B**, respectively. The irregular margins of the cavity are revealed and the frond-like, irregular projections of tissue into the cavity are seen more clearly. There is very slight deviation of the midline structures to the left. Considerable widening of the right sylvian cistern was present, suggesting previous loss of brain substance in this region also.

Comparison with a CT scan obtained 10 months earlier revealed essentially no change during that time.

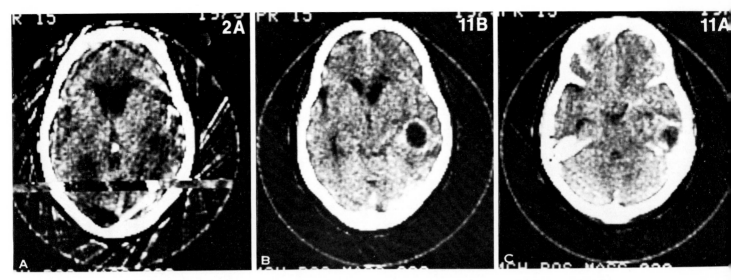

FIG. 21.5. CEREBRAL ABSCESS.

Clinical Features. A 57 y.o. female who, after a respiratory infection with fever and headache 4 weeks earlier, became lethargic and disoriented, with neck rigidity. At another hospital, CSF and blood cultures grew streptococcus fecalis. Electrocardiograms indicated an acute subendocardial anterior septal infarct.

Neurological Examination. When transferred she was lethargic and disoriented. There was severe neck rigidity and minimal weakness of the left extremities.

Skull Examination. The pineal lay 2 mm to the left of the midline 1 day before CT scan.

CT Scan. Abnormal (Fig. 21.5).

Angio. Transfemoral bilateral carotid and vertebral studies revealed a rather diffuse mass lesion in the right temporoparietal region with a suggestion of increased prominence of cerebral vessels. There was a diffuse narrowing of arterial branches in the basal cisterns bilaterally and the narrowed basilar artery was displaced posteriorly from the clivus. These changes were thought to be consistent with widespread meningitis and suggested a right cerebral abscess.

Operation. (Dr. Robert Ojemann.) A right temporal craniotomy and temporal cortical incision revealed a very firm, well-encapsulated abscess, from which pus was aspirated. The abscess was estimated to be 6–8 cm in maximum diameter. It showed a very irregular surface, with large projections anteriorly and medially. Deeply, the abscess extended to become adherent to the ependyma of the right trigone and was adherent to the petrous bone, although the dura here appeared normal. The abscess also extended to the floor of the middle fossa and onto the tentorium. Total excision was accomplished.

Plain and contrast-enhanced CT scans obtained on the day of angiography. 160 x 160 matrix system.

A. Plain scan, showing the pineal displaced 3–4 mm to the left of the midline, and somewhat greater displacement of the third ventricle to the left. A large, amorphous, and somewhat heterogeneous area of reduced absorption (4–14) is shown in the right temporal lobe and extending into the area of the trigone. Extending horizontally through the posterior portion of the scan is a computer artifact, which includes the factitious appearance of displacement of a segment of the right calvarium into the cerebral substance.

B and **C.** Scan following intravenous injection of 300 ml of meglumine diatrizoate 30%.

B. A portion of the abscess capsule is now clearly discriminated (19–33). The contained pus showed low absorption (down to approximately 2 units). Irregular areas of surrounding decreased absorption are consistent with edema. The quadrigeminal plate is visible, showing the brain stem to be slightly displaced and rotated to the left. A slightly widened posterior portion of the left temporal horn is visible. The temporal horn and trigone on the right were obliterated by compression.

C. Section immediately below that in **B**, revealing additional portions of the irregular abscess, with capsular absorption ranging up to 22 and contents ranging down to 5 units. The abscess overlies the anterior portion of the tentorium and petrous bone. It is also shown to extend to the cortical surface at this level. The inferior portions of the ambient cisterns, pontine cistern, and interpeduncular cistern were poorly defined, possibly because of increased absorption values resulting from accumulation of exudate and also compression secondary to mass effect.

Cholesterol Granuloma

For an example of this rare entity, see Figure 11.9.

Tuberculous Granuloma

No proven case of tuberculous granuloma has been encountered in our series to date. Smith et al (61) have presented a case of tuberculoma in the right frontal lobe that produced a moderate local mass effect and showed an irregular but quite well defined margin and an absorption of approximately 6–12 units. The angiogram revealed a large avascular mass. Ethier (personal communication) has described a tuberculoma that exhibited a thin dense ring and a low-density central zone on scans obtained after intravenous injection of 100 ml of Hypaque 60.

CHAPTER 22

Obstructive Hydrocephalus (Nontumorous)

INTRODUCTION

CT scanning provides a relatively simple means of assessment of ventricular size. The low absorption values of CSF (0–8 units) compared with the brain permits quite accurate evaluation of the sizes of the lateral, third, and fourth ventricles, insofar as exclusion of significant dilatation is concerned. However, if the ventricles are normally small or less than usual in size, the phenomenon of partial volume averaging of the absorption values of CSF and of brain in the same tissue block of a CT section will cause the ventricles to appear smaller than they actually are. For a discussion of this phenomenon as it involves the appearance of the transverse dimensions of the lateral ventricles, the reader is referred to Chapter 4, Figures 4.6 and 4.7. Partial volume averaging artifacts may be reduced by using 8-mm thick sections. Certain other limitations of the presently available resolution are apparent; the anterior extremity of the third ventricle is difficult to differentiate from adjacent cerebral structures and from the suprasellar cisterns. The aqueduct of Sylvius is narrow and passes obliquely through scan sections, even those taken at shallow angles to the base line. CSF in this narrow structure therefore occupies only a small fraction of each tissue block, and the aqueduct is not discriminated unless it is grossly enlarged and the scan angle is favorable (Fig. 22.6); the steep scan angle required for generally satisfactory posterior fossa examinations presents an oblique section of the fourth ventricle, which may make assessment of minor alterations in its shape difficult to evaluate. The foramen of Magendie, although usually considerably greater in diameter than the aqueduct, is often not sufficiently clearly demonstrated for useful evaluation.

The above limitations notwithstanding, the general status of the ventricular system is usually more thoroughly demonstrated by CT scanning than by complete cerebral angiography, and this is accomplished more simply and without hazard or discomfort. The method lends itself to serial assessment of ventricular size and therefore to the monitoring of the effectiveness of ventricular shunting. The larger the ventricles, the less the partial volume phenomena and the more accurate the depiction of ventricular size on CT scans.

CT scans are free of the artifactual enlargement of the ventricles that may occur at penumoencephalography and that may be quite marked (33, 56).

In some cases of chronic obstructive hydrocephalus, paraventricular zones of diminished cerebral absorption have been noted. This phenomenon may be related to one or more of the following factors: compensatory transependymal CSF absorption, breakdown of proteins, appearance of neutral fat.

The distribution and degree of ventricular enlargement generally permits indentification of the level of the obstruction. Obstruction at or adjacent to the exit foramina of the fourth ventricle generally causes very marked enlargement of the fourth ventricle, whereas communicating obstructive hydrocephalus, with obstruction of the subarachnoid pathways at the usual levels, generally produces no more than a rather modest enlargement of the fourth ventricle. Well-developed dilatation of the lateral and third ventricles, with a normal or near normal size of the fourth ventricle, generally identifies obstruction at the level of the aqueduct. However, unless the fourth ventricle is included in the scan series, it is not possible to exclude a fourth ventricular level of obstruction by this means (Fig. 22.2).

Once the presence of obstructive hydrocephalus has been established by CT scan, it may be necessary to proceed to angiography or pneumoencephalography. For example, a limited pneumoencephalogram will be advisable to exclude a small mass lesion as a cause of aqueduct stenosis and thereby to confirm the diagnosis of chronic benign aqueductal stenosis. Pneumography will generally be required for further investigation of obstruction in the lower reaches of the posterior fossa, where CT scan resolution is often less than in more superior areas. When penumoencephalography is required following CT scan identification of obstructive hydrocephalus, it is especially important that the greatest detail be obtained. For this reason, the study should include high quality laminography. With the prior information afforded by a CT scan, pneumography can be more specifically directed and smaller volumes of gas may be required.

The capabilities of CT scanning in the differentiation of normal or low-pressure hydrocephalus from cerebral atrophic diseases are of great interest. These different entities are often difficult to differentiate satisfactorily on the basis of clinical features and, hitherto, a battery of tests has generally been required to provide a basis for selection of patients for ventricular shunting. While the reliability of each test is still subject to considerable debate, no single test has proven sufficiently reliable for complete dependence.

Fortunately, the cerebral cisterns and subarachnoid spaces are usually revealed in sufficient detail by CT scanning that the need for penumography, with its attendant morbidity, is obviated in almost all cases of cerebral atrophy in which the accompanying anatomical changes in the subarachnoid spaces and/or ventricles have become established. Even quite minor enlargement of cerebral sulci and of the cerebral cisterns can be demonstrated effectively (see Chapters 5 and 23). In obstructive hydrocephalus, ventricular enlargement is accompanied by generally identifiable compression of the basal cisterns and cerebral sulci. As has been noted previously, from pneumographic studies, symptomatic normal pressure hydrocephalus is usually associated with lateral ventricular dilatation to a greater than 24-mm span of each lateral ventricle at the cella media. Symmetrical ventricular enlargement of greater degree than this is rarely seen in hydrocephalus ex vacuo in the absence of obvious enlargement of the sylvian cisterns and cerebral sulci. These cisterns and sulci are generally inconspicuous or invisible due to compression in obstructive hydrocephalus with this degree of ventricular dilatation or greater. Subarachnoid space obstruction limited to the high cerebral convexity regions (so-called convexity block normal pressure hydrocephalus), which appears to respond less frequently and less markedly to ventricular shunting, may be an exception. Pneumographic studies of this relatively poorly defined entity have often shown some enlargement of the sylvian cisterns and of at least some of the more inferior cerebral sulci. Ventricular enlargement tends to be less than in more caudally situated subarachnoid obstructions, and

these cases may represent combinations of cerebral atrophy and partial CSF absorption defect. Present, very limited experience with CT scanning in cases that appear to fall into this category has shown greater ventricular enlargement relative to subarachnoid space enlargement than is usually seen in "pure" cerebral atrophy and mild to moderate enlargement of sylvian cisterns and a few of a lower cerebral sulci. These cases have shown a mixed pattern (moderate ventricular activity and ventricular persistence of activity, combined with a slow circulation of radionuclide to the parasagittal regions), whereas cases showing typical CT scan features of obstructive hydrocephalus have generally shown typical obstructive patterns on radionuclide cisternography. Marked reduction of the callosal angle, which in our hands has continued to be a useful differentiating feature of obstructive hydrocephalus, can be inferred from CT scans, but accurate measurements are not possible.

Direct information regarding the pattern of CSF circulation that is provided by serial radionuclide cisternography is not available from routine CT scans. However, an interesting variation of CT scanning that does provide information regarding CSF circulation patterns was described by Bergstrom et al at the Tenth Symposium Neuroradiologicum (Montevideo, March 1974). This utilizes a relatively new nonionic water-soluble contrast material (Metrizamide) that can be injected into the lumbar theca. Its distribution within the cranial cavity and its clearance therefrom can be followed by serial CT scans. This method is being studied further and in comparison with radionuclide cisternography by a group in Sweden.

Scan Artifacts Produced by Metallic Shunt Valves

Radiating alternating white and black band artifacts have been encountered regularly in CT scans obtained with the 80 x 80 matrix system, when the scan section included a major segment or all of a Hakim valve, which is 12 mm in length. Such artifacts obscured much of the anatomical detail on the section, although gross ventricular size could usually be identified. These shunt valve artifacts were markedly exaggerated if motion of the head had also occurred. Samples of Hakim valves with plastic rather than metallic casings were supplied by the manufacturer (Cordis Corporation). Scans of these prototype valves were obtained and were found not to produce intracranial scan artifacts (Fig. 22.1, **B** and **C**). The program of the 160 x 160 matrix system subdues such artifacts resulting from large metal objects but does not eliminate them completely. They are still quite striking if combined with head motion (Fig. 22.1, **D** and **E**).

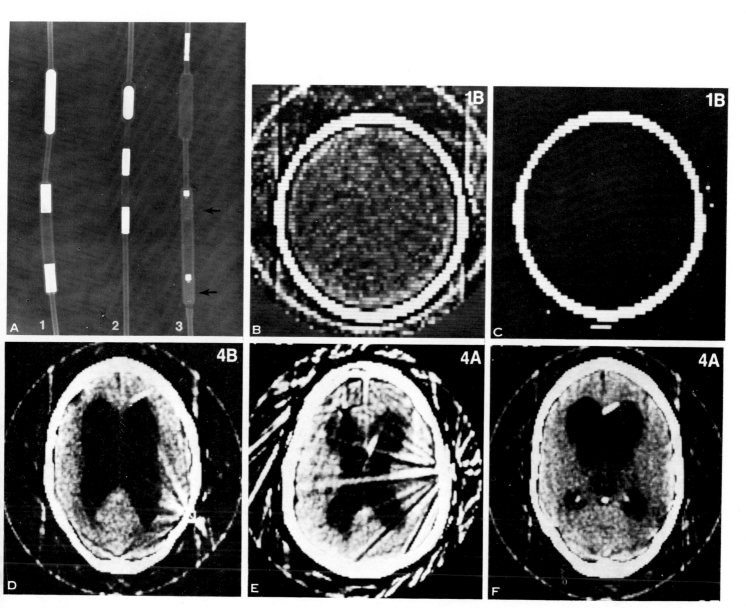

FIG. 22.1.

A. Radiograph of Hakim valves (Cordis Corporation) Adult (*1*) and pediatric (*2*) sizes of currently supplied valves, illustrating the considerable amount of metal in the valve components and pumping chambers. A prototype version (*3*) of the adult Hakim valve is shown, in which the metal casing of the valve unit has been replaced with plastic. The very small amount of metal remaining in the valve (springs (*arrows*) and threaded bases) is shown. The metal plate previously used in the pumping chamber has been replaced. The small amount of metal in a connector is shown at the top of valve *3*.

B. W 20.   **C.** L 20   W M.

Two CRT displays of a portion of a scan series obtained of a glass bottle (simulating the density of the skull) containing water. The prototype plastic-chambered adult and pediatric Hakim valves were placed on the exterior surface of the glass bottle on the right side. Valve-induced artifacts were not observed within the glass bottle on any section. A slight motion was imparted to the bottle, which was relatively loosely supported within the head bag (evidenced by the vertical external black and white streaks through the water bath on either side). An artifactual elevation of absorption values

(inherent in the old program and regularly reproduced by similar phantom studies) is evident as a peripheral ring immediately internal to the narrow black ring of computer undershoot, within the glass bottle. The values in the higher absorption zone ranged up to 3–5 units above the averaged values elsewhere within the internal water. The small amount of metal in the new valves is evidenced by a small zone of high absorption immediately to the right of the glass bottle.

C. The small metallic content of each valve is shown just outside the bottle, on the right side (peak absorption, 26 units).

D. 160 x 160 matrix system. Artifacts radiating into the head from a standard Hakim valve on the right side. There was negligible motion during this scan. Little or no artifact formation has been produced by the red rubber ventricular catheter, shown here entering the right frontal horn.

E. 160 x 160 system. The radiating artifacts from the standard Hakim valve on the right side are much more severe, due to the addition of head motion (evidenced by the streaks in the water field).

F. Scan section immediately below that shown in **D** (same scan pair). The metal of the valve is not included in this section and valve artifacts are not present.

371

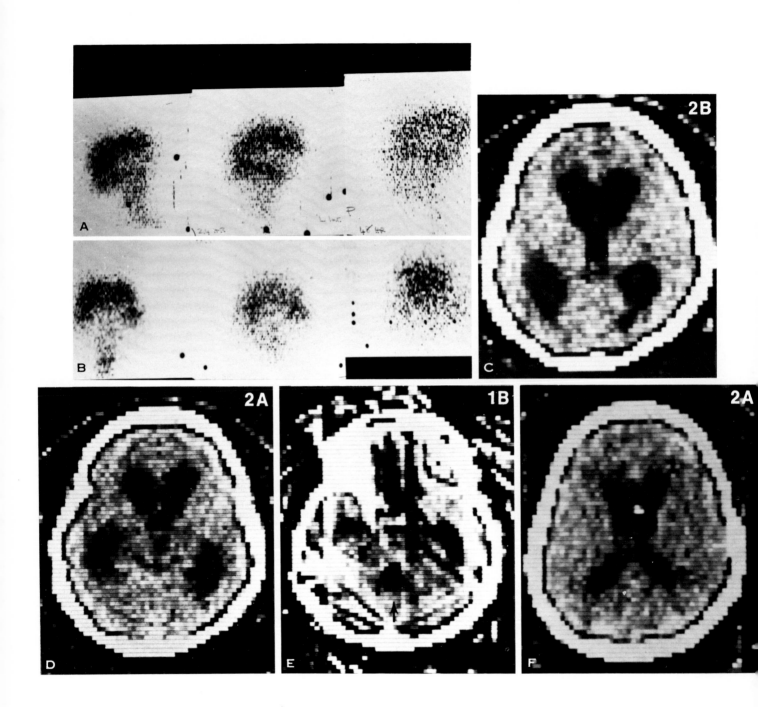

FIG. 22.2. COMMUNICATING OBSTRUCTIVE HYDROCEPHALUS.

Clinical Features. A 30 y.o. female who had suffered a severe subarachnoid hemorrhage 2 months earlier. She had subsequently developed seizures and her mental status deteriorated slowly. She was now severely abulic, without focal neurological signs.

RN Scan. [111]Indium cisternography; abnormal (Fig. 22.2, **A** and **B**).

CT Scan. Abnormal (Fig. 22.2, **C–E**).

Angio. Two months earlier angiography had demonstrated a posterior communicating artery aneurysm.

Operation. (Dr. Robert Ojemann.) Right ventriculoatrial shunt, with a Hakim valve. There was rapid and marked improvement in the patient's mental status.

CT Scan. One day after shunt (Fig. 22.2**F**).

A and **B.** Right lateral and posterior views at 4, 24, and 48 hours after lumbar injection of [111]Indium (*left to right*), respectively. This preoperative study reveals classical features of obstructive communicating hydrocephalus, with marked lateral ventricular enlargement. There is marked activity in the very large lateral ventricles at 4 hours. There is little change at 24 hours. At 48 hours (*right*), most of the activity is still in the lateral ventricles, with little in the subarachnoid spaces.

C–E. Preoperative CT scan, demonstrating well-marked enlargement of the lateral, third, and fourth ventricles. Degradation of scan detail due to motion is shown in **E**, but the enlarged fourth ventricle is visible (*arrow*).

F. Scan obtained 1 day after shunting. There has been a marked decrease in ventricular size. The tip of the shunt tube is shown as a white area centrally, to the right of the septum lucidum.

A further scan was obtained on the second postshunt day (not shown). The ventricles were now of virtually normal size. The rapid return to normal of the lateral ventricles in this young woman with a short history of secondary communicating obstructive hydrocephalus correlated well with the rapid clinical improvement. The appearance of considerable ventricular enlargement, associated with evidence of compression of basal cisterns and the absence of visible cerebral sulci, provides good evidence of the obstructive nature of the process.

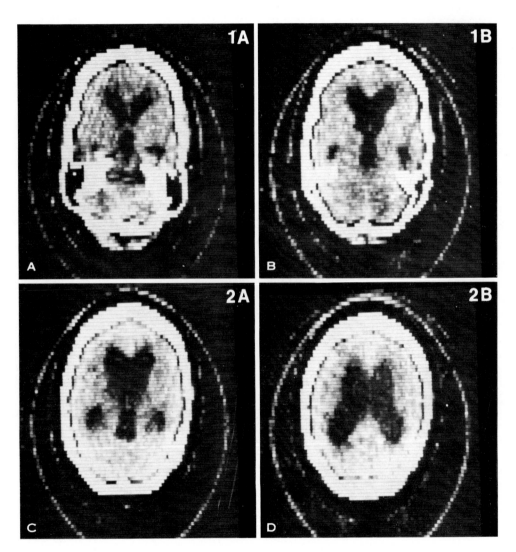

LEGEND FOR FIG. 22.3 A–D ON PAGE 377

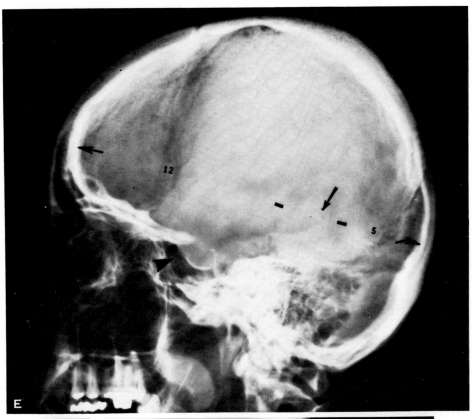

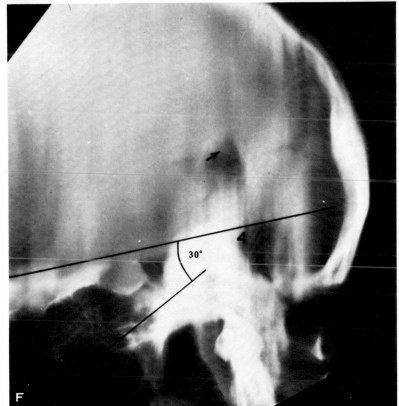

LEGEND FOR FIG. 22.3 E–F ON PAGE 377

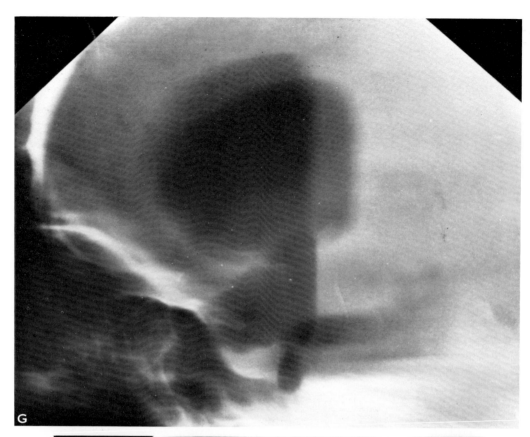

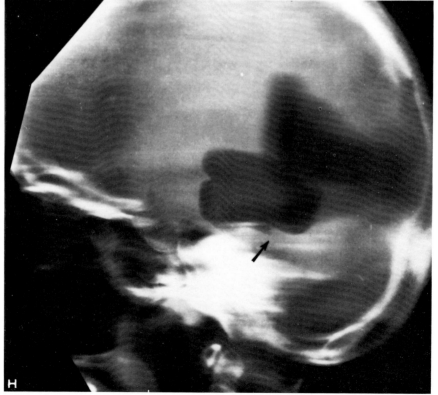

LEGEND FOR FIG. 22.3 E–F ON PAGE 377

FIG. 22.3. BENIGN AQUEDUCTAL STENOSIS.
Clinical Features. A 23 y.o. female with a history of headaches for 8 months and nausea and vomiting for 3 months.
Neurological Examination. Normal, except for papilledema.
Skull Examination. Sellar erosion, consistent with chronic expansion of the third ventricle and raised intracranial tension (Fig. 22.3, **E** and **F**).
CSF. Opening pressure, 300 mm.
RN Scan. Tcp; normal (static and dynamic studies).
CT Scan: Abnormal (Fig. 22.3, **A–D**).
Combined PEG/Ventriculogram. Abnormal (Fig. 22.3, **E–H**).
Operation. (Dr. Michael Scott.) Ventriculoatrial shunt.
A–D. CT scan shortly before pneumography.
A. Lowest 1.3 cm section, 30–35° to RBL. The fourth ventricle is not visualized. A low absorption artifact extends between the anterior portions of the petrous bones. The third ventricle is markedly widened. The inferior portions of enlarged frontal horns and expanded temporal horns are visible.
B. The foramina of Munro are well shown, separated by the anterior columns of the fornix. The enlarged temporal horns are seen in oblique section further posteriorly than in **A**. No abnormal absorption values are visible in the upper portion of the posterior fossa.
C. Severe enlargement of the frontal horns and posterior portions of the temporal horns is shown. The third ventricle is very markedly enlarged and extends far posteriorly, as a diverticulum that appears to surround a posteriorly displaced pineal (small white dot centrally). The subarachnoid spaces are not visualized, indicating generalized compression.

D. Marked enlargement of the bodies and trigones of the lateral ventricles, without visualization of the subarachnoid spaces. Subarachnoid spaces were not visible on more superior scans.
E. Erosion of the lamina dura of the sella, more marked erosion of the tuberculum sellae, mild sellar expansion, and slight truncation of the dorsum are all features consistent with chronic increase in intracranial pressure associated with impingement of an expanded third ventricle upon the sella. These features in a young patient without focal neurological signs permitted the provisional diagnosis of benign aqueductal stenosis. Posterior displacement of the pineal (*arrow*) suggested posterior bulging of a markedly expanded third ventricle.
F. Lumbar injection of gas resulted in filling of a somewhat depressed fourth ventricle, without further ascent in the ventricular system. Gas was arrested at the upper end of the pontine cistern by the downward bulging floor of the third ventricle. Some gas entered expanded subarachnoid spaces dorsal to the midbrain (*arrow*). Pineal calcification lies just above the arrow (midline tomogram).
G. Following ventricular injection of gas, very markedly enlarged frontal horns were shown. The ballooned third ventricle impinges upon the eroded tuberculum sellae and is draped over the slightly eroded superior dorsum.
H. Brow-down lateral projection, showing the stenosed aqueduct (*arrow*) just below a large diverticular posterior expansion of the third ventricle. This diverticulum has occurred below the pineal (midline tomogram).

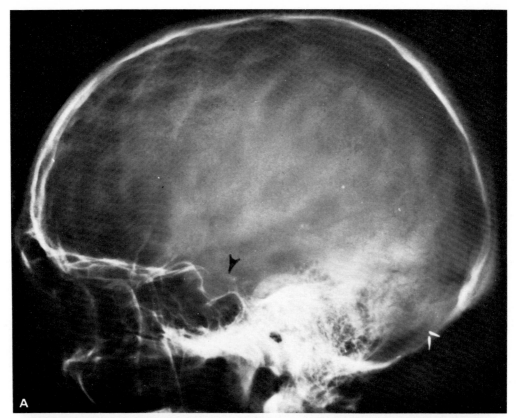

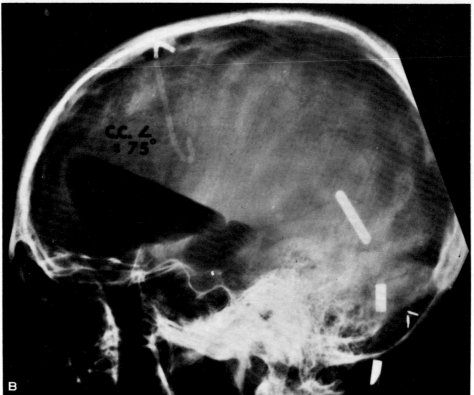

FIG. 22.4. CHRONIC SEVERE OBSTRUCTIVE HY-DROCEPHALUS WITH CERVICO-OCCIPITAL JUNC-TION ARACHNOID CYST.

Clinical Features. A 47 y.o. male who was apparently well until 3 months of progressive spastic paraparesis and mental slowing led to evaluation at another hospital. Angiography and ventriculography there revealed gross enlargement of the fourth, third, and lateral ventricles. At posterior fossa craniotomy, an arachnoid cyst of the cervico-occipital junction was found and partially resected. Over 6 months postoperatively, extreme mental slowing and spastic paraparesis persisted, resulting in further evaluation.

Neurological Examination. Marked slowing of mental re-sponses, blurred and pale optic discs, ataxia of left upper extremity, and severe spastic paraparesis in flexion.

Skull Examination. Truncated dorsum sellae, prominent con-volutional markings over superior convexities, and suboccipital craniotomy defect (Fig. 22.4A).

RN Scan. Normal.

CT Scan. Abnormal (Fig. 22.4, **D–F**).

PEG. Abnormal (Fig. 22.4, **B** and **C**).

Operation. Ventriculoatrial shunt, at which time CSF under markedly increased pressure was found. Over 2 months postoperatively, mental status cleared and spastic paraparesis resolved in large part.

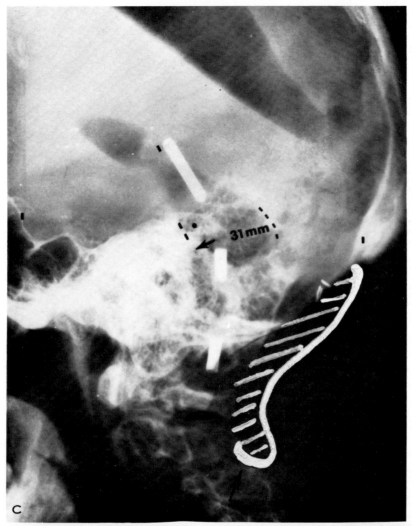

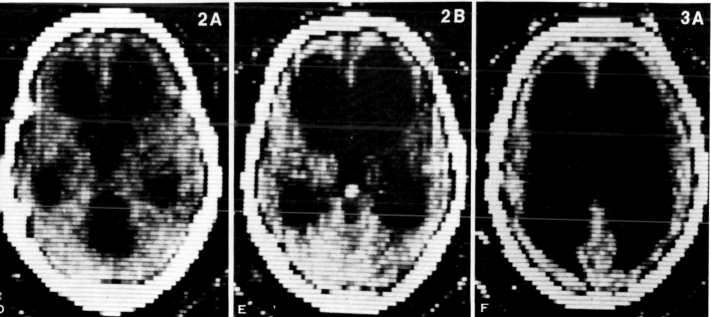

A. Skull x-ray; mildly truncated dorsum, increased convolutional markings over convexities, and suboccipital craniotomy defect.

B. PEG 3 weeks postoperatively; lateral, hanging head; severely expanded lateral and third ventricles, with third ventricle impinging on dorsum sellae. The callosal angle was 75°.

C. PEG 3 weeks postoperatively; lateral upright; greatly expanded fourth ventricle, especially posteroinferiorly. Cervico-occipital subarachnoid cyst is drawn in for clarity. Low basal cisternal obstruction was present. Shunt apparatus is shown.

D and **E.** Very severe enlargement of fourth, third, and lateral ventricles.

F. Marked lateral ventricle enlargement with a very thin cortical mantle. All basal cisterns and superior subarachnoid spaces were markedly compressed in appearance.

Although the clinical history suggested that increased intracranial pressure had existed for only a few months, skull film studies revealed evidence that increased pressure had existed during the growth period (prominence of convolutional impressions in the superior vault regions).

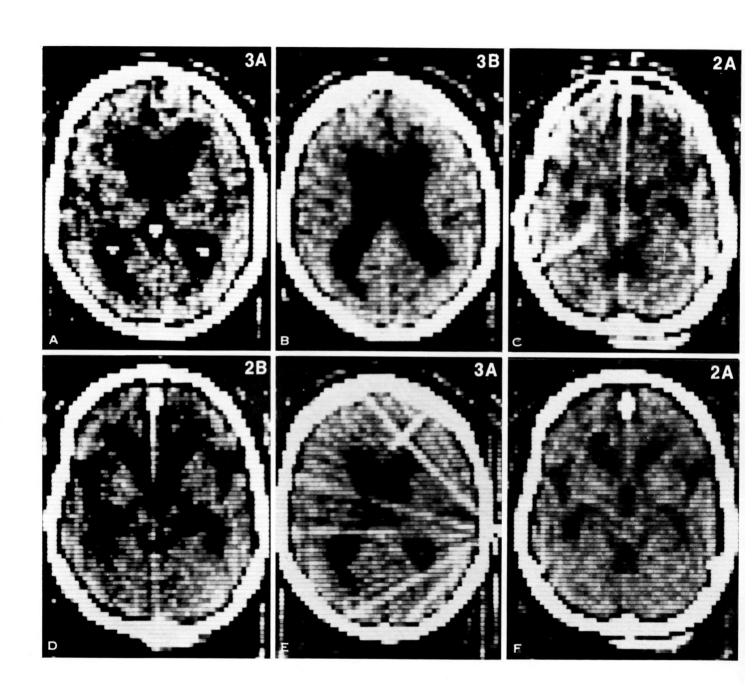

FIG. 22.5. CONVEXITY BLOCK NORMAL PRESSURE HYDROCEPHALUS.

Clinical Features. A 72 y.o. male with slowly progressive gait disturbance over 7 years and mental decline over 1 year. Recent urinary incontinence and progression of gait disturbance to inability to stand without support.

Neurological Examination. Revealed apathetic and at times incoherent responses. Bilateral grasp and suck reflexes were present.

EEG. Bifrontal slowing.

CSF. Opening pressure, 150 mm.

Skull Examination. Normal.

RN Cisternogram. At 4 hours there was activity in enlarged lateral ventricles, persisting at 24 hours, at which time the study was terminated. No activity over cerebral convexities.

CT Scan. Abnormal (Fig. 22.5).

Angio. Lateral ventricular width was 28 mm bilaterally.

PEG. Marked enlargement of fourth, third, and lateral ventricles. The callosal angle was narrowed to 105°. Dilated temporal horns. Large cisterna magna and larger than usual pontine and interpeduncular cisterns. Little gas above the tentorium, except for several dilated inferior frontal sulci. No gas over cerebral convexities.

Operation. (Dr. Robert G. Ojemann.) Ventriculoatrial shunt. The patient was responding slowly at the time of discharge 1 month later.

Several months later, distinct improvement in gait and mentation were being maintained.

A. Moderately severe enlargement of the third and lateral ventricles and moderate widening of the sylvian cisterns. Lower convexity and frontal parasagittal sulci are also enlarged.

B. Higher section through the bodies and trigones of enlarged lateral ventricles. The tops of enlarged sylvian cisterns are seen and the frontal longitudinal fissure is widened slightly. More superior sections (not shown) revealed *no prominent sulci in middle and high convexities.*

C. Section through the enlarged fourth ventricle and enlarged temporal horns. Interpeduncular and suprasellar cisterns are not remarkable, but the inferior portions of gaping sylvian cisterns are well demonstrated. Falx ossification is visible anteriorly.

D. The section passes through huge sylvian cisterns, large ambient cisterns, posterior portions of large temporal horns, and the inferior portions of enlarged frontal horns. A very wide longitudinal fissure and falx ossification are visible anteriorly.

E and F. Nine days after shunting, considerable decrease in lateral ventricular size is shown. There appeared to be slight decrease in size of the third and fourth ventricles. Note the striking artifact due to inclusion of part of the Hakim valve in the section shown in **E.** The shunt tube enters the right frontal horn.

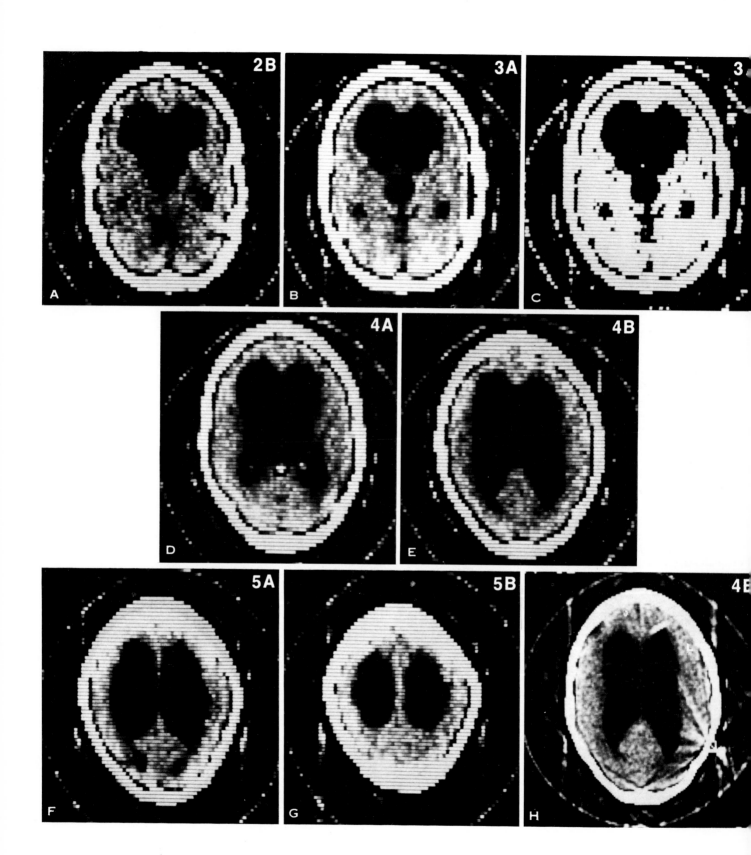

FIG. 22.6. GROSS COMMUNICATING OBSTRUCTIVE HYDROCEPHALUS, IDIOPATHIC NORMAL PRESSURE TYPE.

Clinical Features. A 60 y.o. female, admitted for evaluation of unsteady gait and loss of balance. The patient had noted difficulty with gait originating approximately 20 years earlier, but this had become significantly worse during the past year. She tended to fall backwards and to the right. There had also been increasing urinary incontinence, with rare bowel incontinence.

Neurological Examination. The patient was quite well oriented but had difficulty with recent memory. No abnormality was found in cranial nerve function, except for bilateral hearing loss and left tinnitus. The optic discs were normal. She exhibited a grossly spastic gait and poor balance. There was mild ataxia of both lower extremities. Babinski responses were positive bilaterally. General sensory examination was normal.

Lumbar Puncture. Revealed normal CSF pressure and fluid constituents.

Skull Examination. Normal, except for sclerosis of the walls of the sphenoid sinus and of the right mastoid, consistent with past inflammatory disease.

RN Scan. Tcp; normal.

CT Scan. Grossly abnormal (Fig. 22.6).

Operation. (Dr. Robert G. Ojemann.) Ventriculovenous shunt, with a high-pressure Hakim valve.

The patient showed considerable early improvement in gait and balance.

CT Scans. Postoperative scans were obtained 9 and 21 days after shunting. At 9 days there was no definite change in ventricular size. On the second examination, there was a suggestion of very slight diminution in ventricular size. A further scan 7 months after shunting revealed a distinct but quite modest reduction in lateral ventricular size (Fig. 22.6H).

A–E. Initial CT scan. Marked enlargement of the lateral, third, and fourth ventricles is shown.

B. L 12   W 20.   **C.** L 10   W M. These displays of the same section reveal a 6-mm wide vertical band extending posteriorly from the greatly dilated third ventricle and having absorption characteristics of a CSF-containing space. This appears to be a greatly widened aqueduct of Sylvius. This is only the second case in over 2000 scans with the 80 x 80 matrix system in which it was believed that the aqueduct could be identified.

E–G. The grossly dilated and quite symmetrical lateral ventricles extend far superiorly. The occipital horns are included in sections **E** and **F**.

H. Postshunt scan (160 x 160 matrix system), obtained some 7 months after operation, revealing the distinct but rather modest decrease in size of the lateral ventricles. This section includes a portion of the shunt valve and reveals less intracranial artifact from this cause than is generally seen under similar circumstances with the 80 x 80 matrix system. There was only slight lateral head movement during this scan. The density of the ventricular shunt tube is shown in the anterior portion of the right lateral ventricle.

Although there was evidence that the patient's hydrocephalus had been present for some 20 years, her clinical condition improved considerably a short time after shunting. This occurred in spite of the absence of any definite decrease in ventricular size in the early postoperative scans.

BENIGN INTRACRANIAL HYPERTENSION

Introduction

The ability of CT scanning to exclude with certainty the presence of obstructive hydrocephalus, and its capabilities in revealing the absence of mass effects and of abnormal absorption values associated with focal lesions, render valuable assistance in establishing the diagnosis of pseudotumor cerebri. Further support for the diagnosis is obtained when the lateral ventricles are found to be smaller than expected for the age of the patient. In assessing this feature, partial volume averaging effects must be kept in mind. As has been described earlier (Chapter 4, p. 45, and Fig. 4.6), the width of normally small or smaller than average lateral ventricles cannot be measured accurately from CT scans. Very small lateral ventricles appear almost invisible.

From the foregoing, it will be appreciated that recognition of unusually small lateral ventricles that are due to benign intracranial hypertension will be easier in middle-aged patients than in children, in whom the lateral ventricles may normally appear exceptionally small on CT scans.

In the few cases of benign intracranial hypertension studied by this means, lower than normal absorption values of the cerebrum, associated with increased fluid content, have not been identified.

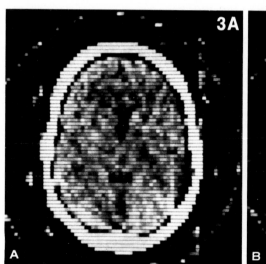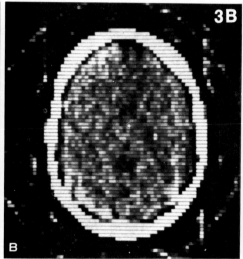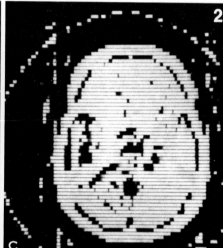

FIG. 22.7. BENIGN INTRACRANIAL HYPERTENSION (PSEUDOTUMOR CEREBRI).
Clinical Features. A 43 y.o. moderately obese female.
Neurological Examination. Normal mental status. Bilateral papilledema, without hemorrhages or exudates. Neurological examination was otherwise normal.
Skull Examination. Normal.
RN Scan. Normal.
Angio. Bilateral carotid angiograms were normal and indicated small lateral ventricles.
CT Scan. (Fig. 22.7).
After initial glycerol therapy, she was treated with a course of prednisone, with improvement of the papilledema. Over a period of 7 months, her status has remained normal (Dr. Vincent Perlo).
A and **B.** These adjacent sections reveal extremely small and relatively poorly defined frontal horns. The third ventricle is barely visible and the trigones are not discriminated, although the quadrigeminal cistern is clearly visible. More superior scan sections did not reveal the bodies of the lateral ventricles.
C. L 12   W M.
The fourth ventricle is not displaced and appears generous in size. No regions of abnormal absorption to suggest focal parenchymal disease were identified at any level. General cerebral absorption ranges appeared normal.

CHAPTER 23

Cerebral Atrophies

INTRODUCTION

The diverse entities that result in cerebral and cerebellar atrophy are collectively the commonest form of intracranial pathology. Until the advent of the EMI Scanner, no noninvasive method existed for the demonstration of the presence, distribution, and severity of the group of diseases causing decrease in brain substance. Computed tomography generally permits highly accurate demonstration of focal and diffuse cerebral atrophy. Ventricular size is demonstrated without the artifactual changes that may be induced by pneumoencephalography. The subarachnoid spaces can be assessed quite completely, without the morbidity associated with gas studies. Although details of anatomical changes are less readily demonstrated in the midbrain and posterior fossa, a generally satisfactory gross assessment can be made if the technical quality of the scan is not appreciably degraded by motion. Demonstration of minute structures and small channels such as the aqueduct cannot, however, match the capabilities of pneumoencephalography.

In general, the difficulties associated with diagnostic evaluation of cerebral and cerebellar atrophic conditions by means of CT scanning involve interpretation of the significance, if any, of the observed morphological changes in relation to the patient's neurological disability. It has become apparent that the normal sylvian cisterns generally are only just recognizable and that the convexity and superior cerebral sulci generally are not visible in normal children and young adults. It remains to be evaluated, on the basis of greater experience, to what extent the more frequent visualization of cerebral sulci, obviously widened cerebral sulci, slightly enlarged-appearing sylvian cisterns, and slight ventricular enlargement, all commonly seen in older adults, represent changes with age that are generally not associated with clinically identifiable neurological disease. It already appears probable that there will not be a high correlation between relatively minor morphological changes and neurological disability.

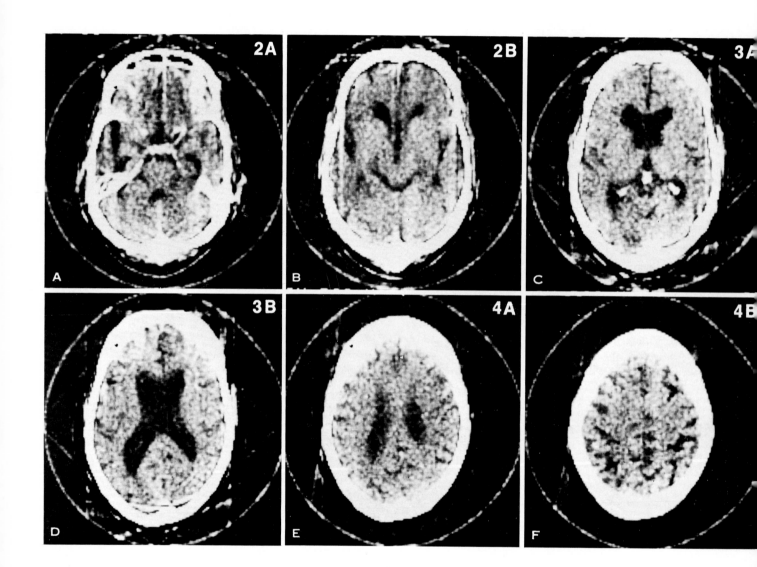

FIG. 23.1. DIFFUSE DEGENERATIVE CEREBRAL DISEASE; PRESENILE DEMENTIA, PROBABLY ALZHEIMER'S DISEASE.

Clinical Features. A 59 y.o. male whose mental deterioration apparently began about 5 years earlier, when he could not continue his work as an accountant. He subsequently failed to hold several jobs because of his inability to master the tasks involved. His family had noted gradual forgetfulness. Traveling abroad, he became separated from his wife and wandered aimlessly for several days. Neurological examination at that time revealed constructional dyspraxia, poor orientation to time, and difficulty with calculations. EEG revealed diffuse temporal slowing, and PEG demonstrated dilated ventricles and enlarged cerebral sulci, consistent with cerebral atrophy. Neurological examination 2 years later revealed a severely demented individual, with visual-spatial disorientation, dyscalculia, very slight dysphasia and impaired verbal capacity, inefficiency of thought, and forgetfulness. Detailed neurological examination was otherwise normal. Lumbar puncture revealed an opening pressure of 115 mm, a protein of 54 mgm %, and normal serology. Recent examination revealed that there had been a gradual worsening of intellectual functions, including progressive impairment of memory.

Neurological Examination. Visual suck response, but no grasp reflex. Flexor plantar responses. Motor, general sensory, and cerebellar tests remained normal.

CT Scan. Abnormal (Fig. 23.1).

A–F. Sequential 13-mm sections from below superiorly.

A. The fourth ventricle is generous in size. Because of a slight canting of the head, the right side of this ventricle is incompletely shown. Just anterolateral to the fourth ventricle, widened fissures are visible between the cerebellar flocculi and the middle cerebellar peduncles, extending mesially and posteriorly from the cerebellopontine angle cisterns. The pontine cistern appears normal. Ossification is visible in the petroclinoid ligaments. In the left temporal region, vertical white and black artifacts are superimposed upon a considerably widened lower sylvian cistern. Somewhat enlarged temporal horns are visible just anterior to the petrous pyramids.

B. There is moderate widening of the left ambient cistern. The quadrigeminal cistern is slightly enlarged. On each side, the inferior portions of the trigones are partly included in the section. The left sylvian cistern is considerably enlarged. There is minor widening of the sulcus between the left superior and middle frontal gyri and minor sulcal widening is present in the mesial aspect of each frontal lobe. The third ventricle is somewhat widened, as is the longitudinal fissure just anterior to it, shown between the lower portions of the somewhat enlarged frontal horns.

C. There is moderate enlargement of the left frontal horn and lesser enlargement of the right. On each side, portions of enlarged sylvian fissures are visible. Slightly widened cingulate sulci are visible, extending from a very slightly widened interfrontal portion of the longitudinal fissure. On each side of the calcified pineal, widened retrothalamic cisterns are visible.

D. The body and trigone of the left lateral ventricle are moderately enlarged and the right lateral ventricle is enlarged to a lesser extent. There is mild widening of many sulci over the lateral portions of each cerebral hemisphere, slightly more pronounced on the left side. The left callosal and right cingulate sulci are widened.

E. Slight but extensive sulcal widening is shown over the cerebral convexities. The parieto-occipital sulci are mildly enlarged also.

F. The superior convexity sulci are moderately to markedly enlarged and there is similar enlargement of mesial sulci bilaterally, particularly in the posterior parietal region.

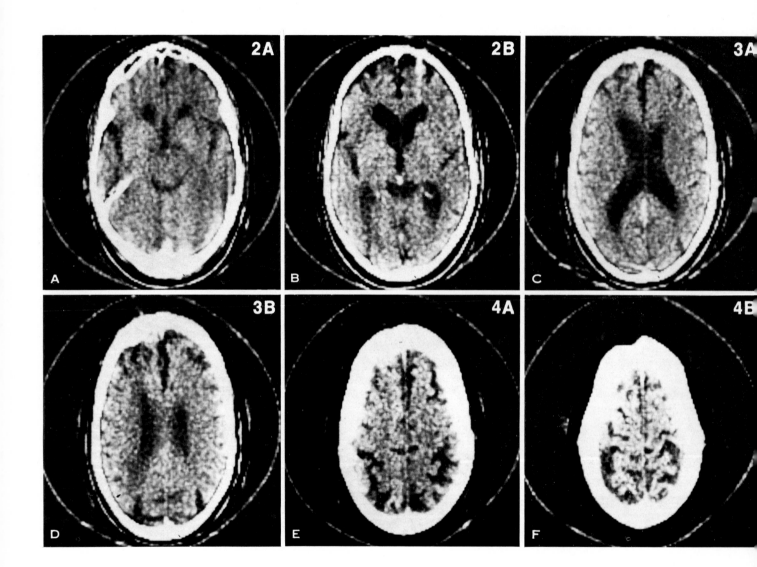

FIG. 23.2. EXTENSIVE SEVERE DEGENERATIVE CERE-BRAL DISEASE, POSSIBLY ALZHEIMER'S DISEASE.
Clinical Features. A 78 y.o. male with "slowness of thinking" for 3–4 years.
Neurological Examination. Poor memory, positive snout and suck reflexes, sensorineural hearing loss in the left ear, and bilateral carotid bruits.
EEG. Abnormal, with generalized slowing, most marked posteriorly and over the left temporal lobe.
Skull Examination. Sclerotic irregular area in the left frontal bone, probably secondary to old depressed skull fracture.
RN Scan. Normal.
CT Scan. Abnormal (Fig. 23.2).
A–F. Sequential 13-mm sections from below superiorly. No abnormality was shown in the lower sections of the posterior fossa.
A. The sylvian cisterns are enlarged bilaterally, the left markedly so. Adjacent to the internal frontal crest, the anterior medial portion of the right superior frontal gyrus is shrunken, with enlargement of the adjacent subarachnoid space.
B. There is moderate enlargement of both frontal horns. There is modest widening of the third ventricle. At this level, there is again considerable widening of the left sylvian cistern and slight enlargement of a portion of the right. There is considerable shrinkage of both superior frontal gyri an-teriorly, with moderate widening of the subarachnoid space anteriorly and in the interfrontal portion of the longitudinal fissure. Gaping of the sulci between the right and left superior and middle frontal gyri is obvious and there is widening of the cingulate and callosal sulci. There is slight widening of the occipital portion of the longitudinal fissure.
C. Moderate enlargement of the lateral ventricles is shown. An asymmetrical appearance of the posterior portions is attributable to slight head canting. Marked widening of the interfrontal portion of the longitudinal fissure is evident. There is moderate widening of the anterior frontal sulci and slight widening of sulci of the inferior cerebral convexities elsewhere.

D. More severe shrinkage of the anterior portions of both frontal lobes is evident at this level, with marked widening of the longitudinal fissure and anterior frontal sulci. Posteriorly, there is evidence of considerable shrinkage of the lateral occipital gyri bilaterally, with marked widening of the sulci between these gyri and the angular gyri. Mesially, there is moderate widening of the calcarine fissures.
E and F. There is very marked shrinkage of the superior parietal lobule, lateral occipital gyri, cuneus, paracentral lobule, precentral, and postcentral gyri of each cerebral hemisphere. Some shrinkage of the cingulate gyri is also shown.

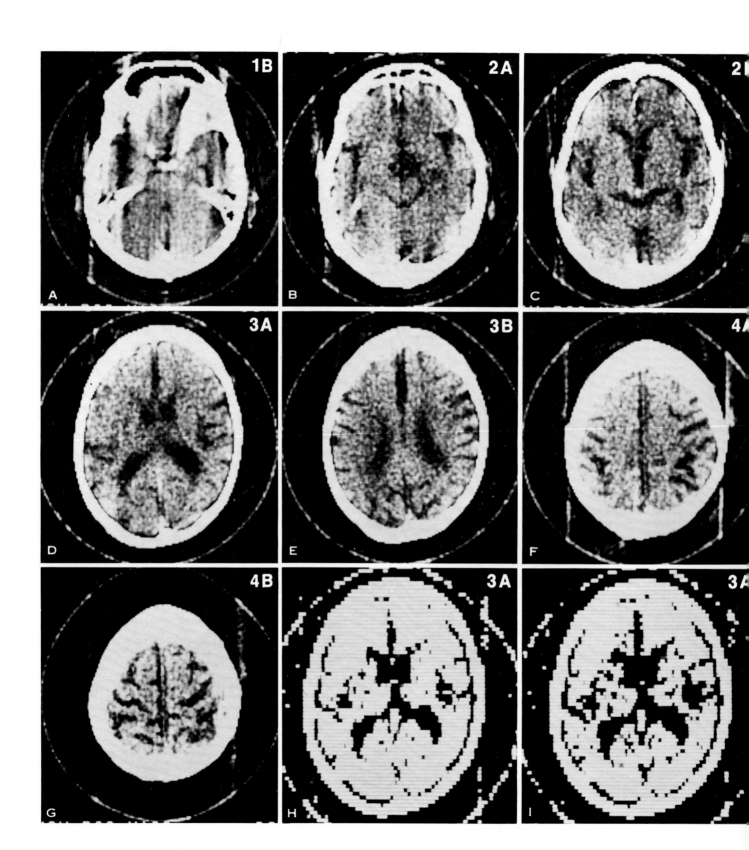

FIG. 23.3. WIDESPREAD, MODERATELY SEVERE CORTICAL ATROPHY, WITH MINOR CHANGES OF CENTRAL ATROPHY. POSSIBLE ETAT LACUNAIRE.

Clinical Features. A 77 y.o. male with longstanding hypertension. He gave a history of a cerebrovascular accident several years previously, with mild left hemiparesis, which resolved. In recent years he had developed increasing difficulty both in walking and in concentrating.

Neurological Examination. Alert, intact memory. Apparent anxiety state, with periods of hyperventilation. Coarse tremor and difficulty initiating movements. Shuffling gait.

Skull Examination. Calcification in carotid siphons, otherwise normal.

CT Scan. Two scans at 6½ months interval; abnormal (Fig. 23.3).

Course. L-Dopa discontinued. Gait, strength, tremor, and confidence improved with reassurance and physiotherapy.

A–G. Sequential 13-mm sections from below superiorly.

A. The base of the skull is slightly asymmetrical in level and the section includes slightly more of the inferior portion of the left frontal lobe and slightly less of the right petrous pyramid than the equivalent structures on the opposite side. The fourth ventricle and other posterior fossa structures appeared normal. An artifact through the left temporal region prevents satisfactory assessment of this region.

B. There is widening of the sylvian cisterns. The ambient and lower quadrigeminal cisterns appear normal.

C. The upper quadrigeminal and retrothalamic cisterns are enlarged. Marked enlargement of both sylvian cisterns is shown. The superior cerebellar cistern is prominent, but not necessarily abnormal. The third ventricle is moderately widened, but the frontal horns (**C** and **D**) appear normal.

D. Portions of somewhat enlarged sylvian fissures are visible bilaterally. What appears to be a modestly enlarged inferior portion of the right central sulcus is visible and the interfrontal portion of the longitudinal fissure is widened. There is mild enlargement of the right trigone, but otherwise the lateral ventricles show only minimal enlargement. The thalamic prominences are visible in the posterior portions of the bodies of the lateral ventricles.

E. There is considerable widening of the longitudinal fissure anteriorly and slight widening posteriorly. There is marked widening of the precentral, central, and postcentral sulci on the right side. A lesser degree of widening appears on the left side. There is moderate shrinkage bilaterally of the lateral occipital and lingual gyri, with widening of the calcarine fissures.

F and G. Quite marked shrinkage of superior parietal lobule, lateral occipital gyrus, and cuneus is shown on both sides. The longitudinal fissure is quite widened, and the falx is shown extending through it.

H. L 10   W M.   I. L 12   W M.
Displays of the same scan, obtained at the earlier CT examination (80 x 80 matrix system). These control settings discriminate well the lateral and third ventricles and the enlarged sylvian cisterns. In addition, small areas of reduced absorption are visible in the left putamen and one small area of reduced absorption is suggested in the right putamen. These small areas showed an absorption range of 8–11, consistent with partial volume representation of small lacunes containing fluid with similar absorption characteristics to those of CSF. In **H**, partial volume representations of the anterolateral portions of the frontal horns are visible.

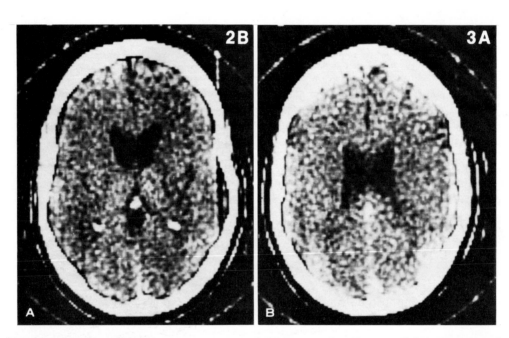

FIG. 23.4.   HUNTINGTON'S CHOREA.

Clinical Features. A 33 y.o. man with an 18-month history consistent with early Huntington's chorea, which had been diagnosed in his grandfather, father, and three brothers.

CT Scan. Abnormal (Fig. 23.4).

CT scan with 160 x 160 matrix system.

A and **B.** There is modest enlargement of the frontal horns and anterior portions of the bodies of the lateral ventricles, with flattening of the caudate surfaces of the lateral ven- tricular walls. The remaining portions of the lateral ven- tricles were of normal size. The third ventricle was mini- mally widened and the fourth ventricle appeared normal (not shown). There was evidence of very slight enlargement of a number of sulci of both frontal lobes, more obvious on sections other than those shown.

The CT findings support the clinical diagnosis of Hunting- ton's chorea.

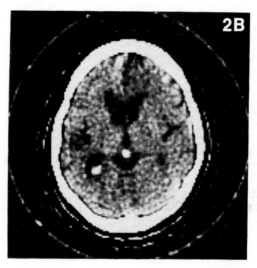

FIG. 23.5. DIFFUSE CORTICAL AND CENTRAL CEREBRAL ATROPHY, OF UNCERTAIN ETIOLOGY. MILD ATROPHY OF CEREBELLAR VERMIS.

Clinical Features. A 67 y.o. hypertensive woman with a history of gradual deterioration in mental functions over approximately 2 years.

Neurological Examination. Alert, but aphasic; language difficulty and memory loss. Blood pressure, 190/100. Hypertensive changes in the fundi. Full visual fields.

There was modest lateral ventricular enlargement, the left slightly more than the right. Mild enlargement of the third ventricle was present. There was moderate enlargement of the sylvian cisterns and superior cerebral sulci. This scan section reveals some enlargement of the quadrigeminal cistern, behind which widened sulci between the folia of the superior vermis are revealed as a ladder-like pattern of CSF absorption, indicating atrophic changes in the superior vermis.

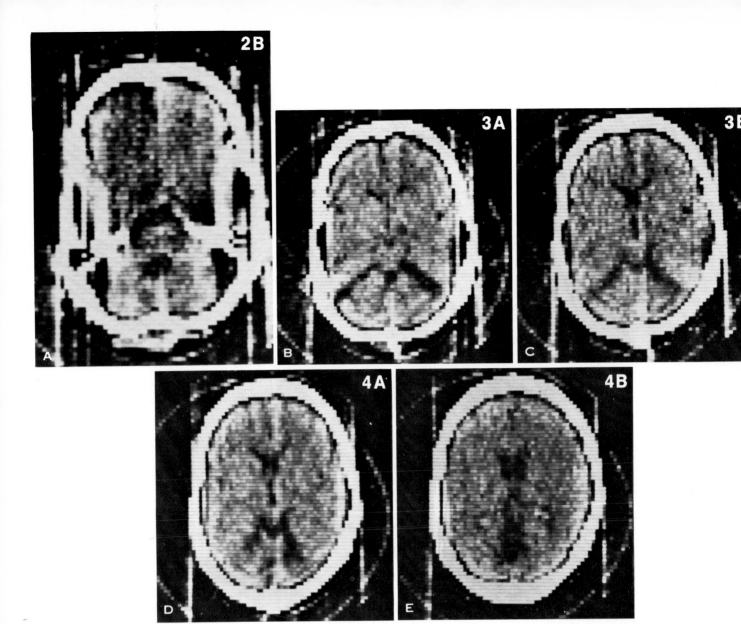

FIG. 23.6 CEREBELLAR DEGENERATION, FAMILIAL; PROBABLY OLIVOPONTOCEREBELLAR DEGENERATION.

Clinical Features. A 60 y.o. male with a 10–12-year history of progressive disturbance of stance and gait. More recent onset of difficulty coordinating fine finger movements, dysarthria, and dysphagia.

Neurological Examination. Severe ataxia of gait, with the patient able to walk only with considerable assistance. Ataxia of arms, diminished upward gaze, extensor plantar responses, and decreased vibratory sensation in the toes. Strength was well preserved. There was a family history of a brother with a similar illness, proven to be olivopontocerebellar degeneration at autopsy.

Skull Examination. Normal.

RN Scan. Normal.

CT Scan. Abnormal (Fig. 23.6).

A–C. Sequential 8-mm sections. **D** and **E.** Thirteen-mm sections, from below superiorly.

A. The fourth ventricle is moderately enlarged. The pons appears somewhat irregular and small, with a correspondingly large-appearing pontine cistern. Head motion during this scan resulted in marked artifacts in both temporal and lateral cerebellar regions. The heterogeneous absorption values in the region of the pons are unreliable and presumed to be artifactual.

B. The subarachnoid spaces over the anterolateral aspects of the cerebellar hemispheres are greatly enlarged, more so on the right. Between the anterior extremities of these subarachnoid spaces is a rectangular central region of CSF absorption, consistent with a markedly enlarged precentral cerebellar fissure. The lower portion of the midbrain is visible immediately anteriorly. Immediately anterior to the midbrain is a partial representation of the interpeduncular cistern, with its crural extensions faintly indicated laterally. Anterior to this, the third ventricle and inferior portions of the frontal horns are visible.

C and **D.** The frontal horns are of normal size. The third ventricle appears minimally widened. Enlarged subarachnoid spaces are shown extending over the anterosuperior aspects of the cerebellar hemispheres. The quadrigeminal cistern is enlarged and a portion of an enlarged superior cerebellar cistern is included in the median area posteriorly. The sylvian cisterns are not enlarged.

E. The section demonstrates a very large superior cerebellar cistern and provides further evidence of reduced volume of the cerebellar vermis. On this section and higher sections (not shown) the lateral ventricles were not unusual in size for the patient's age, and no enlargement of cerebral sulci was demonstrated.

DEMYELINATING DISEASE

Introduction

Although a moderate number of cases of multiple sclerosis has been studied by CT scanning, no definite focal parenchymal absorption abnormality has been recognized. Hillier Baker (personal communications) has observed, in occasional cases of multiple sclerosis, the presence of foci of diminished parenchymal absorption, thought to represent large acute lesions of multiple sclerosis.

In our material, CT scans of patients with advanced multiple sclerosis have not uncommonly revealed evidence of well-developed, irregularly distributed changes of loss of cerebral substance, indicated by regions of enlargement of cerebral subarachnoid spaces and regions of modest ventricular enlargement. A single experience with proven Schilder's disease is illustrated in this section.

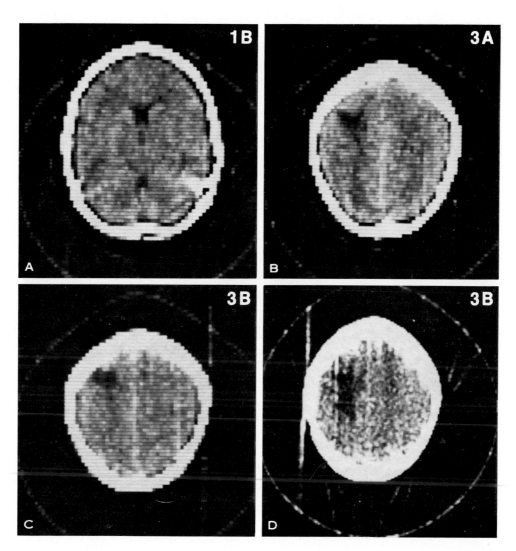

FIG. 23.7. SCHILDER'S DISEASE.
Clinical Features. An 11 y.o. girl who had the sudden onset of weakness of the right arm, followed a few days later by weakness of the right leg, some 3 weeks before the initial CT scan.
Neurological Examination. In addition to the right hemiparesis, disturbance of affect and a Marcus-Gunn phenomenon in the right pupil were noted, indicating multifocal disease.
CT Scan. Both the initial scan and a scan some 5 weeks later, after a small biopsy, were abnormal (Fig. 23.7).
Angio. A left carotid study obtained at another hospital soon after onset indicated the presence of an avascular mass in the middle and higher convexity regions of the left parietal lobe.
Operation. A small biopsy in the region of the lesion that was demonstrated on CT scan revealed the changes of Schilder's disease.

A–C. Scan sections with the 80 x 80 matrix system, showing generous sized but not definitely enlarged ventricles for age (**A**) and a rather well defined focal area of diminished absorption (9–15, 8–16) 2.5 cm in maximum diameter, in the anterior portion of the parietal lobe, involving cortical and subcortical regions. No other evidence of parenchymal disease was identified and the findings raised suspicion of a glioma, although there was not evidence of any contrast enhancement with intravenous Hypaque.
D. CT scan after a small parietal lobe biopsy. The area of diminished absorption (8–16) is considerably larger and more irregular in contour than previously. Adjacent sections (not shown) revealed metal clips at the site of biopsy, and adjacent small areas of modestly increased absorption consistent with small areas of cortical and subcortical hemorrhagic effusion in the region of biopsy. Again, no additional areas of diminished parenchymal absorption were evident in other regions.

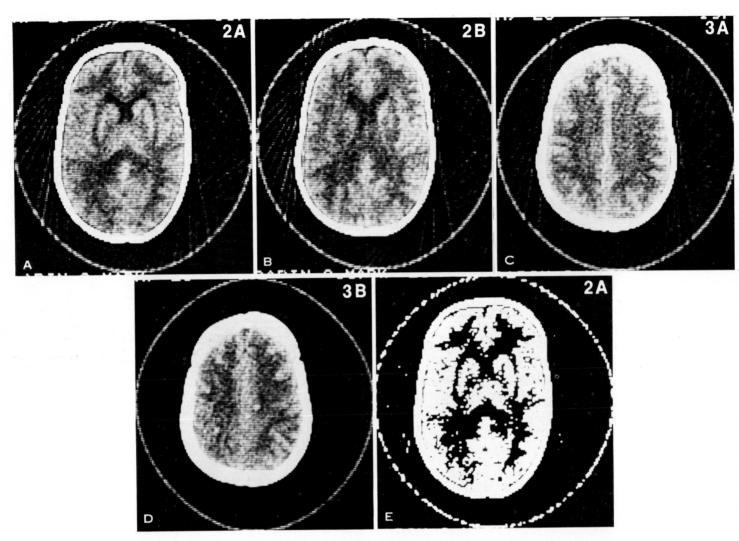

FIG. 23.8. GENERALIZED LEUCODYSTROPHY. (Case contributed by Dr. Leon Menzer, Sabin and Mark P. A., Boston). **Clinical Features.** A 14 y.o. retarded girl in whom increasing head size led to CT examination, for question of hydrocephalus. She was evaluated at another hospital at the age of 4½ months because of poor neurological development from the time of birth. Perinatal history was noncontributory. **Neurological Examinations.** At the age of 4½ months, physical examination was within normal limits. The cry was high pitched. At this time, head circumference and transillumination were normal. The fundi were normal. There was no visual fixation or following. Deep tendon reflexes were hyperactive.
EEG. Normal.
Skull Examination. Normal.
CT Scan. Abnormal (Fig. 23.8).

CT scan obtained at the age of 14 months.

A–D. Serial 8-mm sections from below superiorly. A marked generalized diminution in absorption of white matter is shown throughout both cerebral hemispheres. This change has caused the cerebral cortical convolutions and central grey matter to be thrown into unusual relief. The internal and external capsules are prominently displayed due to the striking reduction in absorption **(A).** Cerebral cortex laterally and mesially does not show evidence of altered absorption and therefore shows marked contrast with the abnormal white matter **(B–D).**
E. L 12   W M.
Same section as in **A.** These control settings reveal clearly the striking diminution in absorption (absorption similar to CSF). The internal and external capsules are visible with considerable clarity. Ventricular size is slightly increased for age, but there is no evidence of obstructive hydrocephalus. The cerebral cisterns and sulci appeared normal throughout.

CHAPTER 24

Developmental Anomalies

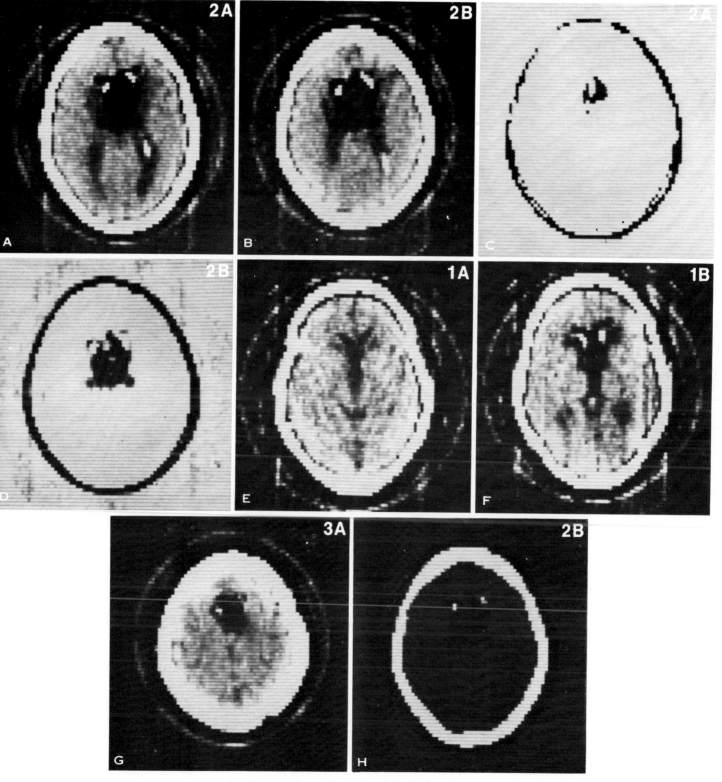

LEGEND FOR FIG. 24.1 A-H ON PAGE 398

FIG. 24.1. AGENESIS OF THE CORPUS CALLOSUM, WITH CORPUS CALLOSUM LIPOMA. (Case contributed by Dr. Thomas M. Lott, University Hospital, Augusta, Georgia.)

Clinical Features. A 51 y.o. female who was first admitted to the University Hospital 9 years earlier with the complaint of intermittent headaches.

Neurological Examination. Normal findings at the previous and present admissions.

Skull Examination. Typical radiolucency of a lipoma in the region of the corpus callosum, with peripheral linear calcifications.

RN Scan. [203]Mercuhydrin; normal.

CT Scan. Abnormal (Fig. 24.1, **A–H**).

Angio. Bilateral carotid studies revealed marked enlargement and tortuosity of an azygos pericallosal artery, with elevation in the region of the calcification. The venous phase showed separation and kinking of the internal cerebral veins. The venous angle was displaced posteriorly, with stretching of the subependymal veins in the anterior caudate region.

Operation. (Dr. Louis O. Manganiello.) Torkildsen shunting at the time of the first admission relieved the headaches.

A–H. CT scan, revealing the various features of the pathology.

A. L 14   W 30.   **B.** L 14   W 20.

These contiguous sections reveal the large, irregular ovoid, low-absorption mass of the lipoma in the region of the corpus callosum (black) and the calcifications (white) towards the right and left periphery of the lipoma. The high density of the Torkildsen shunt tube is visible in the right occipital horn and the lateral ventricles are satisfactorily decompressed.

C. L −50   W M,   **D.** L −20   W 30.

These scans are the same as those in **A** and **B**, respectively, and reveal the very low absorption of the fatty tumor (absorption extending below −50). The oval black zone peripherally represents the much lower absorption of air trapped in the hair between the head bag and the scalp.

E and **F.** L 14   W 20.

Sections below that in **A**, showing the more inferior portions of the lipoma, absence of the septum lucidum, and a widened third ventricle, which extends superiorly to the inferior aspect of the lipoma. There is indication of a large broad suprapineal recess, extending posterior to the calcified pineal, which is included in the same section (**F**).

G. L 18   W 30.

Section immediately above that in **B**, showing the superior portion of the lipoma and additional small calcifications bilaterally. The calcification is evidently within the lateral portions of the lipoma, rather than in a capsule.

H. L 180   W M.

Same section as in **B**, showing the high absorption of the calcifications.

(Illustrations courtesy of Thomas M. Lott, M.D.)

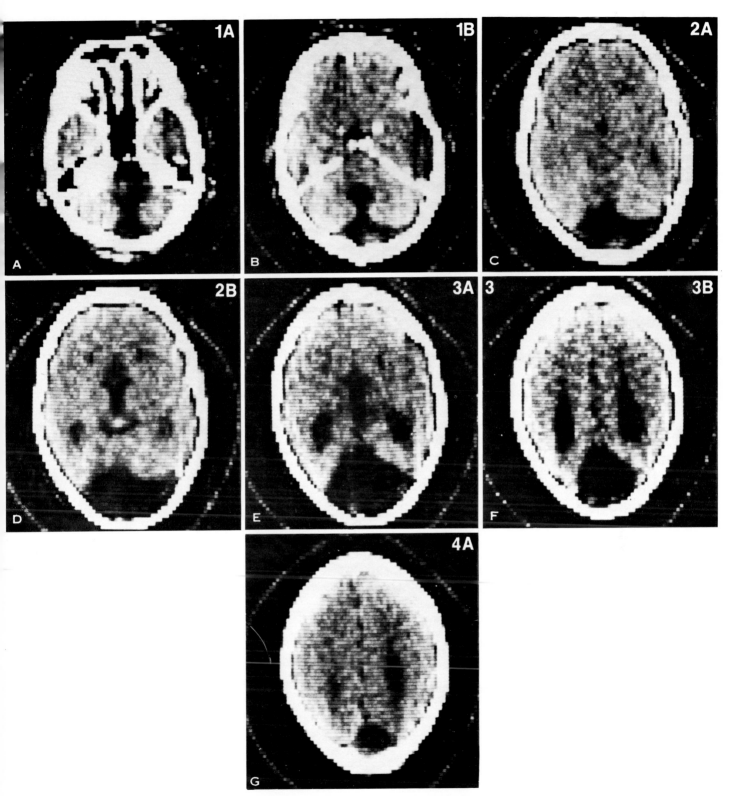

LEGEND FOR FIG. 24.2 A-G ON PAGE 400

FIG. 24.2 DYSGENESIS OF CEREBELLAR VERMIS (VARIANT OF DANDY-WALKER SYNDROME), ASSOCIATED WITH LEPTOMENINGEAL CYST AND AGENESIS OF THE CORPUS CALLOSUM. (Case contributed by Dr. David O. Davis, George Washington University Medical Center, Washington, D. C.)

Clinical Features. A 53 y.o. male with slight unsteadiness of gait. He had otherwise been essentially asymptomatic throughout his life.

A–G. Consecutive scans from below superiorly.

A. A very wide space is shown between the cerebellar hemispheres, communicating anteriorly with a very large fourth ventricle and posteriorly with a generous space in the region of the cisterna magna. The fourth ventricle appears to bulge markedly on both sides, in the area of the lateral recesses.

B. The large size of the upper portion of the fourth ventricle is visible, communicating posteriorly via a broad space between the cerebellar hemispheres, with an extra-axial space showing CSF absorption values. This space is larger than in the subjacent section. The inferior and middle portions of the vermis are absent.

C. The extra-axial cystic space is larger at this level and extends further laterally over the anteriorly displaced right cerebellar hemisphere than over the left. Extending anteriorly from this cystic space to the quadrigeminal cistern is a broad zone of decreased absorption with an irregular, transversely banded appearance, consistent with a dysplastic superior vermis with wide spaces between malformed folia.

D. The extra-axial cyst is still larger at this level. Extending from its anterior aspect to the quadrigeminal cistern is a malformed superior vermis. The quadrigeminal cistern is unusually large. Immediately anterior to the density of a partly calcified pineal is a considerably widened and anteriorly deformed third ventricle. The inferior portions of the trigones of the lateral ventricles are included in this section.

E. The extra-axial cyst exhibits a more triangular configuration at this level. The markedly widened and deformed third ventricle is still visible and the trigones of the lateral ventricles are shown to be enlarged. There is evidence of a deficiency of tissue in the region of the splenium of the corpus callosum.

F. The extra-axial cyst extends above the normal level of the tentorium, between the occipital lobes, which are widely separated. The moderately enlarged lateral ventricles are abnormally separated and, between them, in the median region is a partial volume representation of the broad third ventricle, extending superiorly into the region normally occupied by corpus callosum. This phenomenon can be traced anteriorly to the level of the anterior portions of the lateral ventricles.

G. The leptomeningeal cyst continues to extend superiorly: The enlarged lateral ventricles are still visible. The interrupted low-absorption region extending in the median area from the cyst to the anterior limit of the intracranial scan probably represents a somewhat widened longitudinal fissure, with widened medial hemispheric sulci.

(Illustrations courtesy of David O. Davis, M.D.)

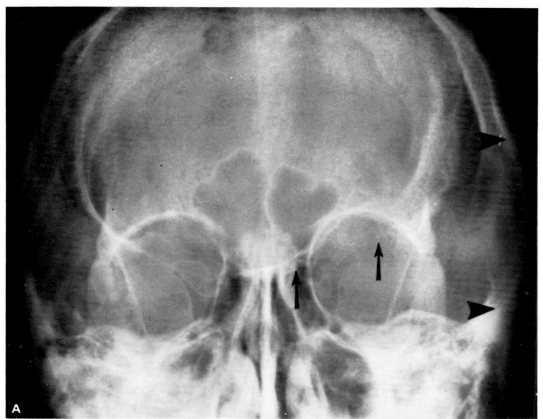

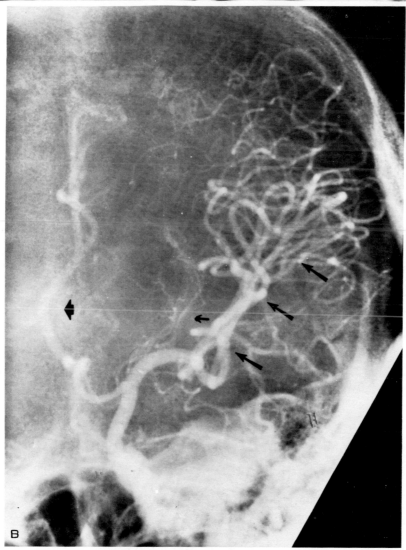

LEGEND FOR FIG. 24.3 A-B ON PAGE 403

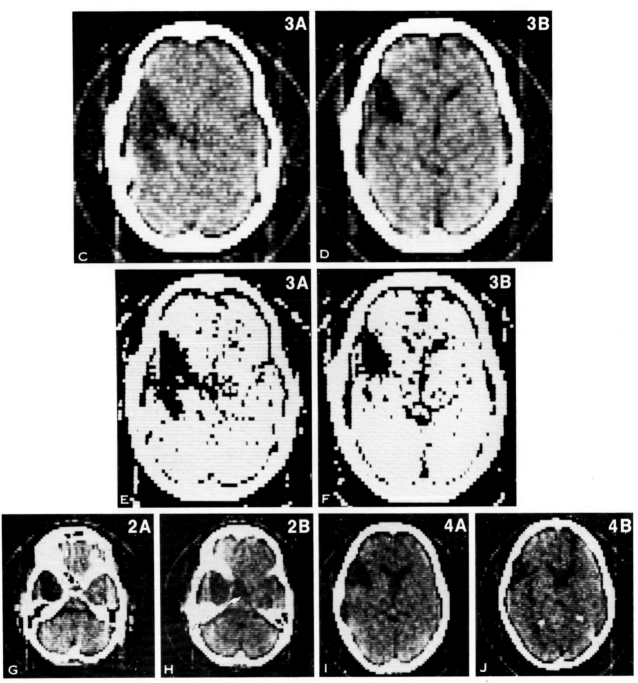

LEGEND FOR FIG. 24.3 A & B ON PAGE 403

FIG. 24.3. DYSGENESIS OF TEMPORAL LOBE, WITH ASSOCIATED ARACHNOID PSEUDOCYST.

Clinical Features. A 69 y.o. male with a past history of atherosclerotic heart disease, congestive heart failure, and carcinoma of the colon. He had had three spells of diplopia and dizziness during the past 2 years. He was admitted for investigation of possible transient ischemic attacks and/or subdural hematoma.

Skull Examination. Abnormal (Fig. 24.3**A**).

RN Scan. Tcp; normal 3 years earlier.

Angio. Transfemoral bilateral carotid and left vertebral studies revealed an extensive left temporal area avascular mass. It could not be determined from the angiogram whether the mass was intra- or extra-axial. (Fig. 24.3**B**).

CT Scan. This was performed after angiography for clarification, which was obtained (Fig. 24.3, **C–J**).

A. Posteroanterior skull projection. The left lesser wing of sphenoid is indistinct and somewhat elevated, and the planum sphenoidale is inclined upwards and to the left (*arrows*). The left superior orbital fissure is much larger than the right and shows an appearance of marginal erosion. The skull is thinned and bulges laterally in the left temporal region (*arrowheads*). The findings are consistent with a large mass in and adjacent to the left middle fossa, which has been present since childhood.

B. Frontal projection of the left carotid angiogram. There is tortuosity and suspicion of minor displacement of the anterior portion of the pericallosal artery to the right (*broad arrow*).

The lenticulostriate arteries are displaced medially (*small arrow*). The middle cerebral artery is elevated and its sylvian branches are considerably displaced medially and also displaced superiorly (*arrows*). The angiogram did not permit differentiation between an intra-axial and extra-axial temporal area mass. A CT scan was therefore obtained for clarification.

C–J. CT scans revealed essentially normal ventricular size for the patient's age. There was slight displacement of midline supratentorial structures to the right (frontal horns, third ventricle, and pineal). The calcified glomus of the left choroid plexus appeared displaced posteromedially. A large region of markedly diminished absorption occupies the area of the left frontal operculum and, in continuity, a considerable portion of the left temporal lobe. The low absorption space measured 2–15 units (2–3 units above the absorption range of CSF, including partial volume representations). Medially, the space extended posteriorly adjacent to the lateral aspect of the putamen and into the region of the inferior left thalamus. Extension inferiorly was to the floor of the middle fossa and suprasellar cisterns. The contours of the fluid-filled space were less regular than is seen in typical leptomeningeal cysts, and irregular encroachment upon the cavity by marginal tissue is apparent. Lateral bulging and thinning of the vault in the left frontotemporal area is visible on the CT scans but is much better appreciated on skull films. The elevation of the left sphenoid ridge is also more reliably identified on the skull examination.

FIG. 24.4. LEPTOMENINGEAL CYST, ASSOCIATED WITH SYRINGOHYDROMYELIA.

Clinical Features. A 9 y.o. girl who was originally seen at the age of 7 weeks for investigation of an abnormally enlarging head. A ventriculovenous shunt was placed. After several revisions during the first 3 years of life, the child developed normally and did well in school studies and sports. About 1 year before the present admission, there was a transient episode of midthoracic back pain following exercise. At this time, it was noted that the shunt tubing was disconnected in the neck and it was presumed that the shunt was not functioning. Three days before admission she complained of headache and pain between her shoulder blades. This was followed by unsteadiness of gait, and the back pain persisted. She noted some weakness of the lower extremities and became unable to walk without support. Mild intermittent headache persisted.

Neurological Examination. Normal appearance of the head and normal visual acuity. Mild papilledema, with a hemorrhage in the left fundus. Bilateral lower extremity weakness, more on the left side. Increased deep tendon reflexes in the lower extremities, with ankle clonus. Bilateral positive Babinski signs and decreased position sense in the feet. Leg weakness increased and a sensory level became apparent below the level of the umbilicus. An emergency positive contrast myelogram demonstrated a complete obstruction opposite the level of the sixth dorsal vertebra.

Skull Examination. At the age of 7 weeks; enlargement and thinning of the cranial vault, with wide bulging fontanels and a shallow posterior fossa. The skull was exceptionally prominent in the parieto-occipital region.

PEG. At the age of 7 weeks; a combined pneumoencephalogram and ventriculogram revealed an enormous infra- and supra-tentorial extra-axial cyst that filled from below, and marked dilatation of the lateral and third ventricles (Fig. 24.4A).

CT Scan. Obtained at the present admission; abnormal (Fig. 24.4, **B–J**).

Operations. (Dr. Robert G. Ojemann.) Ventriculovenous shunt at 7 weeks, with several revisions. Laminography D3–D8, following emergency myelography. Following incision in the dura, marked distention of the spinal cord was found. Below D6, the cord appeared to be normal. In the region of distention, there was poor vascularity over the posterior columns. A cystic cavity was tapped at a depth of 3mm and clear spinal fluid was withdrawn. After removal of 10–12 ml of fluid, it appeared that the cavity was in direct communication with the central canal and presumably with the posterior fossa structures. The dura was left open. After the CT scan, the ventriculovenous shunt was reestablished and connected to a catheter that was placed in the leptomeningeal cyst. Fluid in the cyst appeared clear, but somewhat xanthochromic. It was thought that this finding was due to minor bleeding in the region of the spinal cord puncture and was taken as confirmatory evidence of connection between the cyst and the hydromyelic cavity. It seemed that the cyst had developed increased pressure, causing papilledema, with subsequent decompression of the cyst into the central canal of the spinal cord, causing acute syringohydromelia.

A. Lateral brow-up film from the pneumogram at the age of 7 weeks. The extent of the huge leptomeningeal cyst, as shown by multiple projections in different positions of the head, is

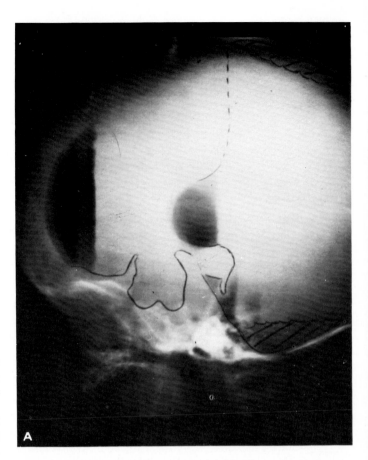

outlined. No cerebral tissue was visible from the point at which the upper vertical *interrupted line* meets the inner skull table, posteriorly down to the foramen magnum. Gas is shown in the portion of the cyst adjacent to the posterior portion of the markedly dilated and rotated third ventricle. The latter impinged upon the planum sphenoidale and sella (*continuous line*). The aqueduct was narrowed and displaced anteriorly beneath the anterior portion of the cyst. The fourth ventricle was displaced markedly anteriorly. The grossly enlarged frontal horns are shown. Leptomeningeal cyst was diagnosed.

B–J. CT scan obtained during the recent admission. The lateral ventricles are small, in spite of the evidence of lack of function of the ventriculovenous shunt. The tip of the shunt tube is shown in the right frontal horn.

B. The fourth ventricle is small and displaced anteriorly, with the cerebellum. The huge cystic space, containing fluid having the absorption characteristics of CSF, is clearly demarcated from the anteriorly displaced cerebellar hemispheres and vermis. Extension above the normal level of the tentorium is demonstrated (**C–E, G,** and **J**).

E. L 16   W 20.

The cyst is shown extending anteriorly to the region of the posterior wall of the third ventricle. The calcified pineal is displaced 6 mm to the right of the midline. The greatly increased sagittal dimension of the posterior half of the skull is evident in this and other sections.

F and **I.** L 11   W M.

These control settings provided the maximum contrast between CSF-containing spaces and cerebral structures. A few small spots of higher absorption scattered through the leptomeningeal cyst presumably represent proteinaceous or hemic aggregates within the cyst fluid.

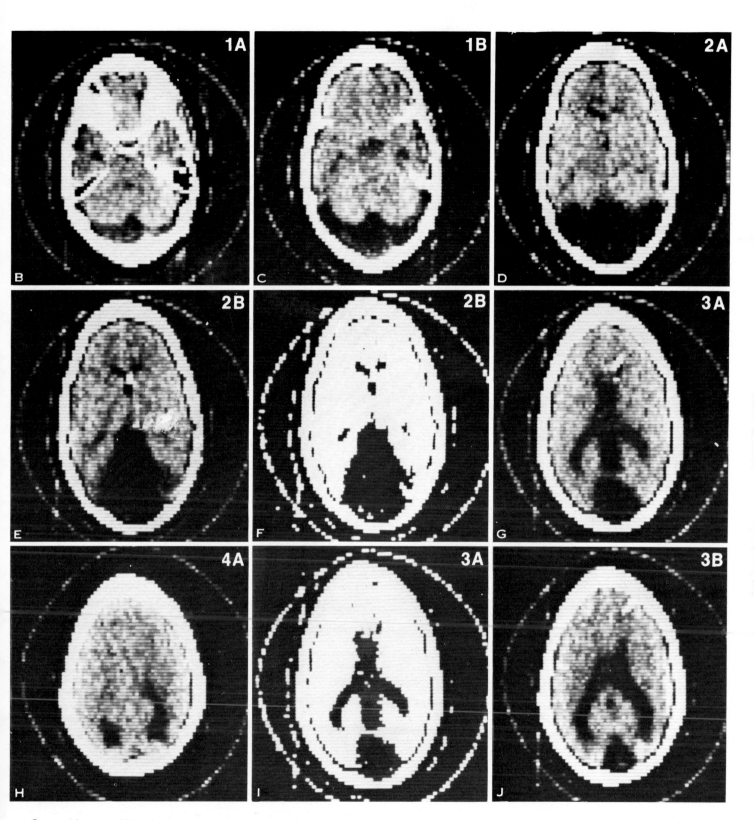

G. L 16 W M.

Between the trigones is a broad cavity, containing fluid with the same absorption as CSF, that appeared to be in continuity with the posterior portions of the lateral ventricles but separated from the cyst at this level by a narrow band of tissue. This may represent a diverticulum of the suprapineal recess or lateral ventricles. In view of the small size of the lateral ventricles in the face of an obstructed ventricular shunt (obstruction confirmed at operation), it was concluded that the ventricular system had developed a communication with the cyst at some earlier time, resulting in CSF absorption from the walls of the cyst but with gradual expansion of the cyst. The large amount of information obtained from the CT scan permitted management of the patient without recourse to angiography and further pneumography.

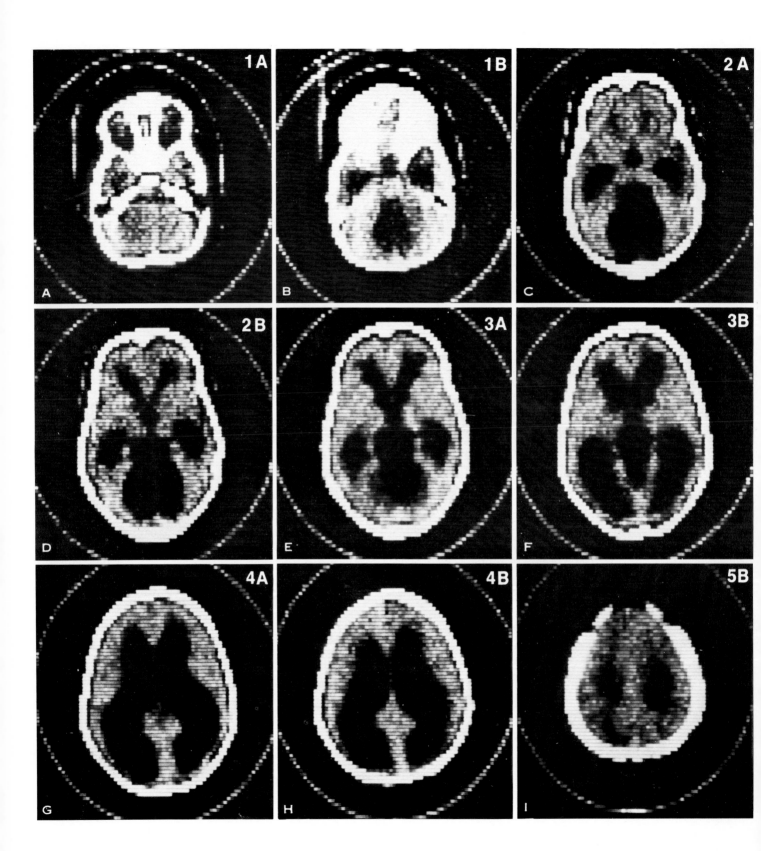

FIG. 24.5. LEPTOMENINGEAL CYST, MASSIVE; INFRA- AND SUPRA-TENTORIAL, AND ASSOCIATED WITH SEVERE OBSTRUCTIVE HYDROCEPHALUS.

Clinical Features. A 12-month-old male, the product of a normal pregnancy. The child appeared completely normal until a few months earlier, when abnormal increase in head size was noted.

Neurological Examination. Head circumference, 51 cm (97th percentile). Bulging brow and a 6-cm diameter tense anterior fontanel. No abnormality noted on transillumination. Alert and playful; no papilledema. Cranial nerve testing and general motor and sensory testing revealed no abnormality.

Skull Examination. Suture diastasis, with increased sutural digitations, enlarged and hydrocephalic configuration of cranial vault, with a large anterior fontanel.

Ultrasound Examination. Suggested a cystic rather than a solid lesion.

CT Scan. Abnormal (Fig. 24.5).

Angio. Large avascular area in the superior cerebellar region, with high position of the straight sinus, forward and downward displacement of the superior cerebellar arteries, and marked lateral ventricular dilatation.

A–H. Consecutive scan sections from below superiorly (8 mm).

A. At this level, no abnormality is visible except for the appearance of the inferior extremities of markedly dilated temporal horns. The fourth ventricle is not visible and is presumably markedly compressed and displaced inferiorly.

B. The inferior portion of a large space containing material of the same absorption as CSF is shown between the cerebellar hemispheres, and the dilated temporal horns are now clearly visible.

C–E. The very large cystic space is shown extending upwards and anteriorly to merge with the posterior wall of an anteriorly displaced and markedly dilated third ventricle. The increased sagittal diameter of the posterior half of the cranium is apparent. There is marked dilatation of the lateral ventricles. The occipital horns are particularly enlarged and extend far superiorly. There is evidence of only a minimal cerebral mantle over these horns (**G** and **H**). Calcar avis indentation is evident mesially (**H**). A large posterior prolongation of the superior portion of the third ventricle is evident between the trigones and occipital horns (**F**), apparently representing a diverticulum of the suprapineal recess.

I. Most superior scan section obtained. The superior extremities of the lateral ventricles are included in this section. Bone defects anteriorly represent the anterior and lateral extremities of the abnormally large anterior fontanel.

The findings are consistent with a very large leptomeningeal cyst, which appears to have originated in the quadrigeminal and superior cerebellar cisterns. Severe obstructive hydrocephalus, due to compression of the aqueduct.

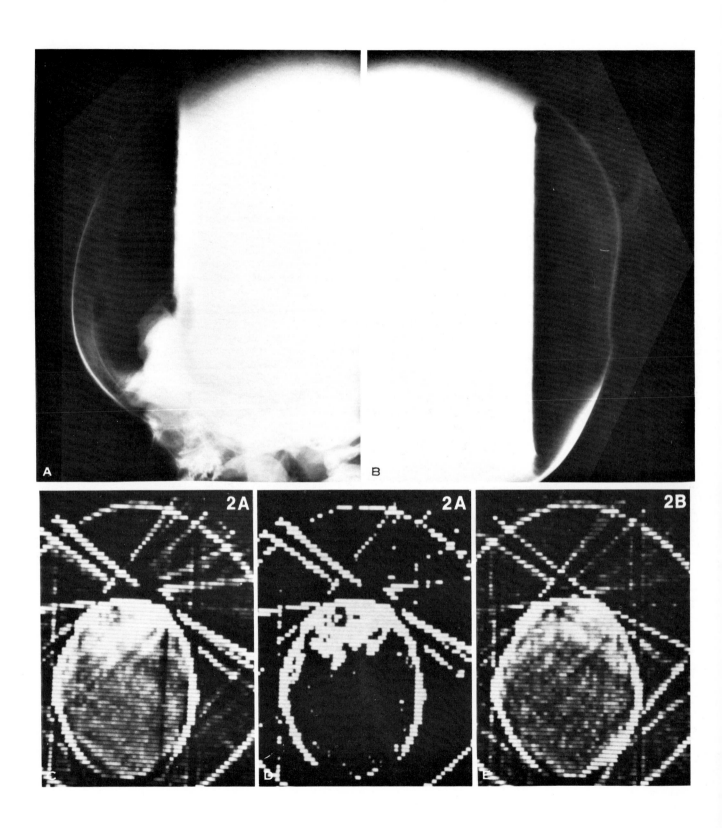

FIG. 24.6. HYDRANENCEPHALY.

Clinical Features. A 10-day-old male infant who presented with an abnormally large head and multiple congenital anomalies.

Skull Examination. Enlarged thin bulging cranial vault, with large fontanels and deficient bone development posteriorly.

CT Scan. Abnormal (Fig. 24.6, C–E).

Ventriculogram. Obtained at the age of 11 weeks. Abnormal (Fig. 24.6, **A** and **B**).

A and **B**. Brow-up and brow-down lateral films, respectively, obtained at ventriculography at the age of 11 weeks. No cerebral mantle is visible from the inferior frontopolar region to, and including, the occipital region. An irregular nodule of soft tissue projects upwards in both inferior frontal regions. The findings are consistent with hydranencephaly with small residues of cerebral tissue in the inferior frontal regions, which may represent anteriorly displaced basal ganglia and/or small portions of the frontal lobes. One-hundred ml of gas were injected for this examination.

C–E. CT scan at 10 days of age. The head could not be maintained in a flexed position and the scan was made parallel to the base line. The lowest scan section was at the level of the orbital roofs. For these reasons, the midbrain and posterior fossa structures were not demonstrated.

C. L 4 W 20 **D.** L 9 W M.

Two respresentations of the same scan, extending through the inferior frontal region. Irregular nodules of tissues are visible in both inferior frontal regions, more extensively on the left side. Absorption of these areas ranged from 9–26 units. No definite cerebral tissue was identified behind or above the inferior frontal regions, and the intracranial space showed a generalized, relatively homogeneous appearance with absorption characteristics of CSF (−2 to +9). The child was sedated with 4 mg of Seconal, but moderate rotary head motion occurred during the scans, as evidenced by the oblique bands in the waterbath portions of the scan. The large area of bone defect posteriorly corresponds with that shown in the plain film examination.

E. Scan section immediately above that in **C** and **D**, showing the extremely irregular nodular cerebral tissues in the anterior and lateral frontal regions. The remainder of the intracranial content has a homogeneous appearance with absorption characteristics of CSF. The grey appearance is due to the low level settings of **C** and **E** (L 4).

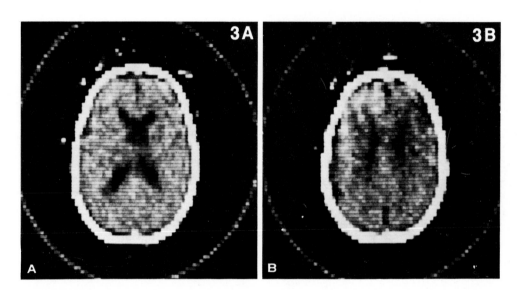

FIG. 24.7. MACRENCEPHALY. (Case contributed by Dr. David O. Davis, George Washington University Medical Center, Washington, D. C.)

Clinical Features. A young child showing delay in achieving milestones and an abnormally large head size (greater than ninety-seventh percentile).

CT Scan. Abnormal (Fig. 24.7, **A** and **B**).

A and **B.** These contiguous scan sections reveal mild and approximately symmetrical enlargement of the lateral ventricles, but ventricular enlargement is insufficient to explain the degree of measured head enlargement. There appears to be slight enlargement of the subarachnoid spaces in the left lateral frontal region and at the frontal poles. The width of the anterior and posterior portions of the longitudinal fissure appears slightly increased. Absorption values of the cerebral grey and white matter were apparently not remarkable. The irregular areas of increased absorption in the left anterior and lateral regions in B appear to be artifactual. The findings are consistent with macrencephaly, which is presently of idiopathic type.

(Illustrations courtesy of David O. Davis, M.D.)

ARNOLD-CHIARI MALFORMATION

CT scanning has no primary place in the diagnosis of Type I Arnold-Chiari malformation, since the presence and degree of caudal malposition of the cerebellar tonsils cannot be established satisfactorily. Associated abnormalities such as obstructive hydrocephalus may be established sufficiently clearly that the use of contrast studies can be limited to the posterior fossa. If high-quality CT scans can be obtained down to the level of the foramen magnum, the value of this method may be somewhat greater in the case of Type II malformations, but it is probable that additional studies will be required to complete the diagnostic evaluation. Theoretically, CT scanning should provide greater assistance in the investigation of Type III malformations, again provided that sufficiently good quality low scans are obtainable. Although we do not have experience with CT scanning in this form of the malformation, the method is known to be capable of producing considerable information concerning the patterns of cerebellar maldevelopment that can be seen in this condition.

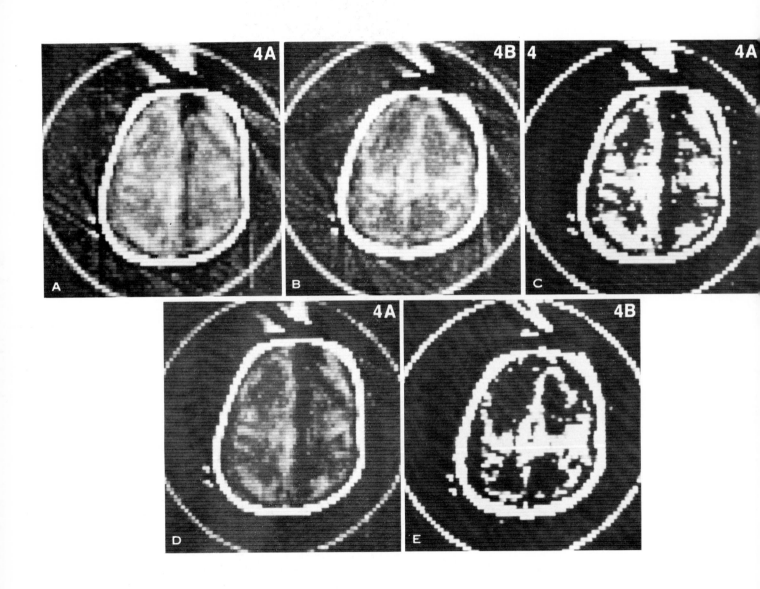

FIG. 24.8. MENKES' SYNDROME (KINKY HAIR DISEASE).

Clinical Features. A 5-month-old Caucasian male who was first admitted to the MGH at the age of 2½ months with generalized seizures. A product of the eighth pregnancy of a 31 y.o. mother, he was delivered at 36 weeks of gestation. Birth weight was 3 lbs., 13 oz. All male siblings (two, of different paternity) had died with a syndrome characterized by retardation, seizures, and enlarging head (no autopsy in either case).

Neurological Examination. At the first admission he was noted to be pale, with sparse and rough-appearing hair, which was very light in color. Head circumference was 37 cm, an increase of 4 cm since birth. He was noted to be very "jittery," with tetany upon tap of the zygoma. Frequent cries, of normal pitch. Increased deep tendon reflexes and positive Babinski responses. Normal transillumination. Seizures were the only manifestation of neurological function above the brain stem. Multiple serum copper measurements showed very low values. Low ceruloplasmin values. Radiographic survey of extremities showed gross periosteal reaction, with metaphyseal spurs and infractions, consistent with Menkes' syndrome. Microscopic examination of the hair showed pylus torti and fractured shafts. An oral absorption test with ^{64}Cu showed less than 0.01% of isotope had been absorbed. Severe persistent hypothermia was present. Head size began to increase rapidly at about 3 months of age and increased quickly to over the ninety-seventh percentile. Subdural taps were unrevealing. Four attempts at ventricular puncture were unsuccessful, indicating "probably normal ventricular size." Head enlargement stabilized on prednisone administration but increased again rapidly when dosage was reduced.

Second Admission. Weight was at the third percentile, height was below the third percentile, and head circumference was above the ninety-seventh percentile. Anterior fontanel was 6 x 6 cm and slightly bulging. Intermittent seizure activity with generalized twitching was noted. Little spontaneous activity. Optic discs appeared normal. Generalized increase in tonus and deep tendon reflexes. Transillumination had changed remarkably, with a mottled pattern over most of the head.

EEG. At first admission. Extremely high voltage slow waves over occipital regions bilaterally.

Skull Examination. Essentially normal at the first admission. Moderate suture diastasis at the second admission.

CT Scan. At the second admission (at 5 months of age). Abnormal (Fig. 24.8).

CT Scan 5 Months Later. Abnormal, with a striking change (Fig. 17.8).

PEG. At 3 months of age. Limited study. Delayed passage of gas superiorly from the fourth ventricle. Normal lateral and fourth ventricular size and position, and normal basal cisterns.

PEG. Repeated 3½ weeks later with 18 ml of oxygen. Gas could not be made to ascend beyond the midaqueduct.

Angio. Multiple attempts at cerebral angiography resulted in only a very limited intracranial study. Abnormally tortuous cerebral arteries were demonstrated.

Treatment. Attempted correction of copper deficiency by oral loading with high-concentration copper, supplemented by parenteral therapy as necessary. Following the later demonstration of massive extracerebral collections (Fig. 17.9), the child's overall condition led to a decision against drainage.

A–E. CT scan obtained at the age of 5 months. At the time of this study, the improved head bag was not yet available. The large size of the available head bag caused additional difficulty in positioning, and the posterior fossa structures could not be studied.

A and B. L 6   W 20.

These adjacent, approximately midcerebral-level sections show grossly abnormal absorption values throughout the cerebral hemispheres. There was a striking diminution in absorption of the cortex (5–12) and of the central grey matter (5–14). The lesser depression of absorption values of the central grey matter compared with the cortex suggests better preservation (better vascular perfusion?). The scan also showed less decrease in absorption of two transverse bands of tissue just behind the midcoronal plane (better preservation of motor cortex and pyramidal fibers?) **(B and E).** Quite large spaces showing CSF absorption values (0–6) were evident over the right frontal pole and lateral surface of the right frontal lobe.

C. L 5   W M.   **D.** L 12   W M.
E. L 6   W M.

Modified displays of the scan sections shown in **A** and **B**, clearly revealing the highly disorganized appearance of the substance of both cerebral hemispheres, with generalized depression of absorption. Also visible are large irregular spaces with CSF absorption values, indicative of irregular and markedly enlarged lateral ventricles that are poorly differentiated from adjacent brain in standard displays, due to the low absorption range of cerebral tissues. A widened space over the left cerebral hemisphere is more clearly visible. This also had CSF absorption values. At the time, it was unclear whether these external CSF absorption spaces represented markedly enlarged subarachnoid spaces or subdural hygromas. In the light of the scan 5 months later (Fig. 17.9), it appears likely that these represent developing subdural hygromas.

SYRINGOMYELIA, HYDROMYELIA, AND SYRINGOBULBIA

In order to achieve high-quality intracranial scans, the EMI scanner was constructed with an equilibrating waterbath, and the present depth of the waterbath is such that scans below the approximate level of the foramen magnum cannot be achieved. Although the diagnosis of syringobulbia is within the capabilities of this scanner, such a case has not yet been seen by us. The demonstration of syringohydromyelia is beyond the present capabilities of this machine.

The ACTA scanner (designed and constructed by Dr. Robert Ledley at Georgetown University) does not em-

ploy an equilibrating waterbath and is capable of scanning the entire body. Scanning times are very similar to those of the EMI scanner. Its capabilities in investigation of cervical intraspinal disease are illustrated by the following two cases (Fig. 24.9), contributed by Giovanni DiChiro, M.D., National Institutes of Health, Bethesda, Maryland.

It is probable that future developments in the field of body scanning will result in additional valuable contributions to neuroradiological diagnosis in the spinal axis in addition to the opening of broad new fields in other radiological realms.

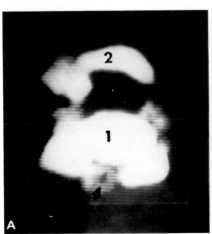 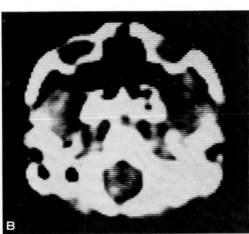 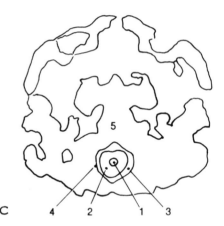

FIG. 24.9.
Case 1. Syringomyelia, verified by surgery (Fig. 24.9A).
Case 2. Syringomyelia and syringobulbia, nonverified (Fig. 24.9, **B** and **C**).
(Cases contributed by Dr. Giovanni Di Chiro, National Institutes of Health, Bethesda, Maryland.)
A. ACTA scan at the level of the 5th cervical vertebra, in a case of syringomyelia confirmed by surgical exploration. The body of the fifth cervical vertebra (1) is visible, behind which can be seen a soft tissue ring representing the spinal cord, within which there is a central region of lower absorption, indicative of a syrinx (*arrow*). The neural arch is absent, due to laminectomy. Part of the mandible is also visible (2).

B. ACTA scan at the level of the foramen magnum in a nonverified case of syringomyelia and syringobulbia. The clinical findings in this patient were strongly suggestive of a syrinx, and a Pantopaque myelogram showed an obvious widening of the cervical spinal cord.
C. Diagrammatic interpretation of the scan shown in **B**: syrinx (*1*); lower medulla oblongata (*2*); subarachnoid space (*3*), which is of varying width around the irregular configuration of the medulla; foramen magnum (*4*); and clivus (*5*). (Reprinted by permission from The New England Journal of Medicine, 292: January 1975.)

CHAPTER 25

Neuroectodermoses

NEUROFIBROMATOSIS

CT scanning represents an extremely useful method of evaluating the protean manifestations of neurofibromatosis as they affect the skull and its contents. Among the many associated abnormalities that may be diagnosed by this means are intraorbital and intracranial neuromas, optic gliomas, single or multiple meningiomas, osseous dysplasias of the cranial vault, orbit, and cranial base, temporal lobe herniation into the orbit and temporal lobe agenesis with associated leptomeningeal pseudocyst formation, and generalized, unilateral, and lobar megaloencephaly.

For examples of various manifestations of neurofibromatosis, the reader is referred to Chapter 9, "Acoustic Neuromas;" Chapter 7, "Meningiomas," Figures 7.4 and 7.5, illustrating multiple meningiomas; Chapter 24, "Developmental Anomalies," Figure 24.3, dysgenesis of temporal lobe with orbital bone defect, and Figure 24.7, macrencephaly; and Chapter 28, "Orbital CT Scanning," Figure 28.22, temporal lobe dysplasia and sphenoid mesodermal defect.

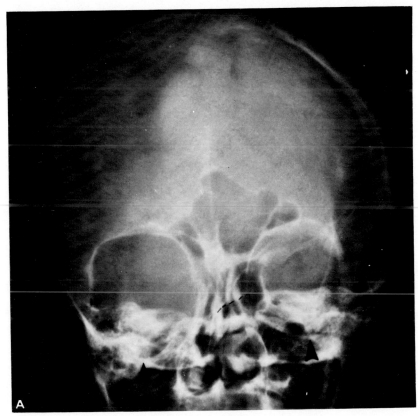

LEGEND FOR FIG. 25.1A ON PAGE 417

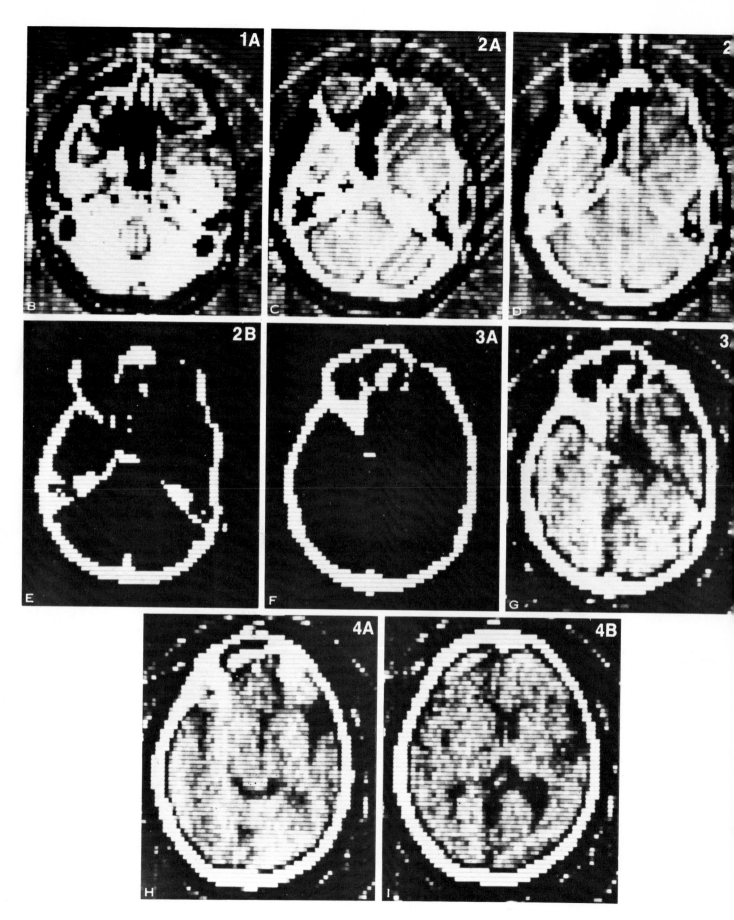

FIG. 25.1. NEUROFIBROMATOSIS, WITH FRONTO-SPHENOIDAL OSSEOUS DYSPLASIA, TEMPORAL LOBE HERNIATION, PULSATING EXOPHTHALMOS, AND BUPHTHALMOS.

Clinical Features. A 55 y.o. female who presented 37 years earlier with a plexiform neuroma of the right eyelids and orbit. This was excised. Cutaneous café au lait spots and an enlarged globe in a deformed orbit were noted. Five years earlier she had undergone excision of neurofibromas of the small bowel. She was noted to have pulsating exophthalmos.

Skull Examination. The cranial vault was markedly asymmetrical. The right hemicranium was very thin and showed a generalized bulging prominence. There was increased prominence of arterial and venous channels over the right hemicranium; the sella was expanded and markedly asymmetrical, with a floor that sloped steeply downwards on the right side. The right orbit was markedly and concentrically enlarged, and its posterior wall was not visible. The general soft tissue density of the right orbit was increased due to exophthalmos (Fig. 25.1A).

CT Scan. Extensive cranial, intracranial, and orbital abnormalities were demonstrated (Fig. 25.1, **B–I**).

A. PA skull film demonstrating the numerous cranial and orbital abnormalities described in the protocol and representing a typical constellation that may be found in neurofibromatosis. Cerebral angiography and pneumoencephalography have previously been used in many such cases for further evaluation of the intracranial features.

B–D. The most inferior pair of scan sections obtained, which reveal considerable enlargement of the right globe (**B**) compared with the left (**C**). The considerable exophthalmos is evident. No bone is visible through much of the area of the posterior wall of the right orbit and the density of the right temporal lobe extends into the posterior portion of the orbit (**C** and **D**).

E and **F.** M settings at high levels, to show only osseous structures. E is the same scan section as in **D**, and F is the next 13-mm section superiorly. These two scan presentations reveal the absence of the posterior wall of the right orbit, part of the medial wall, the entire right side of the planum sphenoidale, and the right anterior clinoid process. Prominence of the right hemicranium is visible in **F**. Thinning of the right hemicranium is visible in **F** and in **G–I**, although the relatively low resolution of the system exaggerates the cranial thickness, which is more clearly visible in plain film skull examination (**A**).

G–I. Consecutive 13-mm sections superiorly. These reveal further evidence of cerebral herniation into the enlarged right orbit and a larger right cerebral hemisphere than left (macrencephaly), in spite of which there is a modest displacement of midline structures to the right (**I**). The lateral and third ventricles are not significantly enlarged, although the right lateral ventricle is a little larger than the left (**I**). These three sections reveal enlarged CSF spaces. The suprasellar cisterns are enlarged to the right (**G**), presumably due to the displacement of the temporal lobe. In addition, there is marked cisternal enlargement in the region of the sylvian cistern and fissure (**H** and **I**). However, a tense-appearing leptomeningeal cyst is not present.

TUBEROSE SCLEROSIS

CT scanning provides a convenient means of surveying the intracranial cavity for the identification of ventricular enlargement secondary to obstructing intraventricular tubers and for the presence of gliomatous changes that may develop. Experience at present is insufficient to evaluate the possibility of increased accuracy in differentiating tubers from gliomas in this condition, a distinction that may be difficult with conventional examinations. The distribution of paraventricular and other calcifications is very accurately identifiable by CT scanning, but the smallest noncalcified tubers projecting into the ventricular system can only be identified by pneumoencephalography, preferably with laminography.

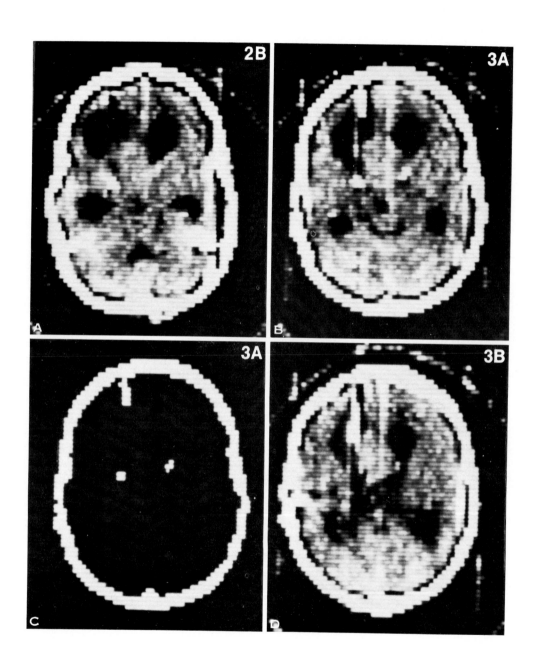

FIG. 25.2 TUBEROSE SCLEROSIS, WITH ASSOCIATED GIANT CELL GLIOBLASTOMA.

Clinical Features. A 12 y.o. girl who presented with multiple stigmata of neurofibromatosis and with diplopia and papilledema.

Skull Examination. Suture diastasis, increased prominence of convolutional impressions superiorly, and sellar enlargement, consistent with very chronic increase in intracranial pressure (2 years earlier).

Angio and Ventriculography. Performed at another hospital 2 years earlier. Revealed obstructive dilatation of the lateral ventricles and a ventriculoperitoneal shunt had been placed. She was now doing well but was referred for further evaluation by CT scan.

CT Scan: Abnormal (Fig. 25.2).

Operation. (Dr. Robert Ojemann.) Radical excision of deeply seated glioma invading the frontal portions of the lateral ventricles.

Histology. Giant cell glioblastoma.

A and **B.** L 16   W 20.

These contiguous 13-mm sections reveal marked enlargement of the frontal and temporal horns, greater on the left side. A large, irregularly rounded mass is shown involving the posteroinferior portions of the frontal horns and the region of the foramina of Munro. The mass is shown to obliterate most of the third ventricle. The high density of a ventricular shunt tube is shown entering the left frontal horn (**B**) and there is a narrow CSF-containing track around the anterior portion of the tube. Bilateral paramedian calcifications, approximately 9 x 12 mm, are shown adjacent to the posterolateral portion of the mass. Plain film examination had revealed only the somewhat larger one on the left side. The mass encroached further on the left lateral ventricle than on the right, and its absorption range was 14–24.

C. L 50   W M.

The left frontal shunt tube and the bilateral calcifications are shown. The left calcification ranged up to 115, and the right ranged to 65 units.

D. Section immediately above that in **B**, showing the shunt tube extending posteriorly adjacent to the mass encroaching upon the frontal horns and anterior bodies of the lateral ventricles.

A diagnosis of glioma was made, primarily on the basis of the size and extent of the single mass. It is not known at present whether there is a useful differential absorption between noncalcified tubers and giant cell astrocytomas that may complicate tuberose sclerosis. The density of the tumor in this case is somewhat greater than is typically seen in plain scans of benign and malignant astrocytomas.

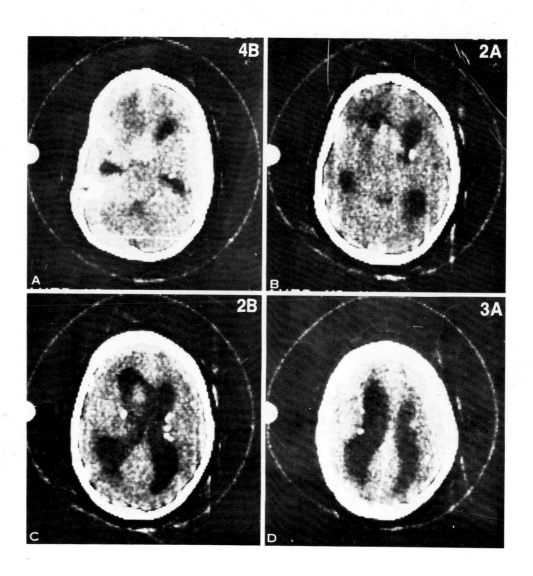

FIG. 25.3. TUBEROSE SCLEROSIS, WITH DEVELOP-MENT OF GLIOMA. (Case contributed by Hillier L. Baker, Jr., M.D., Mayo Clinic.)

Clinical Features. An 8 y.o. girl who had been mentally retarded from birth and who began having mainly tonic seizures at the age of 5. Seizures were frequent and not controlled by medication.

Neurological Examination. Marked mental retardation, with no speech. Chronic bilateral papilledema, without other neurological signs. Papular skin lesions in the malar regions, typical of adenoma sebaceum.

Skull Examination. Suture diastasis of increased intracranial tension. Multiple flecks of cerebral calcification in the paraventricular areas.

Intravenous Pyelography. Multiple bilateral renal masses, consistent with hamartomas.

CT Scan. Abnormal (Fig. 25.3)

Operation. Right frontal exploration revealed an astrocytoma Grade II, involving the frontal lobe and region of the left caudate nucleus. A ventricular shunt was placed and radiation therapy was instituted.

A. L 14   W 30   160 x 160 matrix system.
Section through the frontal horns and fourth ventricle obtained after the more superior contiguous sections shown in 3B–D. The temporal horns are moderately dilated and a tiny calcification is evident at the superior ependymal surface of the right temporal horn. A 2.7 cm diameter region of increased absorption (24) is shown in the region of the apparently obliterated anterior third ventricle. The head is canted up on the left side. A large area of diminished absorption (minimum, 6 units), with poorly defined margins, is shown extending through the left frontal lobe in **A** and **B**.

B. Section slightly higher than that in **A**, showing a large nodular mass (peak, 21) encroaching markedly upon the lumen of the deformed and compressed left frontal horn. The mass extends into the medial portion of the dilated right frontal horn, where there is a small nodular calcification projecting from the ependymal surface in the region of the head of the caudate nucleus. The irregular region of diminished absorption in the left frontal lobe is more obvious in this section.

C. There is quite marked enlargement of both lateral ventricles. The septum lucidum is markedly bowed to the right. The superior portion of the nodular mass visible in **B** is shown projecting freely into the left frontal horn, which is markedly dilated at this level. Four small calcifications are clustered along the ependymal surface of the lateral wall of the right lateral ventricle, and a single calcification is visible in the wall of the left lateral ventricle.

D. Two additional ependymal calcifications are shown in the lateral wall of the left lateral ventricle. A triangular encroachment from the lateral wall of the right lateral ventricle, approximately 4–6 mm in diameter, shows absorption somewhat higher than white matter, without definite evidence of calcification.

This case exhibits calcified and not obviously calcified tubers in the walls of the lateral ventricles and an irregular decreased absorption lesion in the left frontal lobe, indicative of a glioma. The size and configuration of the large increased absorption nodular mass in the area of the anterior portion of third ventricle and left frontal horn is more suggestive of further involvement by glioma than of a giant tuber. Surgery confirmed the presence of glioma in this region as well as in the frontal lobe further anteriorly. In spite of partial volume averaging, the obviously calcified tubers showed values peaking above 40 and 50 units. As expected, there is problem in identifying noncalcified or partly calcified tubers in the cortex, since absorption values of these small lesions tend to be very similar to those of cortex. In this case, there appeared to be multiple small nodules in the cortex of both cerebral hemispheres when these regions were studied with window levels above 20.

(Illustrations courtesy of Dr. Hillier Baker, Jr.)

STURGE-WEBER SYNDROME

The fact that the sensitivity of CT scanning is greater than that of radiographic filming in the identification of calcific absorption values suggests that this method may be useful in the identification of intracranial features of this syndrome, since intracortical calcifications secondary to the cerebral component of the syndrome are usually not visible on skull film examination until the second year of life. In addition, the angiographic abnormalities representing the capillary leptomeningeal angiomatosis may be difficult to identify, particularly when the area involved is relatively small. Under such circumstances, contrast-enhanced CT scans may prove to be a most useful adjunct to diagnostic evaluation.

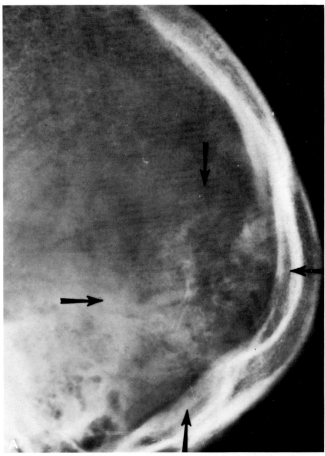

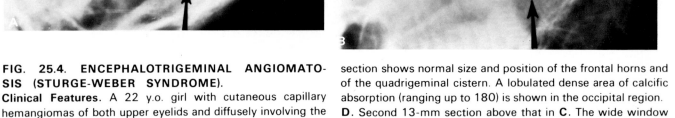

FIG. 25.4. ENCEPHALOTRIGEMINAL ANGIOMATO-SIS (STURGE-WEBER SYNDROME).

Clinical Features. A 22 y.o. girl with cutaneous capillary hemangiomas of both upper eyelids and diffusely involving the face in the trigeminal nerve distribution Left parieto-occipital calcifications. Focal and generalized seizures since the age of 7 and occasional mild bifrontal headaches. The patient was followed at intervals in clinic. A dense right homonymous hemianopsia had recently been discovered. No visual defect had been apparent 5 years earlier. The patient was unclear about the duration of visual difficulty and she was referred for CT scan, to exclude a recent left occipital hemorrhage.

Skull Examination. Typical serpiginous parallel calcifications were demonstrated in the left occipital lobe region, extending slightly into the parietal area. The overlying vault was thickened and slightly flattened (Fig. 25.4, **A** and **B**).

CT Scan. Abnormal (Fig. 25.4, **C**–**F**).

A and **B**. Lateral and AP plain skull examinations, respectively, showing typical intracranial calcifications of the syndrome in the occipital and adjacent parietal lobes (*arrows*).

C–F. CT scan was obtained only after contrast enhancement with 50 ml of Hypaque 60.

C. No ventricular enlargement or mass effect was evident. This

section shows normal size and position of the frontal horns and of the quadrigeminal cistern. A lobulated dense area of calcific absorption (ranging up to 180) is shown in the occipital region.

D. Second 13-mm section above that in **C**. The wide window (75) permitted better differentiation of the calcific areas in the parieto-occipital region from adjacent cerebral cortex and overlying bone.

E. L 60   W M.

Section between those in **C** and **D**, showing the posterior calcifications (25–180) and the slight overlying thickening of the cranial vault.

F. L 60   W M.

Same section as that in **D**. The extension of the calcification into the parietal lobe was much more completely demonstrated by CT scan than by plain films. At this level, partial volume effects resulted in lower absorption (28–80). Small areas ranging in absorption from 20–42 were also noted in this and subjacent scans. Since no plain CT scan was obtained and because the partial volume effects on the highly irregular calcifications were unknown, it was not possible to differentiate between small areas of calcification, areas of blood containing vessels of the angioma, and very small extravasations of blood.

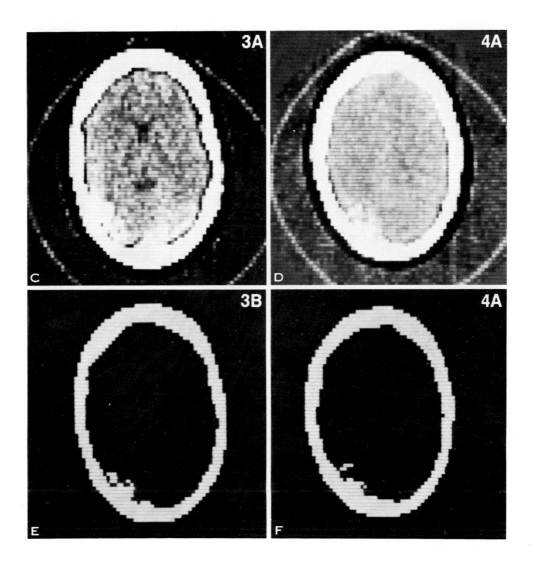

VON HIPPEL-LINDAU DISEASE

Our experience is not sufficient at present to allow assessment of the value of CT scanning in the diagnosis of retinal angiomatosis. Ultrasonic B scanning is likely to be more useful in this regard than is CT scanning, in view of the high resolution depiction of the intrinsic structure of the eye that is possible with the former method.

Small nodules of hemangioblastoma in the cerebellum, occupying only a portion of a CT scan section, are difficult to identify with certainty. The use of large volumes of intravenous contrast material (100–200 ml) may provide definite identification of such small nodules, particularly if 8-mm sections are used with the 160 x 160 matrix system. Low-absorption fluid content of cystic hemangioblastomas may permit identification of quite small cysts, and CT scanning appears to be a useful preliminary method of investigation of cerebellar hemangioblastoma before angiography. Some useful additional information may be obtainable. Cysts containing extensive vascular tumor tissue in their walls should be readily identifiable if they are larger than 1 cm in diameter and if scans of good technical quality are obtained. Both plain and contrast-enhanced scans are desirable, so the latter may be obtained using the circulating contrast material present after angiography, alone or supplemented by additional intravenous contrast medium. Associated obstructive hydrocephalus and its degree should readily be recognized.

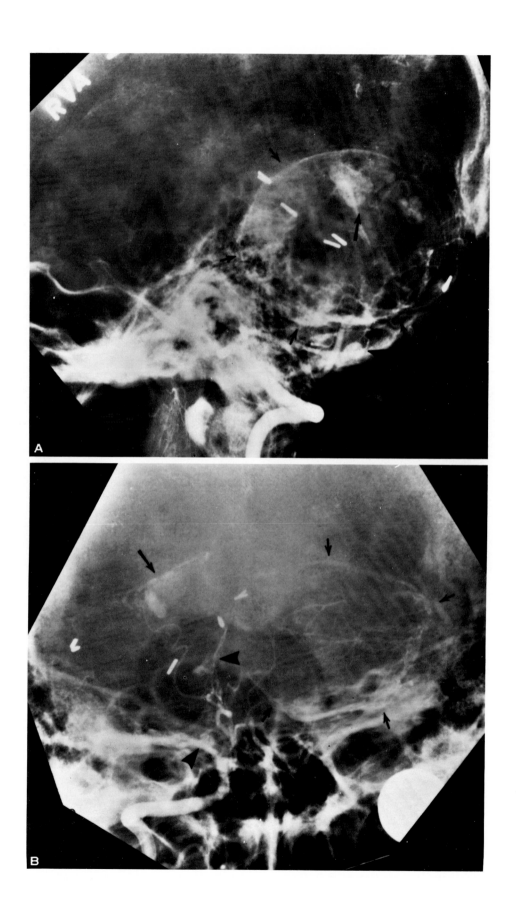

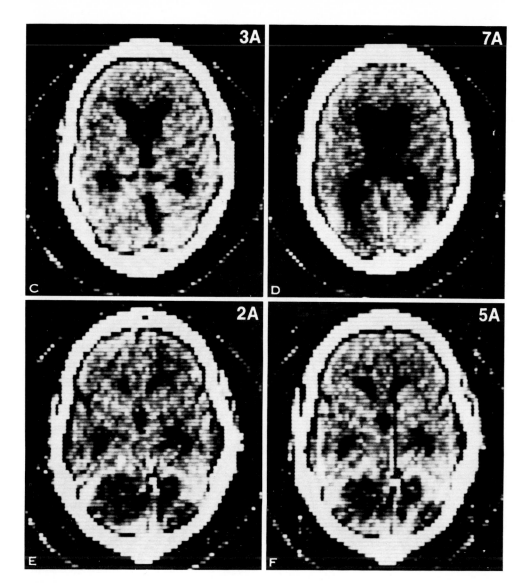

FIG. 25.5. VON HIPPEL-LINDAU DISEASE, WITH MULTIPLE CEREBELLAR AND SPINAL CORD HEMANGIOBLASTOMAS.

Clinical Features. A 30 y.o. male, whose disease was diagnosed at the age of 14. A strong family history of the disease was obtained. Seven years earlier he had undergone enucleation of the left eye after multiple photocoagulation treatments for bilateral retinal angiomatosis. Ten years earlier he had presented with symptoms of increased intracranial pressure and cerebellar signs and underwent removal of a cystic cerebellar hemangioblastoma, with subsequent posterior fossa irradiation. Two years before the present admission he had complained of numbness in the right upper extremity and was studied by vertebral angiography, spinal cord angiography, and myelography.

Angio. Previous vertebral and spinal angiography had demonstrated numerous highly vascular nodules of hemangioblastoma in both of the cerebellar hemispheres, cerebellar vermis, and spinal cord; some of these were associated with small to medium-sized cysts. Repeat transfemoral right vertebrobasilar angiogram after CT scan revealed small nodules of hemangioblastoma in the right cerebellar hemisphere, vermis, and upper cervical spinal cord. In addition, there was a very large ovoid cyst in the left cerebellar hemisphere, with a thin rim of vascular tumor (Fig. 25.5, **A** and **B**).

CT Scan. Abnormal (Fig. 25.5, **C-F**).

A and **B**. Lateral and AP views, respectively, from recent ver-
tebrobasilar angiogram, showing multiple small, highly vascularized nodules of tumor in the cerebellum (*large arrows* and *arrowheads*). A very large cystic mass with a thin vascular wall was shown in the left cerebellar hemisphere (*small arrows*). Previous posterior fossa craniectomy and multiple surgical clips are also visible.

C-F. L 15   W 20.

C and **D**. Scans reveal moderate obstructive dilatation of the lateral and third ventricles. In addition, the superior portion of the large cyst is shown in the cerebellum, just to the right of the midline in **C**.

E and **F**. Plain CT scan and scan after contrast enhancement with 50 ml of Hypaque, respectively, at very similar levels and angles. Both scans show the large ovoid cystic tumor involving the left cerebellar hemisphere and extending several millimeters to the right of the midline. Two smaller cystic lesions are present in the right cerebellar area on these sections, and the high density of several silver clips is shown in the central area of the posterior fossa. Absorption values of the cysts lay in the range of 5–14. It was extremely difficult to identify tumor nodules on both the plain and contrast-enhanced scans, but there appeared to be some increase in density in two areas, consistent with the presence of small vascularized nodules. One of these lies between the two cystic areas in the right cerebellar area. Angiography is clearly overwhelmingly superior to CT scanning in the identification of such small vascularized lesions.

425

CHAPTER 26

Trauma

INTRODUCTION

Computed tomography is extremely effective in the demonstration and differentiation of a wide variety of traumatic effects upon the brain and in the evaluation of later posttraumatic conditions, such as focal or widespread cerebral atrophy, porencephalic cyst formation, and posttraumatric obstructive hydrocephalus. For a consideration of extracerebral and intracerebral hematomas, the reader is referred to the appropriate chapters, and those conditions will not be dealt with in detail here.

The difficulty in differentiation of posttraumatic cerebral edema, hemorrhagic contusion, and frank hematoma formation, alone or in combination, by means of cerebral angiography is well known. Not infrequently, cerebral angiography must be repeated in order to obtain a valid assessment regarding the progression or otherwise of mass effects produced by these conditions if the patient's condition does not improve or worsens.

CT scanning has been found to be very effective in differentiating the presence and extent of low absorption areas in the brain resulting from posttraumatic edema from the focal high absorption of frank intracerebral hematoma. At other times, a patchy appearance of slightly increased absorption within a diffuse area of decreased absorption or a diffuse homogeneous slight elevation in absorption can be identified, indicating a contusion. A series of CT scans, alone or after angiography performed in the acute phase, permits accurate assessment and observation of progress.

Generally, plain film examination will have been obtained, but CT scanning can be useful as a complementary procedure for identifying the presence of de-

pressions of large or even quite small bone fragments. For this purpose, the scans should be studied with the viewer M setting and the window level above that of the highest cortical absorption values (38–40). By this means, even small cortical bone fragments may be identified, in spite of the averaging of bone absorption with adjacent soft tissues. A depressed bone spicule has been identified by Ambrose, in spite of the fact that it lay embedded in the brain, within an intracerebral hematoma. It has been demonstrated that very high window level settings may permit identification of an obliquely running nondepressed fracture, although this is clearly not the definitive method of diagnosis of such fractures.

According to Paxton and Ambrose (51), emergency angiography has been virtually eliminated at Atkinson Morley Hospital by the use of CT scanning in cases of trauma. However, we have found that such patients are frequently unable to cooperate in remaining sufficiently still for satisfactory scans (or are quite combative) unless heavy sedation or general anesthesia is employed. Not infrequently, therefore, such patients have been subjected to emergency angiography to exclude urgent need for surgery, with subsequent CT scanning for additional clarification and for observation of the progress of lesions. Nevertheless, the increasing use of CT and the decreasing use of emergency angiography have been noteworthy in recent months.

It is for study of cranial trauma that the greatest pressures will be generated for improved equipment that is capable of much more rapid scanning. At present, the great potential of the method in the study of such cases is difficult to realize fully.

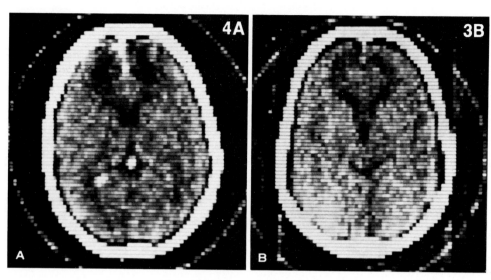

FIG. 26.1. BIFRONTAL CEREBRAL CONTUSION, CONTRECOUP INJURY.

Clinical Features. A 53 y.o. male who was found after apparently having fallen down stairs. A small laceration was present in the right occipital scalp.

Neurological Examination. He was initially drowsy but could be aroused. He had a total amnesia for the event but was otherwise quite well oriented. There was some nuchal rigidity. Lumbar puncture showed an opening pressure of 165 mm, with clear CSF and normal protein. He became more drowsy and his temperature rose to 102°. He was belligerent and confused on the day after injury and developed nystagmus (beating to the left in the primary position).

Skull Examination. Linear vertical fracture of the occipital bone, extending to the foramen magnum.

CT Scan. The scan on the day after admission was technically unsatisfactory because of very extensive motion artifacts. The scan was repeated on the following day, under general anesthesia (Fig. 26.1**A**). He was treated with steroids.

RN Scan. Tcp; on the eighteenth hospital day; normal.

CT Scan. A third CT scan on the twenty-fifth hospital day was again abnormal (Fig. 26.1**B**).

He was discharged on the twenty-sixth hospital day, with abnormal and forgetful behavior with associated gait difficulty.

A. L 15   W 20.

Scan obtained on the second hospital day, under general anesthesia. There was moderate indentation of the anterior aspects of both frontal horns. No ventricular enlargement was present and the ventricular system was otherwise normal. There was no midline dislocation. Immediately anterior to the frontal horns, broad zones of diminished absorption (4–13) are shown extending anteriorly through the front white matter to the medial frontopolar grey matter, which shows locally diminished absorption. There is somewhat better preservation of absorption in the region of the anterior portion of the corpus callosum.

B. L 15   W 20.

CT scan after steroid therapy, obtained the day before discharge. The bilateral anterior frontal paramedian decreased absorption regions are smaller and absorption is higher than previously. At this time there is no evidence of indentation of the anterior aspects of the frontal horns.

In both of the above scans, the diminished absorption of edema extended to involve sections above and below those shown.

Although general anesthesia was necessary for generation of a satisfactory scan in the acute phase because of the patient's confusion and resistive state, the study permitted satisfactory exclusion of intracerebral and extracerebral hematoma, and provided clear evidence of bifrontal contusion, consisting of edema without evident hemorrhagic extravasation. The final scan revealed significant improvement, but still obvious cerebral edema. RN scan 1 week earlier had been negative.

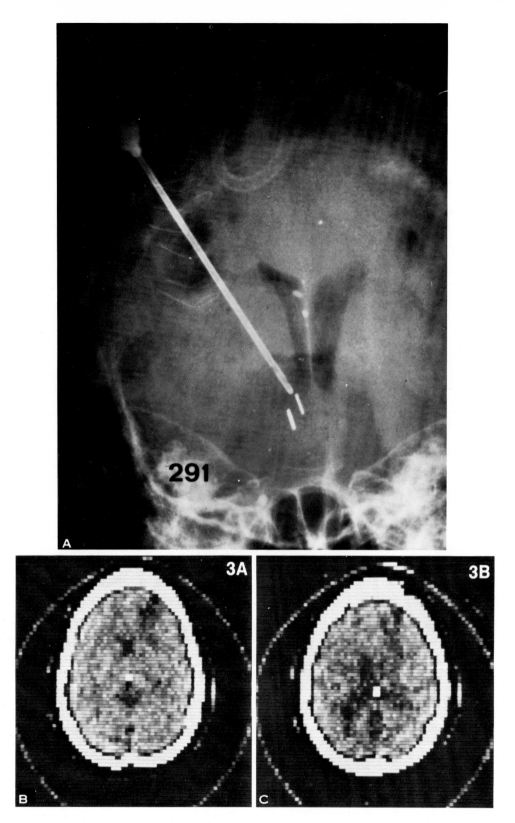

FIG. 26.2. CAUTERY TRACK.
Clinical Features. An 11 y.o. girl who had had resection of a Grade II cerebellar astrocytoma 2 years earlier. She had also received a ventriculoatrial shunt and postoperative radiation. Sixteen months before the present admission, laminectomy had shown intradural metastatic astrocytoma in the spinal canal. She had recently developed frontal headaches, vomiting, and urinary incontinence. Three days before the CT scan, an attempted PEG had failed. Two days before the scan, a right frontal burr hole was made in preparation for a ventriculogram.
CT Scan. Abnormal (Fig. 26.2, **B** and **C**).
A. Brow-up sagittal projection obtained at ventriculography shortly after CT scan. A ventricular needle is shown on the right side. There is a mild compression deformity of the right frontal horn. Also visible are the occipital craniectomy defect, surgical clips, and Pantopaque residues in the posterior fossa.
B and **C.** L 16   W 20.
These contiguous scan sections reveal compression of the body and frontal horn of the right lateral ventricle, slight dislocation of the frontal horns toward the left, and an irregular zone of diminished absorption (8–12) extending from the right frontal horn to the surface of the frontal lobe. A portion of the burr hole is visible in **C**. These findings represent a cauterized tract, made in preparation for ventricular needling, and associated frontal lobe edema from the surgical trauma, 2 days earlier.

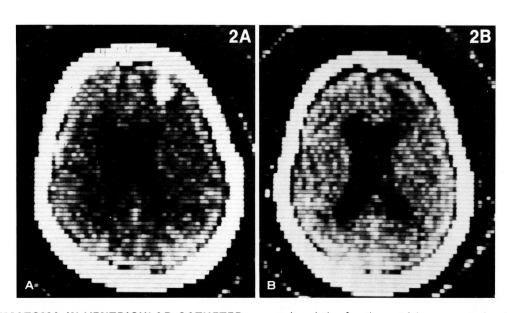

FIG. 26.3. HEMATOMA IN VENTRICULAR CATHETER TRACT.

Clinical Features. A 57 y.o. female who had remained in coma since an automobile accident 1 week before CT scan.

Skull Examination. No evidence of fracture. Pineal midline.

Angio. Bilateral carotid studies, 1 day after injury, suggested slight swelling, consistent with contusion, in both frontal lobes and in the left suprasylvian region. The ventricles did not appear enlarged.

Operation. A right frontal ventricular drainage catheter was placed on the day of injury and removed 24 hours before the CT scan. Lumbar puncture on the day of the scan revealed an opening pressure of 295 mm. At this time, there was evidence of bilateral decortication, with small reactive pupils.

CT Scan. Abnormal (Fig. 26.3).

A and **B**. Adjacent scan sections, showing moderate lateral ventricular enlargement. The third ventricle was slightly wid-ened and the fourth ventricle was not visualized, because of difficulty in obtaining deep insertion of the head into the scanner. An 18-mm rounded area of high absorption, indicative of a small hematoma, is shown in the right frontal lobe (**A**). This is surrounded by a low absorption band, indicative of edema, and the septum lucidum is displaced approximately 6 mm to the left. In **B**, the section lies immediately above the small hematoma and shows only adjacent edema in the region. The findings are consistent with a small hematoma in the ventricular catheter tract, with an area of associated edema and mild focal mass effect upon the ventricular system. The sylvian cisterns and cerebral sulci were not enlarged and the ventricular pattern is consistent with obstructive hydrocephalus. A repeat CT scan 9 days later (not shown) showed partial absorption of the frontal lobe hematoma and still obvious adjacent edema (6–14). No change in ventricular size was noted.

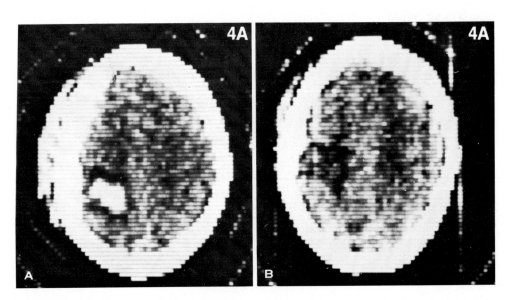

FIG. 26.4. TRAUMATIC INTRACEREBRAL HEMORRHAGE.

Clinical Features. A 20 y.o. man who had undergone surgery for removal of a left parietal epidural hematoma on the day of acute head trauma. Severe residual aphasia and right hemiparesis prompted the initial CT scan 5 days later.

CT Scan. Abnormal (Fig. 26.4A).

CT Scan. Residual changes were present 11 days later (Fig. 26.4B).

A. The typical appearance of a deep superior left parietal intracerebral hematoma, with quite a broad surrounding low absorption zone of edema are shown. There is also a thin left frontoparietal high absorption extracerebral hematoma (ap-

proximately 9 mm in maximum thickness), indicative of residual extradural hematoma. The high absorption of a subgaleal hematoma is visible over the vault in the left frontal and parietal regions.

CT examination can readily provide information regarding associated intra- and extracerebral lesions in acute trauma, provided that scans of satisfactory quality are obtained.

B. Scan 11 days after that illustrated in **A**. The high density hematoma is no longer visible, but a deep parietal region of low absorption remains. This presumably represents liquefied hematoma residues and cerebral edema.

(Reprinted by permission from Radiology, 112: 73–80, 1974.)

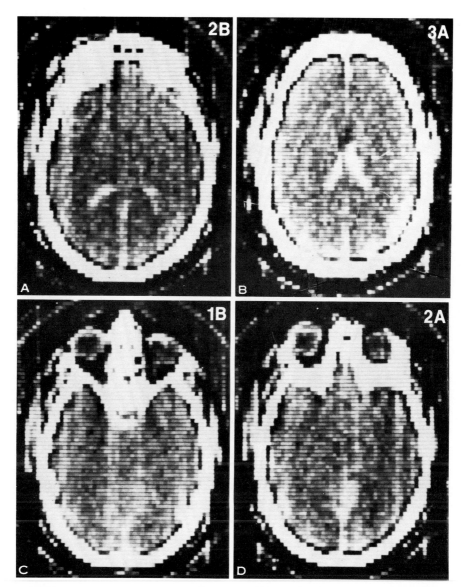

FIG. 26.5. DIFFUSE CEREBRAL SWELLING, INTRA-VENTRICULAR AND SUBARACHNOID HEMORRHAGE AFTER SEVERE TRAUMA.

Clinical Features. A 21 y.o. male who was hit by an automobile while standing in the road.

Neurological Examination. Comatose, with no clear-cut focal neurological signs. Femoral and pelvic fractures were noted.

Skull Examination. A nondepressed linear fracture was present in the left frontotemporal region.

Angio. Unsuccessful because of difficulty in arterial puncture.

CT Scan. Abnormal (Fig. 26.5).

A and **B.** An extensive blood cast is visible in the more posterior portions of each lateral ventricle, larger in volume on the right, and sparing the frontal regions. The lateral and third ventricles are quite small, suggesting the possibility of a mild generalized swelling of the cerebral hemispheres. However, no convincing evidence of abnormal absorption values was detected in either cerebral hemisphere to suggest edema or hemorrhagic contusion.

C and **D.** The high absorption zones in the region of the tentorium and posterior portion of the interhemispheric fissure are indicative of blood clots in these portions of the subarachnoid space.

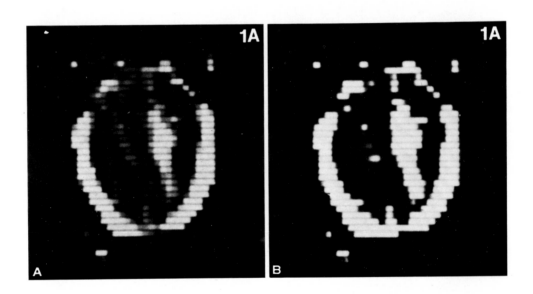

FIG. 26.6. INTRAVENTRICULAR HEMORRHAGE IN A NEONATE.

Clinical Features. A 3-day-old 3 lb. 6 oz. premature male who developed severe respiratory distress leading to coma, shortly after birth. At the time of CT scan, the patient had clinical brain death, with respiration mechanically maintained. The fontanel was bulging and tense. Cerebrospinal fluid was grossly bloody, with a 12% hematocrit.

A. The scan shows blood clot forming a cast of the right lateral ventricle. The anterior and posterior fontanels are visible.
B. L 20   W M.
These settings of the same section more clearly demonstrate the extent of the intraventricular clot. Autopsy confirmed distension of the right lateral ventricle by blood clot.
(Reprinted by permission from Radiology, 112: 73–80, 1974.)

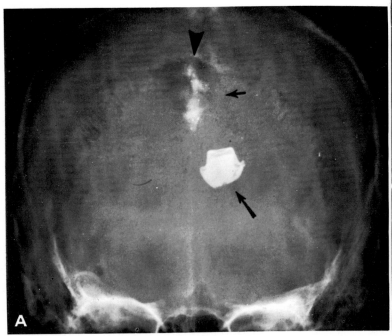

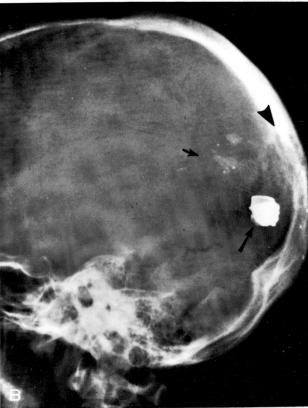

FIG. 26.7. OCCIPITAL GUNSHOT WOUND.

Clinical Features. An 18 y.o. female who was brought to the Emergency Ward after sustaining a gunshot wound of the right occipital region.

Neurological Examination. Alert but disoriented. Able to follow commands. No vision in either eye. Pupils 7 mm and poorly reactive. Small range of ocular motion in all directions. Remaining cranial nerves were intact. General motor and sensory examinations were normal.

Skull Examination. Intracranial bullet and bone fragments (Fig. 26.7, **A** and **B**).

Operation. Debridement of bone fragments.

By the tenth postoperative day, she was able to recognize finger movements in both eye fields and was able to read ¼ inch type. Neuro-ophthalmological examination on the sixteenth day revealed bilateral central inferior visual field defects, consistent with trauma to both occipital lobes above the calcarine fissures.

CT Scan. Abnormal on the twentieth postoperative day (Fig. 26.7, **C–J**).

A. Frontal skull film. **B.** Lateral skull film. The irregularly rounded occipital bone defect extending up to the lambdoid suture is centered slightly to the right of the midline (*arrowhead*). The major bullet fragment is shown lying slightly to the left of the midline in the area of the posterior portion of the left occipital lobe (*large arrow*). Multiple bone fragments, up to a few millimeters in size, and minute metallic particles are shown adjacent to the midline in the occipital region (*small arrows*).

C–J. CT scan obtained on the twentieth postoperative day.

C. The lateral ventricles are normal in size and there is no midline dislocation. There is indication of modest widening of the interfrontal portion of the longitudinal fissure.

D. This more superior scan section shows multiple, small, very dense regions in the area of the cortex of the posterior surfaces of the occipital lobes and extending anteriorly immediately to the right of the normal position of the falx. Immedi-

ately to the left of the region of the falx is a vertical band of absorption extending down to −80, representing computer underswing adjacent to the very high-density material. A 6-mm high absorption focus (+50) is shown in the medial region of the left occipital lobe, indicating presence of a bone fragment that could not be localized readily on skull films.

E. L −20 and +480   W M.

This is the same section as in **D**. The photograph combines the appearance of the display with two widely different level settings, using the persistence of the image on the first level set. With rapid change in level settings, this "double-imaging" can be obtained readily and is useful at times. The combined settings show the black peripheral collection of air in the hair and the white representing the skull vault. Also shown in white is the main bullet fragment, immediately to the left of the midline in the occipital region, with small black regions representing adjacent computer underswing artifact.

F. L 270   W M.

Only the main bullet fragment and the vault are shown as white.

G. L 15   W 10.

Section between those shown in **C** and **D**. Most of the main bullet fragment lay in this section and caused severe artifacts (radiating black and white streaks), which almost completely obscured intracranial detail.

H. L 300   W M.

Same scan as in **G**. At this high setting, the computational artifacts are no longer visible and the metallic and bone fragments are shown in the occipital lobes.

I. L 28   W M.

Same scan as in **D**, **E**, and **F**. Metal fragments to the left of the midline, just internal to the vault, measure 480, and bone fragments bilaterally measure up to 120 units.

J. L 20   W 20.

The most superior section obtained, which passes through the region of occipital bone defect, slightly to the right of the midline. Most of the metallic and bone fragments are below

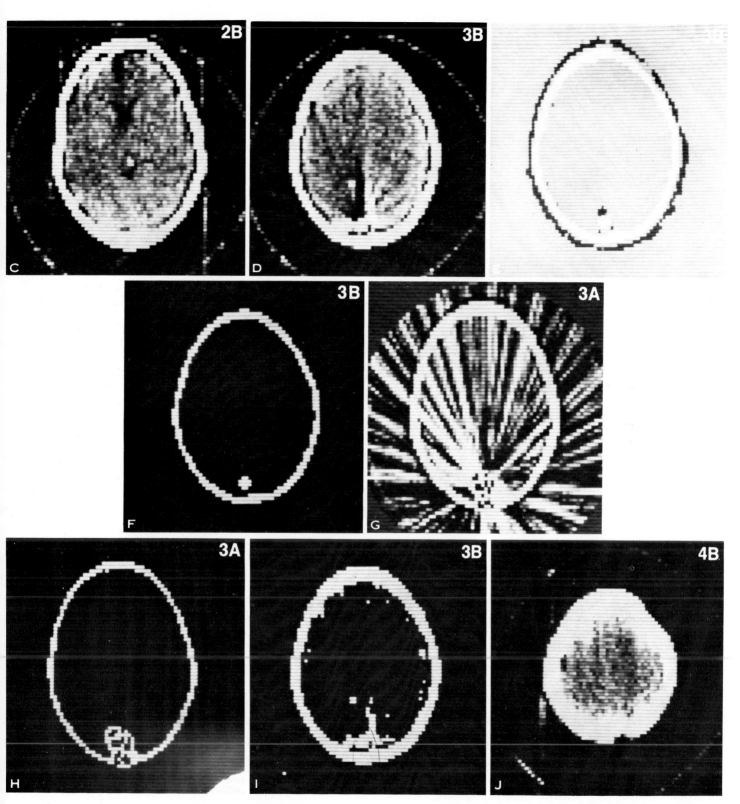

this scan level, because of the obliquity of the section.

In addition to providing information regarding the general anatomical status of cerebral structures, the study was able to exclude the possibility of significant late intracranial hematoma formation and to identify more completely the presence and distribution of metallic and bone fragments within the brain. In the 160 x 160 system, artifacts produced by major metal structures are subdued by arbitrarily assigning the value 800 units to objects (such as metal shunt valves, large surgical clips, and metallic foreign bodies) even though their actual absorption extends very much higher than this.

435

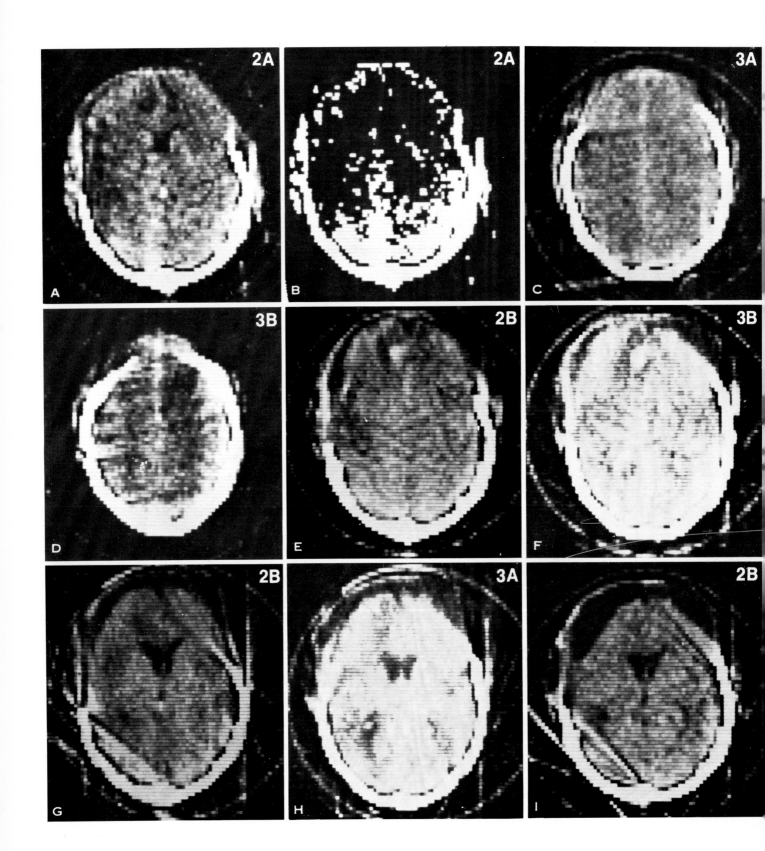

FIG. 26.8. SEVERE CRANIOCEREBRAL INJURY, WITH DEPRESSED FRACTURE, EXTENSIVE CEREBRAL CONTUSION, AND SUBSEQUENT SUBDURAL HYGROMAS.

Clinical Features. A 30 y.o. resident physician, transferred by helicopter from an outlying hospital after an aircraft accident earlier that evening.

Neurological Examination. Comatose, with decerebrate posturing on the right and decorticate movements of the left upper extremity. Left pupil slightly larger than the right, both regular and reactive. Eyes were deviated to the right. The fundi appeared normal. A large depressed fracture of the left frontotemporal area was present, with extruding brain.

Operation. Immediate surgery, with removal of much depressed bone in the left frontotemporal region. There was bleeding from a dural laceration and underlying cortex. Debridement of necrotic and contaminated brain to a depth of 4½ inches. Wide bifrontal decompressive craniectomy, with section of the frontal portion of the falx. Burr holes were placed in the left parietal, right frontal, and right temporal regions. There was no extracerebral hematoma, but contused brain was noted at each site.

CT Scan. Initial examination 3 days after injury (Fig. 26.8, **A–D**).

CT scans were repeated 8, 26, and 33 days after injury (Fig. 26.8, **E** and **F**; **G** and **H**; **I**, respectively). During this period, there was very slight return of cerebral function.

A–D. Initial scan, obtained 3 days after injury. The wide bifrontal craniectomy is visible, with considerable bulging of the cerebral hemispheres through the decompression (**C**). Extensive irregular and rather patchy diminution of absorption is shown through the frontal, temporal, and parietal lobes, with minimal extension into the occipital lobes. The diminished absorption of cerebral edema was most striking in the left frontotemporal regions (8–12, **A**) and right frontal region (10–12, **D**). The anterior portions of the frontal horns are compressed. There was no significant lateral displacement of midline structures (**A**). The general decrease in absorption of the cerebral cortex, of a rather patchy nature, is brought out in

B (same section as **A**, at L   18   W   M). There is some depression of large residual cranial fragments (**C** and **D**). No frank hematomas are visible intracranially, although a few small islands of greater density in the lateral left frontal region are consistent with small extravasations of blood (contusion). Sanguineous collections are shown in the scalp layers bilaterally, but there is no evidence of an intracranial extracerebral collection.

E and **F.** CT scan 8 days after injury. Although diminished absorption of cerebral edema is still present, particularly in the left temporal and both anterior frontal regions, edema is slightly less. Immediately to the left of the midline in the anterior frontal region is a 12 x 15-mm region of increased absorption, indicating a small local hematoma surrounded by edema. A small amount of blood clot is present in the region of the left occipital horn and patchy increase in density suggests smaller clots extending anteriorly into the body of the ventricle. There is a low absorption extracerebral collection over both frontal lobes and internal to the bifrontal skin flap. The lateral ventricles are now not visible except where there is intraventricular blood, indicating considerable diffuse cerebral swelling with ventricular compression.

G and **H.** CT scan obtained 26 days after injury. Although extensive diminution in absorption is still visible through most of the frontal lobes, indicating residual edema and/or ischemic brain, the lateral ventricles are now larger than at the first examination. Developing posttraumatic atrophy or very early obstructive communicating hydrocephalus may be a factor. The median frontal hematoma has undergone considerable absorption. Low absorption bifrontal extracerebral collections, consistent with hygroma formation, are still apparent.

I. CT scan 33 days after injury. The lateral ventricles had increased slightly in size in the interval (more obvious on higher sections) and the third ventricle appears slightly wider. There is still no evidence of significant obstructive hydrocephalus. Diminished absorption values are still present throughout the cortex and white matter of the left temporal and both frontal lobes. The bilateral hygromas are larger and the frontal lobes have become slightly concave beneath these collections, which showed an absorption range of 3–6.

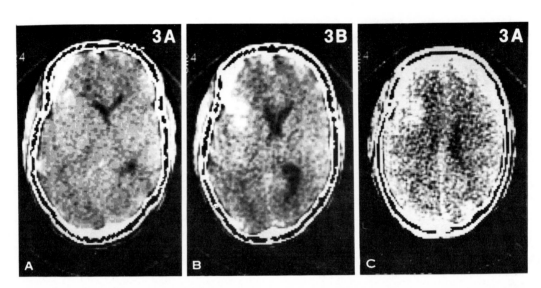

FIG. 26.9. SCALP HEMATOMA, DEPRESSED FRAC-TURE, ACUTE SUBDURAL HEMATOMA AND SEVERE CEREBRAL CONTUSION.

Clinical Features. An 18 y.o. man who sustained head injury in an automobile accident.

Neurological Examination. Semicomatose, with bilateral positive Babinski signs.

Skull Examination. Depressed left frontotemporal skull fracture.

CT Scan. Abnormal (Fig. 26.9).

A–C. Consecutive 13-mm sections from below superiorly. 160 x 160 matrix system.

A. A high-absorption region indicative of a scalp hematoma is demonstrated in the left lateral frontal and temporo-parietal regions, beneath the anterior portion of which is a concave depression of the cranial vault. In the more anterior lateral frontal region is a homogeneous crescentic region of increased absorption (21–46), indicative of an acute subdural hematoma. A few millimeters internal to the posterior portion of the latter is a small irregular region of increased absorption, indicative of intracerebral hemorrhage. There is considerable displacement of the frontal horns to the right and marked compression of the more posterior portions of the left lateral ventricle. The pineal is faintly visible and is displaced approximately 4 mm to the right. There is evidence of a smaller scalp hematoma on the right side.

B. The bilateral scalp hematomas and the left frontal sub-dural hematoma are again visible. An irregular larger region of parenchymal hemorrhage is shown in the left lateral and central frontal regions (absorption, 21–36).

C. Section immediately above that in **B**, showing the very patchy distribution of blood (21–32) in the superior portion of the markedly hemorrhagic contusion.

This case illustrates well the potential of CT in demonstrating and differentiating multiple forms of traumatic lesion, even when they occur in close proximity.

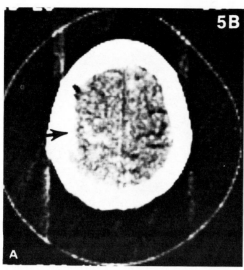
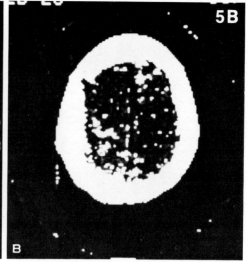

FIG. 26.10. CRANIOCEREBRAL TRAUMA, WITH PARIETAL FRACTURE, SUPERFICIAL CEREBRAL CONTUSION, AND SMALL EXTRACEREBRAL HEMORRHAGES.

Clinical Features. A 66 y.o. man who was admitted because of progressive right hemiparesis, headache with nausea, and vomiting and increasing dysarthria following a fall in which he hit the left parieto-occipital region 2 days earlier.

Neurological Examination. Revealed the patient to be alert and well oriented. He had a right hemiparesis involving the arm more than the leg, mild right hemisensory impairment, and asteriognosis of the right hand.

Skull Examination. A linear fracture was shown running obliquely in the left parietal region.

Angio. Small traumatic middle meningeal artery aneurysm, without evidence of epidural hematoma. Suggestion of minor left posterior suprasylvian mass effect, suggestive of contusion.

CT Scan. Abnormal (Fig. 26.10), 1 day after angiography and 3 days after head injruy.

Over the next few days, his neurological status fluctuated, with prominent confusion and disorientation. Gastrointestinal hemorrhage was followed by neurological deterioration and cardiopulmonary arrest 2 weeks after the CT scan.

Autopsy. Beneath the left parietal skull fracture was a 3½-cm dural laceration, with a small amount of subjacent epidural and subdural blood, mainly over the left parietal cortex. Parenchymal hemorrhages (contusion) extending internally from the pial surface were noted, involving especially the left postcentral gyrus and with some involvement of the precentral gyrus.

A. Scan section through the superior portions of the cerebral hemispheres, at a relatively shallow angle. 160 x 160 matrix system. A region of increased absorption (20–36), consistent with hemorrhage, is shown in a serpiginous configuration, apparently representing the contour of a gyrus (*arrow*). This appears to be the postcentral gyrus and corresponds well with the position of the parietal skull fracture and the hemorrhagic parenchymal lesion involving the region of the postcentral gyrus at autopsy. The sulci on either side are evidently compressed, in contrast with the corresponding sulci of the right cerebral hemisphere, which are slightly enlarged secondary to cerebral atrophy. Immediately posterior to the serpiginous high absorption configuration is a less dense, poorly marginated rounded zone and similar smaller, irregularly rounded zones of slightly increased absorption are visible immediately to the right of the longitudinal fissure in the superior frontal and posterior parietal regions. No hemorrhagic parenchymal lesions were noted in the right cerebral hemisphere at autopsy, and these islands of increased absorption presumably represent the subarachnoid hemorrhage observed.

B. L 25   W M.

Same section as in **A,** for better contrast of the multiple zones of abnormally increased absorption. A 1-cm ovoid superficial parenchymal hemorrhage was also noted in this region. Small collections of subarachnoid blood were noted over the superior portions of the right cerebral hemisphere.

CHAPTER 27

CT Scans with Intravascular Contrast Medium

GENERAL CONSIDERATIONS

Injection of contrast medium, either intravenously, or intra-arterially for angiography, will increase absorption values of normal and pathological tissues in subsequent scans in proportion to the vascularity of the tissues, the permeability of the blood-brain barrier, and the blood concentration of iodine. If a plain CT scan is not obtained (preferably first, since it requires many hours for near-complete elimination of iodine from the circulation), it may be more difficult to evaluate the nature of pathology. Without a plain scan as a base line, the possible contribution of contrast medium to absorption values cannot be determined, and differentiation between densely compacted tissue, extravasated blood, and psammomatous calcifications will be conjectural.

Enhancement of the absorption of very vascular neoplasms has been shown to persist for many hours after injection of 40–50 ml of Conray 60 or Hypaque 60. Extravascular diffusion of contrast medium may contribute to prolonged persistence of increased absorption in a wide variety of pathological conditions. Gado (25A) has studied the increase in absorption produced by a variety of malignant gliomas and a variety of meningiomas after the injection of intravenous contrast medium. In the same cases, he also determined the increased absorption produced in the blood by withdrawing and scanning blood samples. In this way, a tissue to blood ratio of contrast enhancement was obtained. Expressed in percentages, the ratios varied from 17.9 to 110% in the gliomas and up to 130% in the meningiomas. The unrealistically high values indicated that a major portion of the contrast enhancement of tumor tissue was due to extravascular diffusion of contrast medium resulting from impairment of the blood-brain barrier. Although it is to be expected that abnormal vascularity of lesions would be more readily identified by CT contrast enhancement than by angiography, the lack of

consistent relationship between the degree of contrast enhancement and angiographically shown vascularity supports the concept that extravascular diffusion is occurring. Gado obtained additional confirmation of the occurrence of the latter when later scans in some patients revealed a changing tissue to blood ratio. Normally occurring extravascular diffusion of contrast medium into the dura explains both the well-known prolonged angiographic opacification of the falx and tentorium and the marked and prolonged CT contrast enhancement of these structures.

Gado (25A) has also noted a strong relationship between the occurrence of contrast enhancement in intracranial tumors and the appearance of increased activity in these tumors on radionuclide scanning. Also, in his series of twenty-three non tumor cases that did not show contrast enhancement on CT scanning, radionuclide scans were negative except in five cases, which were all cases of cerebral infarction.

Undoubtedly, higher accuracy in the identification of pathological changes and in differential diagnosis will be possible when a contrast-enhanced scan is obtained after a plain scan. Some lesions may have a general absorption range so similar to that of normal brain that the lesions cannot be identified with certainty on plain scan, whereas even minor vascularity of the lesion (in angiographic terms) will result in obviously abnormal absorption in the contrast-enhanced scan.

Rarely, it may happen that a lesion that has a clearly identifiable lower absorption than the brain, and that is associated with very slight vascularity, may be obscured more or less completely when its absorption is increased after contrast enhancement. In a case of moderately extensive cerebral infarction exhibited by Ethier (25), a clearly apparent and typical appearance of reduced absorption in the parietal lobe was converted to a homogeneous absorption level completely indistinguishable from adjacent normal brain after intravenous injec-

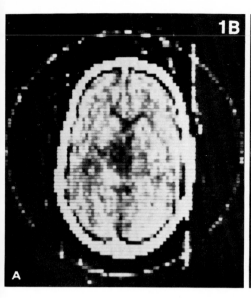
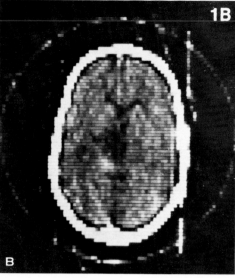
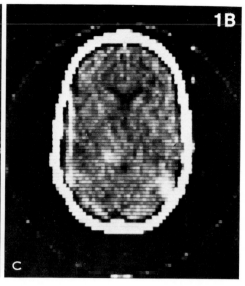

FIG. 27.1. THALAMIC AND MIDBRAIN GLIOMA (NONVERIFIED). (Case contributed by Leon Menzer, M.D., Sabin and Mark, P.A. Boston).

Clinical Features. A 13 y.o. girl with a 4-year history of slowly progressive quadriparesis.

RN Scan. Approximately 1 month before CT scan; increased uptake in the area of the "diencephalon."

Angio. and PEG. One month before CT scan; said to show only ventricular enlargement.

CT Scan. Abnormal (Fig. 27.1).

A. Plain CT scan. W 10. A well-defined area of diminished absorption (11–15) is shown in the region of the left thalamus, extending into the genu and posterior limb of the internal capsule anteriorly and into the region of the left cerebral peduncle posteriorly. Laterally, the lesion becomes less regular and appears to extend into the temporal lobe. The frontal horn is displaced anteromedially and the third ventricle is displaced 6 mm to the right.

B. Plain CT scan. Same section as in **A.** Higher L, W 20. These control settings again show the area of diminished absorption presumed to be attributable to a glioma originating in the thalamus. In addition, a localized area of greater than normal absorption (approximately 22–28) is shown in the left cerebral peduncle more clearly than in **A.**

C. CT scan section very similar to that in **A** and **B,** after intravenous injection of 40 ml of Hypaque 60 M, with similar control settings to those in **B.** There is no definite change in the appearance of the high absorption zone in the left cerebral peduncle. However, the large low absorption region previously visible has now become almost invisible. True, there is a focal, abnormal-appearing heterogeneity of absorption values in the region of the thalamus and medial portion of the lenticular nucleus, but these features and the slight ventricular displacements could be overlooked readily in a scan of slightly less than optimal quality. The area of increased absorption presumably represents a small area of hemorrhagic extravasation in the tumor.

This case serves to illustrate the errors in diagnosis that could occur if only contrast-enhanced CT examinations are performed.

(Illustrations courtesy of Dr. Leon Menzer.)

---

tion of Hypaque 60. Another case in point is illustrated in Fig. 27.1.

The disadvantages of the regular use of contrast enhancement must be given due weight. Firstly, the use of 50–200 ml of intravenous contrast medium changes the nature of CT scanning from completely innocuous to one carrying a small but defined risk of reaction, which, although the risk is miniscule, may lead to death even when the most modern resuscitative measures are applied promptly. Secondly, repeating the CT scan in whole or only in part on the same day or later considerably increases the scheduling problems that are likely to remain severe until CT scanners are widely available in given communities.

The problem of time has been eased somewhat by the advent of the higher resolution 160 x 160 matrix system, since this allows viewing of the scan a few seconds after completion of the study. This permits the physician to determine whether abnormalities shown are such as to make the obtaining of a contrast-enhanced scan highly important. If it is so decided, the selection of the appropriate levels for the additional study is easier and more precise reproduction of scan level and angle is possible than with the old system, with which it was usually necessary to recall the patient at some later time for supplementary contrast-enhanced scan (vide Chapter 3, "Patient Scheduling").

Nevertheless, the frequent use of additional contrast-enhanced scans pre-empts a considerable amount of time that would otherwise be available for additional patients in each day's schedule. This problem is an extension of that created by the need to decide between the use of CT scanning as a rapid "survey" method as contrasted with a more individualized and time-consuming form of study, which is hopefully to be a definitive diagnostic method in a high percentage of cases.

A reasonable compromise may be to arrange for the physician to review the clinical history, findings, and results of antecedent studies in sufficient detail that a routine examination of three scan sequences can be employed with reasonable security, in the knowledge that immediate viewing of the scan results by the physician before the patient leaves the scanner couch can serve to indicate the need for additional plain scan levels and/or an additional, but limited, contrast-enhanced scan. It must be understood that plain scans may appear negative in occasional cases of small neoplasms and vascular malformations. An approach of this type has been used by Ambrose (1) and by Paxton and Ambrose (51), who have used contrast enhancement in all tumor suspects. Ethier has advocated the use of relatively large volumes of intravenous Hypaque 60 M, following studies of the effectiveness of 50 and 100 ml of this contrast medium and of the serum plasma diatrizoate levels that were produced. He has found that a plasma diatrizoate level of approximately 300 mg/100 ml has been significantly more effective than were lower levels in revealing tumors that were not discriminated or were marginally visible on plain scans. These were presumably poorly vascularized neoplasms. He has observed that a dosage of 1.2 ml of Hypaque 60 M per kilogram is required to produce such plasma levels. He has also noted that the plasma level of diatrizoate falls to approximately 50% of the initial level about 30–50 minutes after injection, and therefore he uses an infusion pump to obtain a slow continuous injection after the initial intravenous injection in order to maintain a constant blood level of the contrast medium. He has termed the high-dosage contrast enhancement technique "computed angiotomography" (24). This technique is said to be employed in 30–40% of CT scans performed at the Montreal Neurological Institute. At Stanford University Hospital all serious tumor suspects are given intravenous contrast infusion, and 52% of all CT scans performed receive contrast enhancement.

Cattell et al (11) have investigated the mean plasma concentration and ranges of values obtained after intravenous injection of 20, 40, and 80 ml of Hypaque (45%) in normal subjects. They describe an initial rapid fall in plasma concentration, due to mixing in the vascular compartment. This phase is essentially complete at 10 minutes (during which time approximately 12% of the contrast medium has been excreted in the urine). A second phase with a slower fall in plasma concentration was noted, corresponding with mixing of contrast material with extracellular fluid. A third phase exhibited a very gradual decrease in plasma concentration over several hours, resulting from urinary excretion. These

workers have found initial plasma concentrations of 220–240 mg/100 ml, following injection of 40 ml of 45% Hypaque. Plasma levels fell to approximately 100 mg/100 ml by 30 minutes. Eighty ml of the contrast material gave plasma concentrations of 350–490 mg/100 ml, decreasing to 220–250 at 30 minutes. Cumulative urinary excretion as a percentage of injected dose was 45% at 3 hours, 83% at 6 hours, and 94–100% at 24 hours.

Following the recent introduction of the 160 x 160 matrix system, our use of supplementary contrast-enhanced scans has increased considerably, as was anticipated. Drip infusion contrast enhancement is now being employed in many cases, using meglumine diatrizoate injection (300 ml) (42.3 grams iodine per 300 ml).

High doses of iodine result in a striking increase in absorption of the normal larger vascular structures, such as the great vein of Galen and dural sinuses, of the falx and tentorium (Fig. 19.5), and of many vascularized lesions or those with increased capillary permeability (vide Figs. 7.9, 8.4, and 19.4).

The time course of changes in blood iodine concentration after intravenous bolus injection or infusion of contrast medium is well documented in the radiologic literature. Corresponding changes in terms of EMI absorption units are less thoroughly worked out. Preliminary data (W. Marshall and W. Scott, unpublished data) for change in the EMI absorption unit values of blood samples were obtained before and after intravenous infusion of contrast in patients. Three-hundred ml of Hypaque 30 were infused intravenously over 12–22 minutes, with 25-ml blood samples being drawn before and immediately after the completion of the infusion. The blood samples were scanned at 120 kV in 2.5-cm inner diameter plastic tubes. The average preinfusion absorption value of 28 units increased to an average postinfusion value of 51 units for an average increase of 23 units. The variation between patients was a minimum increase of 15 units and a maximum increase of 30 units.

In addition to contrast enhancement, a further variation of technique worthy of additional study is the reduction of kilovoltage to 100 or even lower in order to increase significantly the absorption produced by circulating iodine. A limiting factor in this regard is the further quantum noise that would be produced unless the scan time were significantly increased. No doubt future improvement may permit greater latitude in this regard.

Pathological conditions in which additional information from contrast enhancement is especially likely to be helpful are the following.

In intracranial neoplasms in general, increased detectability and increased specificity of tumor diagnosis can be expected in proportion to the vascularity of the tumor and permeability of the blood-brain barrier (Fig. 27.3).

1. **Gliomas.** Recognition of a neoplastic pattern of

abnormal absorption is rendered easier if and when absorption is increased by injection of contrast medium. It has been said that there is generally no increase in absorption in astrocytoma Grades I and II and that a variably extensive and marked increase in absorption may be seen in glioblastoma multiform (51). Our early experience suggests that this may not be true if larger doses than 60–100 ml of contrast medium are used. In proportion to the degree and extent of tumor vascularity, there may be more complete differentiation of tumor and associated edema. Gliomas with highly vascularized peripheral contours may be rendered extremely dense; there is better differentiation of relatively or completely avascular areas representing necrotic changes within malignant tumors. It may be possible to achieve recognition of smaller gliomas by the use of contrast enhancement in patients who present with minimal symptoms and signs. While further information is needed, it appears likely that CT scanning with the addition of contrast enhancement will be more sensitive than is angiography in identification of the grade of malignancy.

2. **Metastatic neoplasms.** It has been demonstrated that, very occasionally, even moderate-sized metastatic nodules may be invisible until scanned with contrast enhancement (24). Our experience indicates that small vascularized metastatic nodules may be completely obscured by absorption averaging with surrounding large volumes of edema on plain scans, with clear discrimination of the nodules after contrast enhancement.

3. **Meningiomas.** Meningiomas showing relatively little absorption differential from the brain tend to become very dense with contrast enhancement. The full extent of the lesion will then be more clearly apparent. However, if a meningioma can be identified with confidence on the basis of plain film and CT examinations and if the patient is an operative candidate, angiography will be needed in any case, and there is therefore little or no practical value in supplementary scans with contrast enhancement.

4. **Pituitary adenomas** with suprasellar extension. Since these tumors are often sufficiently vascular that blushes are visible on angiography, contrast enhancement will tend to improve CT recognition of these lesions, which may be difficult to identify unless the suprasellar mass is quite large. The striking increase in density frequently seen strongly suggests a component of extravascular diffusion. However, complete plain film examination, pneumography with laminography, and cavernous sinography will commonly be required for definitive evaluation. The presence and extent of important cystic changes may be shown more clearly when the solid areas are enhanced.

5. **Acoustic neuromas.** Since these may not be identified directly on plain CT scan (and deformity and displacement of the fourth ventricle may be so minimal as to be unidentifiable), examination with contrast enhancement, especially with the higher doses, is extremely important. If the neuroma can be identified clearly by this means, a good quality CT scan may permit operation without recourse to angiography, pneumoencephalography, or positive-contrast cisternography.

6. **Pineal area tumors.** The addition of contrast-enhanced scans may be quite helpful in evaluating the full size and configuration of tumors of this region and in classifying the general type of tumor present.

7. **Miscellaneous primary neoplasms.** Medulloblastomas, cavernous hemangiomas, and choroid plexus papillomas are tumors that are sufficiently vascular that contrast enhancement will be of great assistance in recognition and determination of their extent.

8. **Aneurysms and arteriovenous malformations.** The minimum size of such lesions recognizable in CT scans of a given technical quality will be reduced by the use of contrast enhancement, particularly with high dosage.

9. **Infarctions.** Our experience of contrast-enhanced scans in cerebral infarction is small. Not surprisingly, in view of the frequency with which angiographic hypervascularity can be identified in an area of infarction, a clear-cut increase in absorption has been identified after intravenous contrast injection in the region of previously low absorption. A study of the distribution of such increase in vascularity relative to the area of low absorption in infarcts of various types and of various ages is desirable. With the use of high intravenous doses, the sensitivity of CT scanning in the detection of small recent infarcts may be improved significantly. The possibility of recognizing diffusion of contrast medium from the microvasculature into the ischemic zone is intriguing. Contrast enhancement may be helpful in differentiating absorption variations due to neoplasm from those of ischemic disease.

10. **Inflammatory diseases.** Experience of contrast enhancement in inflammatory disease is still very limited. The combination of plain and contrast-enhanced CT scans is likely to increase accuracy of detection and discrimination of such lesions. Improved recognition of abscess capsules was expected and has been observed (Fig. 21.2).

ESTIMATION OF REGIONAL CEREBRAL BLOOD VOLUME

The finding that the absorption of cerebral cortex and, to a lesser degree, of central grey matter rises after intravascular injection of contrast media raises consideration of the possibility of using CT to calculate the blood volume per unit of tissue in these regions. With a knowledge of the blood iodine levels from blood samples obtained during CT scanning (Fig. 27.2), and of the CT absorption values of an appropriate range of iodinated contrast medium concentrations, it is theoretically pos-

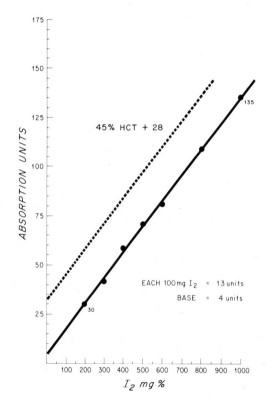

FIG. 27.2 Various dilutions of meglumine diatrizoate (Renografin) in distilled water were prepared and scanned in 2-cm diameter plastic tubes. The absorption values obtained are shown plotted against iodine concentration in milligrams per 100 ml (*solid line*). It is shown that each 100 mg/100 ml of iodine results in an increment of 13 EMI units. The base of the contrast medium contributes 4 units to the total absorption. Given concentrations of contrast medium in whole blood will give absorption values representing the sum of the concentration of contrast medium and of the blood. Therefore, with knowledge of the patients hematocrit, scans of blood samples withdrawn after injection of contrast medium and homogeneous distribution through the blood pool will provide identification of the concentration of circulating iodine. The interrupted line represents the peak EMI values obtained at given concentrations of iodine in blood of 45% hematocrit.

sible to derive the regional blood volume by measuring the increase in absorption values produced by contrast injection after a plain scan. Serious practical difficulties exist at present, but these may be overcome in the future. Present limitations include the standard deviation in the absorption measurements obtained with the present 160 x 160 matrix system, which is only slightly better than the guaranteed accuracy of $\pm$ ½% (close to $\pm$ 2.5 EMI units). The observed increase in absorption in cerebral cortex after injection of 300 ml of Renografin 30% has ranged between approximately 1 and 3 units. Increases of 3 units have been observed sufficiently frequently that we have reasonable confidence that this represents a real change, but the increase is not suffi-

cient for satisfactory reliability of blood volume estimation with the present system. Although the relationship of large systemic vessel hematocrit and EMI absorption values has been determined (chapter 15), the hematocrit of blood in the cerebral microvasculature is apparently lower, and a correction factor will probably be required for attempted cerebral blood volume measurements (31B). When, in addition, it is realized that it is impossible to be certain that the full thickness of the CT section is occupied by the tissue being studied or that there has not been a slight but significant change in the plane of the scan section between the plain and contrast-enhanced studies, it is apparent that practicality depends on future improvements in the method.

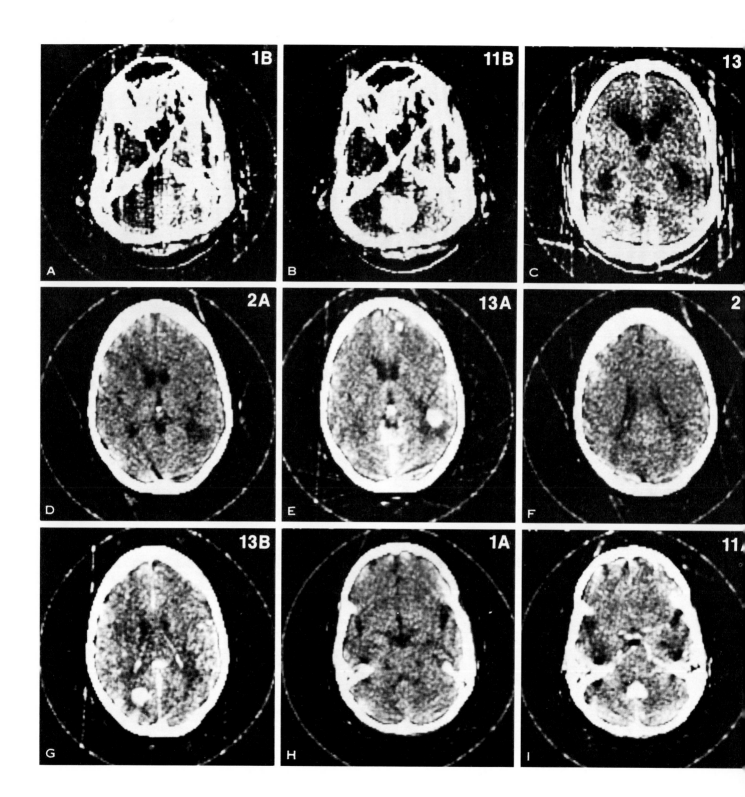

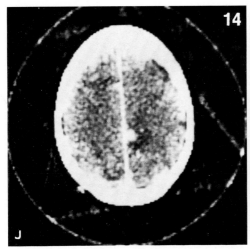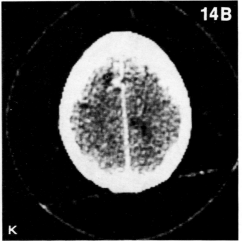

FIG. 27.3 ILLUSTRATION OF INCREASED DETECTABILITY OF NEOPLASM BY THE USE OF CONTRAST ENHANCEMENT.

A. This plain 8-mm scan through the midcerebellum reveals slight upward tilting of the left side of the head relative to the right side and an artifact involving most of the left half of the posterior fossa, where there is a generally decreased absorption and vertically oriented alternating bands of greater and lesser absorption. The presence of this artifact make assessment of the remainder of the posterior fossa very difficult. Although the fourth ventricle was not identified with certainty and there was enlargement of the third and lateral ventricles, an unequivocal focal lesion of the posterior fossa could not be identified on the plain scan.

B. Scan at an almost identical level to that in **A**, following drip infusion of over 200 ml of meglumine diatrizoate 30%. A very large irregularly rounded neoplastic mass, centered in the region of the cerebellar vermis, is very visible. Surgery revealed a solid hemangioblastoma.

C. Moderate enlargement of the lateral and third ventricles was visible on higher sections. *This section shows a relatively diffuse increase in absorption posteriorly, representing a commonly seen contrast enhancement of the tentorium, and adjacent portions of superior cerebellar and inferior cerebral gray matter.* Enhancement of vessels coursing in both ambient cisterns is also visible.

D–K. L 15   W 30   160 x 160 matrix system. Multiple metastases from ductal carcinoma of the breast.

D. Plain scan. An irregular region of diminished absorption is shown in and lateral to the area of the right trigone, with a suggestion of a nodular component anteriorly, with absorption similar to normal brain.

E. Scan at the same level after intravenous injection of 300 ml of meglumine diatrizoate 30%. Marked enhancement of the absorption of a metastatic nodule is evident at the site of the abnormality noted in **A**. In addition, a 7-mm diameter nodule is now visible in the anterior portion of the right frontal lobe. No parenchymal abnormality is visible at this site in the plain scan, although there is a suggestion of a slight mass effect upon the right frontal horn.

F. Plain scan. **G.** Corresponding section after intravenous contrast enhancement. A small irregular area of reduced absorption is visible behind the left trigone on the plain scan, but an unequivocal nodular mass is detected only after intravenous injection. Note the enhancement of the noncalcified portions of the choroid plexuses of the lateral ventricles, of the great vein of Galen, and of the straight sinus.

H. Plain scan. **I.** Contrast-enhanced scan. The plain scan raises suspicion of compression of the midline fourth ventricle from the posterior aspect, but no definite focal mass is visible. After enhancement, a very obvious tumor nodule is visible.

J and **K.** Contrast-enhanced scans at more superior levels, showing very small nodules surrounded by some edema immediately adjacent the the right and left sides of the contrast-enhanced falx.

CHAPTER 28

Orbital CT Scanning

INTRODUCTION

During the time that the 80 x 80 matrix system was employed, it was apparent that CT had significant potential in the evaluation of suspected orbital disease. The study of some 70 cases established that the method was capable of contributing significantly to the management of many orbital problems, and our preliminary assessment has been reported (31, 40). Other workers have also reported encouraging preliminary evaluations (5, 36).

The recent advent of a finer matrix (160 x 160 system) has been of particular importance in orbital CT scanning, because it allows greatly improved demonstration of details of the relatively small anatomical structures of this region. Further experience with the new matrix will be required for determination of the precise place of CT scanning in the study of orbital disease and the extent to which it may be capable of replacing other methods, such as hypocycloidal tomography, ultrasonography, venography, and carotid angiography. The established short-comings of orbital venography in the identification and localization of intraorbital tumors make it likely that the CT will result in diminishing use of venography in investigation of such lesions. However, since 20 to 25% of mass lesions of the orbit are vascular anomalies and, therefore, are optimally demonstrated by venography (for venous malformations) and carotid angiography (for arteriovenous malformations and fistulae), angiographic methods will remain the most definitive forms of investigation in a significant percentage of cases.

As in other regions, plain film studies, including laminography, remain an essential preliminary form of study and are complementary to both CT and ultrasonography. Preliminary findings indicate that CT and ultrasonography are in many respects complementary. The high resolution of B-mode ultrasonography allows demonstration of details of the structures of the globe itself that are beyond the capability of present day CT. On the other hand, ultrasonography fails to provide detail in the region of the orbital apex, a region in which CT is effective. In the remainder of the retro-orbital space, both methods are capable of yielding important and useful information. CT examination has the important additional advantage of routinely demonstrating intracranial structures in orbital examinations. The method is capable, therefore, of providing significant information in those primary orbital lesions that extend into the cranial cavity and in primary intracranial lesions that extend to involve orbital structures.

Almost all of the investigations to date on the capability of CT evaluation of orbital disease have been performed with scanning equipment designed for other purposes, i.e., intracranial studies, and using only minor modifications of technique. Our preliminary tests, using smaller collimators that provide 4-mm scan sections, which are more suitable for examination of the smaller anatomical structures within the orbit, indicate that quantum noise is excessive in these thin sections, when the standard algorithm is employed. Increasing the duration of· the scans offsets this disadvantage but increases the probability of patient motion during the examination. Significantly improved detail of orbital structures may be demonstrated by careful attention to technique, the use of 3- and 4-mm tissue sections, and modifications of the computer program, as has been demonstrated already by Sadek Hilal and his coworkers at the Neurological Institute of New York. Undoubtedly, as the great advantages of such modifications are documented, interest in further equipment modifications directed to more effective orbital and suprasellar CT examinations will be forthcoming, and the present place of ultrasonography of the orbit will be challenged even more effectively. The novel method of thin section scanning by overlapping thicker CT sections and the display of these thin sections in transverse, coronal, and sagittal orientations, developed by Glenn et al. (Chapter 4, 53) (27 B), should prove to be of great value in orbital studies.

TECHNIQUE OF ORBITAL CT SCANNING

Positioning

The construction of the EMI scanner, which was primarily designed for intracranial examination, is not ideal for examination of the orbits. It may not be possible to insert the adult head sufficiently deeply into the waterbox to allow optimal coverage of the entire orbital region. Consideration of the anatomy of the orbit leads to a choice of scan plane parallel to RBL. If a lesion of the optic nerve is suspected, a scan angle parallel to the course of the optic nerves is more appropriate. This will be achieved by extending the head so that the scan angle is 5–10° to RBL. The depth of the waterbox may prevent the lower portions of the orbit from being brought into the scan plane unless the head is extended. This contrasts with the head flexion that is normally employed for intracranial examination. The construction of the scanner commonly prevents a uniform and close fit of the latex cap over the eyes, except in young children. Therefore, an air gap of varying depth is usually present between the eyes and the cap. However, this does not seem to affect adversely the quality of the scan of the greater portion of the globe and the posterior orbital structures.

Very accurate positioning of the head is important. The inferior orbital line (line tangent to the inferior orbital margins) should be precisely parallel to the head box portal and, therefore, to the plane of the scanning beam. If the head is canted so that one orbit lies higher than the other orbit, the globes will appear to be asymmetrical in size on individual sections, and proptosis can be simulated. With correct positioning and orbits of equal vertical dimension, the orbital roofs will be symmetrically displayed in the superior orbital scan section. If the head has been canted or if the vertical orbital dimensions are asymmetrical, the orbital roofs will be unequally included in the superior scan section. A review of plain film orbital studies is required for satisfactory evaluation of positioning, in addition to its fundamental importance in diagnostic evaluation of CT findings. As retro-orbital osseous structures such as the anterior clinoids and petrous pyramids are included in the orbital CT studies, these can provide additional information regarding cranial positioning and anatomical symmetry.

Immobilization

Immobilization of the head is very important in achieving scans of high quality. As most adult patients and older children with orbital disease are able to cooperate satisfactorily, use of the dental fixation device (Chapter 3) has been very important in orbital studies. Sedation or general anesthesia is necessary for infants and young children. As the eyes must remain closed be-

neath the latex cap, it is not possible for the patient to fixate during the scans. It seems helpful to instruct the patients to move the eyes as little as possible during the scan, although movement of the globes does not seem to degrade detail in the retro-orbital regions. At times, pressure on the eylids may cause discomfort to a patient with severe proptosis. Rarely, very severe proptosis may preclude CT examination, as may an unusually large cranium or very prominent nose. Eventually, demand will likely stimulate modifications of equipment that will overcome such problems.

Since this was written, EMI Ltd. has announced an optional retrofit modification of their cranial scanner, details of which will be described in December 1975. This modification involves replacement of the water box by another equilibrating medium and permits scan sequence times as short as 1½ minutes. Orbital scanning may well be facilitated by these changes.

Section Thickness

The use of 8-mm sections has been routine. Collimators for 4-mm sections have been constructed. Tests are in progress to determine whether the use of 4-mm sections will require a prolongation of scan time in order to achieve satisfactory photon yield for accurate absorption measurements.

Using 8-mm sections and starting at the floor of the orbit, the entire orbit is examined with the use of two scan sequences (four sections). As noted earlier, intracranial structures in these planes are also scanned, and the scan sections are appropriate for evaluation of retro-orbital intracranial structures and lesions. After each scan sequence, the patient's head is adjusted 15 mm. It has recently been determined that a change of approximately 12 mm in head position is required in order to avoid tissue gaps between scan pairs when the 8-mm collinators are used (see page 27 and Fig. 5.1). It has been our practice to complete orbital examinations by obtaining 1 or 2 contiguous scan sequences at higher levels, using 13-mm sections. By this means, a survey of the lateral ventricles and lower portions of the cerebral hemispheres is obtained.

Photographic and Analytical Considerations

Absorption Measurements. The osseous walls of the orbits are readily identified. Owing to the very thin and curving configuration of bone in certain areas (notably the medial wall and portions of the floor), the window level settings must often be quite low to reveal these bone regions, which are best studied with the M setting of window width. An additional important factor in producing factitiously low absorption values for portions of the orbital walls is the presence of air in the adjacent paranasal sinuses and fat within the orbit. Since the true (full volume) values of these substances are very low, −500 and −50, respectively, only a small amount of these substances in a matrix block with bone will reduce considerably the apparent absorption of the bone. Similar considerations apply to absorption measurements of smaller anatomical structures, such as the extraocular muscles and optic nerves, and of smaller lesions within the orbit. Accurate absorption measurements of such small structures and lesions are not to be expected when averaging with orbital fat in the same tissue section has occurred. Useful absorption measurements can be obtained, however, in the more central regions of larger structures, such as the globes, and of larger lesions. Identification of the structure or lesion in sections above and below that being analyzed provides assurance of the validity of the absorption measurements.

Spatial Measurements: Minification Factor on Polaroid Film. The diameter of the outline of the water field (D) is measured on the Polaroid film. The actual diameter of this area of the waterbath is currently 21.8 cm. Thus, D/21.8 represents the minification factor. This is 1/3.3 with the 160 x 160 matrix system on our equipment (see Chapter 4, pp. 45–46).

Routine Photographic Settings. Owing to the high contrast between retrobulbar fat, the globe, optic nerve, extraocular muscles, and many lesions in the posterior orbit, a window width of 75 is generally the optimal setting for general recording. Optimal level settings vary with individual cases and sections, but settings between −10 and +10 generally serve to demonstrate the optic nerve to best advantage.

Absorption Values of Normal Intraorbital Structures

Globe. The globe exhibits a dense rim formed by the sclera, choroid, and retina, with a peak absorption of approximately 35 units.

Lens. When movement of the globe during the scan has not been excessive, the lens can be identified as an ovoid region, which, like the rim of the globe, has a considerably higher density than the aqueous and vitreous humors. The lens is sometimes observed to be of considerably higher density in older individuals than in younger patients, and calcification in the lens has been identified (a case of congenital blindness).

Optic Nerves. As the thickness of the normal optic nerve does not exceed 6 mm, and the standard section thickness at present is 8 mm, a variable amount of retrobulbar fat will be included in the sections showing the optic nerve, and the calculated absorption will be factitiously low. Measured absorption of normal optic nerves has been in the range of 8–18 units, and it is likely that the true absorption of these nerves is similar to that of cerebral white matter (11 or 12–17 or 18 units).

Extraocular Muscles. Although these were usually poorly visualized with 80 x 80 matrix system, they are quite commonly visible, particularly the medial and lateral recti, with the high resolution system. Their small size relative to section thickness militates against obtaining useful absorption measurements of these structures. The confluence of the extraocular muscles at the aponeurotic ring sometimes gives rise to a small, localized rounded density at the orbital apex in the region of the superior orbital fissure. This must be differentiated from a pathological mass.

Retrobulbar Fat. Full volume measurement of this fat extends down to below −50. Owing to partial volume averaging, full demonstration of the region of retro-orbital fat requires window level settings up to approximately 0 units on some sections.

Contrast Enhancement of Orbital Scans

The place of intravenous contrast enhancement in CT examination of the orbit is still under preliminary evaluation. Except in the case of arteriovenous malformation (Fig. 28.17), the lesions examined in this series have all seemed to be capable of satisfactory evaluation on plain scans, and contrast enhancement was not frequently employed in this series. Ambrose et al (5) have followed plain scans of the orbit with contrast scans routinely but have not indicated what significant additional information was gained thereby. It must be noted that partial volume effects tend to be striking in the orbit, due to the large section thickness, relative to the size of anatomical structures and smaller lesions, and due to the wide difference between the absorptions of fat and paranasal sinus air and those of lesions. Thus, very slight changes in section position between plain and enhanced scans will tend to produce appreciable changes in measured absorption, independent of the effect of contrast medium. It is therefore more difficult to identify an increase in absorption due to the effect of circulating contrast medium (intrinsic vascularity of lesions and/or absence of capillary barrier to contrast medium) than in the case of intracranial lesions, which tend to be larger at the time of examination.

At the very least, it is advisable to use contrast enhancement after plain CT scans whenever a vascular lesion is suspected or when the plain scan is negative or equivocal. In the latter situation, the increased absorption that may be produced by contrast medium may overcome the obscuring effect of partial volume averaging of the lesion or of extraocular muscles by orbital fat, and small lesions may become visible for the first time.

Clinical Material

Normal Orbits. The CT appearance of the normal orbit was studied in 30 cases scanned with the 80 x 80 matrix system and in 10 cases studied with the 160 x 160 matrix system in patients who were examined for intracranial disease and had no evidence of orbital disease. The material was selected on the basis of scan sections of 8-mm thickness and scan angles similar to those routinely employed for the orbit.

Orbital Pathology. A total of 120 CT studies in patients with definite clinical evidence of intraorbital disease were reviewed, and the initial 55 cases were studied in detail.

Orbital Disease with Normal CT Scans. Thirteen of 55 patients in this group (23.6%) were scanned for evaluation of exophthalmos, optic atrophy, or ptosis. The commonest reason for investigation in this group was unilateral exophthalmos. There were 8 cases of exophthalmos in which no CT scan abnormality could be demonstrated, except for slight anterior displacement of the globe. Three of these cases were proven to have hyperthyroidism and one had hypothyroidism. Four others had no identifiable endocrinological abnormality (euthyroid Graves' disease?). Proptosis improved with ACTH therapy in one case and without therapy in another. The CT scans in the two other cases appeared to be normal but one of these appeared to have a retrobulbar mass on ultrasound B scan. Neither case was proven by exploratory surgery. A case of ptosis and a patient with a clinical diagnosis of orbital edema had normal CT scans, but neither of these was pursued with other tests. Three patients with optic atrophy had normal-appearing optic nerves on CT scans.

In this initial group of 55 patients, all of whom were scanned with the earlier matrix, CT accuracy in demonstration of disease was 76.4% which compares with the CT scan accuracy of 76.5% reported by Ambrose et al (5) in a series of 24 patients scanned with the 160 x 160 matrix system.

Endocrine Exophthalmos. To date in our series, we have infrequently identified abnormality of CT scans other than the exophthalmos itself. However, Baker (6) found a poorly defined diffuse increase in absorption (8–16) in the retrobulbar fat in three of nine cases of endocrine exophthalmos studied at the Mayo Clinic. The scans of the remaining 6 cases revealed only proptosis. W. Marshall and W. R. Scott (unpublished data) have observed poorly defined areas of increased absorption (−5 to +18) in the posterior orbital regions in 7 of 10 patients with thyrotoxic exophthalmopathy studied with CT scans (Fig. 28.23) (see comment at the end of Fig. 28.24 legend).

Recent improvements in ultrasonographic equipment (12) have resulted in the identification of abnormalities in even the milder forms of orbital involvement in Graves' disease (65). According to these authors, these changes are consistent with "erosion" of the peripheral portions of the retrobulbar fat, associated with a variable degree of thickening of the extraocular muscles, which in turn is secondary to deposition of mucoproteins or of mucopolysaccharides, round cell infiltration, and/or edema. Occasionally, perineural inflammation is indicated by duplication echoes of the optic nerve outline. The changes caused by other forms of orbital myositis and by orbital pseudotumor may cause diagnostic difficulty, but the frequent finding of bilateral changes may serve to distinguish Graves' disease. A detailed comparative study of B-mode ultrasonography and CT scanning in this group of diseases is clearly highly desirable now that the 160 x 160 matrix system is available.

Orbital Disease with Abnormal CT Scans. The 41 cases in this group (76.4%) showed CT scan abnormalities indicative of the pathology. In general, the detected abnormalities were accurately localized by CT examination. In a preliminary report on the use of the 160 x 160 matrix system in the diagnosis of orbital space-occupying lesions, Ambrose et al (5) have reported a CT scan accuracy in 24 patients of 76.5%. Venography provided the same percentage accuracy, and axial hypocycloidal tomography had a very similar accuracy in their series (75%). Ultrasonic examination provided an accuracy of 62.5%. In several patients, CT examination provided the strongest evidence of abnormality, but these authors emphasized that a combination of the above techniques was required for successful preoperative diagnosis in all patients. In this respect, the two most complementary procedures were orbital venography and ultrasonic examination. The authors comment that one result of the use of CT examination in combination with the other techniques has been a decrease in the number of patients investigated by carotid angiography.

SUMMARY OF CASE MATERIAL IN THIS SERIES

Retrobulbar Tumor

A. Primary tumors.
1. Lymphoma.
   Discrete retrobulbar masses, with a tissue density measuring −4 to +34, were shown in two patients with known lymphoma who developed proptosis. The proptosis improved with radiotherapy (Fig. 28.6)
2. Plasmacytoma.
   A large mass with a tissue density measuring 20–32 was shown within the muscle cone and was proven to be a plasmacytoma by biopsy (Fig. 28.8). This lesion decreased in size with radiotherapy.
3. Lymphangioma.
   A large retrobulbar mass was shown, with irregular areas of increased density that measured between 18 and 30 units. At operation, the tumor was completely removed and proved to be a lymphangioma with areas of hemorrhage. The globe was displaced anteriorly and laterally (Fig. 28.9). A similar proven case was also

studied by CT scanning, with demonstration of a retrobulbar mass on the left side, with a tissue density of −2 to 30 units, which was also surgically removed. (A recently examined case of lymphagioma is illustrated in Fig. 28.10).

4. Cavernous hemangioma.
There were two cases of cavernous hemangioma that extended from the temporal wall of the orbit. The tissue density ranged from 0–26 units (Fig. 28.11).

5. Rhabdomyosarcoma.
A large retrobulbar mass was shown, with a tissue density of 10–30 units in the lower outer quadrant of the left orbit in a case of incompletely excised embryonal rhabdomyosarcoma. This mass produced severe proptosis (Fig. 28.12).

B. Secondary tumors.
1. Carcinoma.
A moderate-sized discrete mass extended from the temporal wall of the orbit in a 73-year-old man with a swollen eye and chronic sinusitis. The tissue density measured 0–25 units, and this proved to be an anaplastic carcinoma on biopsy. Another patient, with a known carcinoma of the breast, had considerable destruction of the sphenoid and frontal bone on the right side, which appeared as thinned bone on the CT scan. A flat dense mass with a density of 10–20 units was shown in relation to the eroded thinned temporal wall of the orbit in the retrobulbar space. Skull radiographs showed considerable erosive changes of bone at this site. A third patient had a small soft tissue mass in the orbital apex on the right side due to a carcinoma, with a density range of 12–18 units. The site of the primary tumor was unknown.

2. Neuroblastoma.
A 21-month-old infant with disseminated neuroblastoma and proptosis showed bilateral abnormal soft tissue densities measuring 14–18 units in the retrobulbar spaces (Fig. 28.15).

Tumor in the Lacrimal Region

1. Lymphoma.
A 3-cm mass was shown in the lacrimal area and appeared to extend posteriorly to the retrobulbar space. Proptosis was present. The tissue density measured 21–26 units. Biopsy confirmed a reticulum cell sarcoma (Fig. 28.7).

2. Mixed tumor.
A mass in the lacrimal gland on the right side, with a tissue density of 8–10 units, proved to be a mixed tumor at surgery.

Congenital Blindness

A 53-year-old woman, who was studied for a recurrent glioma of the frontal lobe, had congenital blindness. Her CT scans demonstrated dense calcification of both lenses in addition to a recurrent frontal lobe tumor.

Arteriovenous Malformation

A 26-year-old girl with a known arteriovenous malformation of the left orbit and eyelid was studied by plain CT scans and after intravenous injection of 50 ml of Hypaque. The dilated abnormal vessels were shown anterior and posterior to the globe on the plain scans. With intravenous Hypaque, further densities were shown anterior and posterior to the globe as well as in the orbital apex, representing the abnormal dilated vessels, which were rendered denser by the contrast medium injection (Fig. 28.17).

Bone Lesions

There was one case of a large osteoma in the right ethmoid sinus that encroached on the globe and slightly displaced it laterally and anteriorly (Fig. 28.18).

A patient with neurofibromatosis had a demonstrated absence of the lesser and greater wings of the sphenoid with enlargement of the right orbit. The right optic globe was enlarged and displaced anteriorly. The right temporal lobe herniated forward in the superior portion of the right orbit (Fig. 25.1). A more recently studied case of neurofibromatosis with orbital defect is illustrated in Fig. 28.22.

Trauma

Two children who were struck in the eye showed large masses in the retrobulbar space with densities measuring 16–20 units, thought to be due to hematomas that were producing exophtalmos. One of these cases showed a decrease in the size of the mass and degree of exophthalmos when the CT scan was repeated 4 weeks later (Fig. 28.19). The exophthalmos in the second case also decreased over a period of 6 weeks, and no surgical intervention was needed.

Another case had a penetrating wound with a draining fistula and a mass due to abscess formation around a wooden splinter in the retrobulbar space. The mass density measured 25–60 units. The splinter was not separately visible on CT scan.

A fragment of glass was easily localized in the prosterior orbit (Fig. 28.5).

Inflammation

A patient thought to have optic neuritis demonstrated a slight enlargement of the optic nerve at the orbital apex. Another case with proven retrobulbar abscess, which had been partially drained, demonstrated considerable distortion of the tissues in the retrobulbar space, with a density range of 10–18 units and which was thought to be due to a mixture of pus and blood.

A third case also had abnormal tissue densities in the retrobulbar space, measuring 10–15 units, and believed to be due to inflammatory changes.

Granuloma.

A large mass in the right lacrimal area with a range of 17–30 units was studied with and without intravenous Hypaque. There was no definite change in the density of the lesion with Hypaque. The histological diagnosis was nonspecific granuloma (Fig. 28.20).

Pseudotumor

This case showed no definite abnormality in the retrobulbar space, although there was an area of increased density anterior to the globe with a tissue density of −8 to +10 units, suggesting a mass extending from the lacrimal gland. The globe was displaced anteriorly.

Epidermoid Cyst

A nonspecific mass in the outer canthus and the left upper lid in a 15-year-old girl measured 7 x 13 mm in size and had a tissue density of 15–20 units. The tissue diagnosis was epidermoid cyst.

Meningioma

Of six cases of middle fossa meningioma, two showed extension of the tumor to the apex of the retro-orbital space. The tumor density was 13–27 units. One case had an increased thickness of bone about the lesser and greater wings of the sphenoid from which the meningioma arose.

Postoperative Changes after Eye Surgery

Two cases were studied by CT scanning 5 and 15 days after eye surgery for drainage of a retrobulbar abscess and after an intracapsular cataract extraction, respectively, to rule out retrobulbar hemorrhage. The first case showed considerable tissue density changes from 10–18 units, which were thought to be due to residual pus and inflammation, without evidence of hematoma (tissue density of a hematoma is in the range of 25–40 units).

The second case also showed retrobulbar tissue changes of 10–20 units, compatible with edema and inflammatory changes related to a recent operation, but showed no densities in the range of hematoma.

The third case was scanned to rule out a recurrent melanoma of the orbit six years after the right eye was enucleated for this condition. A well-positioned prosthesis was shown in the right orbit, having a density range of 27–80 units with no evidence of any abnormal tissue in the retrobulbar space.

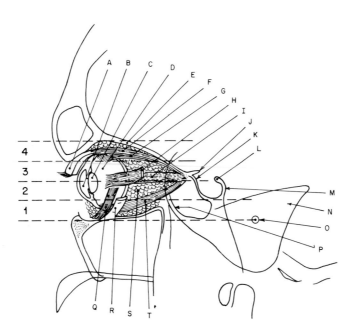

FIG. 28.1. This diagram shows the position of Reid's base line (a line drawn from the external auditory canal to the lower rim of the orbit) with the orbit divided into four sections, 8 mm apart.
A, eyelid; *B,* anterior chamber; *C,* lens; *D,* posterior chamber; *E,* roof of the orbit; *F,* levator palpebrae superioris; *G,* superior rectus muscle; *H,* lateral rectus muscle; *I,* optic nerve; *J,* anterior clinoid process; *K,* tuberculum sellae; *L,* posterior clinoid process; *M,* dorsum sellae; *N,* petrous bone; *O,* external auditory canal; *P,* anterior border of the middle fossa; *Q,* inferior oblique muscle; *R,* zygomatic rim of orbit; *S,* retrobulbar fat; *T,* inferior rectus muscle.

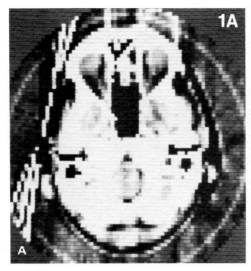
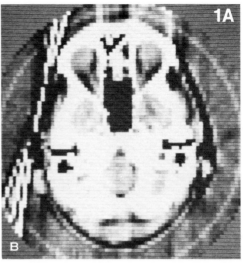

FIG. 28.2.
A. W 50. **B.** W 75. 80 x 80 system, 13-mm section.
Normal appearance of the orbits, in a scan obtained at approximately 30° to RBL, as part of an intracranial study. The scan section passes obliquely through the superior orbital margin, the superior portions of the globes, and the optic nerves. The posterior and medial surfaces of the globes and the optic nerves are well contrasted against the low absorption of orbital fat. The inferior portion of the frontal sinuses, the ethmoid sinuses, and the sphenoid sinus are visible in the median area. The section passes just above the foramen magnum posteriorly.

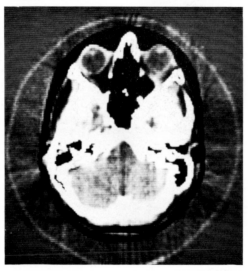

FIG. 28.3. Scan section at approximately 10° to RBL. 160 x 160 matrix system. This 13-mm section includes the equators of the globes. Improved anatomical detail compared with the 80 x 80 system is striking. The dense walls of the globes contrast with the lower absorption of the aqueous and vitreous. The globes evidently moved little during this scan and the relatively high density of each lens stands out quite clearly. On the left side, a narrow band representing the lateral rectus is visible arching posteriorly and medially from the lateral portion of the globe to merge with the lateral wall of the orbit posteriorly. This portion of the muscle cone is outlined by a very narrow strip of fat externally. In other normal orbits, the lateral portion of the muscle cone lies closer to the lateral orbital wall, when it is barely distinguishable from the orbital wall on wide window displays. The same is true of the medial portion of the muscle cone, and these variations appear to be due both to individual anatomical variations and variations in the position of the scan section relative to the medial and lateral recti. The fat within the muscle cone regularly serves to indicate the inner surfaces of these muscles on scans of good quality with the high resolution system. On the right side, the retrobulbar fat is partly replaced by a portion of a retrobulbar mass, which is producing moderate proptosis. The structures of the nose and the air within the ethmoid and sphenoid sinuses are visible centrally. Air is shown in the mastoids and in the right external auditory canal and middle ear. The prominences of the frontal processes of the zygoma form the anterior limit of the lateral wall of each orbit in this section. Most of the zygomatic arch is included on the right side and, deep to this, the section passes through the muscles of the infratemporal fossa.

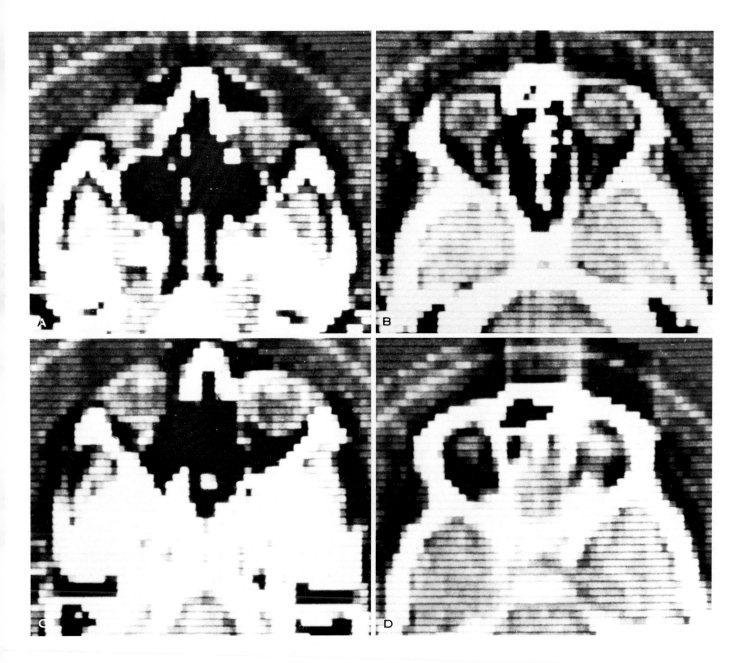

FIG. 28.4. Normal series of contiguous 8-mm sections through the orbits. L 0   W 75   80 x 80 matrix system.

A. The lowest section achieved passed above the floor of the orbit and through the inferior portions of the globes, which therefore appear small. The large black areas posterior to the globes are the superior recesses of the maxillary sinuses. Nasal structures and the sphenoid sinus are present in the median portions of the section, which includes the zygomatic processes on each side, and the muscles of the infratemporal fossae are shown deep to these processes.

B. The next section superiorly is close to the equators of the globes and includes the greater portion of each optic nerve. The optic nerves in the more posterior portions of the orbits are clearly contrasted against the low absorption of the retrobulbar fat. The extraocular muscles are not discriminated in this scan or in the other sections in the series.

C. The next superior scan section includes the equatorial region of each globe and shows the higher absorption of the lens on each side. There is slight tilting of the head, and the anterior portion of the optic nerve is visible only on the left side. The dense wall of each globe is visible here, as in **B**.

D. This section is through the superior portion of each orbit, just below the orbital roof. Only a small segment of the upper portion of each globe is included. The right orbit was slightly inferior to the left, relative to the scan plane in this examination. The anterior clinoid processes and region of the tuberculum sellae are included here, in addition to the dorsum and petrous apices.

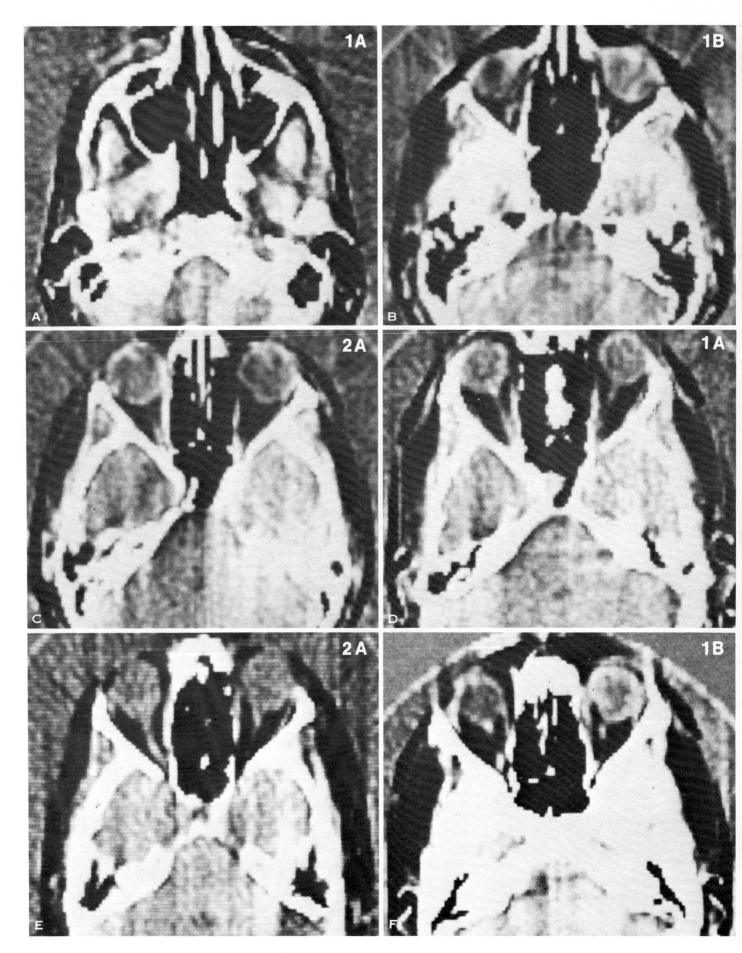

See legend for fig 28.5. A–F on page 458

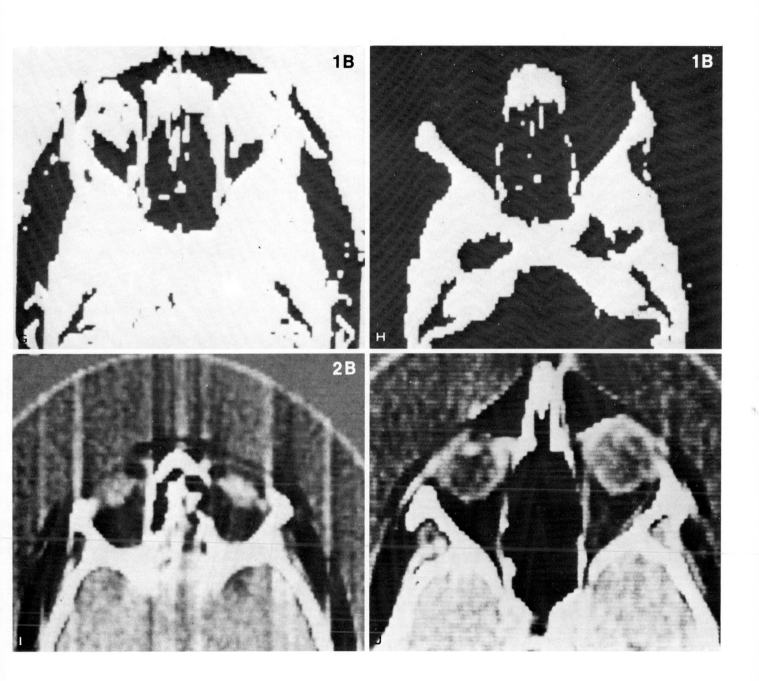

See legend for fig 28.5. G–J on page 458

FIG. 28.5. Composite series of normal orbital scans. L 0 to −10   W 75. 8-mm sections between 0° and 10° to RBL. 160 x 160 matrix system.

A. Section through the region of the orbital floors and including the superior portions of the maxillary sinuses. Portions of the orbital floors are visible anteriorly, but these lie above the scan plane centrally and posteriorly. The zygomatic arches are visible bilaterally. The muscles of the infratemporal fossae are shown between the zygomatic processes and lateral walls of the antra. The nasal fossae and the upper portion of the nasopharynx are visible centrally.

B. The section passes through the inferior portions of the globes. Due to slight inferior tilting of the right orbit relative to the scan plane, a more superior section of the right globe is shown, as compared with the left. A portion of the inferior segment of the muscle cone is contrasted with the retro-orbital fat on the left side. The section passes through the sphenoid sinus.

C. Section in the region of the equators of the globes, showing the dense ocular rim and density of the lens. There is very slight tilting of the orbits relative to the scan plane, and the quality of the scan is better on the left side, where the optic nerve is visible at the orbital apex.

D. Scan section just above the equators of the globes. The optic nerves are quite clearly visible on each side. On the right side, the faint narrow strip of the lateral rectus is just visible, partly separated from the lateral wall of the orbit by the lower absorption of a little fat. Further posteriorly, this strip merges with the orbital wall. On the left side, part of the medial rectus is visible, separated from the medial wall of the orbit as it extends towards the globe.

E. Similar plane of section to that in **D,** in another patient. The section passes just above the equators of the globes. The density of the ocular rim is not clearly shown, but the section very clearly demonstrates the left optic nerve. The anterior portion of the lateral rectus is clearly visible just behind the globe, where it is outlined by fat medially and laterally. Further posteriorly, it merges with the lateral wall of the orbit. On both sides, there is a hint of the medial recti, which are not clearly distinguished from the medial orbital walls. On the left side, the most anterior portion of the lateral rectus is just visible within the orbital fat, adjacent to the globe.

F. Scan section similar to that in **E,** in another patient. On both sides, the anterior portions of the medial and lateral recti can be seen. The small areas of greater absorption in the region of each orbital apex may represent portions of the optic nerves and/or a portion of the attachment of the muscle cone.

G. L −10   W M.

Same section as in **F.** These settings provide maximum contrast to show most of the retrobulbar fat in this section. The anterior extremities of the optic nerves are visible adjacent to the globes. The small regions of higher absorption in the orbital apices referred to in **F** are more clearly visible, as are the medial and lateral recti on the left side.

H. L 50   W M.

Same section as in **F** and **G,** with settings to discriminate the orbital walls. Due to partial volume effects at this high window level, portions of the very thin medial orbital walls are not discriminated from the orbital fat laterally and air in the ethmoid sinuses mesially.

I. Scan section through the superior portions of the orbits, including a small portion of the globes. The low absorption of the orbital fat is not encroached upon by abnormal tissue. The anterior clinoid processes are included posteriorly but are not well discriminated at these control settings.

J. Section showing the lateral rectus on the right side with exceptional clarity. The muscle is of normal thickness. A portion of the medial rectus of the right orbit is visible just behind the globe. Further posteriorly, it merges with the medial wall of the orbit. The right optic nerve is incompletely included in the section and is barely visible, with a factitiously narrow appearance.

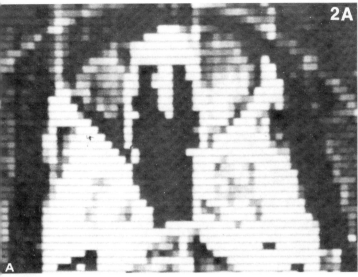

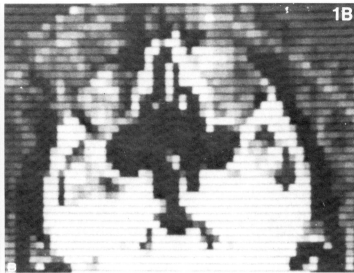

FIG. 28.6. LYMPHOBLASTIC LYMPHOMA.

Clinical Features. A 67 y.o. female known to have lymphoblastic lymphoma for 12 years, proved by lower extremity biopsies. Previous lesions had regressed with radiation therapy. She had noted right-sided exophthalmos during the previous 4–6 months.

A. L 10   W 40.

Scan section through the middle thirds of the orbits. The right globe is displaced forwards by a mass in the retrobulbar space,

extending from the medial wall almost to the lateral orbital wall. The mass (24–34 units) replaces most of the retrobulbar fat and extends anteriorly to overlap the posterior portion of the globe.

B. L 10   W 75.

This section is immediately below that shown in **A**. The proptosis appears more marked in this section and the wide extent of the retrobulbar mass is again shown.

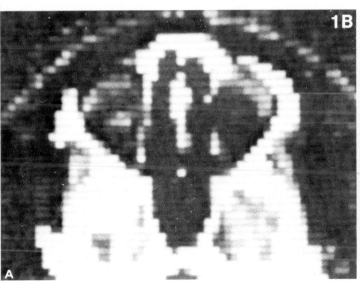

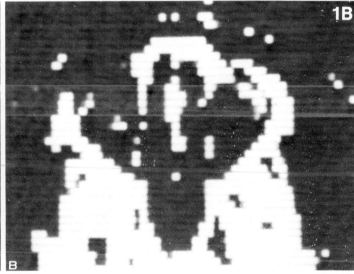

FIG. 28.7. RETICULUM CELL SARCOMA, INVOLVING THE LACRIMAL GLAND.

Clinical Features. A 54 y.o. female who presented with right-sided proptosis. The anterior portion of the mass was palpable. Ultrasonography indicated a mass lesion in the superior temporal quadrant of the right orbit that did not appear to extend into the retrobulbar space.

Orbital exploration revealed a reticulum cell sarcoma.

A. L 18   W 40.

Section through the superior portions of the orbits. The right orbit was tilted somewhat below the level of the left orbit, so that the superior orbital margin was included on the right but

not on the left. The upper third of the left globe is included in the section, but no portion of the right globe is shown, due to a combination of head tilt and depression of the right globe. An arcuate band of increased absorption (21–26), approximately 6 mm in width, is shown in the anterosuperior portion of the right orbit. The mass was shown to extend into the lateral portion of the orbit, but it did not appear to extend into the retrobulbar region.

B. L 20   W M.

Same section as in **A**. The mass in the lacrimal gland area is shown lying immediately posterior to the superior orbital margin.

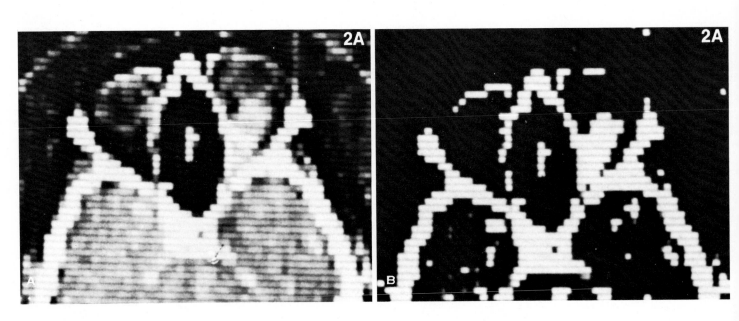

FIG. 28.8. PLASMACYTOMA.

Clinical Features. A 55 y.o. man who had noted progressive right exophthalmos for 3 months. Movements of the eye were restricted in all directions of gaze. The right eye protruded 8 mm beyond the left.

Orbital exploration revealed a plasmacytoma.

A. L 10   W 40.

This section, near the equator of the globe, shows the marked right proptosis. An ovoid mass (20–32 units) is shown extending from the orbital apex anteriorly to the posterior aspect of the globe. Its contact with the medial wall of the orbit is more extensive than with the lateral wall.

B. L 20   W M.

Same section as in **A.** The mass is maximally contrasted with the orbital contents.

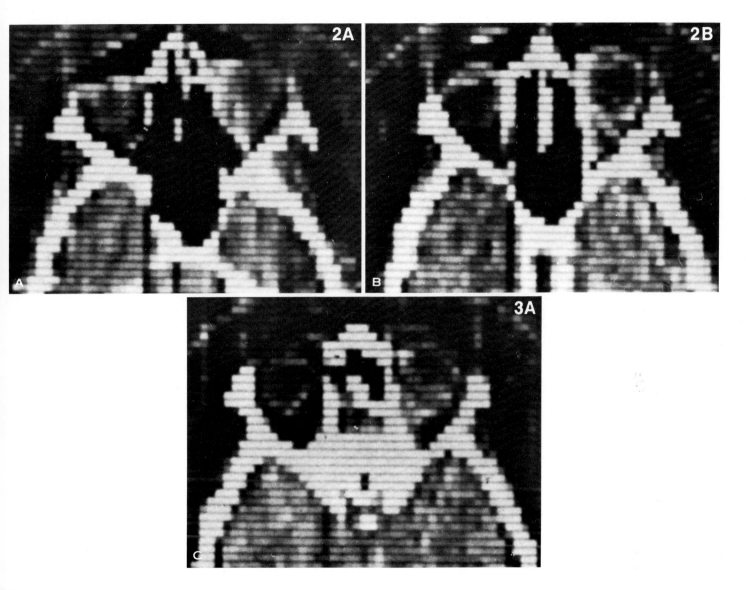

FIG. 28.9. LYMPHANGIOMA.
Clinical Features. An 8 y.o. girl who suddenly developed
right-sided exophthalmos.
Orbital exploration resulted in complete removal of a lymphangioma containing areas of hemorrhage.

A–C. Contiguous 8-mm sections from below superiorly. An irregular mass occupies much of the retrobulbar space. Its absorption (peak, 30) is not homogeneous, and there is a suggestion of a multilocular character. Part of the orbital apex (**C**) and part of the lateral retrobulbar region do not appear to be involved by the mass, which is more extensive along the medial wall of the orbit. Proptosis is evident but does not appear to be marked.

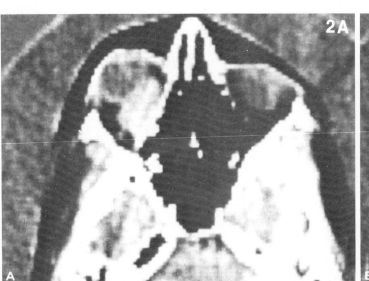

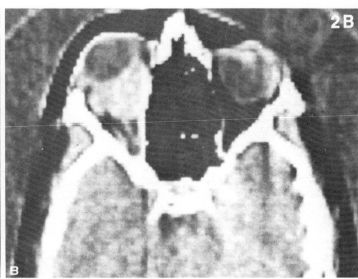

FIG. 28.10. LYMPHANGIOMA.

Clinical Features. A 20 y.o. female who had had a lymphangioma of the left orbit proven by biopsy 7 years earlier. Progressive proptosis and diplopia had been followed by a recent further proptosis and sudden onset of pain in the orbit, suggesting hemorrhage into the mass.

A and **B.** L 10   W 75   160 x 160 matrix system.

Contiguous 8-mm sections. The marked left proptosis is obvious.

A. This section, which is inferior to **B**, passes through the inferior portion of the right globe. The inferiorly displaced left globe is sectioned at a somewhat higher plane. A large ovoid mass is shown extending through the retrobulbar space, predominantly in the medial side of the orbit.

B. The section immediately above that in **A** extends through the equatorial portion of the right globe, in which the density of the lens is clearly visible. The left orbital mass is more extensive in this section and almost reaches the lateral orbital wall. The region of the orbital apex is spared, and the optic nerve is shown extending from the posterior aspect of the sharply defined rounded mass to the apex. Lateral to the optic nerve the lateral rectus is visible, contrasted on each side with fat. On both sections, the medial portion of the mass showed higher absorption values (peak, 30), suggesting the presence of hemorrhage in this portion of the mass.

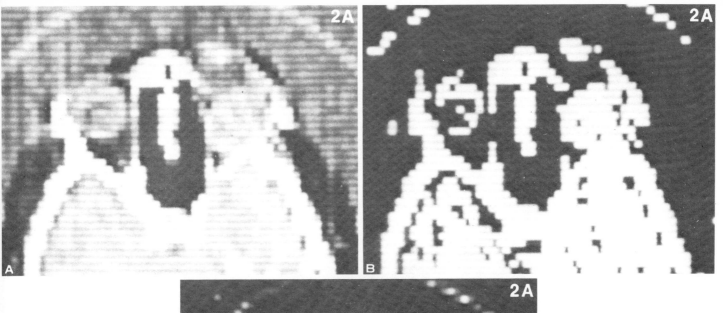

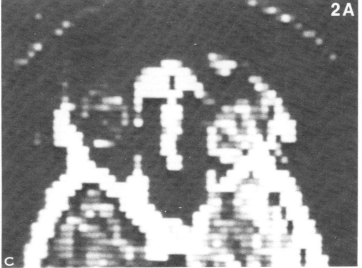

FIG. 28.11. CAVERNOUS HEMANGIOMA.

Clinical Features. A 51 y.o. woman with a history of right-sided exophthalmos for 2–4 years. The eye was displaced anterosuperiorly, and there was increased orbital resistance. The orbit was explored and a cavernous hemangioma was excised.

A. L 0   W 75.
Section that extends through the left globe slightly above its equator. The right globe is displaced markedly anteriorly and somewhat superiorly, so that it is sectioned at a somewhat lower level than is the left globe. A large rounded mass fills most of the right retrobulbar space (peak absorption, 26 units).

B. L 11   W M.
Same section as in **A**. These control settings show the blurred region of the right lens anteriorly, a portion of the superior orbital margin laterally, and the rounded mass posteriorly.

C. Same section as in **A**, with higher window level and lower window width settings to bring out the multilocular appearance of the hemangioma.

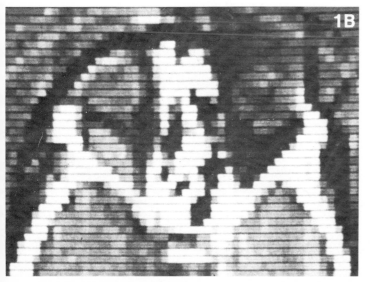

FIG. 28.12. RHABDOMYOSARCOMA.

Clinical Features. A 75 y.o. man who had a longstanding history of recurrent paranasal sinus infections presented with proptosis and left periorbital swelling.
Exploration of the orbit resulted in a diagnosis of rhabdomyosarcoma.

L 10   W 75.
An ovoid mass with a homogeneous appearance and an absorption range of 10–30 is shown involving the lateral portion of the retrobulbar space and extending to the region of the orbital apex. Retrobulbar fat is interposed between the anterior aspect of the mass and the posterior surface of the bulb.

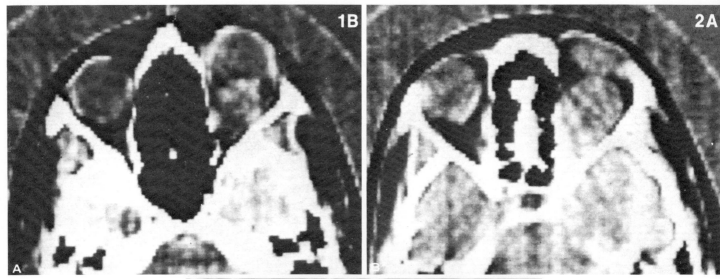

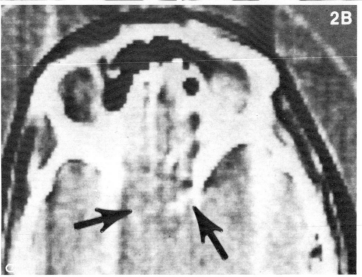

FIG. 28.13. OPTIC GLIOMA.
Clinical Features. A 26 y.o. female who had presented 3 years earlier with increasing right-sided proptosis of 1 year's duration. Vision was normal on the left and considerably impaired on the right, with a contracted visual field. The neurological examination was otherwise normal.
Skull Examination. Enlargement of the right optic foramen was present.
RN Scan. An area of increased activity was demonstrated in the right retro-orbital region. A frontal craniotomy was performed and a biopsy confirmed optic nerve glioma. She was then given radiation therapy, which resulted in a decrease in exophthalmos from 7 to 4 mm. There was no further deterioration in vision of the right eye over the next 2 years.
A CT scan was performed because of increasing exophthalmos (Fig. 28.13).

A–C. 160 x 160 matrix system. Contiguous scans from below superiorly.
A. Marked right proptosis is evident, with a large rounded area of increased absorption in the central portion of the retrobulbar space.
B. This section shows the maximum dimensions of the very large rounded mass occupying most of the retrobulbar space and extending to the posterior surface of the globe, which is displaced inferiorly.
C. Section through the most superior portions of the orbits, showing the superior portion of the very large right intraorbital mass. The scan passes through the plane of the anterior clinoid processes. The normal appearance of the suprasellar cisterns is replaced by a poorly defined but apparently quite extensive region of increased absorption, indicative of an extensive suprasellar extension of the glioma (*arrows*).

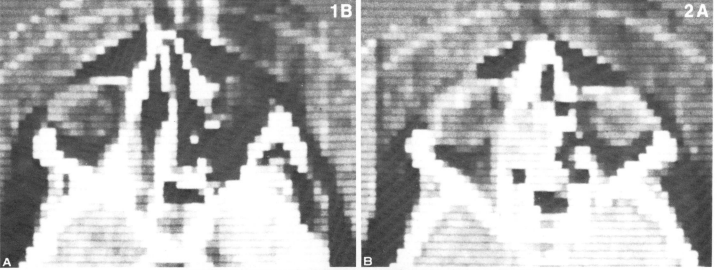

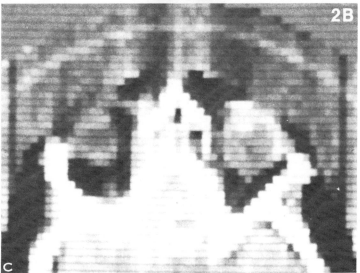

FIG. 28.14. METASTATIC BREAST CARCINOMA.
Clinical Features. A 57 y.o. woman who had a history of breast carcinoma that had been treated by left radical mastectomy 2 years earlier. She had recently developed left facial weakness. There were 4 mm of left proptosis and limitation of adduction, elevation, and depression of the left eye. Skull examination, including hypocycloidal tomography, showed partial destruction of the walls of the left paranasal sinuses and cribriform plate. There was evidence of a mass with the nasal fossae and left ethmoid sinus.
Biopsy of the tumor within the nasal fossa revealed a poorly differentiated metastatic breast carcinoma.

A–C. Contiguous 8-mm sections from below superiorly. Soft tissue encroachment upon the nasal fossae, ethmoid and sphenoid sinuses is visible. There is indication of direct extension of tumor from the nasal fossae and paranasal sinuses through the medial wall of the left orbit into the medial portion of the retrobulbar space and into the left orbital apex. There is evidence of minor proptosis (**B**).

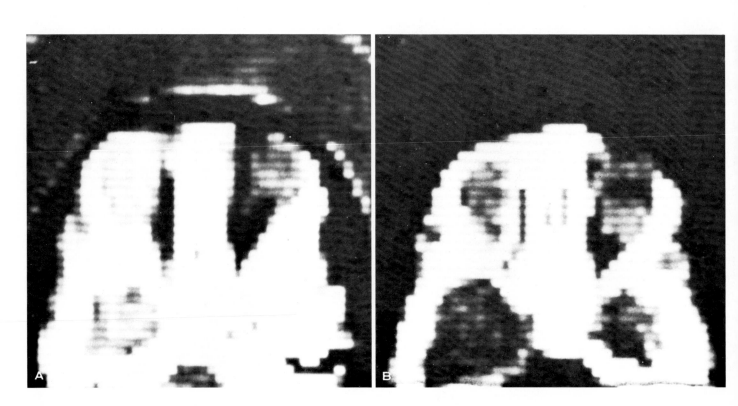

FIG. 28.15. NEUROBLASTOMA.
Clinical Features. A 21-month-old child, with known disseminated neuroblastoma, who developed bilateral proptosis.
A and **B**. Contiguous sections, showing a diffuse replacement of retrobulbar fat in the left orbit that obscures most of the contour of the globe. On the right side, there is a more discrete, moderately large mass in the anterior portion of the retrobulbar space and extending lateral to the globe. Absorption of the masses ranged from 14–18 units. The right orbit is tilted inferiorly relative to the left, so that, in **B**, only the medial and lateral extremities of the superior orbital margin are shown, whereas the entire left superior orbital margin is included in the section.

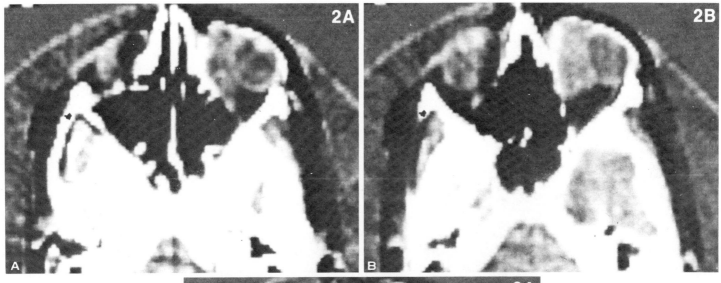

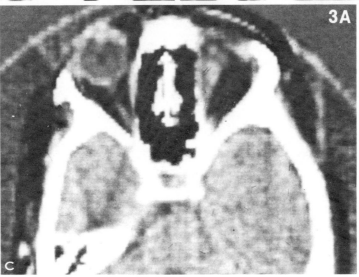

FIG. 28.16. ADENOCARCINOMA, SEBACEOUS GLAND TYPE.

Clinical Features. A 59 y.o. female who was seen 3 years earlier with a painless, fixed hard mass in the medial portion of the right lower eyelid. Biopsy indicated an adenocarcinoma and she received radiation therapy (5600 R). She had had 4 months of diplopia and progressive exophthalmos and blurred vision of the right eye before CT scan. Examination revealed 5 mm of exophthalmos, with normal pupillary function and full visual field. There was marked restriction of extraocular movement in all directions.

Skull Examination; including basal hypocycloidal laminography of the region of the orbits, revealed destruction of the medial wall of the right orbit in its middle and anterior thirds, extending from roof to the ethmoidomaxillary plate. There was an increase in the density of the right ethmoid sinus adjacent to the orbit.

CT Scan. Abnormal (Fig. 28.16).

Biopsy of the orbital mass and a virtually en bloc dissection were carried out, with right orbital exenteration, partial maxillectomy, ethmoidectomy, sphenoidectomy, and frontal sinusotomy, with subsequent skin grafting.

A–C. Contiguous 8-mm sections from below superiorly. 160 x 160 matrix system.

A. L 5   W 75.

The section shows marked lateral displacement of the right globe, due to a large medially situated intraorbital mass (10–30) extending from the anterior orbit to the orbital apex.

B. L 5   W 75.

This section reveals the greater dimensions of the mass, which lies medial to the displaced globe and somewhat overlapping it. The lesion does not extend posteriorly to the orbital apex.

C. L 10   W 75.

The section passes above the right globe (right side of the head is canted inferiorly relative to the left). A triangular superior portion of the mass is shown lying adjacent to the medial wall of the orbit, the density of which is reduced in the anterior two thirds, apparently due to destruction of the medial orbital wall by the tumor, with beginning encroachment upon the ethmoidal sinus. The posterior extremity of the right optic nerve is shown. The entire length of the left optic nerve is visible. The section passes through the left globe slightly above the exact equator. The anterior extremities of the left medial and lateral rectus muscles are just visible.

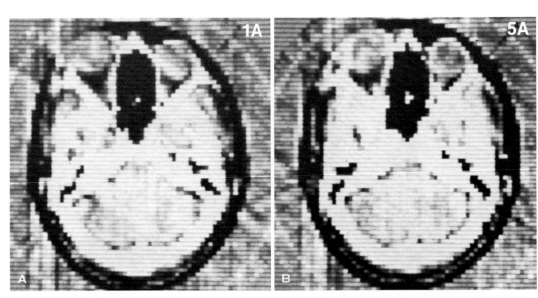

FIG. 28.17. A–B

FIG. 28.17. ARTERIOVENOUS MALFORMATION OF THE ORBIT AND UPPER EYELID.

Clinical Features. A 28 y.o. woman whose left upper eyelid had become progressively thickened and ptotic during a period of 4 years. A vascular malformation in the superior portion of the left orbit had been diagnosed and two operations had been performed previously, in unsuccessful attempts to obliterate the lesion.

A. L −7 W 75.

Plain CT scan, showing focal areas of increased absorption superimposed upon the left globe, which is proptosed. Areas of increased absorption are evident in the region of each orbital apex, more obvious on the right side. These presumably represent the posterior portions of the muscle cones and optic nerves.

B. L −7 W 75.

Scan after intravenous injection of 50 ml of Hypaque 60 M. The plane of the scan section is similar to but not identical with that in **A**. However, there appears to be an increase in the absorption of the densities previously noted, superimposed upon the left globe. These areas of increased absorption show irregular contours and now appear to be more extensive (20–40 units), consistent with the presence of an irregular vascular lesion over the superior portion of the left globe. The areas of absorption in the region of each orbital apex also appear to have increased in density. A broad band of increased absorption of the densities previously noted, superimposed represent the superior rectus and superior oblique muscles.

C and **D.** Orbital angiogram, with magnification and subtraction. An extensive arteriovenous malformation is shown in the left orbit, lying in the superior two thirds of the orbit and extending to involve markedly the upper eyelid. The malformation is supplied mainly by considerably enlarged branches of the ophthalmic artery. The angiogram is far more informative than is the CT examination, as expected with this type of vascular lesion.

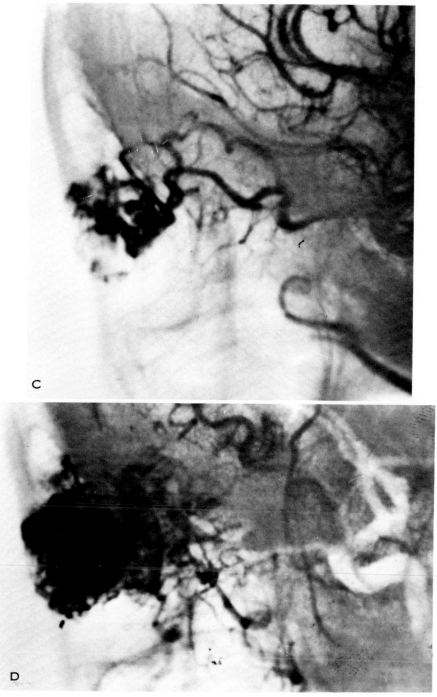

FIG. 28.17. C–D

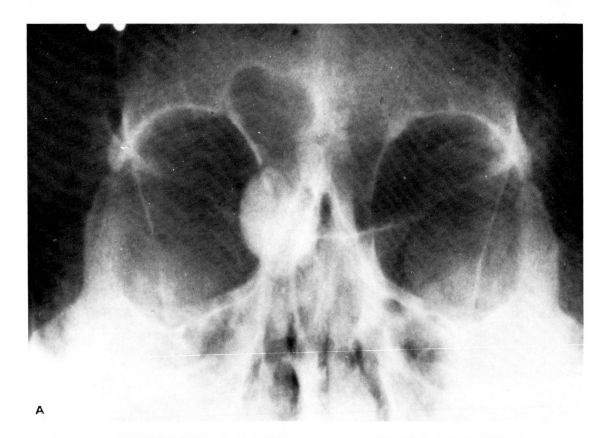

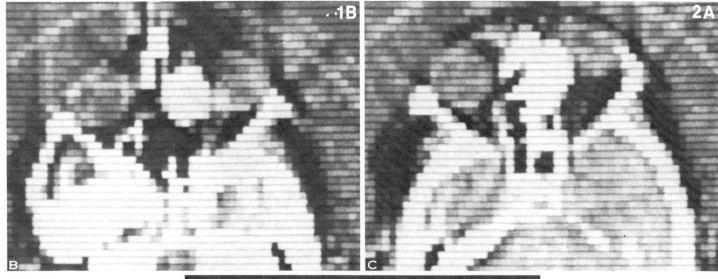

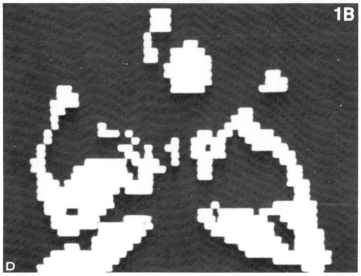

FIG. 28.18. OSTEOMA OF THE RIGHT ETHMOID SINUS.

Clinical Features. A 77 y.o. man with longstanding proptosis of the right eye. Radiography of the skull revealed a large compact osteoma arising from the right ethmoid sinus and projecting into the right orbit.

A. Posteroanterior skull radiograph, showing the large, compact osteoma in the right ethmoid region, projecting into the orbit.

B. L 10   W 75.

CT scan through the middle third of the orbit, showing the high density of the osteoma, its relationship to the ethmoid sinus and right orbit, and the lateral displacement of the right globe, which is proptosed.

C. L 0   W 75.

Section immediately above that in **B**, showing a broader cross section of the osteoma. The right globe is somewhat depressed and therefore is sectioned at a higher level than is the left globe.

D. L 150   W M.

Same section as in **B**. The osteoma and thicker segments of normal bone remain white. Thinner sections of bone, particularly those adjacent to low absorbing air in the paranasal sinuses and fat in the retrobulbar spaces, are not differentiated at this window level, due to marked downward partial volume averaging. Thus, most of the medial walls of the orbits and the thinner curving lateral orbital bone are not visible.

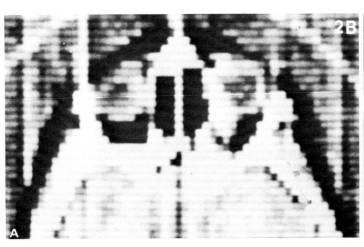

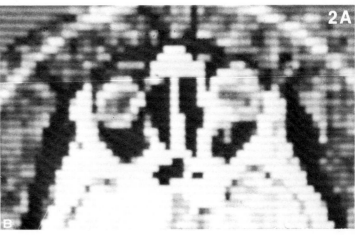

FIG. 28.19. RETROBULBAR HEMATOMA (PRE-SUMED).

Clinical Features. A 9 y.o. boy who was hit in the right eye by a blunt object 1 month before the first CT scan. He developed sudden exophthalmos, with markedly impaired vision and limited ocular movement.

A. L 0   W 40.

Initial CT scan. The section passes above the equators of the globes and reveals a quite large ovoid zone of increased absorption (peak, approximately 40) in the right orbit, medial to the globe and extending to involve much of the medial portion of the retrobulbar space.

B. L 0   W 30.

CT scan obtained 1 month after that shown in **A**. The plane of the scan section is quite similar to but not identical with that shown in **A**. However, comparison of the entire sequence of sections from both examinations indicated that the presumed hematoma had become smaller in the interval. It was also now less dense (peak, 30). The exophthalmos had correspondingly become less, and vision and ocular movement had improved.

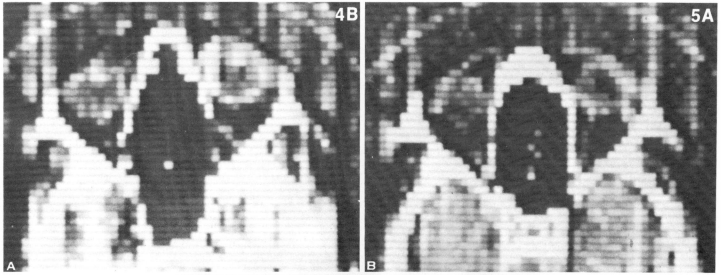

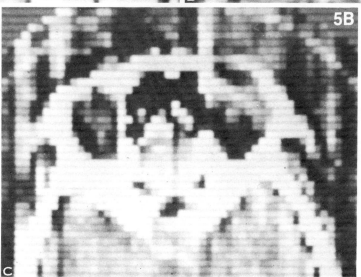

FIG. 28.20. GRANULOMA (IDIOPATHIC INFLAMMATION) OF LACRIMAL GLAND.

Clinical Features. A 67 y.o. man who had complained of chronic irritation in the right eye for more than 1 month, associated with edema of the right upper lid. A nontender movable mass was palpated within the right lacrimal fossa. There was no limitation of ocular motility.

Orbital exploration revealed a markedly enlarged lacrimal gland. Microscopic examination revealed intense lymphocytic infiltration in the gland. No evidence of sarcoidosis or infection was found in the lesion, which was diagnosed as an idiopathic granuloma of the lacrimal gland.

A–C. Contiguous 8-mm sections from below superiorly.

A. Section through the equatorial region of the right globe, indicating modest proptosis. The density of the lens is clearly visible. No abnormality is evident in the retrobulbar space.

B. Section through the upper third of the right globe. A small irregular area of increased absorption is evident adjacent to the lateral portion of the ocular rim. The optic nerve is visible and there is again no evidence of retrobulbar abnormality.

C. Section through the superior portion of the orbit, above the globe. A broad arcuate band of abnormal absorption is present extending across the anterior superior portion of the right orbit and broadening as it approaches the superior orbital margin. This region of increased absorption (17–30) corresponds well with the grossly enlarged lacrimal gland mass found at surgical exploration.

Repeat scans after injection of approximately 50 ml Hypaque 60 M showed no definite change in absorption of the lesion.

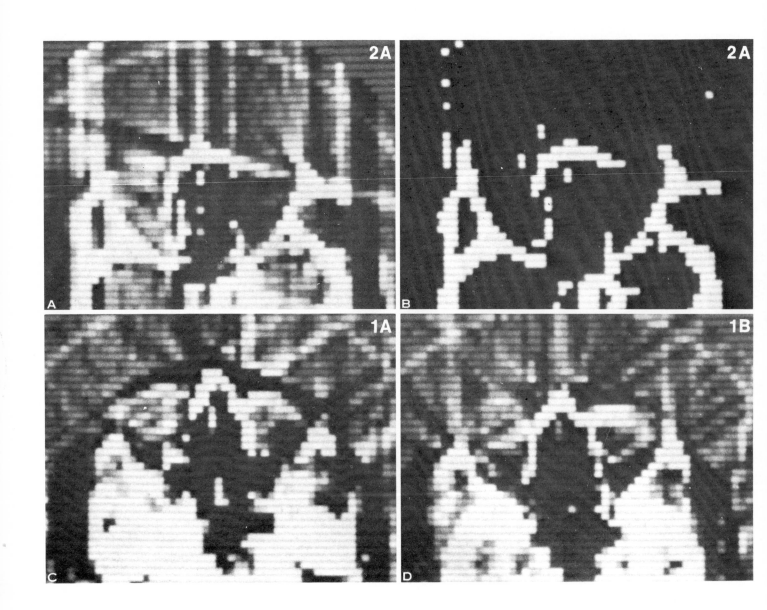

FIG. 28.21. MENINGIOMA, EXTENSIVE; LARGELY EN PLAQUE, WITH INFILTRATION THROUGH BONE INTO THE ORBIT AND TEMPORAL FOSSA.

Clinical Features. A 64 y.o. woman who first noted ptosis of the left upper eyelid nearly 3 years earlier, followed by some swelling of the eyelid. Six months before CT scan, she first noted diplopia on upward gaze. Proptosis of the left eye had been present for 3 months. She had no headaches, change in mental status, or seizures.

Examination showed a 7-mm exophthalmos on the left, with a hard, rubbery nontender fullness in the left temporal region. There was increased left orbital resistance, with no bruit. There was moderate limitation of upward and downward gaze of the left eye, with normal lateral gaze. The left pupil was slightly larger than the right and reacted less briskly. Visual fields were full. The remainder of the neurological examination was within normal limits.

Skull Examination. In addition to increased soft tissue density in the left orbital region, there was destruction of the lateral wall of the left orbit. Hypocycloidal laminography revealed a granular hyperostosis involving the anterolateral wall of the left middle fossa and extending to the greater and lesser wings of the sphenoid, associated with evidence of soft tissue mass projecting external to the skull in the temporal fossa. The findings were considered most likely due to meningioma, with an osteoblastic metastasis a less likely possibility.

RN Scans. Tcp dynamic scan revealed increased activity in the region of the left orbit, and static imaging showed evidence of increased activity in the region of the lateral wall of the left orbit. Tcd scan also showed extensive increase in activity in the left orbital region.

CT Scan. Abnormal (Fig. 28.21).

Angio. A transfemoral left carotid study, including selective external, internal, and common carotid series, the day after the CT scan, revealed a vascular mass in the area of the left pterion and adjacent portion of the greater wing of the sphenoid, with elevation of the middle cerebral artery and posterior dislocation of its anterior branches. A diffuse tumor blush was present, and the findings were indicative of meningioma. The internal cerebral vein lay in the midline and no tumor vessels were noted within the left orbit.

Operation. Left frontotemporal craniotomy, with excision of extensive meningioma that had widely infiltrated bone anteriorly and laterally in the middle fossa. A quite vascular mass of tumor of the anterior wall of the middle fossa invaginated the anterior portion of the left temporal lobe, and tumor had infiltrated into the temporal muscle. The tumor straddled the superior orbital fissure and widely involved the lateral wall of the orbit, with extension into the orbit. A plane of cleavage between the meningioma and extraocular muscles was found, and extensive resection resulted in a widely decompressed orbit. A large fascial graft was inserted to cover the large dural defect. The involved temporal muscle was excised.

A–D. Plain CT scan.

A. A broad zone of increased absorption (0–11) is shown extending along the lateral wall of the lower portion of the orbit from the apex to the lateral orbital rim and projecting markedly into the retrobulbar space. Scan detail is degraded by patient motion, but there is an indication of a slight thickening of the lateral wall of the left orbit with minor encroachment upon the orbital space, and there is a suggestion of a slight thickening of the anterior wall of the left middle fossa.

B. L 40   W M. Same section as in **A.**

C and **D.** L 5   W 50.

These two sections are below that shown in **A** and **B** and demonstrate the considerable left proptosis. The mass in the region of the lateral wall of the left orbit is less obvious on these sections, but there is again indication of encroachment upon the left orbital space from the lateral aspect. Both **C** and **D** indicate the presence of a soft tissue mass of quite high absorption extending into the left temporal fossa. More superior scan sections indicated the presence of a poorly localized mass effect in the left frontotemporal region but failed to reveal clearly the intracranial portion of the meningioma.

This study would doubtless have been more informative had the 160 x 160 matrix system been available at the time and if a supplementary contrast-enhanced study had been obtained.

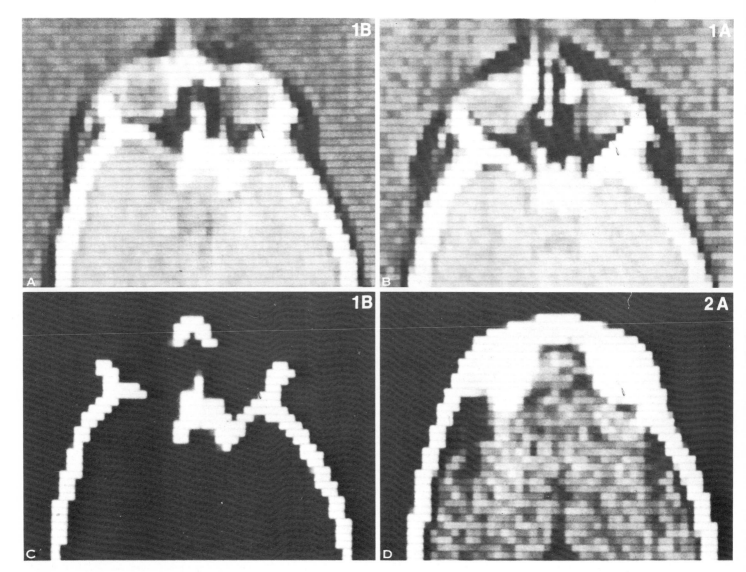

FIG. 28.22. NEUROFIBROMATOSIS, ASSOCIATED WITH MESODERMAL DEFECT INVOLVING THE GREATER WING OF SPHENOID, AND TEMPORAL LOBE DYSPLASIA.

Clinical Features. An 18-month-old boy with multiple café au lait spots who developed a progressive ptosis and thickening of the lateral portion of the left upper eyelid. No exophthalmos was evident, but the left eye pulsated synchronously with the carotid pulse. No intraocular or optic nerve abnormalities were evident.

(For another example of orbitotemporal dysplasia associated with neurofibromatosis, see Fig. 25.1).

A and **B.** L −5   W   75.

Contiguous scan sections demonstrating forward and lateral bulging of the anterior wall of the left middle fossa. Anteriorly, this encroaches upon the central and lateral portions of the retrobulbar space. The left globe appears generally enlarged compared with the right, and it appears to project further anteriorly. The latter is presumably due to the thickened left upper eyelid, which is not clearly distinguished from the anterior portion of the globe. In **A,** abnormally low absorption is evident in the medial half of the anteriorly bulging middle fossa.

C. L 45   W M.

These control settings reveal more clearly the defect of the medial half of the posterior wall of the left orbit. The thin medial walls of both orbits are not seen, owing to marked partial volume effects.

D. L 15   W 20.

Scan section immediately above that in **C,** at the level of the orbital roofs. An abnormally large space with the absorption characteristics of CSF (0–10) is shown extending from the irregular and abnormally small anterior portion of the left temporal lobe to the posterior orbital wall. This is consistent with an arachnoid pseudocyst secondary to defective development of the anterior portion of the temporal lobe. There also appears to be an enlarged subarachnoid space in the region of the anterior portion of the right temporal lobe, and the trigones of the lateral ventricles are larger than expected for the patient's age.

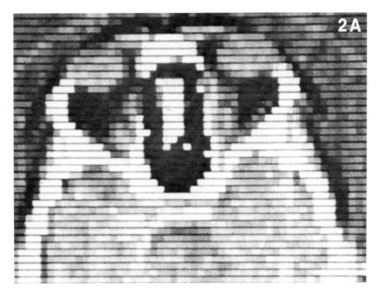

FIG. 28.23. THYROTOXIC EXOPHTHALMOPATHY.
Clinical Features. A 71 y.o. man on medical therapy for thyrotoxicosis with bilateral exophthalmos. Neurological examination was normal.
L 5 W 50.
The scan demonstrates bilateral proptosis (note the relative positions of the anterior portions of the globes and the lateral portions of the superior orbital margins). The retrobulbar spaces are enlarged. There is an abnormal, poorly marginated increase in absorption involving the orbital apices and adjacent portions of the retrobulbar spaces, particularly medially. On the right side, a normal lateral rectus muscle density is visible. The left lateral rectus is not visible, and there is no abnormal absorption in the lateral retrobulbar space on the left side.

This type of increase in absorption in the retrobulbar space, usually less obvious, has been observed in 7 of 10 patients with thyrotoxic exophthalmopathy studied by W. Marshall and W. R. Scott (unpublished data), and suggests thickening of the apex of the muscle cone.

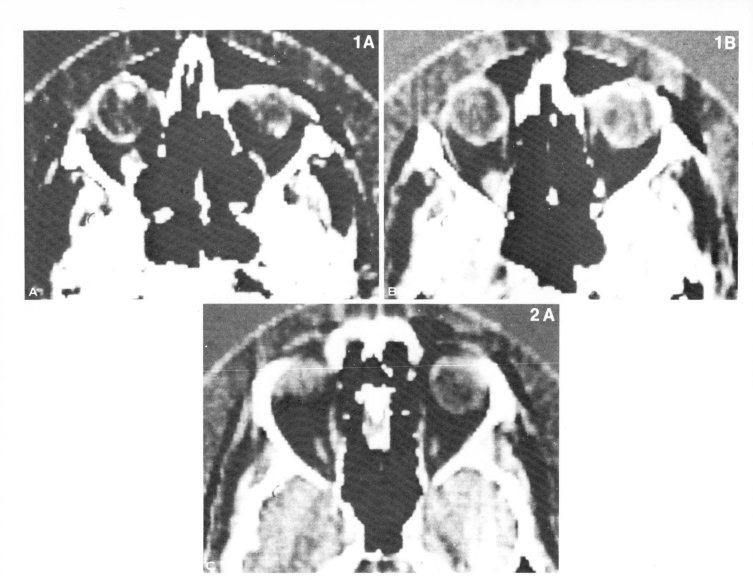

FIG. 28.24. ENDOCRINE EXOPHTHALMOS, PRESUMED ORBITAL GRAVES' DISEASE.

Clinical Features. A 47 y.o. male with a history of thyrotoxicosis, treated with radioactive iodine 2 years previously and now euthyroid. He had noted progressive eyelid swelling and left exophthalmos over the past year. Examination revealed the proptotic eye to be deviated downward, and there was marked increase in orbital resistance, without tenderness on palpation, palpable mass, or bruit.

Skull Examination; including orbital and optic canal projections; normal.

Ultrasonography. B-mode study revealed enlargement of the extraocular muscles of the left eye, interpreted as probably representing orbital Graves' disease.

CT Scan. Abnormal (Fig. 28.24).

Orbital Venography. Frontal vein injection resulted in filling of normal-appearing ophthalmic veins on the right, but there was no filling of veins in the left orbit.

Owing to the prominence of the patient's nose, the lower portion of the orbit could not be inserted into the scanner. 160 x 160 matrix system.

A. L 12   W 40.

The lowest CT section obtained, which was at the level of the equator of the left globe, the dense lens of which is clearly shown. An irregular focal area of increased absorption (16–38) projects anteriorly from the region of the apex of the left orbit.

B. L −2   W 75.

Section immediately superior to that in **A,** showing the increase in absorption (peak, 25) filling the left orbital apex, consistent with thickening of the apex of the muscle cone. Further anteriorly are visible the medial and lateral rectus muscles, which may be slightly thickened in these regions. No abnormality is visible in the right orbit, in which the anterior portion of the medial rectus is visible. This section is through the equator of the right globe, and the lens is quite clearly visible. It is difficult to estimate the degree of proptosis in **A** and **B,** owing to the difference in position of the globes relative to the sections.

C. L 8   W 75.

The lower position of the left globe results in the section passing through its superior portion, whereas the section passes only slightly above the equator of the right globe. On both sides, the posterior portions of the optic nerves are shown, and the retrobulbar space appears normal on both sides at this level of section. The left medial rectus appears thickened.

Sadek Hilal and Stephen Trokel have demonstrated distinct thickening of the lateral and medial recti and of the more posterior portions of the superior extraocular muscles (superior rectus, superior oblique, and levator palpebrae superioris) in ophthalmic Graves' disease. These investigators have employed 3- and 4-mm collimators and a modified computer program for improved anatomical detail in and behind the orbit. The tissue thickenings observed in the posterior orbit in Figures 28.3 and 28.4 are presumed to represent thickening of the posterior portions of the extraocular muscles.

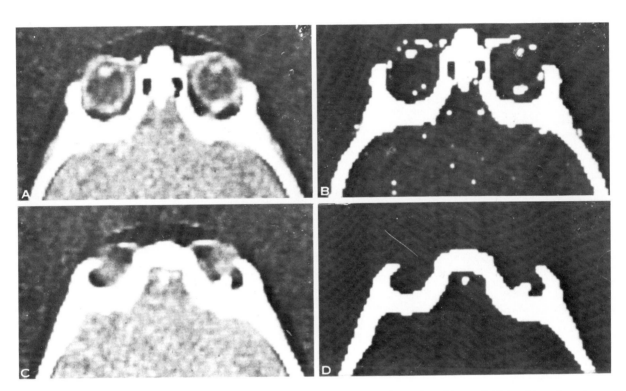

FIG. 28.25. Orbital foreign body. Orbital scans; 8-mm sections, 160 x 160 matrix system.

A. Section including the equators of the globes. Posteriorly, the sections extend just above the optic nerves. On the right side, a very high density region lies adjacent to the sclera, immediately above the optic nerve. This is discriminated better in **B**, which is a photograph taken at L   6   W M.

C. Section immediately above that in **A** and also photographed at L   0   W   75. The section includes portions of the superior segments of the globes. Above and behind the right

globe is an irregular object of high absorption, immediately below the orbital roof. This is discriminated more clearly in **D**, photographed at L   70   W M, which shows the foreign body projecting from the posterosuperior portion of the orbital roof. Maximum absorption of the foreign body was over 500 units, consistent with the leaded glass foreign body removed at surgery (Dr. A. Grove). The glass fragment measured 11 x 6 x 4 mm and was embedded in the periosteum of the orbital roof, but not in the bone.

Bibliography

1. Ambrose, J. Personal communication.
2. Ambrose, J. Computerized transverse axial scanning (tomography). Part 2. Clinical application. Brit J Radiol 46: 1023–1047, 1973.
3. Ambrose, J. Computerized x-ray scanning of the brain. J Neurosurg 40: 679–695, 1974.
4. Ambrose, J., and Hounsfield, G. Computerized transverse axial tomography. Brit J. Radiol 46: 148–149, 1973.
5. Ambrose, J., Lloyd, G., and Wright, J. A preliminary evaluation of fine matrix computerized axial tomography (Emiscan) in the diagnosis of orbital space-occupying lesions. Brit J Radiol 47: 747–751, 1974.
6. Baker, H. Personal communication.
7. Baker, H., Campbell, J., and Houser, D. Computer assisted tomography of the head. Mayo Clin Proc 49: 17–27, 1974.
7A. Baker, H. L., Campbell, J. K., Houser, O. W., et al. Early experience with the EMI scanner for study of the brain. Radiology 116: 327–333, 1975.
8. Baker, H. L., Kearns, T. P., Campbell, J. K., et al. Computerized transaxial tomography in neuro-ophthalmology. Am J Ophthalmol 78: 285–294, 1974.
9. Barnett, H. J. M., Foster, J. B., and Hudgson, P. Syringomyelia. London, W. B. Saunders Company Ltd., 1973.
10. Bergstrom, K., Carlsson, C., Cronqvist, S., et al. Preliminary Experience with the EMI Scanner. Presented at the X Symposium Neuroradiologicum, Montevideo, Uruguay, March 1974.
11. Cattell, W. R., Fry, I. K., Spencer, A. G., et al. Excretion urography. Part I. Factors determining the excretion of Hypaque. Brit J Radiol 40: 561–580, 1967.
12. Coleman, D. J., Jack, R. L., and Franzen, L. A. High resolution B-scan ultrasonography of the orbit. I. The normal orbit. II. Hemangioma of the orbit. III. Lymphoma of the orbit. IV. Neurogenic tumors of the orbit. Arch Ophthalmol 88: 355–380, 1972.
13. Coleman, D. J., Jack, R. L., Franzen, L. A., et al. High resolution B-scan ultrasonography. V. Eye changes of Graves' disease. VI. Pseudotumors of orbit. Arch Ophthalmol 88: 465–480, 1972.
13A. Computer Tomography of Brain Lesions. Acta Radiol Supp 346. Ed. Erik Lindgren, Stockholm, 1975.
13B. Cormack, A. M. Representation of a function of its line integrals, with some radiological applications. J Appl Physics 34: 2722–2727, 1963.
14. Crowther, A., DeRosier, D. J., and Klug, A. The reconstruction of a three-dimensional structure from projections and its application to electron microscopy. Proc. Roy. Soc. London A 317: 319–340, 1970.
15. Davis, D. O., and Pressman, B. D. Computerized tomography of the brain. Radiol Clin North Am 12(2): 297–313, 1974.
15A. Davis, K. R., Taveras, J. M., New, P. F. J., Schnur, J. A., and Roberson, G. H. Cerebral Infarction: Diagnosis by Computed Tomography Analysis and Evaluation of Findings. Am J Roentgenol Radium Ther Nucl Med, in press.
16. Di Chiro, G. Axial transverse encephalography. Am J Roentgenol Radium Ther Nucl Med 92: 441–447, 1964.
16A. Di Chiro, G. Of CAT and other beasts. Editorial. Am J Roentgenol Radium Ther Nucl Med 122 (3): 659–661, 1975.
17. Di Chiro, G., and Fisher, R. L. Contrast radiography of the spinal cord. Arch Neurol 11: 125–143, 1964.
18. Di Chiro, G., Schellinger, D., Axelbaum, S. P., et al. Computerized axial tomography in syringomyelia. N Engl J Med 292: 13–16, 1975.
19. du Boulay, G. Help! Brit J Radiol Special Issue 46: 783–792, 1973.
20. Editorial: Computer assisted tomography. Brit J Med 22: 623–624, 1974.
21. Editorial: New, P. F. J. Computer assisted tomography. J Am Med Assoc, 232: 941–943, 1975.
22. Editorial: Computer-assisted tomography of the brain. Lancet, 1052–1054, 1974.
23. Ellertsson, A. B. and Greitz, T., Myelocystographic and fluorescein studies to demonstrate communication between intramedullary cysts and cerebrospinal fluid space. Acta Neurol Scand 45: 418–439, 1969.
24. Ethier, R. "Computerized Angio Tomography." Presented at the First International Symposium on Computed Tomography, Montreal Neurological Institute, Montreal, Canada, May 31–June 1, 1974.
25. Ethier, R. Scientific Exhibit, "Computerized Axial Tomography." First International Symposium on Computerized Tomography, Montreal Neurological Institute, Montreal, Quebec, Canada, May 31–June 1, 1974.
25A. Gado, M. H. Mechanisms and Implications of Contrast Enhancement in Cranial Computed Tomography. Presented at Workshop on Reconstruction Tomography in Diagnostic Radiology and Nuclear Medicine, San Juan, Puerto Rico, April 17–19, 1975.
26. Gawler, J., et al. Orbital scanning. Brit J Ophthalmol, in press.
27. Gawler, J., DuBoulay, G. H., Bull, J. W. D., et al. Computer-assisted tomography (EMI scanner). Its place in investigation of suspected intracranial tumours. Lancet 2: 419–423, 1974.
27A. Glenn, W. V., Jr., Johnston, R. J., Morton, P. W., et al. Reconstruction and Display of Sagittal and Coronal Planes from Overlapped Transverse CT Images. Presented at the CT International Symposium and Course, Hamilton, Bermuda, March 9–14, 1975.
27B. Glenn, W. V., Jr., Johnston, R. J., Morton, P. E., et al. Image generation and display techniques for CT scan data: Thin transverse and reconstructed coronal and sagittal planes (1975 Memorial Award Lecture, 23rd Annual Meeting of the Association of University Radiologists, San Diego, Calif.). Invest Radiol Vol. 10, 1975.
28. Goitein, M. Three-dimensional density reconstruction from a series of two-dimensional projections. Nucl Inst Meth 101: 509–518, 1972.
29. Gordon, R., Bender, R., and Herman, G. Algebraic reconstruction techniques (ART) for three-dimensional electron microscopy and X-ray photography. J Theor Biol 29: 471–481, 1970.
30. Gregg, E. C. Tomography with monoenergetic photons. AAPM Quart Bull 7: 96–97, 1973.
30A. Greitz, T. and Hindmarsh, T. Computer assisted tomography of intracranial and CSF circulation using a watersoluble contrast medium. Acta Radiol Diag 15: 497–507, 1974.
31. Grove, A. S., Jr., New, P. F. J., and Momose, K. J. Computerized tomographic (CT/EMI) scanning for orbital evaluation. Trans Am Acad Ophthalmol Otolaryngol 79(1): 137–149, 1975.
31A. Grove, A. S., Jr. Evaluation of exophthalmos. N Engl J Med

292(19): 1005–1013, 1975.

31B. Grubb, R. L., Jr., Phelps, M. E., and Ter-Pogossian, M. M. Regional cerebral blood volume in humans. Arch Neurol 28: 38–44, 1973.

32. Hounsfield, G. H. Computerized transverse axial scanning (tomography). Part 1. Description of system. Brit J Radiol 46: 1016–1022, 1973.

32A. Hounsfield, G. H. Personal communication.

33. Huber, P., and Rivoir, R. The influence of intraventricular pressure on the size and shape of the anterior part of the third ventricle. Neuroradiology 5: 33–36, 1973.

33A. Huckman, M. S., Fox, J., and Topei, J. The validity of criteria for the evaluation of cerebral atrophy by computed tomography. Radiology 116: 85–92, 1975.

33B. Kistler, J. P., Hochberg, F. H., Brooks, B. R., et al. Computerized axial tomography: Clinicopathologic correlation. Neurology 25(3): 201–209, 1975.

34. Kuhl, D. E., and Edwards, R. G. Reorganizing transverse section scan data as a rectilinear matrix using digital processing. J Nucl Med 7: 332, 1966.

35. Kuhl, D. E., and Edwards, R. Q. Reorganizing data from transverse section scans of the brain using digital processing. Radiology 91: 975–983, 1968.

36. Lambert, V. L., Zelch, J. V., and Cohen, D. N. Computed tomography of the orbits. Radiology 113: 351–354, 1974.

37. Ledley, R. S., Di Chiro, G., Lussenhop, A. J., et al. Computerized transaxial x-ray tomography of the human body. Science 186: 207–212, 1974.

38. McCullough, E. C., Baker, H. L., Houser, W. O., et al. An evaluation of the quantitative and radiation features of a scanning x-ray transverse axial tomograph: The EMI scanner. Radiology 111: 709–715, 1974.

39. McDonald, J. V. Midline Hematomas Simulating Tumors of the Third Ventricle. Neurology 12: 805–809, 1962.

39A. McKusick, K. A., New, P. F. J., Pendergrass, H. P., et al. Impact of computerized axial tomography upon radionuclide brain scanning in non-neoplastic disease (abst.) J Nucl Med 15: 515, 1974.

40. Momose, K. J., New, P. F. J., Grove A. S., Jr., et al. The use of computed axial tomography in ophthalmology. Radiology 115: 361–368, 1975.

41. New, P. F. J. Computed Tomography: Experience at the Massachusetts General Hospital. *Cerebral Vascular Diseases*. Ed. by J. P. Whisnant and B. A. Sandok, 203–221. New York, Grune and Stratton, Inc., 1975.

42. New, P. F. J. Computed Tomography: A Major Diagnostic Advance. Hosp Prac 10(2): 55–64, 1975.

43. New, P. F. J., Scott, W. R., Davis, K. R., and Schnur, J. A. Computed tomographic aspects of intra- and extra-vascular blood. Presented at the First International Symposium on Computed Tomography. Montreal Neurological Institute, Montreal, Canada, May 31–June 1, 1974, Radiology, in press.

44. New, P. F., Scott, R., Schnur, J. A., et al. Computerized axial tomography with the EMI scanner. Radiology 110: 109–123, 1974.

45. New, P. F., Scott, W. R., Schnur, J. A., et al. The Impact of Computerized Axial Tomography upon Neuroradiological Practice. Read at the X Symposium Neuroradiologicum, Montevideo, Uruguay, March 1974.

46. New, P. F. J., Scott, W. R., Schnur, J. A., et al. Computed tomography (CT) with the EMI scanner in the diagnosis of primary and metastatic intracranial neoplasms. Radiology 114: 75–87, 1975.

47. New, P. F. J., Scott, W. R., Schnur, J. A., et al. Computed tomography: Immobilization of the head by dental holder. Radiology 114: 474–476, 1975.

48. Oldendorf, W. H. Isolated flying spot detection of radiodensity discontinuities displaying the lateral structural pattern of a complex object. IRE Transactions on Biomedical Electronics. Vol. BME 8, no. 1, January 1961.

49. Ommaya, A. K. Computerized axial tomography of the head. The EMI scanner, a new device for direct examination of the brain "in vivo." Surg Neurol 1(4): 217–222, 1973.

50. O'Brien, M. D., Waltz, A. G., and Jordan, M. M. Ischemic Cerebral Edema. Arch Neurol 30: 456–460, 1974.

51. Paxton, R., and Ambrose, J. The EMI scanner. A brief review of the first 650 patients. Brit J Radiol 47: 530–565, 1974.

51A. Pendergrass, H. P., McKusick, K. A., New, P. F. J., et al. Relative efficacy of radionuclide imaging and computed tomography of the brain. Radiology 116: 363–366, 1975.

52. Perry, B. J., and Bridges, C. Computerized transverse axial scanning (Tomography: Part 3). Radiation dose considerations. Brit J Radiol 46: 1048–1051, 1973.

53. Peters, T. M., Smith, P. R., and Gibson, R. D. Computer aided transverse body-section radiography. Brit J Radiol 46: 314–317, 1973.

54. Phelps, M. E. Personal communication.

54A. Phelps, M. E., Hoffman, E. J., and Ter-Pogossian, M. M. Attenuation coefficients of various body tissues, fluids and lesions at photon energies of 18 and 136 keV. Radiology, in press.

55. Potter, G. *Sectional Anatomy and Tomography of the Head*. New York, Grune and Stratton, Inc., 1971.

56. Probst, F. P. Gas distension of the lateral ventricles at encephalography. Acta Radiol 14(1): 1–4, 1973.

57. Purnell, E. W. Ultrasonic interpretation of orbital disease. In *Ophthalmic Ultrasound*. Ed. by K. A. Gitter, A. H. Keeney, L. E. Sarin, et al., 249–255. St. Louis, C. V. Mosby, 1969.

57A. Radon, J. Uber die Bestimmung von Funktionen durch ihre Integralwerte längs gewissbr Mannigfaltigkeiten. Ber Verh Sachs Akad Wiss 67: 262–277, 1917.

57B. Sackett, J. F., Messina A. V., and Petito, C. K. Computed tomography and magnification vertebral angiotomography in the diagnosis of colloid cysts of the third ventricle. Radiology 116: 95–100, 1975.

58. Schellinger, D., Di Chiro, G. Axelbaum, S. P., et al. Early clinical experience with the ACTA scanner. Radiology 114: 257–261, 1975.

59. Scott, W. R., New, P. F. J., Davis, K. R., et al. Computerized axial tomography of intracerebral and intraventricular hemorrhage. Radiology 112: 73–80, 1974.

60. Shields, R. A., Isherwood, I., and Pullan, B. R. The use of an off-line static display system with a computerised axial tomographic unit. Brit J Radiol 47: 893–895, 1974.

61. Smith, D., Davis, D., Pressman, B., et al. Computerized Axial Tomography of the Brain (EMI Scan). Scientific Exhibit, Congress of Neurological Surgeons, 24th Annual Meeting, Vancouver, British Columbia, September 23–27, 1974.

61A. Smith, P. R., Peters, T. M., Muller, H. R., et al. Towards the assessment of the limitations on computerized axial tomography. Neuroradiology 9: 1–8, 1975.

62. Sternick, E. S., Ting, J. Y., and Hughes, M. An on-line computer method for obtaining densities of internal anatomical structures using a dual probe scanner. AAPM Quart Bull 7: 104, 1973.

63. Taveras, J. M., Davis, K. R., and New, P. F. J. Diagnosis of Cerebral Infarction with the EMI Scanner. Presented at the First International Symposium on Computed Tomography, Montreal Neurological Institute, Montreal, Canada, May 31–June 1, 1974.

64. Thieme, G. A., Hendlee, W. R., Carson, P. L., et al. Determination of cross-sectional anatomy by transmission scanning. AAPM Quart Bull 7: 94, June, 1973.

65. Werner, S. C., Coleman, D. J., and Franzen, L. A. Ultrasonographic evidence of a consistent orbital involvement in Graves's disease. N Engl J Med 290: 1447–1450, 1974.

List of Abbreviations

Angio   — angiography
AVM   — arteriovenous malformation
cm   — centimeter
CP   — cerebellopontine
CSF   — cerebrospinal fluid
CT   — computed tomography or computed tomo-
          graphic
EEG   — electroencephalogram(y)
L   — viewer level (setting)
M   — viewer window MEASURE setting
MGH   — Massachusetts General Hospital
ml   — milliliter
mm   — millimeter
PEG   — pneumoencephalogram(y)
PICA   — posterior inferior cerebellar artery
RBL   — Reid's anatomical base line
RN   — radionuclide
Tcd   — ^{99m}technetium diphosphonate
Tcp   — ^{99m}technetium pertechnetate
W   — viewer window (setting)
y.o.   — year-old

Subject Index*

---

*Page numbers in boldface type refer to illustrations.

Index of Personal Names

The authors acknowledge in the following Index of Personal Names the persons not listed in the Bibliography who, through their individual and collective experiences, have made contributions to the field and ultimately to the knowledge that has been presented in this volume.

Alfidi, Ralph, 6
Altemus, L. R., 355
Ambrose, James, ix, 4, 5, 6, 55, 187, 235, 263, 287, 332, 333, 362, 426, 442, 451
Aronow, Saul, ix
Baker, Edward P., 242
Bresnan, Michael J., 360
Cares, Herbert, 225, 365
Cavalho, Angelina, 264
Chapman, Paul H., 139. 193, 256, 293, 306
Conway, Melvin E., 52
Crowell, Robert M., 137, 149, 291, 366
Deck, Michael D. F., 259
Eisenberg, Howard, 223
Golden, J., 157
Hanberry, J., 182

Harwood-Nash, Derek C., 330
Hatton, John, ix
Hilal, Sadek, 448
Hochberg, Fred H., ix
Hounsfield, Godfrey, ix, 3, 5, 6, 28, 35, 37, 57, 263
Kistler, J. Philip, ix
Kjellberg, Raymond N., 185, 213, 220, 318
Kornblith, Paul L., 142, 153
Lott, Thomas M., 398
Manganiello, Louis O., 398
Marshall, W., 442, 451, 477
Mendelsohn, George, 301
Menzer, Leon, 225, 365, 396, 441
Ojemann, Robert G., 135, 143, 165, 169, 173, 176, 191, 207, 211, 217, 219, 241, 253, 271,

297, 313, 337, 368, 373, 381, 383, 404, 419
Perlo, Vincent, 384
Poletti, Charles, 225, 262
Richardson, Allan, 6
Richardson, E. P., ix
Roberson, Glenn, ix
Schechter, M., 5
Scott, Michael, 126, 163, 289, 320, 377
Strand, Roy, 145, 158, 361
Sweet, William H., ix, 140, 142, 146, 152, 155, 179, 181, 203, 232, 236, 283, 364
Tarlov, Edward, 175, 215, 278, 281, 303
Taveras, Juan, ix, 6
Thompson, C. J., 48, 51
Wepsic, James, 167, 228, 240, 295, 309